Molecular Diagnostics

Fundamentals, Methods and Clinical Applications

Second Edition

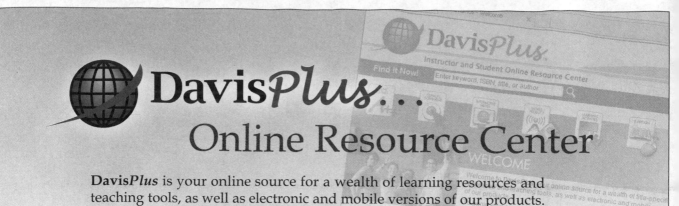
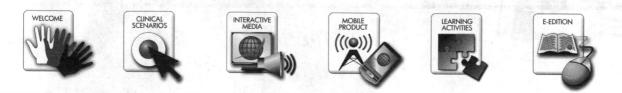
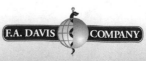

Molecular Diagnostics

Fundamentals, Methods and Clinical Applications

Second Edition

Lela Buckingham, PhD, MB, DLM (ASCP)
Unit Director, Molecular Oncology
Department of Pathology
Rush Medical Laboratories
Rush University Medical Center
Chicago, Illinois

F.A. Davis Company • Philadelphia

F.A. Davis Company
1915 Arch Street
Philadelphia, PA 19103
www.fadavis.com

Senior Acquisitions Editor: Christa A. Fratantoro
Manager of Content Development: George W. Lang
Developmental Editor: Julie Munden
Manager of Art & Design: Carolyn O'Brien

As new scientific information becomes available through basic and clinical research, recommended treatments and drug therapies undergo changes. The author(s) and publisher have done everything possible to make this book accurate, up to date, and in accord with accepted standards at the time of publication. The author(s), editors, and publisher are not responsible for errors or omissions or for consequences from application of the book, and make no warranty, expressed or implied, in regard to the contents of the book. Any practice described in this book should be applied by the reader in accordance with professional standards of care used in regard to the unique circumstances that may apply in each situation. The reader is advised always to check product information (package inserts) for changes and new information regarding dose and contraindications before administering any drug. Caution is especially urged when using new or infrequently ordered drugs.

Library of Congress Cataloging-in-Publication Data

Buckingham, Lela.
  Molecular diagnostics : fundamentals, methods, and clinical applications /
Lela Buckingham. — 2nd ed.
      p. ; cm.
  Includes bibliographical references and index.
  ISBN-13: 978-0-8036-2677-5
  ISBN-10: 0-8036-2677-0
  1. Molecular diagnosis. I. Title.
  [DNLM: 1. Molecular Diagnostic Techniques—methods. 2. Nucleic
Acids   analysis. QY 25]
  RB43.7.B83 2012
  616.9'041—dc23

                                    2011024996

To my brother, John.

Preface

Molecular Technology has been incorporated into diagnostic testing in a relatively short period. Programs that educate clinical laboratory professionals have had to integrate molecular diagnostic testing into their curricula just as rapidly despite a lack of formal resources. This textbook was written to address these concerns.

The primary audience for this text is students enrolled in Clinical Laboratory Science/Medical Technology programs at all levels. The textbook explains the principles of molecular technology that are used for diagnostic purposes. Examples of applications of molecular-based assays are included in the text as well as case studies that illustrate the use and interpretation of these assays in patient care.

This textbook is also appropriate for those in other health-related disciplines who have to understand the purpose, principle, and interpretation of molecular diagnostic tests that they will be ordering and assessing for their patients.

Students who are first learning about molecular-based assays will find this text useful for explaining the principles. Practitioners who are performing and interpreting these assays can use this text as a resource for reference and troubleshooting and to drive the implementation of additional molecular-based assays in their laboratory.

An Instructor's Resource package has been developed for educators who adopt this text for a course. These resources, which include a Brownstone test generator, image bank, and PowerPoint presentation, are available on CD-ROM and on Davis*Plus* at http://davisplus. fadavis.com. Educators should contact their F.A. Davis Sales Representative to obtain access to the Instructor's Resources.

Lela Buckingham, PhD, MB^{CM}, DLM^{CM} (ASCP)

Reviewers

Denise Anamani, MA, CLSp(MB), I(ASCP)
Lecturer
University of Connecticut
Allied Health Sciences
Storrs, Connecticut

Amy R. Groszbach, MLT, CLSp(MB)
Education Specialist II
Mayo Clinic, Molecular Genetics Laboratory
Department of Laboratory Medicine and Pathology
Rochester, Minnesota

April L. Harkins, PhD, MT(ASCP)
Assistant Professor
Marquette University
Clinical Laboratory Science
Milwaukee, Wisconsin

Rick Intres, PhD
Director
Berkshire Medical Center
Pathology Department
Pittsfield, Massachusetts

Kathy Kenwright, MS, MT(ASCP)SI
Assistant Professor
University of Tennessee Health Science Center
Clinical Laboratory Science
Memphis, Tennessee

Hamida Nusrat, PhD, in Microbiology and Immunology
Lecturer
San Francisco State University
CLS Internship Program
San Ramon, California

Rodney E. Rohde, BS, MS, PhD, SV, SM, MP
Associate Professor
Texas State University–San Marcos
Clinical Laboratory Science
San Marcos, Texas

Acknowledgments

Thanks and gratitude are extended to all who helped in the completion of the second edition of this work. The useful input provided by the reviewers who gave their valuable time during the production of the second addition is greatly appreciated. It is only necessary to observe the citations and references following each chapter to appreciate the amount of scientific discovery applied, often in novel and creative ways to medical laboratory science.

I owe thanks to my colleagues at Rush University Medical Center, Dr. John Coon and Dr. Robert DeCresce in the Department of Pathology, and Dr. Wei-Tong Hsu, Dr. Kamaljit Singh, Dr. Mary Hayden, and Dr. Elizabeth Berry-Kravis for help and support in their areas of expertise. I would also like acknowledge the residents, fellows, medical laboratory scientists, and students who provided suggestions for the second edition, particularly, Alexandra Vardouniotis, Mezgebe Gebrekiristos, and Christine Braun with whom I worked with and from whom I learned from every day.

This book was originally envisioned by my co-author for the first edition, Dr. Maribeth Flaws. Thanks to her for initiating this project. Thanks to Dr. Herb Miller and the Medical Laboratory Science faculty in the Rush University College of Health Sciences for the opportunity to participate in clinical science education. I greatly appreciate the guidance and support of the staff at F.A. Davis, especially Christa A. Fratantoro and my patient and well-organized developmental editor, Julie Munden.

Finally, I would like to thank fellow members of the Association for Molecular Pathology, a vibrant and resourceful organization dedicated to education and policy in the practice of Molecular Diagnostics. This organization has provided an outlet for contextual information, training, and sanction to further this ever-advancing field of study.

Lela Buckingham

Contents

Fundamentals of Nucleic Acid Biochemistry: An Overview

Chapter 1

DNA

OBJECTIVES

• Diagram the structure of nitrogen bases, nucleosides, and nucleotides.

• Describe the nucleic acid structure as a polymer of nucleotides.

• Demonstrate how deoxyribonucleic acid (DNA) is replicated such that the order or sequence of nucleotides is maintained (semi-conservative replication).

• Explain the reaction catalyzed by DNA polymerase that results in the phosphodiester backbone of the DNA chain.

• Note how the replicative process results in the antiparallel nature of complementary strands of DNA.

• List the enzymes that modify DNA, and state their specific functions.

• Illustrate three ways in which DNA can be transferred between bacterial cells.

• Define recombination, and sketch how new combinations of genes are generated in sexual and asexual reproduction.

When James Watson coined the term "molecular biology,"[1] he was referring to the biology of deoxyribonucleic acid (DNA). Of course, there are other molecules in nature. However, the term is still used to describe the study of nucleic acids. In the medical laboratory, molecular techniques are designed for the handling and analysis of the nucleic acids, DNA and **ribonucleic acid (RNA)**. Protein analysis and that of carbohydrates and other molecular species remain, for the most part, the domain of the chemistry laboratory. Molecular techniques are, however, being incorporated into other testing venues such as cell surface protein analysis, in situ histology, and tissue typing. The molecular biology laboratory, therefore, may be a separate entity or part of an existing molecular diagnostics or molecular pathology unit.

Nucleic acids offer several characteristics that support their use for clinical purposes. Highly specific analyses can be carried out without requiring extensive physical or chemical selection of target molecules or organisms, allowing specific and rapid analysis from limiting specimens. Furthermore, information carried in the sequence of the nucleotides that make up the DNA macromolecule is the basis for normal and pathological **traits** in all organisms from microorganisms to humans and, as such, provides a powerful means of predictive analysis. Effective prevention and treatment of disease will result from the analysis of these sequences in the medical laboratory.

DNA

DNA is a macromolecule of carbon, nitrogen, oxygen, phosphorous, and hydrogen atoms. It is assembled in units of **nucleotides** that are composed of a phosphorylated ribose sugar and a **nitrogen base**. There are four nitrogen bases that make up the majority of DNA found in all organisms. These are **adenine**, **cytosine**, **guanine**, and **thymine**. Nitrogen bases are attached to a **deoxyribose** sugar, which forms a polymer with the deoxyribose sugars of other nucleotides through a **phosphodiester bond**. Linear assembly of the nucleotides makes up one strand of DNA. Two strands of DNA comprise the DNA double helix.

In 1871, Johann Friedrich Miescher published a paper on **nuclein**, the viscous substance extracted from cell nuclei. In his writings he made no mention of the function of nuclein. Walther Flemming, a leading cell biologist, describing his work on the nucleus in 1882 admitted

that the biological significance of the substance was unknown. We now know that the purpose of DNA, contained in the nucleus of the cell, is to store information. The information in the DNA storage system is based on the order or sequence of nucleotides in the nucleic acid polymer. Just as computer information storage is based on sequences of 0 and 1, biological information is based on sequences of A, C, G, and T. These four building blocks (with a few modifications) account for all of the biological diversity that makes up life on earth.

DNA Structure

The double helical structure of DNA (Fig. 1-1) was first described by James Watson and Francis Crick. Their molecular model was founded on previous observations of the chemical nature of DNA and physical evidence, including diffraction analyses performed by Rosalind

---

Historical Highlights

Johann Friedrich Miescher is credited with the discovery of DNA in 1869.[2] Miescher had isolated white blood cells out of seepage collected from discarded surgical bandages. He found that he could extract a viscous substance from these cells. Miescher also observed that most of the nonnuclear cell components could be lysed away with dilute hydrochloric acid, leaving the nuclei intact. Addition of extract of pig stomach (a source of pepsin to dissolve away contaminating proteins) resulted in a somewhat shrunken but clean preparation of nuclei. Extraction of these with alkali yielded the same substance isolated from the intact cells. It precipitated upon the addition of acid and redissolved in alkali. Chemical analysis of this substance demonstrated that it was 14% nitrogen and 2.5% phosphorus, different from any group of biochemicals then known. He named the substance "nuclein." (Analytical data indicate that less than 30% of Miescher's first nuclein preparation was actually DNA.) He later isolated a similar viscous material from salmon sperm and noted: "If one wants to assume that a single substance . . . is the specific cause of fertilization, then one should undoubtedly first of all think of nuclein."

Franklin.[3] The helical structure of DNA results from the physicochemical demands of the linear array of nucleotides. Both the specific **sequence** (order) of nucleotides in the strand as well as the surrounding chemical microenvironment can affect the nature of the DNA helix.

Nucleotides

The four nucleotide building blocks of DNA are molecules of about 700 kilodaltons (kd; one dalton is equal to the atomic mass of 1/12 of the [12]carbon isotope). Each nucleotide consists of a five-carbon sugar, the first carbon of which is covalently joined to a nitrogen base and the fifth carbon to a phosphate moiety (Fig. 1-2). A nitrogen base bound to an unphosphorylated sugar is a **nucleoside**. **Adenosine** (**A**), **guanosine** (**G**), **cytidine** (**C**), and **thymidine** (**T**) are nucleosides. If the ribose sugar is phosphorylated, the molecule is a nucleoside mono-, di-, or triphophosphate, or a nucleotide. For example, adenosine with one phosphate is adenosine monophosphate (AMP). Adenosine with three phosphates is adenosine

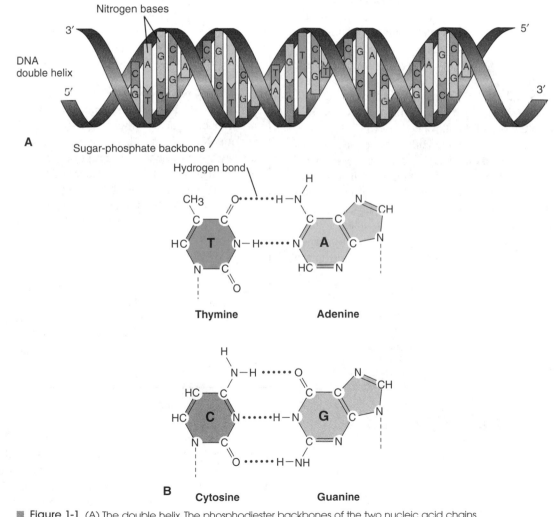

■ **Figure 1-1** (A) The double helix. The phosphodiester backbones of the two nucleic acid chains form the helix. Nitrogen bases are oriented toward the center where the hydrogen bonds with homologous bases to stabilize the structure. (B) Two hydrogen bonds form between adenine and thymine. Three hydrogen bonds form between guanine and cytosine.

triphosphate (ATP). Nucleotides can be converted to nucleosides by hydrolysis. The five-carbon sugar of DNA is deoxyribose, which is ribose with the number 2 carbon of deoxyribose linked to a hydrogen atom rather than a hydroxyl group (see Fig. 1-2). The hydroxyl group on the third carbon is important for forming the phosphodiester bond that is the backbone of the DNA strand.

Nitrogen bases are planar carbon-nitrogen ring structures. The four common nitrogen bases in DNA are adenine, guanine, cytosine, and thymine. Amine and ketone substitutions as well as the single or double bonds within the rings distinguish the four bases that comprise the majority of DNA (Fig. 1-3). Nitrogen bases with a single ring structure (thymine, cytosine) are **pyrimidines**. Bases with a double ring structure (guanine, adenine) are **purines**.

Numbering of the positions in the nucleotide molecule starts with the ring positions of the nitrogen base, designated C or N 1, 2, 3, etc. The carbons of the ribose sugar are numbered 1' to 5', distinguishing the sugar ring positions from those of the nitrogen base rings (Fig. 1-4).

The nitrogen base components of the nucleotides form **hydrogen bonds** with each other in a specific way. Guanine forms three hydrogen bonds with cytosine. Adenine forms two hydrogen bonds with thymine (see Fig. 1-1B). Hydrogen bonds between nucleotides are the key to the specificity of all nucleic acid–based tests used in the molecular laboratory. Specific hydrogen bond formation is also how the information held in the

Advanced Concepts

The double helix first described by Watson and Crick is DNA in its hydrated form (B-form) and is the standard form of DNA.[4] It has 10.5 steps or pairs of nucleotides (bp) per turn. Dehydrated DNA takes the A-form with about 11 bp per turn and the center of symmetry along the outside of the helix rather than down the middle as it is in the B-form. Both A- and B-form DNA are right-handed helices. Stress and torsion can throw the double helix into a Z-form. Z-DNA is a left-handed helix with 12 bp per turn and altered geometry of the sugar-base bonds. Z-DNA has been observed in areas of chromosomes where the DNA is under torsional stress from unwinding for transcription or other metabolic functions.

Watson-Crick base pairing (purine:pyrimidine hydrogen bonding) is not limited to the ribofuranosyl nucleic acids—those found in our genetic system. Natural nucleic acid alternatives can also display the basic chemical properties of DNA (and RNA). Theoretical studies have addressed such chemical alternatives to DNA and RNA components. An example is the pentopyranosyl-(2'→4') oligonucleotide system that exhibits stronger and more selective base pairing than DNA or RNA.[5] Study of nucleic acid alternatives has practical applications. For example, protein nucleic acids, which have a carbon-nitrogen peptide backbone replacing the sugar-phosphate backbone,[6,7] can be used in the laboratory as alternatives to DNA and RNA hybridization probes.[8] They are also potential enzyme-resistant alternatives to RNA in antisense RNA therapies.[9]

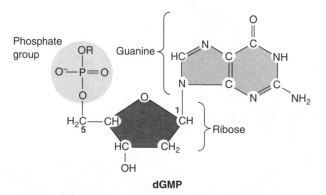

dGMP

■ **Figure 1-2** The nucleotide deoxyguanosine 5' phosphate, or guanosine monophosphate (dGMP). It is composed of deoxyribose covalently bound at its number 1 carbon to the nitrogen base, guanine, and at its number 5 carbon to a phosphate group. The molecule without the phosphate group is the nucleoside deoxyguanosine.

linear order of the nucleotides is maintained. As DNA is polymerized, each nucleotide to be added to the new DNA strand hydrogen bonds with the **complementary** nucleotide on the parental strand (A:T, G:C). In this way the parental DNA strand can be replicated without loss of the nucleotide order. Base pairs (bp) other than A:T and G:C or **mismatches** (e.g., A:C, G:T, A:A) can distort the DNA helix and disrupt the maintenance of sequence information.

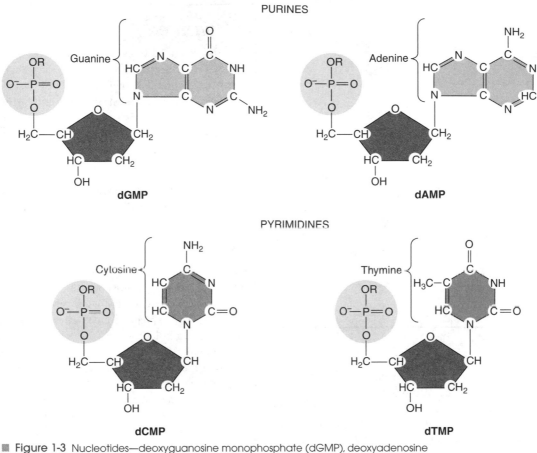

PURINES

dGMP

dAMP

PYRIMIDINES

dCMP

dTMP

■ **Figure 1-3** Nucleotides—deoxyguanosine monophosphate (dGMP), deoxyadenosine monophosphate (dAMP), deoxythymidine monophosphate (dTMP), and deoxycytidine monophosphate (dCMP)—differ by the attached nitrogen bases. The nitrogen bases, guanine and adenine, have purine ring structures. Thymine and cytosine have pyrimidine ring structures. Uracil, the nucleotide base that replaces thymine in RNA, has the purine ring structure of thymine minus the methyl group and hydrogen bonds with adenine.

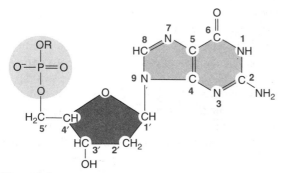

■ **Figure 1-4** Carbon position numbering of a nucleotide monophosphate. The base carbons are numbered 1 through 9. The sugar carbons are numbered 1' to 5'. The phosphate group on the 5' carbon and the hydroxyl group on the 3' carbon form phosphodiester bonds between bases.

Substituted Nucleotides

Modifications of the nucleotide structure are found throughout nature. Methylations, deaminations, additions, substitutions, and other chemical modifications generate nucleotides with new properties. Changes such as methylation of nitrogen bases have biological consequences for gene function and are intended in nature. Changes can also be brought about by environmental insults such as chemicals or radiation. These changes can affect gene function as well, resulting in undesirable effects such as cancer.

Due to their specific effects on enzymes that metabolize DNA, modified nucleosides have been used effectively for clinical applications (Fig. 1-5). The anticancer

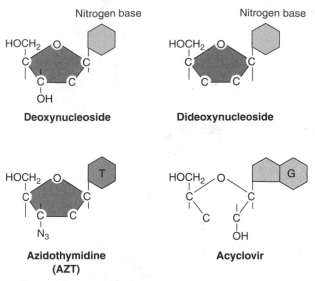

■ **Figure 1-5** Substituted nucleosides used in the clinic and the laboratory.

Advanced Concepts

In addition to the four commonly occurring nucleotide bases, modified bases are also often found in nature. Base modifications have significant effects on phenotype. Some modified bases result from damage to DNA; others are naturally modified for specific functions or to affect gene expression, as will be discussed in later sections.

---

drugs, 5-bromouridine (5BrdU) and cytosine arabinoside (cytarabine, ara-C), are modified thymidine and cytosine nucleosides, respectively. Azidothymidine (Retrovir, AZT), cytosine, 2' ,3'-dideoxy-2'-fluoro (ddC), and 2', 3'-dideoxyinosine (Videx, ddI), drugs used to treat patients with human immunodeficiency virus (HIV) infections, are modifications of thymidine and cytosine and a precursor of adenine, respectively. An analog of guanosine, 2-amino-1,9-dihydro-9-[(2-hydroxyethoxy) methyl]-6*H*-purin-6-one (Acyclovir, Zovirax), is a drug used to combat herpes simplex virus and varicella-zoster virus.

In the laboratory, nucleosides can be modified for purposes of labeling or detection of DNA molecules,

---

Advanced Concepts

Modified nucleotides are used in bacteria and viruses as a primitive immune system that allows them to distinguish their own DNA from that of the host or invaders (**restriction modification [rm] system**). Recognizing its own modifications, the host can target unmodified DNA for degradation.

---

sequencing, and other applications. The techniques used for these procedures will be discussed in later chapters.

Nucleic Acid

Nucleic acid is a macromolecule made of nucleotides bound together by the phosphate and hydroxyl groups on their sugars. A nucleic acid chain grows by the attachment of the 5' phosphate group of an incoming nucleotide to the 3' hydroxyl group of the last nucleotide on the growing chain (Fig. 1-6). Addition of nucleotides in this way gives the DNA chain a polarity; that is, it has a 5' phosphate end and a 3' hydroxyl end. We refer to DNA as oriented in a *5' to 3' direction*, and the linear sequence of the nucleotides, by convention, is read in that order.

DNA found in nature is mostly double-stranded. Two strands exist in an opposite 5' to 3'/3' to 5' orientation held together by the hydrogen bonds between their

---

Advanced Concepts

The sugar-phosphate backbones are arranged at specific distances from one another in the double helix (see Fig. 1-1). The two regions formed in the helix by the backbones are called the **major groove** and **minor groove**. The major and minor grooves are sites of interaction with the many proteins that bind to specific nucleotide sequences in DNA (binding or **recognition sites**). The double helix can also be penetrated by **intercalating agents**, molecules that slide transversely into the center of the helix. **Denaturing agents** such as formamide and urea displace the hydrogen bonds and separate the two strands of the helix.

Growing strand

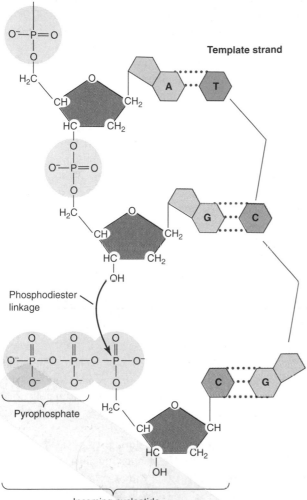

Figure 1-6 DNA replication is a template-guided polymerization catalyzed by DNA polymerase.

respective bases (A with T and G with C). The bases are positioned such that the sugar-phosphate chain that connects them (**sugar-phosphate backbone**) is oriented in a spiral or helix around the nitrogen bases (see Fig. 1-1).

PO 5′ **G T A G C T C G C T G A T** 3′ OH
HO 3′ **C A T C G A G C G A C T A** 5′ OP

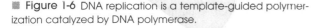

Figure 1-7 Homologous sequences are not identical and are oriented in opposite directions.

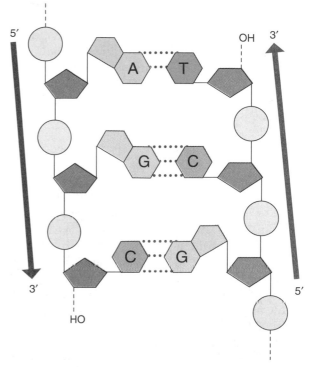

Figure 1-8 DNA synthesis proceeds from the 5' phosphate group to the 3' hydroxyl group. The template strand is copied in the opposite (3' to 5') direction. The new double helix consists of the template strand and the new daughter strand oriented in opposite directions from one another.

The DNA double helix represents two versions of the information stored in the form of the order or sequence of the nucleotides on each chain. The sequences of the two strands that form the double helix are complementary, not identical (Fig. 1-7). They are in **antiparallel** orientation with the 5' end of one strand at the 3' end of the other (Fig. 1-8). The formation of hydrogen bonds between two complementary strands of DNA is called **hybridization**. Single strands of DNA with identical sequences will not hybridize with each other. In later sections we will appreciate the importance of this when designing assays.

DNA Replication

DNA has an antiparallel orientation because of the way it is replicated. As DNA synthesis proceeds in the 5' to 3' direction, DNA polymerase, the enzyme responsible for polymerizing the nucleotides, uses a guide, or **template**, to determine which nucleotides to add. The enzyme reads the template in the 3' to 5' direction. The resulting double strand, then, will have a parent strand in one orientation and a newly synthesized strand in the opposite orientation.

As Watson and Crick predicted, **semi-conservative** replication is the key to maintaining the sequence of the nucleotides in DNA through new generations. Every cell in a multicellular organism or in a clonal population of unicellular organisms carries the same genetic information. It is important that this information, in the form of the DNA sequence, be transferred faithfully at cell division. The replication apparatus is designed to copy the DNA strands in an orderly way with minimal errors before each cell division.

The order of nucleotides is maintained during DNA replication because each strand of the parent double helix is the template for a newly replicated strand. In the process of replication, DNA is first unwound from the helical duplex so that each single strand may serve as a template for the addition of nucleotides to the new strand (see Fig. 1-6). The new strand is elongated by hydrogen bonding of the proper incoming nucleotide to the nitrogen base on the template strand and then a nucleophilic attack of the deoxyribose 3' hydroxyl oxygen on a phosphorous atom of the phosphate group on the hydrogen-bonded nucleotide triphosphate. Orthophosphate is

Historical Highlights

A few years after solution of the double helix, the mechanism of semi-conservative replication was demonstrated by Matthew Meselson and Franklin Stahl,[11] using the technique of equilibrium density centrifugation on a cesium gradient. They prepared "heavy" DNA by growing bacteria in a medium containing the nitrogen isotope ^{15}N. After shifting the bacteria into a medium of normal nitrogen (^{14}N), they could separate hybrid ^{14}N:^{15}N DNA molecules synthesized as the bacteria replicated. These molecules were of intermediate density to the ones from bacteria grown only in ^{14}N or ^{15}N. They could differentiate true semi-conservative replication from **dispersive** replication by demonstrating that approximately half of the DNA double helices from the next generation grown in ^{14}N were ^{14}N:^{15}N and half were ^{14}N:^{14}N.

Historical Highlights

Before the double helix was determined, Erwin Chargaff[10] made the observation that the amount of adenine in DNA corresponded to the amount of thymine, and the amount of cytosine to the amount of guanine. Upon the description of the double helix, Watson proposed that steps in the ladder of the double helix were pairs of bases, thymine with adenine and guanine with cytosine. Watson and Crick, upon publication of their work, suggested that this arrangement was the basis for a copying mechanism. The complementary strands could separate and serve as guides or templates for producing like strands.

released with the formation of a phosphodiester bond between the new nucleotide and the last nucleotide of the growing chain. The duplicated helix will ultimately consist of one template strand and one newly synthesized strand.

DNA replication proceeds through the DNA duplex with both strands of DNA replicating in a single pass. DNA undergoing active replication can be observed by electron microscopy as a forked structure, or **replication fork**. Note, however, that the antiparallel nature of duplex DNA and the requirement for the DNA synthesis apparatus to read the template strand in a 3' to 5' direction are not consistent with copying of both strands simultaneously in the same direction. The question arises as to how one of the strands of the duplex can be copied in the same direction as its complementary strand that runs antiparallel to it.

This problem was addressed in 1968 by Okazaki and Okazaki,[12] who were studying DNA replication in *Escherichia coli*. In their experiments, small pieces of DNA, about 1000 bases in length, could be observed by density gradient centrifugation in actively replicating DNA. The fragments converted into larger pieces with time, showing that they were covalently linked together shortly after synthesis. These small fragments, or

Okazaki fragments, were the key to explaining how both strands were copied at the replication fork. The two strands of the parent helix are not copied in the same way. While DNA replication proceeds in a continuous manner on the 3' to 5' strand, or the **leading strand**, the replication apparatus jumps ahead a short distance (~1000 bases) on the 5' to 3' strand and then copies backward toward the replication fork. The 5' to 3' strand copied in a discontinuous manner is the **lagging strand** (Fig. 1-9).[13]

Another requirement for DNA synthesis is the availability of a deoxyribose 3' hydroxyl oxygen for chain growth. This means that DNA cannot be synthesized de novo, as a preceding base must be present to provide the hydroxyl group. This base is provided by another enzyme component of the replication apparatus, **primase**.[14] Primase is a ribonucleic acid (RNA) synthesizing enzyme that lays down short (6–11 bp) RNA **primers** required for priming DNA synthesis. Primase must work repeatedly on the lagging strand to prime synthesis of each Okazaki fragment.

Polymerases

The first purified enzyme shown to catalyze DNA replication in prokaryotes was designated DNA polymerase I (pol I). DNA polymerases II (pol II) and III were later characterized, and it was discovered that DNA polymerase III (pol III) was the main polymerizing enzyme during bacterial replication (Table 1.1). The other two polymerases were responsible for repair of gaps and discontinuities in previously synthesized DNA. It not surprising that pol I was preferentially purified in those early studies. In in vitro studies where the enzymes were first described, pol II and pol III activity was less than 5% of that of pol I. In vivo, pol III functions as a multisubunit

Advanced Concepts

The DNA replication complex (**replisome**) contains all the necessary proteins for the several activities involved in faithful replication of double-stranded DNA. **Helicase** activity in the replisome unwinds and untangles the DNA for replication. Primase functions either as a separate protein or in a primase-helicase polyprotein in the replisome. Primase activity is required throughout the replication process to prime the discontinuous synthesis on the lagging DNA strand. The *E. coli* primase, DnaG, transcribes 2000–3000 RNA primers at a rate of 1 per second in the replication of the *E. coli* genome. Separate polymerase proteins add incoming nucleotides to the growing DNA strands of the replication fork. The details of synthesis of the lagging strand are not yet clear, although recent evidence suggests discontinuous replication proceeds by a ratcheting mechanism, with replisome molecules pulling the lagging strand in for priming and copying.[15] Once DNA is primed and synthesized, **RNAse H**, an enzyme that hydrolyzes RNA from a complementary DNA strand, removes the primer RNA from the short RNA-DNA hybrid, and the resulting **gap** is filled by gap-filling DNA polymerase.

holoenzyme. The holoenzyme works along with a larger assembly of proteins required for priming, initiation, regulation, and termination of the replication process (Fig. 1-10). Two of the 10 subunits of the holoenzyme are catalytic DNA polymerizing enzymes, one for leading and one for lagging strand synthesis.[16]

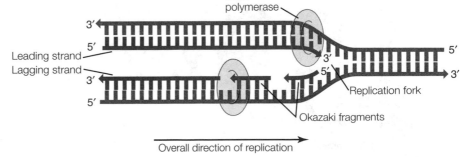

■ **Figure 1-9** Simultaneous replication of both strands of the double helix. Both strands are read in the 3' to 5' direction. The lagging strand is read discontinuously, with the polymerase skipping ahead and reading back toward the replication fork on the lagging strand.

Overall direction of replication

Table 1.1 **Examples of Polymerases Classified by Sequence Homology**

Family	Polymerase	Source	Activity
A	Pol I	*E. coli*	Recombination, repair, replication
A	T5 pol, T7 pol	T5, T7 bacteriophage	Replication
A	Polγ	Mitochondria	Replication
B	Pol II	*E. coli*	Repair
B	Archael	*P. furiosus*	Replication, repair
B	φ29 pol, T4 pol	φ29, T4 bacteriophage	Replication
B	Polα Polδ, Polε	Eukaryotes	Repair
B	Viral pols	Various viruses	Repair
C	Pol III core	*E. coli*	Replication
C	dnaE, dnaE$_{BS}$	*B. subtilis*	Replication
X	Polβ	Eukaryotes	Repair, replication
?	Polη, Polι	Eukaryotes	Bypass replication
?	Polκ	Eukaryotes	Bypass replication, cohesion
?	Pol IV, Pol V	*E. coli*	Bypass replication
?	Rev1, Rad30	*S. cerevisiae*	Bypass replication, uv-induced repair
?	Rad 6, Polξ	*S. cerevisiae*	

Most DNA polymerases have more than one function, including, in addition to polymerization, pyrophosphorolysis and **pyrophosphate** exchange, the latter two activities being a reversal of the polymerization process. DNA polymerase enzymes thus have the capacity to synthesize DNA in a 5' to 3' direction and degrade DNA in both a 5' to 3' and 3' to 5' direction (Fig 1-11). The catalytic domain of *E. coli* DNA pol I can be broken into two fragments, separating the two functions, a large fragment carrying the polymerase activity and a small fragment carrying the exonuclease activity. The large fragment without the exonuclease activity (**Klenow fragment**) has been used extensively in the laboratory for in vitro DNA synthesis.

One purpose of the **exonuclease** function in the various DNA polymerases is to protect the sequence of nucleotides, which must be faithfully copied. Copying errors will result in base changes, or **mutations**, in the DNA. The 3' to 5' exonuclease function is required to assure that replication begins or continues with a correctly base-paired nucleotide. The enzyme will remove a mismatch (e.g., A opposite C instead of T on the template) in the primer sequence before beginning polymerization. During DNA synthesis, this exonuclease

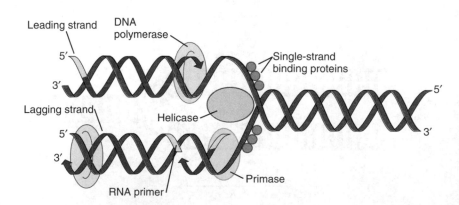

■ Figure 1-10 DNA polymerase activity involves more than one protein molecule. Several cofactors and accessory proteins are required to unwind the template helix (purple), prime synthesis with RNA primers (gray), and protect the lagging strand (dark gray).

Advanced Concepts

Genome sequencing has revealed that the organization of the proteins in and associated with the holoenzyme is similar in bacteria of the *Bacillus/Clostridium* group and in the unrelated thermophile, *Thermotoga maritima*. The conserved nature of the polymerase complex suggests a limited range of possible structures with polymerase activity. It also explains how a bacterial polymerase can replicate DNA from diverse sources. This is important in the laboratory where prokaryote polymerases are used extensively to copy DNA from many different organisms.

Historical Highlights

At a conference on the chemical basis of heredity held at Johns Hopkins University in June 1956, Arthur Kornberg, I. Robert Lehman, and Maurice J. Bessman reported on an extract of *E. coli* that could polymerize nucleotides into DNA in vitro.[13] It was noted that the reaction required preformed DNA and all four nucleotides along with the bacterial protein extract. Any source of preformed DNA would work—bacterial, viral, or animal. At the time it was difficult to determine whether the new DNA was a copy of the input molecule or an extension of it. During the next 3 years, Julius Adler, Sylvy Kornberg, and Steven B. Zimmerman showed that the new DNA had the same A-T to G-C base pair ratio as the input DNA and was indeed a copy of it. This ratio was not affected by the proportion of free nucleotides added to the initial reaction, confirming that the input or template DNA determined the sequence of the nucleotides on the newly synthesized DNA.

function gives the enzyme the capacity to **proofread** newly synthesized DNA, that is, to remove a misincorporated nucleotide by breaking the phosphodiester bond and replace it with the correct one.

During DNA replication, *E. coli* DNA pol III can synthesize and degrade DNA simultaneously. At a **nick**, or discontinuity, in one strand of a DNA duplex, the enzyme can add nucleotides at the 3' end of the nick while removing nucleotides ahead of it with its 5' to 3' exonuclease function (Fig. 1-12). This concurrent synthesis and hydrolysis then move the nick in one strand of the DNA forward in an activity called **nick translation**. The polymerization and hydrolysis will proceed for a short distance until the polymerase is dislodged. The nick can then be reclosed by DNA **ligase**, an enzyme that forms phosphodiester bonds between existing DNA strands.

Nick translation is often used in vitro as a method to introduce labeled nucleotides into DNA molecules. The resulting labeled products are used for DNA detection in hybridization analyses.

One type of DNA polymerase, **terminal transferase**, can synthesize polynucleotide chains without a template. This enzyme will add nucleotides to the end of a DNA strand in the absence of hydrogen base pairing with a template. The initial synthesis of a large dA-dT polymer by terminal transferase was a significant event in the

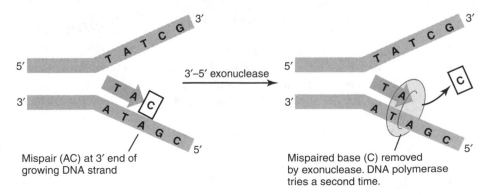

■ **Figure 1-11** DNA polymerase can remove misincorporated bases during replication using its 3' to 5' exonuclease activity.

Mispair (AC) at 3' end of growing DNA strand

3'–5' exonuclease

Mispaired base (C) removed by exonuclease. DNA polymerase tries a second time.

Advanced Concepts

Like prokaryotes, eukaryotic cells contain multiple polymerase activities. Two polymerase protein complexes, designated α and β, are found in the nucleus and one, γ, in the mitochondria. The three polymerases resemble prokaryotic enzymes, except they have less demonstrable exonuclease activity. A fourth polymerase, δ, originally isolated from bone marrow, has 3' to 5' exonuclease activity. Polymerase α, the most active, is identified with chromosome replication, and β and δ are associated with DNA repair.

Advanced Concepts

After replication, distortions in the DNA duplex caused by mismatched or aberrantly modified bases are removed by the 5' to 3' exonuclease function of repair polymerases such as DNA pol I. This activity degrades duplex DNA from the 5' end and can also cleave diester bonds several bases from the end of the chain. It is important for removing lesions in the DNA duplex such as **thymine** or **pyrimidine dimers**, which are boxy structures formed between adjacent thymines or cytosines and thymines on the same DNA strand that are induced by exposure of DNA to ultraviolet light. If these structures are not removed, they can disrupt subsequent transcription and replication of the DNA strand.

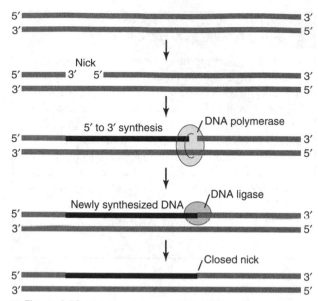

■ **Figure 1-12** Nick translation of DNA. DNA polymerase extends the 3' end of a nick in double-stranded DNA with a newly synthesized strand (gray) while digesting the original strand from the 5' end. After polymerization, the nick is closed by DNA ligase.

are based on similarities in protein structure. Polymerases in the A and B families are most useful for biotechnological engineering, as the polymerase activity of these enzymes is contained in a **monomeric**, or single, protein. Chemical manipulation of the amino acid structure produces polymerases with characteristics that are useful in the laboratory. These include altered **processivity** (staying with the template longer to make longer products), **fidelity** (faithful copying of the template), and **substrate specificity** (affinity for altered nucleotides).[19]

history of DNA polymerase studies.[17] Terminal transferase is used in the laboratory to generate 3'-labeled DNA species.

DNA polymerases play a central role in modern biotechnology. Cloning as well as some amplification and sequencing technologies all require DNA polymerase activity. The prerequisite for specific polymerase characteristics has stimulated the search for new polymerases and the engineering of available polymerase enzymes. Polymerases from various sources were classified into families (A, B, C, X) based on sequence structure.[18,19] A short summary is shown in Table 1.1. Other classifications

Advanced Concepts

Polymerases replicate DNA under different cellular conditions, as shown in Table 1.1. A large part of DNA synthesis activity in the cell occurs after replication of the cellular DNA is complete. New information as to the nature of these enzymes indicates that polymerases can participate in cohesion (holding together) of sister chromatids to assure proper recombination and segregation of chromosomes.[20]

Enzymes That Metabolize DNA

Once DNA is polymerized, it is not static. The information stored in the DNA must be tapped selectively to make RNA and, at the same time, protected from damage. Protective systems in prokaryotes eliminate foreign DNA, such as infecting **bacteriophages** or other viruses. Enzymes that modify and digest foreign DNA prevent infection. In sexually reproducing organisms, mixing of parental DNA generates genetic diversity (hybrid vigor) in the offspring. This process requires cutting and reassembly of the DNA strands in advance of cell division and **gamete** formation. A host of enzymes performs these and other functions during various stages of the cell cycle. Some of these enzymes, including DNA polymerase, have been isolated for in vitro manipulation of DNA in the laboratory. They are key tools of recombinant DNA technology, the basis for commonly used molecular techniques.[21]

Restriction Enzymes

Genetic engineering was stimulated by the discovery of deoxyriboendonucleases, or **endonucleases**. Endonucleases break the sugar-phosphate backbone of DNA.

   Restriction enzymes are endonucleases that recognize specific base sequences and break or restrict the DNA polymer at the sugar-phosphate backbone. These enzymes were originally isolated from bacteria, where they function as part of a primitive defense system to cleave foreign DNA entering the bacterial cell. The ability of the cell to recognize foreign DNA depended on both DNA sequence recognition and methylation. Restriction enzymes are named for the organism from which they were isolated. For example, *Bam*HI was isolated from *Bacillus amyloliquefaciens* H, *Hind*III from *Haemophilus influenzae* Rd, *Sma*I from *Serratia marcescens* Sb_b, and so forth.

   Restriction endonucleases have been classified into four types. Type I restriction enzymes have both nuclease and methylase activity in a single enzyme. They bind to host-specific DNA sites of 4–6 bp separated by 6–8 bp and containing methylated adenines. The site of cleavage of the DNA substrate can be over 1000 bp from this binding site. An example of a type I enzyme is *EcoK* from *E. coli* K 12. It recognizes the site:

$$5' - A^{Me} C N N N N N G T\ \ \ G C$$
$$T\ \ \ G N N N N N N C A^{Me}\ C G - 5'$$

where N represents nonspecific nucleotides and the adenine residues are methylated (A^{Me}).

   Type III restriction enzymes resemble type I enzymes in their ability to both methylate and restrict (cut) DNA. Like type I, they are complex enzymes with two subunits. Recognition sites for these enzymes are asymmetrical, and the cleavage of the substrate DNA occurs 24–26 bp from the site to the 3' side. An example of a type III enzyme is *Pst*IIII from *P. stuartii*.[22] It recognizes the site:

$$5'\ C T G A T\ \ G$$
$$G A C T A^{Me} C\ \ 5'$$

where the adenine methylation occurs on only one strand. The enzyme cuts the DNA 25–26 bp 3' to the recognition site.

   Type IV restriction enzymes have similar subunit structures and enzyme requirements. Type IV enzymes have cutting and methyltransferase functions. An example of type IV restriction enzymes is *Bse*MII from *Bacillus stearothermophilus*. The *Bse*MII target sequence is:

$$5'\ C T C A G$$
$$G A G T C\ 5'$$

The restriction endonuclease function of *Bse*MII cuts one strand of DNA 10 bp following the recognition sequence. *Bse*MII also has a methylation function, adding methyl groups to both of the adenine residues in the target sequence.[23]

   Type II restriction enzymes are those used most frequently in the laboratory. These enzymes do not have inherent methylation activity. They bind as simple dimers to symmetrical DNA recognition sites. These sites are **palindromic** in nature; that is, they read the same 5' to 3'

Advanced Concepts

There are of several types of endonucleases. Some prefer single-stranded and some prefer double-stranded DNA. Repair endonucleases function at areas of distortion in the DNA duplex such as baseless (apurinic or apyrimidic) sites on the DNA backbone, thymine dimers, or mismatched bases. As the chemical structure of DNA is the same in all organisms, most enzymes are active on DNA from diverse sources.

Advanced Concepts

Type II restriction enzyme recognition sequences in DNA are generally areas of bilateral rotational symmetry around an axis perpendicular to the DNA helix. The enzymes bind to the recognition site, which is usually 4–8 bp in length, as dimers to form a complex with twofold symmetry. The enzymes then cleave the DNA backbone at sites symmetrically located around the same twofold axis.

Advanced Concepts

Some type II enzymes have characteristic activity. Type IIS restriction endonucleases (e.g., *Fok I*, *Alw1*) recognize 5 to 7 bp nonpalindromic sequences and cut DNA within 20 bases of the recognition site. Type IIM restriction enzymes (e.g., *Bis1I*, *Dpn1*) cut methylated DNA. Methylation-specific enzymes are a useful tool in detecting methylation in DNA.

on both strands of the DNA (Fig. 1-13), referred to as **bilateral symmetry**. Type II restriction enzymes cleave the DNA directly at the binding site, producing fragments of predictable size.

Type II restriction enzymes have been found in almost all prokaryotes, but none, to date, have been found in eukaryotes. The specificity of their action and the hundreds of enzymes available that recognize numerous sites are key factors in the ability to perform DNA recombination in vitro. Cutting DNA at specific sequences is the basis of many procedures in molecular technology, including mapping, cloning, genetic engineering, and mutation analysis. Restriction enzymes are frequently used in the medical laboratory, for example, in the analysis of gene rearrangements and in mutation detection.

Although all type II restriction enzymes work with bilateral symmetry, their patterns of **double-stranded breaks** differ (see Fig. 1-13). Some enzymes cut the duplex with a staggered separation at the recognition site, leaving 2–4 base single-strand **overhangs** at the ends of the DNA. The single-strand ends can hybridize with **complementary** ends on other DNA fragments, directing the efficient joining of cut ends. Because of their ability to form hydrogen bonds with complementary overhangs, these cuts are said to produce "**sticky ends**" at the cut site. Another mode of cutting separates the DNA duplex

at the same place on both strands, leaving flush, or **blunt**, ends. These ends can be rejoined as well, although not as efficiently as sticky ends.

Restriction enzymes can be used for mapping a DNA fragment, as will be described in later sections. The collection of fragments generated by digestion of a given DNA fragment—for example, a region of a human chromosome—with several restriction enzymes will be unique to that DNA. This was the basis for forensic

Advanced Concepts

The advantage of blunt ends for in vitro recombination is that blunt ends formed by different enzymes can be joined, regardless of the recognition site. This is not true for sticky ends, which must have matching overhangs. Sticky ends can be converted to blunt ends using DNA polymerase to extend the recessed strand in a sticky end, using the nucleotides of the overhang as a template or by using a single-strand exonuclease to remove the overhanging nucleotides. Synthetic short DNA fragments with one blunt end and one sticky end (**adaptors**) can be used to convert blunt ends to specific sticky ends.

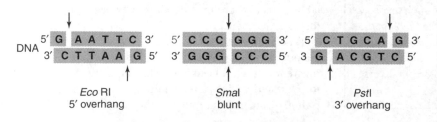

■ Figure 1-13 Restriction enzymes recognize symmetrical DNA sequences and cut the sugar-phosphate background in different ways. Exposed single-stranded ends are "sticky" ends that can hybridize with complementary overhangs.

identification and paternity testing using restriction fragment analysis of human DNA.

DNA Ligase

DNA ligase catalyzes the formation of a phosphodiester bond between adjacent 3'-hydroxyl and 5'-phosphoryl nucleotide ends. Its existence was predicted by the observation of replication, recombination, and repair activities in vivo. These operations require reunion of the DNA backbone after discontinuous replication on the lagging strand, strand exchange, or repair synthesis. In 1967, five separate laboratories discovered DNA ligase.[24] The isolated enzyme could catalyze end-to-end cleavage of separated strands of DNA.

Other DNA Metabolizing Enzymes

Other Nucleases

In contrast to endonucleases, exonucleases degrade DNA from free 3' hydroxyl or 5' phosphate ends. Consequently, they will not work on closed, circular DNA. These enzymes are used, under controlled conditions, to manipulate DNA in vitro,[27] for instance, to make stepwise deletions in linearized DNA or to modify DNA ends after cutting with restriction enzymes. Exonucleases have different substrate requirements and will therefore degrade specific types of DNA ends.

Exonuclease I from *E. coli* degrades single-stranded DNA from the 3' hydroxyl end into mononucleotides. Its activity is optimal on long, single-stranded ends, slowing significantly as it approaches a double-stranded region.

Advanced Concepts

DNA ligase can join both DNA and RNA ends.[26] RNA ligase, first found in phage T4–infected bacteria, has the same activity. DNA ligases are more efficient in joining DNA ends and have been found in a wide variety of bacteria. The ability to convert open or nicked circles of DNA to closed circles, to protect free DNA ends, to extend DNA into an overhanging template, and to recover transformation-capable DNA after nicking are all activities of **DNA ligase** that led to its discovery and isolation.

Exonuclease III from *E. coli* removes 5' mononucleotides from the 3' end of double-stranded DNA in the presence of Mg^{2+} and Mn^{2+}. It also has some endonuclease activity, cutting DNA at apurinic sites. Exo III removes nucleotides from blunt ends, recessed ends, and

---

Historical Highlights

The initial analysis of the reaction joining separate DNA helices was performed with physically fractured DNA with no complementary bases at the ends of the fragments. The joining reaction required the chance positioning of two adjacent ends and was, therefore, not very efficient. A better substrate for the enzyme would be ends that could be held together before ligation, that is, by hydrogen bonds between single strands. H. Gobind Khorana showed that short synthetic segments of DNA with single-strand complementary overhangs joined into larger fragments efficiently.[25] Several investigators noted the increased efficiency of joining of ends of DNA molecules from certain bacterial viruses. These ends have naturally occurring single-stranded overhangs. It was also observed that treatment of DNA ends with terminal transferase to add short runs of A's to one fragment and T's to another increased the efficiency of joining ends of any two treated fragments. Although not yet available when ligase activity was being studied, the single-strand overhangs left by some restriction enzymes were better substrates for DNA ligase than blunt ends due to hydrogen bonding of the complementary single-stranded bases.

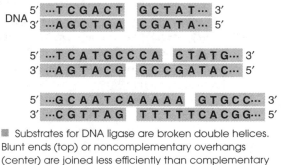

■ Substrates for DNA ligase are broken double helices. Blunt ends (top) or noncomplementary overhangs (center) are joined less efficiently than complementary overhangs (bottom). Also note the complementary overhangs in Figure 1-13.

nicks but will not digest 3' overhangs. Exo III has been used in the research setting to create nested deletions in double-stranded DNA or to produce single-stranded DNA for dideoxy sequencing.

Exonuclease VII from *E. coli* digests single-stranded DNA from either the 5' phosphate or 3' hydroxyl end. It is one of the few enzymes with 5' exonuclease activity. Exo VII can be employed to remove long single strands protruding from double-stranded DNA.

Nuclease Bal31 from *Alteromonas espejiani* can degrade single- and double-stranded DNA from both ends. Because its activity at 20°C is slow enough to control with good resolution, it has been useful in research applications to make nested deletions in DNA.

Mung bean nuclease from Mung bean sprouts digests single-stranded DNA and RNA. Because it leaves double-stranded regions intact, it is used to remove overhangs from restriction fragments to produce blunt ends for cloning.

S1 nuclease from *Aspergillus oryzae* is another single-strand–specific nuclease. It hydrolyzes single-stranded DNA or RNA into 5' mononucleotides. It also has endonuclease capability to hydrolyze single-stranded regions such as gaps and loops in duplex DNA. It was used in early RNAse protection assays of gene expression. It is also used for nuclease mapping techniques.[28]

recBC nuclease from *E. coli* is an ATP-dependent single- and double-stranded DNA nuclease. Although it has no activity at nicks (short, single-strand gaps) in the DNA, it digests single-stranded DNA from either the 3' hydroxyl or the 5' phosphate end. It has some endonuclease activity on duplex DNA, generating short fragments, or **oligonucleotides**.

Micrococcal nuclease digests single- and double-stranded DNA and RNA at AT- or AU-rich regions. Although this enzyme can digest duplex DNA, it prefers single-stranded substrates. It is used in the laboratory to remove nucleic acid from crude extracts and also for analysis of chromatin structure.[29]

Deoxyribonuclease I (DNAse I) from bovine pancreas digests single- and double-stranded DNA at pyrimidines to oligodeoxyribonucleotides; so, technically, it is an endonuclease. It is used in both research and clinical laboratories to remove DNA from RNA preparations. DNAse I has also been used to detect exposed regions of DNA in DNA protein-binding experiments.

DNA pol I from *E. coli* has exonuclease activity. Formerly called exonuclease II, this activity is responsible for the proofreading function of the polymerase.

As nucleases are natural components of cellular lysates, it is important to eliminate or inactivate them when preparing nucleic acid specimens for clinical analysis. Most DNA isolation procedures are designed to minimize both endonuclease and exonuclease activity during DNA isolation. Purified DNA is often stored in **TE buffer** (10 mM Tris-HCl, pH 8.0, 0.1 mM EDTA) to chelate cations required by nucleases for activity.

Helicases

DNA in bacteria and eukaryotes does not exist as the relaxed double helix shown in Figure 1-1 but as a series of highly organized loops and coils. Release of DNA for transcription, replication, and recombination without tangling is brought about through cutting and reclosing of the DNA sugar-phosphate backbone. These functions are carried out by a series of enzymes called helicases.

As described with restriction endonucleases, the DNA double helix can be broken apart by the separation of the sugar-phosphate backbones in both strands, a **double-strand break**. When only one backbone is broken (a single-strand break, or nick), the broken ends are free to rotate around the intact strand. These ends can be digested by exonuclease activity or extended using the intact strand as a template (nick translation). The nicking and reclosing of DNA by helicases relieve topological stress in highly compacted, or supertwisted, DNA as required, for example, in advance of DNA replication or transcription. Helicases are of two types: topoisomerases and **gyrases**. Topoisomerases interconvert topological isomers or relax supertwisted DNA. Gyrases (type II topoisomerases) untangle DNA through double-strand breaks. They also separate linked rings of DNA (**concatamers**).

Topoisomerases in eukaryotes have activity similar to that in bacteria but with different mechanisms of cutting and binding to the released ends of the DNA. Because of their importance in cell replication, topoisomerases are the targets for several anticancer drugs, such as camptothecin, the epipodophyllotoxins VP-16 and VM-26, amsacrine, and the intercalating anthracycline derivatives doxorubicin and mitoxantrone. These topoisomerase inhibitors bring about cell death by interfering with the breaking and joining activities of the enzymes, in some cases trapping unfinished and broken intermediates.

Methyltransferases

DNA methyltransferases catalyze the addition of methyl groups to nitrogen bases, usually adenines and cytosines in DNA strands. Most prokaryotic DNA is methylated, or **hemimethylated** (methylated on one strand of the double helix and not the other), as a means to differentiate host DNA from nonhost and to provide resistance to restriction enzymes. Unlike prokaryotic DNA, eukaryotic DNA is methylated in specific regions. In eukaryotes, DNA binding proteins may limit accessibility or guide methyltransferases to specific regions of the DNA.

In eukaryotic cells, there are two main types of methyltransferases. Maintenance methyltransferases work throughout the life of the cell and methylate hemimethylated DNA. In contrast, de novo methyltransferases work only during embryonic development and may be responsible for the specific methylation patterns in differentiated cells.

Advanced Concepts

Enzymatic interconversion of DNA forms was first studied in vitro by observing the action of two *E. coli* enzymes, topoisomeraseI[30] and gyrase,[31] on circular plasmids. Topo I can relax supercoils in circular plasmid DNA by nicking one strand of the double helix. Gyrase, also called topoisomerase II, can introduce coiling by cutting both strands of the helix, passing another part of the duplex through, and re-ligating the cut strand.

Advanced Concepts

Both DNA and RNA helicases have been identified in molds, worms, and plants.[32–35] These enzymes may function in the establishment of local chromosome architecture as well as the regulation of transcription.

Advanced Concepts

Cytosine methyltransferases are key factors in vertebrate development and gene expression. These enzymes catalyze the transfer of an activated methyl group from *S*-adenosyl methionine to the 5 position of the cytosine ring (producing 5-methyl cytosine). Methylation marks DNA for recognition by or resistance to enzymes such as nucleases or architectural proteins in higher eukaryotes. Methylation is the source of DNA **imprinting**, a system that provides a predetermined program of gene expression during development. A specific methyl transferase, Dmnt1, prefers hemimethylated DNA, indicating a mechanism for keeping methylation patterns in the genome.[36] Defects in methylation have been observed in cancer cells,[37] some disease states,[38] and clones,[39] To date, three DNA cytosine methyltransferases have been cloned: DNMT1, DNMT3a, and DNMT3b.[40,41]

Recombination in Sexually Reproducing Organisms

Recombination is the mixture and assembly of new genetic combinations. Recombination occurs through the molecular process of **crossing over**, or physical exchange between molecules. A **recombinant** molecule or organism is one that holds a new combination of DNA sequences.

Based on Mendel's laws, each generation of sexually reproducing organisms is a new combination of the parental genomes. The mixing of genes generates genetic diversity, increasing the opportunity for more robust and well-adapted offspring. The beneficial effect of natural recombination is observed in **heterosis**, or hybrid vigor, observed in genetically mixed or hybrid individuals compared to purebred organisms.

Sexually reproducing organisms mix genes in three ways. First, at the beginning of **meiosis**, duplicated chromosomes line up and **recombine** by crossing over, or breakage and reunion of the four DNA duplexes (Fig. 1-14). This generates newly recombined duplexes with genes from each duplicate. Then, the recombined

Historical Highlights

Early studies of recombination were done with whole organisms. Mendel's analysis of peas (*Pisum* species)[42] established the general rules of recombination in sexually reproducing organisms. Mendel could infer the molecular exchange events that occurred in the plants by observing the phenotype of progeny. These observations had been made before, with quantitative predictions of the probability of phenotypes. Mendel proposed that traits are inherited in a particulate manner rather than blending, as was previously thought.

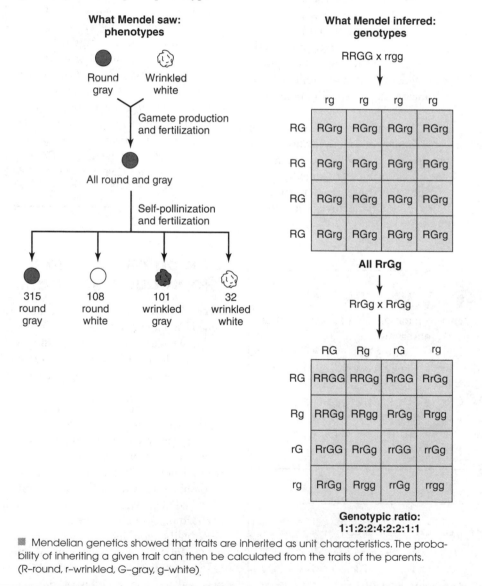

■ Mendelian genetics showed that traits are inherited as unit characteristics. The probability of inheriting a given trait can then be calculated from the traits of the parents. (R–round, r–wrinkled, G–gray, g–white).

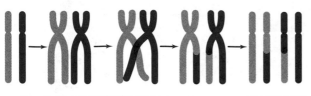

Genetic recombination by crossing over   Recombinant
chromosomes

■ **Figure 1-14** Generation of genetic diversity by crossing over of homologous chromosomes.

duplexes are randomly assorted into gametes (Fig. 1-15) so that each gamete contains one set of each of the recombined parental chromosomes. Finally, the gamete will merge with a gamete from the other parent carrying its own set of recombined chromosomes. The resulting offspring will contain a new set or recombination of genes of both parents. The nature of this recombination is manifested in the combinations of inherited traits of subsequent generations.

Recombinant DNA technology is a controlled mixing of genes. Rather than relying on natural mixing of whole genomes, single genes can be altered, replaced, deleted, or moved into new genomes. This directed diversity can produce organisms with predictable traits, as natural purebreds, but with single-gene differences. The ability

to manipulate single traits has implications not only in the laboratory but also potentially in the treatment and prevention of disease; for example, through gene therapy.

Recombination in Asexual Reproduction

Movement and manipulation of genes in the laboratory began with the study of natural recombination in asexually reproducing bacteria. Genetic information in asexually reproducing organisms can be recombined in three ways: conjugation, transduction, and transformation (Fig. 1-16).

Conjugation

Bacteria that participate in **conjugation** are of two types, or sexes, termed F+ and F–. For conjugation to occur, F– and F+ cells must be in contact with each other. The contact requirement can be demonstrated by physically separating F+ and F' cells, in which case mating does not occur (Fig. 1-17). Microscopically, a filamentous bridge is observed between mating bacteria. Work by J. Lederberg and William Hayes demonstrated polarity in the

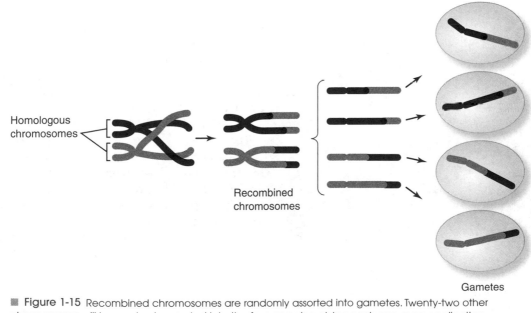

Homologous
chromosomes

Recombined
chromosomes

Gametes

■ **Figure 1-15** Recombined chromosomes are randomly assorted into gametes. Twenty-two other chromosomes will be randomly assorted into the four gametes, giving each one a new collection of recombined chromosomes.

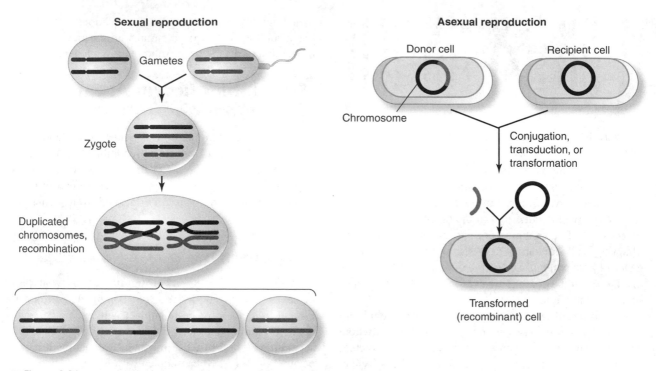

■ Figure 1-16 Recombination in sexual (left) and asexual (right) reproduction.

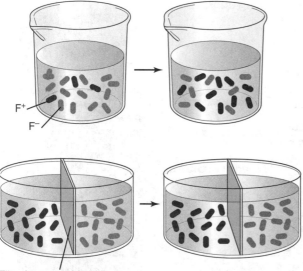

■ Figure 1-17 Conjugating cells must be in physical contact with each other (top) for successful transfer of the F+ phenotype. If cells are separated by a membrane (bottom), F– bacteria do not become F+.

conjugation process; that is, genetic information could move from F+ to F– bacteria but not from F– to F+ bacteria. The explanation for this was soon discovered. The F+ bacteria had a "**fertility factor**" that not only carried the information from one cell to another but also was responsible for establishing the physical connection between the mating bacteria. The fertility factor was transferred from F+ to F– bacteria in the mating process so that afterward the F– bacteria became F+ (Fig. 1-18).

The F factor was shown to be an extrachromosomal circle of double-stranded DNA carrying the genes coding for construction of the mating bridge. Genes carried on the F factor are transferred across the bridge and simultaneously replicated so that one copy of the F factor remains in the F+ bacteria and the other is sent into the F– bacteria. After mating, both bacteria are F+. The F factor may be lost or cured during normal cell division, converting an F+ bacteria to the F– state.

The F factor can also insert itself into the host chromosome through a crossover or recombination event. Embedded in the chromosome, the F factor maintains its ability to direct mating and can carry part or all of the

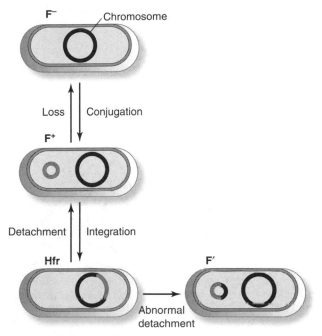

■ Figure 1-18 Fertility (the ability to donate genetic information) is controlled by the F factor (purple). The F factor can exist by itself or be integrated into the host chromosome (large black circle).

Historical Highlights

Historically, recombination was studied through controlled mating and propagation of organisms. George Beadle[43] and others confirmed the connection between the units of heredity and physical phenotype using molds (*Neurospera crassa*), bacteria, and viruses. Joshua Lederberg and Edward L. Tatum[44] demonstrated that bacteria mate and exchange genetic information to produce recombinant offspring and proved that genetic exchange between organisms was not restricted to the sexually reproducing molds. These early studies first demonstrated the existence of recombination in *E. coli*.

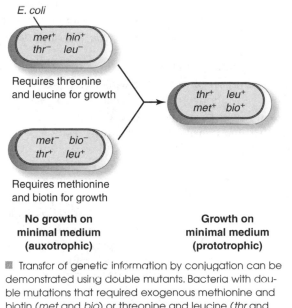

■ Transfer of genetic information by conjugation can be demonstrated using double mutants. Bacteria with double mutations that required exogenous methionine and biotin (*met* and *bio*) or threonine and leucine (*thr* and *leu*) cannot grow on a medium without addition of these nutrients (minimal medium). When these strains are mixed together, however, growth occurs. The resulting bacteria have acquired the normal genes (+) through transfer or conjugation.

insert that information into the recipient chromosome, forming a recombinant or new combination of genes of the Hfr and F– bacteria. Hfr bacteria were used in the first mapping studies.

Transduction

In the early 1960s, Francois Jacob and Elie Wollman[45] studied the transmission of units of heredity carried by viruses from one bacterium to another (**transduction**). Just as animal and plant viruses infect eukaryotic cells, bacterial viruses, or **bacteriophages**, infect bacterial cells. The structure of bacteriophage T4 is one example of the specialized protein coats that enable these viruses to insert their DNA through the cell wall into the bacterial cell (Fig. 1-19). Alfred Hershey and Martha Chase confirmed that the DNA of a bacterial virus was the carrier of its genetic determination in the transduction process.[46] Hershey and Chase used ^{35}S to label the viral protein and ^{32}P to label the viral DNA. The experiment showed that viral protein remained outside of the cell

host chromosome with it across the mating bridge into F– bacteria. Strains with chromosomally embedded F factors are called **Hfr** bacteria (for high frequency of recombination). When the embedded F factor in these rarely occurring strains pulls host chromosomal information into recipient bacteria, another recombination event can

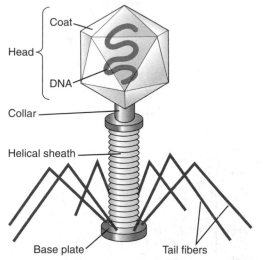

■ Figure 1-19 Bacteriophage T4 infects specific strains of *E. coli*. It has specialized structures. The tail fibers find the bacterial surface and allow contact of the tail plate and injection of the DNA in the viral head through the sheath into the bacterium.

while viral DNA entered the cell. Furthermore, ^{32}P-labeled DNA could be detected in new viruses generated in the transduction process (Fig. 1-20).

Methods soon developed using bacteriophages to move genetic information between bacteria by growing the phage on one strain of bacteria and then infecting a second strain with those viruses. Transduction is also useful in determining gene order. Seymour Benzer used transduction of the T4 bacterial virus to fine-map genes.[47]

Transformation

Although conjugation and transduction were the methods for the initial study of the connection between DNA and phenotype, **transformation**, which had first been observed in 1928 by Frederick Griffith,[48] is the basis for modern-day recombinant techniques. Griffith was investigating virulence in *Diplococcus* (now known as *Streptococcus*) *pneumoniae*. He had two strains of the bacteria: one with a rough colony type that was avirulent and one with a smooth colony type that was virulent. Griffith intended to use these strains to develop a protective vaccine (Fig. 1-21). He knew that the live smooth-type bacteria were lethal in mice and the live rough-type were not. If he first killed the smooth-type bacteria by boiling them, virulence was lost and they were no longer lethal to mice. Surprisingly, when he mixed killed smooth-type and live rough-type bacteria, virulence returned. Furthermore, he could recover live smooth-type bacteria from the dead mice. He concluded that something from the dead smooth-type bacteria had "transformed" the rough-type bacteria into virulent smooth-type.

What Griffith had observed was the transfer of DNA from one organism to another without the protection of a conjugative bridge or a viral coat. Fifteen years later, Oswald T. Avery, Colin MacLeod, and M.J. McCarty identified the transforming material as DNA.[49,50] They prepared boiled virulent bacterial cell lysates and sequentially treated them with recently discovered enzymes (Fig. 1-22). **Protease** and **ribonuclease** treatment, which degraded protein and RNA, respectively, did not affect the transformation phenomenon that Griffith had demonstrated earlier. Treatment with **deoxyribonuclease**, which degrades DNA, however, prevented transformation. They concluded that the "transforming factor" that Griffith had first proposed was DNA. The transduction experiment of Alfred Hershey and Martha Chase also confirmed their findings that DNA carried genetic traits.

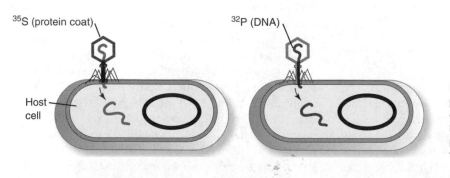

■ Figure 1-20 Radioactive (purple) protein does not enter the host cell during transduction (left). Radioactive DNA, however, does enter (right) and is passed to subsequent generations of viruses.

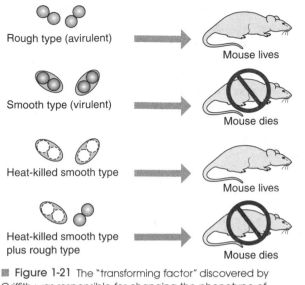

Figure 1-21 The "transforming factor" discovered by Griffith was responsible for changing the phenotype of the avirulent rough-type bacteria to that of the virulent smooth-type.

Rough type (avirulent) — Mouse lives
Smooth type (virulent) — Mouse dies
Heat-killed smooth type — Mouse lives
Heat-killed smooth type plus rough type — Mouse dies

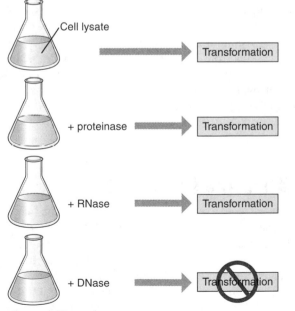

Cell lysate — Transformation
+ proteinase — Transformation
+ RNase — Transformation
+ DNase — Transformation

Figure 1-22 Avery, MacLeod, and McCarty showed that destruction of protein or RNA in the cell lysate did not affect the transforming factor. Only destruction of DNA prevented transformation.

Advanced Concepts

Investigators performing early transformation studies observed the transfer of broken chromosomal DNA from one population of bacterial cells to another. Naked DNA transferred in this way is very inefficient, however. Unprotected DNA is subject to physical shearing as well as chemical degradation from naturally occurring nucleases, especially on the broken ends of the DNA molecules. Natural transformations are much more efficient, because the transforming DNA is in the form or circles or otherwise protected, especially on the ends.

Plasmids

DNA helices can assume both linear and circular forms. Most bacterial chromosomes are in circular form, in contrast to chromosomes in higher organisms, such as fungi, plants, and animals, which are mostly linear. A bacterial cell can contain, in addition to its own chromosome complement, extrachromosomal entities, or **plasmids** (Fig. 1-23). Most plasmids are double-stranded circles,

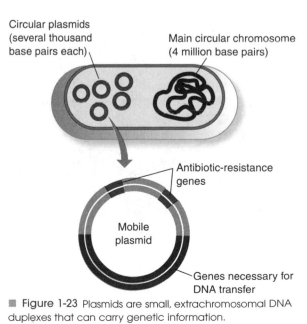

Circular plasmids (several thousand base pairs each) — Main circular chromosome (4 million base pairs) — Antibiotic-resistance genes — Mobile plasmid — Genes necessary for DNA transfer

Figure 1-23 Plasmids are small, extrachromosomal DNA duplexes that can carry genetic information.

2000–100,000 bp (2–100 kilobase pairs) in size. Plasmids can carry genetic information, but due to their size and effect on the host cell, they carry only a limited amount of information.

The plasmid DNA duplex is compacted, or supercoiled. Breaking one strand of the plasmid duplex, or nicking, will relax the supercoil (Fig. 1-24), whereas breaking both strands will linearize the plasmid. Different physical states of the plasmid DNA can be resolved by distinct **migration** characteristics during gel electrophoresis.

Plasmids were found to be a source of resistant phenotypes in multidrug-resistant bacteria.[51] The demonstration that multiple drug resistance in bacteria can be eliminated by treatment with acridine dyes[52] was the first indication of the **episomal** (plasmid) nature of the resistance factor, similar to the F factor in conjugation. (Acridine dyes induce the loss of **episomes**.) In resistant bacteria, plasmids carrying the genes for inactivation or circumvention of antibiotic action were called resistance transfer factors (RTF), or **R factors**. R factors promote resistance to such common antibiotics as chloramphenicol, tetracycline, ampicillin, and streptomycin. Another class of plasmid, **colicinogenic factors**, carries resistance to **bacteriocins**, toxic proteins manufactured by bacteria.

The acquisition of the resistance genes from host chromosomes of unknown bacteria is the presumed origin of these resistance factors.[53] Drug-resistance genes are commonly gained and lost from episomes in a bacterial population. Two different R factors in a single cell can undergo a recombination event, producing a new, recombinant plasmid with a new combination of resistance genes.

Plasmids were initially classified into two general types: large plasmids and small plasmids. Large plasmids include the F factor and some of the R plasmids, carry genes for their own transfer and propagation, and are self-transmissible. Large plasmids occur in small numbers, one or two copies per chromosome equivalent. Small plasmids are more numerous in the cell—about 20 copies per chromosomal equivalent—however, they do not carry genes directing their maintenance. They rely on high numbers for distribution into daughter cells at cell division or uptake by host cells in transformation.

Compared with fragments of DNA, plasmids are more efficient vehicles for the transfer of genes from one cell to another. Upon cell lysis, supercoiled plasmids can enter other cells more efficiently. Plasmids are used in recombinant DNA technology to introduce specific traits. By manipulation of the plasmid DNA in vitro, specific genes can be introduced into cells to produce new phenotypes or recombinant organisms. The ability to express genetic traits from plasmids makes it possible to manipulate phenotype in specific ways. As will be described in later chapters, plasmids play a key role in the development of procedures used in molecular analysis.

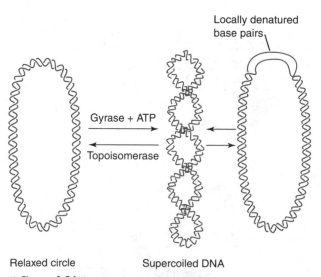

Figure 1-24 Supercoiled plasmids can be relaxed by nicking (left) or by local unwinding of the double helix (right).

Locally denatured base pairs

Gyrase + ATP

Topoisomerase

Relaxed circle   Supercoiled DNA

Advanced Concepts

The circular nature of R factors was demonstrated by buoyant density centrifugation.[54] Plasmid DNA has a density higher than that of the host chromosome and can be isolated from separate, or **satellite**, bands in the gradient. Examination of the fractions of the higher-density DNA revealed small circular species. These circles were absent from drug-sensitive bacteria.

Advanced Concepts

Plasmids are found not only in bacteria but in multicellular plants and animals as well. Some viruses, such as the single-stranded DNA virus M13, have a transient plasmid phase in their life cycle. Laboratory techniques requiring single-stranded versions of specific DNA sequences have been based on the manipulation of the plasmid (duplex circle) phase of these viruses and isolation of the single-stranded, recombinant circles from the virus. This technology was used in methods devised to determine the order or sequence of nucleotides in the DNA chain.

• STUDY QUESTIONS •
DNA Structure and Function

1. What is the function of DNA in the cell?

2. Compare the structure of the nitrogen bases. How do purines and pyrimidines differ?

3. Write the complementary sequence to the following:

   5' AGGTCACGTCTAGCTAGCTAGA 3'

4. Which of the ribose carbons participate in the phosphodiester bond?

5. Which of the ribose carbons carries the nitrogen base?

6. Why does DNA polymerase require primase activity?

DNA Replication

1. What is the covalent bond between nucleotides catalyzed by DNA polymerase?

2. Is DNA replication conservative or semi-conservative?

3. What is the lagging strand in DNA synthesis?

4. Short pieces of DNA involved in DNA synthesis in replicating cells are called _____ fragments.

5. Name the function of the following enzymes:
   polymerase
   helicase
   primase
   exonuclease
   endonuclease

Restriction Enzyme Analysis

1. A plasmid was digested with the enzyme *Hpa*II. On agarose gel electrophoresis, you observe three bands: 100, 230, and 500 bp.
   a. How many *Hpa*II sites are present in this plasmid?
   b. What are the distances between each site?
   c. What is the size of the plasmid?
   d. Draw a picture of the plasmid with the *Hpa*II sites.
      A second cut of the plasmid with *Bam*H1 yields two pieces, 80 and *x* bp.
   e. How many *Bam*H1 sites are in the plasmid?
   f. What is *x* in base pairs (bp)?

2. How would you determine where the *Bam*H1 sites are in relation to the *Hpa*II sites?

3. The plasmid has one *Eco*R1 site into which you want to clone a blunt-ended fragment. What type of enzyme could turn an *Eco*R1 sticky end into a blunt end?

Recombination and DNA Transfer

1. Compare how DNA moves from cell to cell by (a) conjugation, (b) transduction, and (c) transformation.

2. Bacteria with phenotype A+ are mixed with bacteria with phenotype A– in a culture. Some of the A– bacteria become A+. When A+ bacteria are removed from the culture and A– bacteria only are grown in the A+ cell culture medium, they all remain A–. What type of transfer occurred in the mixed culture?

3. What was the rationale for labeling bacteriophage with ^{35}S and ^{32}P in the Hershey and Chase "blender" experiment?

4. A plasmid that carries genes for its own transfer and propagation is called _____.

5. What enzymes can convert a supercoiled plasmid to a relaxed circle?

References

1. Watson J. Molecular Biology of the Gene. New York: W.A. Benjamin, Inc., 1965.
2. Mirsky AE. The discovery of DNA. *Scientific American* 1968;218(6):78–88.
3. Crick F, Watson J. DNA structure. *Nature* 1953;171:737–738.
4. Watson J, Hopkins N, Roberts J, et al. The Molecular Biology of the Gene, 4th ed. Redwood City, CA: Benjamin/Cummings, 1987.
5. Eschenmoser A. Chemical etiology of nucleic acid structure. *Science* 1999;284:2118–2124.
6. Egholm M, Buchardt O, Christensen L, et al. PNA hybridizes to complementary oligonucleotides obeying the Watson-Crick hydrogen-binding rules. *Nature* 1993;365:566–658.
7. Demidev VV, Yavnilovich MV, Belotserkovskii BP, et al. Kinetics and mechanism of polyamide ("peptide") nucleic acid binding to duplex DNA. *Proceedings of the National Academy of Sciences* 1995;92:2637–2641.
8. Ray A, Norden B. Peptide nucleic acid (PNA): Its medical and biotechnical applications and promise for the future. *FASEB Journal* 2000;14 (9):1041–1060.
9. Dean D. Peptide nucleic acids: Versatile tools for gene therapy strategies. *Advanced Drug Delivery Reviews* 2000;44(2–3):81–95.
10. Chargaff E. Chemical specificity of nucleic acids and mechanisms of their enzymatic degradation. *Experimentia* 1950;6:201–209.
11. Meselson M, Stahl FW. The replication of DNA in *Escherichia coli*. *Proceedings of the National Academy of Sciences* 1958;44:671–682.
12. Okazaki R, Okazaki T, Sakabe K, et al. In vivo mechanism of DNA chain growth. *Cold Spring Harbor Symposium on Quantitative Biology* 1968;33:129–144.
13. Kornberg A. The synthesis of DNA. *Scientific American* 1968;219:64–78
14. Akabayov B, Lee S-J, Akabayov SR, Rekhi S, Zhu B, Richardson CC. DNA recognition by the DNA primase of Bacteriophage T7: A structure-function study of the zinc-binding domain. *Biochemistry* 2009;48:1763–1773.
15. Panday M, Syed S, Donmez I, Patel G, Ha T, Patel SS. Coordinating DNA replication by means of priming loop and differential synthesis rate. *Nature* 2009;462:940–943.
16. Dervyn E, Suski C, Daniel R, et al. Two essential DNA polymerases at the bacterial replication fork. *Science* 2001;294:1716–1719.
17. Schachman HK, Adler J, Radding CM, et al. Enzymatic synthesis of deoxyribonucleic acid. VII. Synthesis of a polymer of deoxyadenylate and deoxythymidylate. *Journal of Biological Chemistry* 1960;235:3242–3249.
18. Ito J, Braithwaite DK. Compilation and alignment of DNA polymerase sequences. *Nucleic Acids Research* 1991;19(15):4045–4057.
19. Braithwaite DK, Ito J. Complication, alignment, and phylogenetic relationships of DNA polymerases. *Nucleic Acids Research* 1993;21:787–802.
20. Wang Z, Castano IB, De Las Penas A, et al. Pol K: A DNA polymerase required for sister chromatid cohesion. *Science* 2000;289:774–779.
21. Hamilton SC, Farchaus JW, Davis MC. DNA polymerases as engines for biotechnology. *BioTechniques* 2001;31(2):370–383.
22. Sears A, Peakman LJ, Wilson GG, Szczelkun MD. Characterization of the Type III restriction endonuclease PstII from Providencia stuartii. *Nucleic Acids Research* 2005;33:4775–4787.
23. Jurenaite-Urbanaviciene S, Kazlauskiene R, Urbelyte V, et al. Characterization of BseMII, a new type IV restriction–modification system, which recognizes the pentanucleotide sequence 5'-CTCAG(N)10/8. *Nucleic Acids Research* 2001;29:895–903.
24. Lehman IR. DNA ligase: Structure, mechanism, and function. *Science* 1974;186(4166):790–977.
25. Sgaramella V, Van de Sande JH, Khorana HG. Studies on polynucleotides, C: A novel joining reaction catalyzed by the T4-polynucleotide ligase. *Proceedings of the National Academy of Sciences* 1971;67(3):1468–1475.

26. Kleppe K, Van de Sande JH, Khorana HG. Polynucleotide ligase–catalyzed joining of deoxyribo-oligonucleotides on ribopolynucleotide templates and of ribo-oligonucleotides on deoxyribopolynucleotide templates. *Proceedings of the National Academy of Sciences* 1970;67(1):68–73.

27. Gray HB, Lu T. The BAL 31 nucleases (EC 3.1.11). *Methods in Molecular Biology* 1993;16:231–251.

28. Berk AJ, Sharp PA. Sizing and mapping of early adenovirus mRNAs by gel electrophoresis of S1 endonuclease-digested hybrids. *Cell* 1977;12(3): 721–732.

29. Kornberg RD. Structure of chromatin. *Annual Review of Biochemistry* 1977;46:931–954.

30. Wang J. Interaction between DNA and an *Escherichia coli* protein omega. *Journal of Molecular Biology* 1971;55(3):523 533.

31. Gellert M, Mizuuchi K, O'Dea MH, et al. DNA gyrase: An enzyme that introduces superhelical turns into DNA. *Proceedings of the National Academy of Sciences* 1976;73(11):3872–3876.

32. Matzke MA, Matzke AJM, Pruss G, et al. RNA-based silencing strategies in plants. *Current Opinions in Genetic Development* 2001;11(2):221–227.

33. Vance V, Vaucheret H. RNA silencing in plants: Defense and counterdefense. *Science* 2001;292 (5525):2277–2280.

34. Cogoni C, Macino G. Post-transcriptional gene silencing across kingdoms. *Current Opinions in Genetic Development* 2000;10(6):638–643.

35. Plasterk R, Ketting R. The silence of the genes. *Current Opinions in Genetic Development* 2000;10(5):562–567.

36. Reik W, Dean W, Walter J. Epigenetic reprogramming in mammalian development. *Science* 2001;293:1089–1093.

37. Esteller M, Corn PG, Baylin SB, et al. A gene hypermethylation profile of human cancer. *Cancer Research* 2001;61:3225–3229.

38. Jones P, Takai D. The role of DNA methylation in mammalian epigenetics. *Science* 2001;293:1068–1070.

39. Kang Y, Koo DB, Park JS, et al. Aberrant methylation of donor genome in cloned bovine embryos. *Nature Genetics* 2001;28(2):173–177.

40. Bestor T, Laudano A, Mattaliano R, et al. CpG islands in vertebrate genomes. *Journal of Molecular Biology* 1987;196(2):261–282.

41. Okano M, Xie S, Li E. Cloning and characterization of a family of novel mammalian DNA (cytosine-5) methyltransferases. *Nature Genetics* 1998;19(3):219–220.

42. Mendel G . Versuche über Pflanzen-Hybriden (1865). In Peters JA, ed. Classic Papers in Genetics. vol. iv. Englewood Cliffs, NJ: Prentice-Hall, 1959.

43. Beadle GW. Genes and the chemistry of organism. *American Scientist* 1946;34:31–53.

44. Lederberg J, Tatum, EL. Sex in bacteria: Genetic studies, 1945–1952. *Science* 1953;118(3059): 169–175.

45. Jacob F, Wollman E. Viruses and genes. *Scientific American* 1961;204:92–110.

46. Hershey AD, Chase M. Independent function of viral protein and nucleic acid in growth of bacteriophage. *Journal of General Physiology* 1952;26:36–56.

47. Benzer S. The fine structure of the gene. *Scientific American* 1962;206(1):70–84.

48. Griffith F. Significance of pneumococcal types. *Journal of Hygiene* 1928;27:113–159.

49. Avery O, MacLeod CM, McCarty M. Studies on the chemical nature of the substance-inducing transformation of pneumococcal types. I. Induction of transformation by a DNA fraction isolated from pneumococcal type III. *Journal of Experimental Medicine* 1944;79:137–158.

50. Hotchkiss RD. The genetic chemistry of the pneumococcal transformations. *The Harvey Lectures* 1955;49:124–144.

51. Clowes R. The molecule of infectious drug resistance. *Scientific American* 1973;228(4):19–27.

52. Watanabe T, Fukasawa T. Episome-mediated transfer of drug resistance in Enterobacteriaceae. II. Elimination of resistance factors with acridine dyes. *Journal of Bacteriology* 1961;81:679–683.

53. Watanabe T. Episome-mediated transfer of drug resistance in Enterobacteriaceae. VI. High frequency resistance transfer system in *E. coli.* *Journal of Bacteriology* 1963;85:788–994.

54. Moller JK, Bak AL, Christiansen G, et al. Extra-chromosomal DNA in R factor harboring Enterobacteriaceae. *Journal of Bacteriology* 1976;125:398–403.

Chapter *2*

RNA

OBJECTIVES

- Compare and contrast the structure of RNA with that of DNA.

- List and compare the different types of RNA.

- Describe the cellular processing of messenger RNA.

- List several types of RNA polymerases, their substrates, and products.

- Recognize the reactions catalyzed by ribonucleases and RNA helicases and their roles in RNA metabolism.

- Describe how ribonucleotides are polymerized into RNA (transcription) and the relation of the sequence of the RNA transcript to the DNA sequence of its gene.

- Describe gene regulation using the Lac operon as an example.

- Define epigenetics and list examples of epigenetic phenomena.

Ribonucleic acid (RNA) is a polymer of nucleotides similar to DNA. It differs from DNA in the sugar moieties, having **ribose** instead of deoxyribose and, in one nitrogen **base** component, having **uracil** instead of thymine (thymine is 5-methyl uracil; Fig. 2-1). Furthermore, RNA is synthesized as a single strand rather than as a double helix. Although RNA strands do not have complementary partner strands, they are not completely single-stranded. Through internal homologies, RNA species fold and loop upon themselves to take on a double-stranded character that is important for its function. RNA can also pair with complementary single strands of DNA or RNA and form a double helix.

There are several types of RNAs found in the cell. Ribosomal RNA, messenger RNA, transfer RNA, and small nuclear RNAs have distinct cellular functions. RNA is copied, or transcribed, from DNA.

Transcription

DNA can only store information. In order for this information to be utilized, it must be transcribed and then translated into protein, a process called **gene expression**. A specific type of RNA, messenger RNA (mRNA), carries the information in DNA to the ribosomes where it is translated into protein.

Transcription is the copying of one strand of DNA into RNA by a process similar to that of DNA replication. This activity, catalyzed by **RNA polymerase**, occurs mostly in interphase. While a single type of RNA polymerase catalyzes synthesis of all RNA in most prokaryotes, there are three types of RNA polymerases in eukaryotes: RNA polymerase Pol I, Pol II and Pol III. Pol I and III synthesize non-coding RNA.[1] Pol II is responsible for synthesis of **messenger RNA** (mRNA), the type of RNA that carries genetic information to be translated into protein. Evidence suggests that transcription takes place at discrete stations of the nucleus into which the DNA molecules move.[2] One of these sites, the **nucleolus**, is the location of ribosomal RNA synthesis.

Advanced Concepts

Evolutionary theory places RNA as the original genetic material from which DNA has evolved. In most organisms, RNA is an intermediate between the storage system of DNA and the proteins responsible for phenotype. One family of RNA viruses, the retroviruses, which include leukemia viruses and the human immunodeficiency virus, have RNA genomes and, in order to replicate using host cell machinery, must first make a DNA copy of their genome by **reverse transcription**.

Advanced Concepts

DNA must be released locally from histones and the helix unwound in order for transcription to occur. These processes involve the participation of numerous factors, including DNA binding proteins, transcription factors, histone modification enzymes, and RNA polymerase.

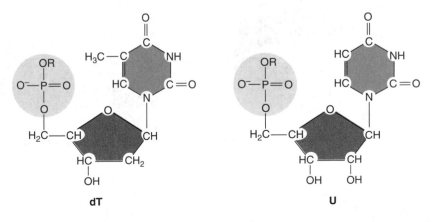

■ **Figure 2-1** Uracil (U), the nucleotide base that replaces thymine in RNA, has the purine ring structure of thymine (dT) minus the methyl group. Uracil forms hydrogen bonds with adenine.

Transcription Initiation

RNA polymerase and its supporting accessory proteins assemble at a start site in DNA, a specific sequence of bases called the **promoter**. Sites for initiation of transcription (RNA synthesis) greatly outnumber DNA initiation sites in both prokaryotes and eukaryotes. There are also many more molecules of RNA polymerase than DNA polymerase in the cell. Although functionally catalyzing the same reaction, RNA polymerases in prokaryotes and eukaryotes differ and work with different supporting proteins to find and bind to DNA in preparation for transcription. In prokaryotes, a basal transcription complex comprised of the large and small subunits of RNA polymerase and additional sigma factors assembles at the start site. The eukaryotic transcription complex requires RNA polymerase and up to 20 additional factors for accurate initiation. Initiation of RNA synthesis is regulated in all organisms so that genes are transcribed as required by specific cell types. The regulation of transcription differs in prokaryotes and eukaryotes (see below).

Transcription Elongation

RNA polymerases in both eukaryotes and prokaryotes synthesize RNA using the base sequence of one strand of the double helix (the **antisense strand**) as a guide (Fig. 2-2). The **sense strand** of the DNA template has a sequence identical to that of the RNA product (except for the U for T substitution in RNA), but it does not serve as the template for the RNA.

RNA polymerases work more slowly than DNA polymerases (50–100 bases/sec for RNA synthesis vs. 1000 bases/sec for DNA replication) and with less fidelity. The DNA double helix is locally unwound into single strands to allow the assembly and passage of the transcription machinery, forming a transcription bubble.

Unlike DNA synthesis, RNA synthesis does not require priming. The first ribonucleoside triphosphate retains all of its phosphate groups as the RNA is polymerized in the 5' to 3' direction. Subsequent ribonucleoside triphosphates retain only the **alpha phosphate**, the one closest to the ribose sugar. The other two phosphate groups are released as orthophosphate during the synthesis reaction.

Transcription Termination

RNA synthesis terminates differently in prokaryotes and eukaryotes. In prokaryotes, RNA synthesis is responsive to protein products, such that high levels of a gene product induce termination of its own synthesis. This synthesis is

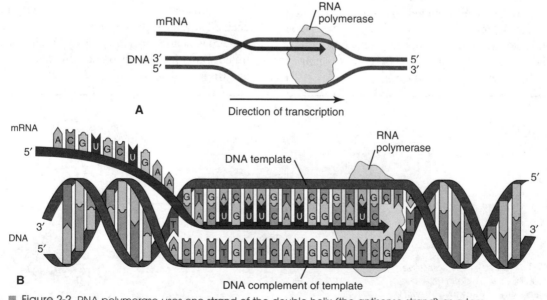

■ **Figure 2-2** RNA polymerase uses one strand of the double helix (the antisense strand) as a template for synthesis of RNA. About 10 base pairs of DNA are unwound or opened to allow the polymerase to work.

accomplished in some genes by interactions between RNA polymerase and termination signals in the DNA template. In other genes, an additional transcription complex factor, **rho**, is required for termination. Rho is a helicase enzyme that associates with RNA polymerase and inactivates the elongation complex at a cytosine-rich termination site in the DNA.[3,4] Rho-independent termination occurs at G:C-rich followed by A:T-rich regions in the DNA. The G:C bases are transcribed into RNA and fold into a short double-stranded **hairpin**, which slows the elongation complex. The elongation complex then dissociates as it reaches the A:T-rich area.

In eukaryotes, mRNA synthesis, catalyzed by pol II, proceeds along the DNA template until a **polyadenylation signal** (polyA site) is encountered. At this point, the process of termination of transcription is activated. There is no consensus sequence in DNA that specifies termination of transcription. As the polymerase proceeds past the polyA site, the nascent mRNA is released by an endonuclease associated with the carboxy terminal end of pol II. RNA synthesized beyond the site trails out of the polymerase and is bound by another exonuclease that begins to degrade the RNA 5' to 3' toward the RNA polymerase.

When the exonuclease catches up with the polymerase, transcription stops.

Pol I terminates transcription just prior to a site in the DNA (Sal box) with the cooperation of a termination factor, TTF1.[5] The pol III termination signal is a run of adenine residues in the template. Pol III transcription termination requires a termination factor.

Types/Structures of RNA

There are several types of RNAs found in the cell. Ribosomal RNA, mRNA, transfer RNA, and small nuclear RNAs have distinct cellular functions.

Ribosomal RNA

The largest component of cellular RNA is **ribosomal RNA** (rRNA), comprising 80% to 90% of the total cellular RNA. The various types of ribosomal RNAs are named for their sedimentation coefficient (S) in density gradient centrifugation.[6] rRNA is an important structural and functional part of the ribosomes, cellular organelles where proteins are synthesized (Fig. 2-3).

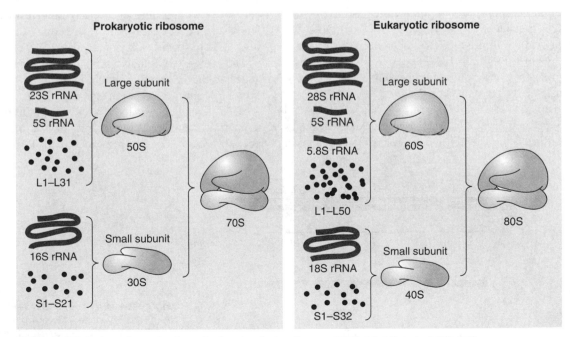

■ **Figure 2-3** Prokaryote and eukaryote ribosomal subunits are of similar structure but different size. Ribosomal RNAs (left) are assembled with 52 or 82 ribosomal proteins (center) to make the subunits that will form the complete ribosome in association with mRNA.

In prokaryotes, there are three rRNA species, the 16S found in the ribosome small subunit and the 23S and 5S found in the ribosome large subunit, all synthesized from the same gene. In eukaryotes, rRNA is synthesized from highly repeated gene clusters. Eukaryotic rRNA is copied from DNA as a single 45S precursor RNA (pre-ribosomal RNA) that is subsequently processed into 18S of the ribosome small subunit and 5.8S and 28S species of the large subunit. Another rRNA species, 5S, found in the large ribosome subunit in eukaryotes, is synthesized separately.

Messenger RNA

Messenger RNA (mRNA) is the initial connection between the information stored in DNA and the translation apparatus that will ultimately produce the protein products responsible for the phenotype dictated by the chromosome. In prokaryotes, mRNA is synthesized and simultaneously translated into protein. Prokaryotic mRNA is sometimes **polycistronic**; that is, coding for more than one protein on the same mRNA. Eukaryotic mRNA, in contrast, is monocistronic, having only one protein per mRNA. Eukaryotes can, however, produce different proteins from the same DNA sequences by starting the RNA synthesis in different places or by processing the mRNA differently. In eukaryotes, copying of RNA from DNA and protein synthesis from the RNA are separated by the nuclear membrane barrier. Eukaryotic mRNA undergoes a series of post-transcriptional processing events before it is translated into protein (Fig. 2-4).

The amount of a particular mRNA in a cell is related to the requirement for its final product. Some messages are transcribed constantly and are relatively abundant in

> ### *Advanced Concepts*
>
> The secondary structure of rRNA is important for the integrity and function of the ribosome. Not only is it important for ribosomal structure, it is also involved in the correct positioning of the ribosome on the mRNA and with the transfer RNA during protein synthesis.[7,8]

the cell (**constitutive** transcription), whereas others are transcribed only at certain times during the cell cycle or under particular conditions (**inducible**, or regulatory, transcription). Even the most abundantly transcribed mRNAs are much less plentiful in the cell than rRNA.

Messenger RNA Processing
Polyadenylation

Study of mRNA in eukaryotes was facilitated by the discovery that most messengers carry a sequence of **polyadenylic acid** at the 3' terminus, a **polyA tail**. The run of adenines was first discovered by hydrogen bonding of mRNA to polydeoxythymine on poly(dT) cellulose.[9] Polyuridine or **polythymine** residues covalently attached to cellulose or sepharose substrates are often used to specifically isolate mRNA in the laboratory.

The polyA tail is not coded in genomic DNA. It is added to the RNA after synthesis of the pre-mRNA. A protein complex recognizes the RNA sequence, AAUAAA, and cleaves the RNA chain 11–30 bases 3' to that site. The enzyme that cuts pre-mRNA in advance of polyadenylation has not been identified. Recent studies

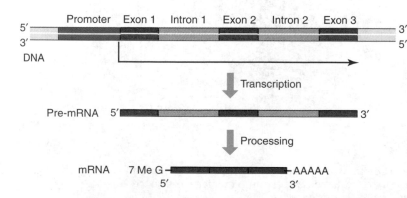

■ **Figure 2-4** DNA (top) and heteronuclear RNA (middle) contain intervening (intron) and expressed (exon) sequences. The introns are removed and the mature RNA is capped and polyadenylated during processing (bottom).

Historical Highlights

A DNA copy (complementary DNA, copy DNA [cDNA]) of mature mRNA can be made by reverse transcription of mRNA (synthesis of DNA from the mRNA template). Compared with the original gene on the chromosome, the cDNA version of eukaryotic genes is smaller than the chromosomal version. Restriction enzyme mapping confirms that this is not due to premature termination of the genomic transcript. The entire functional gene is present in the shorter sequence because cDNA versions of eukaryotic genes can be expressed (transcribed and translated) into complete proteins. The chromosomal version of the gene must, therefore, have extra sequences inserted between the protein coding sequences. Direct location and size of these **intervening sequences** were first demonstrated by electron microscopy of hybrids between mRNA and cDNA[10] using the method of R loop mapping developed by White and Hogness.[11] In these experiments, mRNA and duplex genomic DNA were incubated together at conditions under which the more stable RNA-DNA hybrids are favored over the DNA duplexes. The resulting structures released loops of unpaired DNA (introns). The DNA duplexed with RNA corresponded to the coding sequences (exons).

Advanced Concepts

About 30% of the mRNAs, notably histone mRNAs, are not polyadenylated.[14] The function of the polyA tail, or functional differences between polyA+ and polyA– mRNA, is not clear. The **polyA tail** may be involved in movement of the mRNA from the nucleus to the cytoplasm, association with other cell components, maintenance of secondary structure, or stability of the molecule.

where p represents a phosphate group and N represents any nucleotide.

The cap confers a protective function as well as serves as a recognition signal for the translational apparatus. Caps differ with respect to the methylation of the end nucleotide of the mRNA. In some cases, 2' O-methylation occurs not only on the first but also on the second nucleotide from the cap. Other caps methylate the first three nucleotides of the RNA molecule.

Splicing

Prokaryotic structural genes contain uninterrupted lengths of **open reading frame**, sequences that code for amino acids. In contrast, eukaryotic coding regions are interrupted with long stretches of noncoding DNA sequences called **introns**. Newly transcribed mRNA, heteronuclear RNA (hnRNA), is much larger than mature mRNA because it still contains the intervening sequences. Labeling studies demonstrated that the hnRNA is capped and tailed and that these modifications survive the transition from hnRNA to mRNA, which is simply a process of removing the **intervening sequences** from the hnRNA. Introns are removed from hnRNA by **splicing** (Fig. 2-5). The remaining sequences that code for the protein product are **exons**.

Although removal of all nuclear introns requires protein catalysts, some introns are removed without the participation of protein factors in a self-splicing reaction. The discovery of self-splicing was the first demonstration that RNA could act as an enzyme.

Inspection of splice junctions from several organisms and genes has demonstrated the following consensus

suggest that a component of the protein complex related to the system that is responsible for removing the 3' extension from pretransfer RNAs may also be involved in generation of the 3' ends on mRNA.[12,13] The enzyme **polyadenylate polymerase** is responsible for adding the adenines to the end of the transcript. A run of up to 200 nucleotides of polyA is typically found on mRNA in mammalian cells.

Capping

Eukaryotic mRNA is blocked at the 5' terminus by an unusual 5'-5' pyrophosphate bridge to a methylated guanosine.[15] The structure is called a **cap**. The cap is a 5'-5' pyrophosphate linkage of 7-methyl guanosine to either 2' O-methyl guanine or 2' O-methyl adenine of the mRNA,

$$^{7\text{-methyl}}G^{5'} + ppp\ ^{5'} + G\ \text{ or }\ A\ ^{2'O\text{-methyl}}\ pNpNpNp$$

Advanced Concepts

Caps are present on all eukaryotic mRNA bound for translation, with the exception of some mRNA transcribed from mitochondrial DNA. Capping occurs after initiation of transcription, catalyzed by the enzyme guanylyl transferase. This enzyme links a guanosine monophosphate provided by guanosine triphosphate to the 5' phosphate terminus of the RNA with the release of pyrophosphate. In some viruses, guanosine diphosphate provides the guanidine residue and monophosphate is released. Caps of mRNA are recognized by ribosomes just before translation.[16]

Advanced Concepts

There are four types of introns—group I, group II, nuclear, and tRNA—depending on the mechanism of their removal from hnRNA. Group I introns are found in nuclear, mitochondrial, and chloroplast genes. Group II introns are found in mitochondrial and chloroplast genes. Group I introns require a guanosine triphosphate molecule to make a nucleophilic attack on the 5' phosphate of the 5' end of the intron. This leaves a 3' OH at the end of the 5' exon (splice donor site), which attacks the 5' end of the next exon (splice acceptor site), forming a new phosphodiester bond and releasing the intervening sequence. Group II introns are removed in a similar reaction initiated by the 2' OH of an adenosine within the intron attacking the 5' phosphate at the splice donor site. When the 3' OH of the splice donor site bonds with the splice acceptor site of the next exon, the intervening sequence is released as a lariat structure (see Fig. 2-4). This lariat contains an unusual 2', 3', and 5' triply linked nucleotide, the presence of which proved the mechanism. Removal of nuclear introns occurs by the same transesterification mechanism, except this reaction is catalyzed by specialized RNA-protein complexes (small nucleoprotein particles). These complexes contain the small nuclear RNAs U1, U2, U4, U5, and U6.

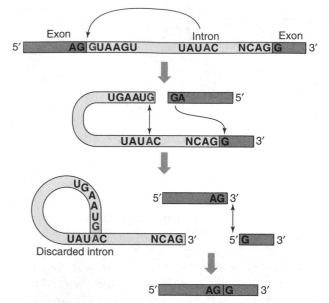

■ **Figure 2-5** RNA splicing at the 5' splice site (AGGUAAGU), branch (UAUAC), and 3' splice site (NCAGG) consensus sequences. The intron (light gray) is removed through a transesterification reaction involving a guanine nucleotide of the 5' site and an adenine in the branch sequence. The product of this reaction is the discarded intron in a lariat structure. Another transesterification reaction connects the exons.

sequences for the donor and acceptor splice junctions of group I, II, and nuclear introns[17]:

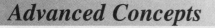

$$A\,G\,//G\,U\,A\,A\,G\,U \qquad Y\,N\,C\,U\,R\,\underline{A}\,C \qquad Y_N\,N\,C\,A\,G\,//G$$
(intron)

| splice donor site | branch point | splice acceptor site |

The branch point sequence YNCURAC is variable in mammals but almost invariant in the yeast *Saccharomyces cervisiae* (UACUA<u>A</u>C).

Why are eukaryotic genes interrupted by introns? Splicing may be important for timing of translation of mRNA in the cytoplasm. One theory holds that introns evolved as a means of increasing recombination frequency within genes as well as between genes without breaking coding sequences. The discontinuous nature of eukaryotic genes may also protect the coding regions from genetic damage by toxins or radiation.

Alternative splicing modifies products of genes by alternate insertion of different exons. For example, the production of calcitonin in the thyroid or calcitonin

Advanced Concepts

The splicing of transfer RNA (tRNA) transcripts involves breakage and reunion of the RNA chain. Endonucleases cleave the tRNA precisely at the intron ends. The resulting tRNA ends, a 2', 3' cyclic phosphate and a 5' OH, are then ligated in a complex reaction that requires ATP, followed by further base modification in some tRNAs.

Advanced Concepts

Small nuclear RNAs serve mostly a structural role in the processing of mRNA. Several of a family of proteins (**Sm proteins**) assemble into a (60 Aδ by 30–40 Aδ) doughnut-shaped complex that interacts with the U-rich regions of poly (U) RNAs.[19,20]

U1 RNA is complementary to sequences at the splice donor site, and its binding distinguishes the sequence GU in the splice site from other GU sequences in the RNA. U2 RNA recognizes the splice acceptor site. In lower eukaryotes, another protein, splicing factor 1,[21] binds to the branch point sequence, initiating further protein assembly and association of U4, U5, and U6, with the looped RNA forming a complex called the **splicesosome**, in which the transesterification reaction linking the exons together takes place.

gene-related peptide in the brain depends on the exons included in the mature mRNA in these tissues.[18] Alternative splicing has been found in over 40 different genes.

Abnormalities in the splicing process are responsible for several disease states. Some β-thalassemias result from mutations in splice recognition sequences of the β-globin genes. Certain autoimmune conditions result from production of antibodies to RNA protein complexes. Auto-antibodies against U1 RNA, one of the small nuclear RNAs required for splicing, are associated with systemic lupus erythematosus.

Small Nuclear RNA

Small nuclear RNA (snRNA) functions in splicing in eukaryotes. Small nuclear RNA stays in the nucleus after its transcription by RNA polymerase I or III. These RNAs sediment in a range of 6–8S. Small nuclear RNAs isolated from hepatoma and cervical carcinoma cell lines are summarized in Table 2.1.

Transfer RNA

Translation of information from nucleic acid to protein requires reading of the mRNA by **ribosomes**, using adaptor molecules or **transfer RNA** (tRNA). Transfer RNAs are relatively short, single-stranded polynucleotides of 73–93 bases in length, MW 24–31,000. There is at least one tRNA for each amino acid.

Eight or more of the nucleotide bases in all tRNAs are modified, usually methylated, after the tRNA synthesis. Most tRNAs have a guanylic residue at the 5' end and the sequence CCA at the 3' end. Through intrastrand hybridization, tRNAs take on a cruciform structure of four to five double-stranded stems and three to four

Advanced Concepts

Mitochondria contain distinct, somewhat smaller, tRNAs.[22]

Table 2.1 **Small Nuclear RNA Isolated from HeLa Cervical Carcinoma and Novikoff Hepatoma Cells[17]**

Species (HeLa)	Species (Novikoff)	Approximate Length (Bases)
SnA	U5	180
SnB		210
SnC	U2	196
SnD	U1B	171
SnE/ScE (5.8S rRNA)	5.8S	
SnF	U1A	125
SnG/ScG (5S rRNA)	5S I and II	
SnG'	5S III	120
SnH	4.5S I, II and III	96
SnI (tRNA)		
SnK		260
SnP		130
ScL (viral 7S)		260
ScM		180
ScD		180

single-stranded loops (Fig. 2-6). The CCA at the 3' end of the tRNA is where the amino acid will be covalently attached to the tRNA. A seven-base loop (the TψC loop, where ψ stands for the modified nucleotide pseudouridine) contains the sequence 5'-TψCG-3'. The variable loop is larger in longer tRNAs. Another seven-base loop (the anticodon loop) contains the three-base pair **anticodon** that is complementary to the mRNA codon of its cognate amino acid. An 8-12–base loop (D loop) is relatively rich in dihydrouridine, another modified nucleotide. X-ray diffraction studies of pure crystalline tRNA reveal that the cruciform secondary structure of tRNA takes on an additional level of hydrogen bonding between the D loop and the TψC loop to form a γ-shaped structure (see Fig. 2-6).

Micro RNAs

Micro RNAs (**miRNA**) are regulatory RNAs, 17–27 nucleotides (nt) in length, derived from endogenous RNA **hairpin** structures (RNA folded into double-stranded states through intrastrand hydrogen bonds). Micro RNAs were discovered in the worm *Caenorhabditis elegans*.

Advanced Concepts

The tRNA genes contain 14–20 extra nucleotides in the sequences coding for the anticodon loop that are transcribed into the tRNA. Enzymes that recognize other tRNA modifications remove these sequences (introns) by a cleavage-ligation process. Intron removal, addition of CCA to the 3' end, and nucleotide modifications all occur following tRNA transcription. Enzymatic activities responsible for intron removal and addition of CCA may also ontribute to intron removal and polyA addition to mRNA.

Historical Highlights

In 1964, Robert Holley and colleagues at Cornell University solved the first tRNA sequence. The sequence was that of alanine tRNA of yeast.[23] Yeast tRNA[ala] is 76 bases long; 10 of these bases are modified.

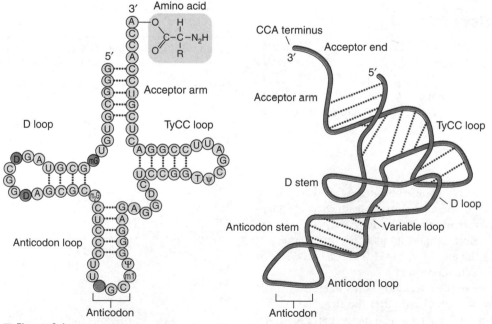

■ **Figure 2-6** Alanine tRNA is an example of the general structure of tRNA, which is often depicted in a cruciform structure (left). The inverted "L" (right) more accurately depicts the structure formed by intrastrand hydrogen bonding.

Two 22-nt RNAs were shown to contribute to temporal progression of cell fates by triggering down regulation of target mRNAs.[24–26] These RNA species were also called small temporal RNA (stRNA).

Functionally, miRNAs control gene expression by pairing with partially complementary sequences in mRNAs and inhibit translation. Many miRNAs have been identified in eukaryotic cells and viruses.[27,29–32] Bacteria have genes that resemble miRNA precursors; however, the full miRNA system has not been demonstrated in bacteria. The true number of these RNAs may amount to thousands per genome.

Micro RNAs perform diverse functions in eukaryotic cells affecting gene expression, cell development, and defense. Because production of miRNAs is strictly regulated as to time or stage of cell development, finding them is a technical challenge. Many of these species are only present in virally infected cells or after introduction of foreign nucleic acid by transformation. Novel approaches will be required for discovery of rare miRNAs expressed in specific cell types at specific times.

Small Interfering RNA

Small interfering RNAs (siRNA) are the functional intermediates of **RNA interference** (RNAi, discussed later in this chapter), a defense in eukaryotic cells against viral invasion. In a process that is not yet completely understood, double-stranded RNA (dsRNA) species are believed to originate from transcription of inverted repeats or by the activity of cellular or viral RNA-directed RNA polymerases. Biochemical analysis of RNA interference has revealed that these 21–22 nucleotide dsRNAs, also called small intermediate RNAs, are derived from successive cleavage of dsRNAs that are 500 or more nucleotide **base pairs** in length.[33] The ribonuclease III enzyme, dicer, is responsible for the generation of siRNA and another small RNA, micro RNA (see below), from dsRNA precursors.[34]

Other Small RNAs

Since the late 1990s a growing variety of small RNAs (sRNA) have been described in prokaryotes and eukaryotes, including tiny noncoding RNAs (tncRNA, 20–22b),[39] small modulatory RNA (smRNA, 21–23b),[40] small nucleolar RNAs (snoRNA),[41] tmRNA,[42] guide RNA (gRNA),[43,44] and others. In addition to RNA synthesis and processing, these molecules influence numerous cellular processes, including plasmid replication, bacteriophage development, chromosome structure, and

---

Historical Highlights

In 1993, a small non-protein-coding RNA was discovered in the worm *Caenorhabditis elegans*.[24,26] Discovery of this RNA, *lin-4*, was followed by other small RNAs necessary for proper gene expression in the worm. One of these tiny RNAs, *let-7*, was found to be evolutionarily conserved and in 2001, multiple transcripts similar to *lin-4* and *let-7*, termed microRNA, were cloned from several sources, including human cells.[27] To date, over 650 mature miRNA sequences have been identified in humans. These tiny transcripts have great potential in the clinical laboratory to aid in diagnosis and prognostic predictions for complex diseases such as diabetes, cardiovascular disease, and cancer.[28]

Advanced Concepts

The first demonstration of directed RNAi in the laboratory occurred in the experiments of Fire et al. with *C. elegans*.[35] These investigators injected dsRNA into worms and observed dramatic inhibition of the genes that generated the RNA. Since then, siRNAs have been introduced into plants and animals, including human cells growing in culture. Injection of long dsRNA kills human cells, but gene silencing can be achieved by introduction of the siRNAs or plasmids coding for the dsRNA. Libraries of siRNAs or DNA plasmids encoding them have been made that are complementary to over 8000 human genes.[36] These genetic tools have potential applications not only in identifying genes involved in disease but also as treatment for some of these diseases, particularly cancer where overexpression or abnormal expression of specific genes is part of the tumor phenotype.[37,38]

development. These small, untranslated RNA molecules have been termed sRNAs in bacteria and noncoding RNAs (ncRNAs) in eukaryotes.

RNA Polymerases

RNA synthesis is catalyzed by RNA polymerase enzymes (Table 2.2). One multisubunit prokaryotic enzyme is responsible for the synthesis of all types of RNA in the prokaryotic cell. Eukaryotes have three different RNA polymerase enzymes. All of these enzymes are DNA-dependent RNA polymerases, that is, they require a DNA template. In contrast, **RNA-dependent RNA polymerases** require an RNA template.

Bacterial RNA polymerase consists of five subunits, two α and one of each β, β', and σ (Fig. 2-7).[45]

Table 2.2 RNA Polymerases

Enzyme	Template	Product
E. coli RNA polymerase II	DNA	mRNA
RNA polymerase I	DNA	rRNA
RNA polymerase II	DNA	mRNA
RNA polymerase III	DNA	tRNA, snRNA
Mitochondrial RNA polymerase	DNA	mRNA
Mammalian DNA polymerase α	DNA	primers
HCV RNA polymerase	RNA	Viral genome
Dengue virus RNA polymerase	RNA	Viral genome
PolyA polymerase	None	PolyA tails

In eukaryotes, there are three multisubunit, nuclear, DNA-dependent RNA polymerases: RNA polymerase I, II, and III (Table 2.3). A single-subunit mitochondrial RNA polymerase, imported to organelles, is also encoded in the nucleus. The three RNA polymerases in eukaryotic cells were first distinguished by their locations in the cell. RNA polymerase I (pol I) is found in the nucleolus. RNA polymerase II (pol II) is found in the nucleus. RNA polymerase III (pol III), one of the first nucleic acid polymerases discovered, is also found in the nucleus and sometimes the cytoplasm.

Advanced Concepts

The nucleotide sequence of mRNA can be altered after RNA synthesis in a process called **RNA editing**. It occurs in humans through two mechanisms. In one, such enzymes as cytidine deaminase and adenosine deaminase convert C to U and A to inosine (read as G), respectively. These enzymes recognize specific sequences in the mRNA. The other mechanism involves guide RNA (gRNA), a small nuclear RNA that hydrogen bonds to the mRNA transcript and mediates addition or removal of bases from the mRNA. The former substitution mechanism is responsible for RNA editing of the APOB gene so that different versions are made in the liver and intestines.

Advanced Concepts

Burgess et al.[46] showed that the $\alpha2,\beta,\beta'$ core enzyme retained the catalytic activity of the $\alpha2,\beta',\sigma$ complete, or **holoenzyme**, suggesting that the **sigma factor** played no role in RNA elongation. In fact, the sigma factor is released at RNA initiation. The role of the sigma factor is to guide the complete enzyme to the proper site of initiation on the DNA.

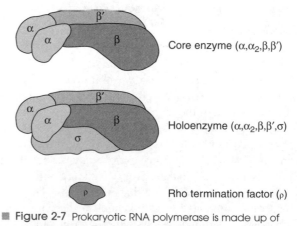

■ **Figure 2-7** Prokaryotic RNA polymerase is made up of separate proteins. The four subunits that make up the core enzyme have the capacity to synthesize RNA. The sigma cofactor aids in accurate initiation of RNA synthesis. The rho cofactor aids in termination of RNA synthesis.

Table 2.3 **Cellular Location and Activity of RNA pol I, II, and III in Eukaryotes**

Type	Location	Products	α-Amanitin
I	Nucleolus	18s, 5.8s, 28s rRNA	Insensitive
II	Nucleus	mRNA, snRNA	Inhibited
III	Nucleus	tRNA, 5s rRNA	Inhibited by high concentration

Advanced Concepts

The three polymerases were also distinguished by their differential sensitivity to the toxin α-amanitin.[47–49] This toxin is isolated from the poisonous mushroom *Amanitaphalloides*. Pol II is sensitive to relatively low amounts of this toxin, pol III is sensitive to intermediate levels, and pol I is resistant. α-amanitin has been invaluable in the research setting to determine which polymerase activity is responsible for synthesis of newly discovered types of RNA and to dissect the biochemical properties of the polymerases.[50–52]

Advanced Concepts

The most well-studied eukaryotic RNA polymerase is pol II from the yeast *Saccharomycescervisiae*. It is a 0.4 megadalton complex of 12 subunits. The yeast enzyme works in conjunction with a large complex of proteins required for promoter recognition and melting, transcription initiation, elongation and termination, and transcript processing (splicing, capping, and polyadenylation).

The differential drug sensitivity, cellular location, and ionic requirements of the three eukaryotic RNA polymerases were used to assign the polymerases to the type of RNA they synthesize. Pol I synthesizes rRNA (except 5S rRNA). Pol II synthesizes mRNAs and snRNAs. Also called RNA polymerase b (Rpb), pol II is the central transcribing enzyme of mRNA in eukaryotes. Pol III synthesizes tRNAs, 5S rRNA, and some snRNAs.

RNA viruses carry their own **RNA-dependent RNA polymerases**. Hepatitis C virus and Dengue virus carry this type of polymerase to replicate their RNA genomes. RNA-dependent RNA polymerase activity has also been found in lower eukaryotes.[53] The purpose of these enzymes in cells may be associated with RNAi and gene silencing.

PolyA polymerase is a template-independent RNA polymerase. This enzyme adds adenine nucleotides to the 3' end of mRNA.[54] The resulting polyA tail is important for mRNA stability and translation into protein (see Chapter 3, "Proteins").

Other RNA-Metabolizing Enzymes

Ribonucleases

Ribonucleases degrade RNA in a manner similar to the degradation of DNA by deoxyribonucleases (Table 2.4). There are several types of ribonucleases, generally classified as endoribonucleases and exoribonucleases.

Endocucleases include RNase H, which digests the RNA strand in a DNA/RNA hybrid; RNase I, which cleaves single-stranded RNA; and RNase III, which digests double-stranded RNA. RNase P removes precursor nucleotides from tRNA molecules. RNase A, RNase T1, and RNase T2 cleave single-stranded RNA at specific residues. A combination of RNase A, T1, and T2 is used in some laboratory procedures investigating gene expression and transcript structure. An endoribonuclease formed by cleavage and polyadenylation specific factor (CPSF) and other factors that bind to the polyA site, are required for proper termination of RNA synthesis in mammals.[55,56] Along with RNA polymerase II subunits and other proteins, this activity cuts the nascent RNA transcript before addition of the polyA tail by polyA polymerase. Regulatory RNAs (microRNA and siRNA) are digested by special RNA endonucleases that recognize double-stranded RNA.

Exonribonucleases digest single-stranded RNA from the 3' or 5' ends. This group of enzymes inlcudes polynucleotide phosphorylase (PNPase), RNase PH, RNase II, RNase R, RNase D, RNase T, and others. Like the endoribonuclease RNase P, RNase D is involved in the 3'-to-5' processing of pre-tRNAs.

Table 2.4 **RNases Used in Laboratory Procedures**[82]

Enzyme	Source	Type	Substrate
RNAse A	Bovine	Endoribonuclease	Single-stranded RNA 3'+ to pyrimidine residues
RNAse T1	*Aspergillus*	Endoribonuclease	3' Phosphate groups of guanines
RNAse H	*E. coli*	Exoribonuclease	RNA hybridized to DNA
RNAse CL3	*Gallus*	Endoribonuclease	RNA next to cytidylic acid
Cereus RNAse	*Physarum*	Endoribonuclease	Cytosine and uracil residues in RNA
RNAse Phy M	*Physarum*	Endoribonuclease	Uracil, adenine, and guanine residues in RNA
RNAse U2	*Ustilago*	Endoribonuclease	3' Phosphodiester bonds next to purines
RNAse T2	*Aspergillus*	Endoribonuclease	All phosphodiester bonds, preferably next to adenines
S1 nuclease	*Aspergillus*	Exoribonuclease	RNA or single-stranded DNA
Mung bean nuclease	Mung bean sprouts	Exoribonuclease	RNA or single-stranded DNA
RNAse Phy I	*Physarum*	Exoribonuclease	Guanine, adenine, or uracil residues in RNA

RNases are ubiquitous, stable enzymes that degrade all types of RNA. Some RNases are secreted by higher eukaryotes, possibly as an antimicrobial defense mechanism.[57,58] They are of particular concern in laboratories where RNA work is performed as they are very resistant to inactivation. Special precautions are used to protect RNA from degradation by these enzymes (see Chapter 16, "Quality Assurance and Quality Control in the Molecular Laboratory").

RNA Helicases

RNA synthesis and processing require the activity of helicases to catalyze the unwinding of double-stranded RNA. These enzymes have been characterized in prokaryotic and eukaryotic organisms. Some RNA helicases work exclusively on RNA. Others can work on DNA:RNA heteroduplexes and DNA substrates. Another activity of these enzymes is in the removal of proteins from RNA-protein complexes.

Regulation of Transcription

Gene expression is a key determinant of phenotype. The sequences and factors controlling when and how much protein is synthesized are equally as important as the DNA sequences encoding the amino acid makeup of a protein. Early studies aimed at the characterization of gene structure were confounded by phenotypes that resulted from aberrations in gene expression rather than in protein structural alterations.

Advanced Concepts

With advances in crystallography, the molecular mechanisms of RNA synthesis are being revealed. During transcription, DNA enters a positively charged cleft between the two largest subunits of the RNA polymerase. At the floor of the cleft is the active site of the enzyme to which nucleotides are funneled through a pore in the cleft beneath the active site (pore 1). In the active site, the DNA strands are separated and the RNA chain is elongated, driven by cleavage of phosphates from each incoming ribonucleoside triphosphate. The resulting DNA-RNA hybrid moves out of the active site nearly perpendicular to the DNA coming into the cleft. After reaching a length of 10 bases, the newly synthesized RNA dissociates from the hybrid and leaves the complex through an exit channel. Three protein loops— "rudder," "lid," and "zipper"— are involved in hybrid dissolution and exit of the RNA product.[59,60]

Advanced Concepts

There are two major groups of RNA helicases defined by the amino acid sequence of their conserved regions. DEAD-box helicases (DEAD = asp-glu-ala-asp) are typified by the yeast translation initiation factor e1F4A, which unwinds messenger RNA at the 5' untranslated end for proper binding of the small ribosomal subunit. DEAD-box proteins are not strong helicases and may be referred to as unwindases or RNA **chaparones**.[61] The DEAH-box helicases (asp-glu-ala-his) (DExDH-box helicases) resemble DNA helicases. They act on mRNA and snRNA during splicing. They may also be required for ribosome biosynthesis. In addition to RNA unwinding, protein dissociation, splicing, and translation, RNA helicases also participate in RNA turnover and chromatin remodeling.

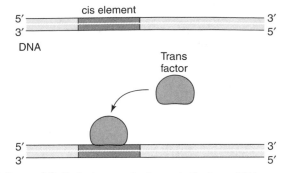

■ Figure 2-8 Cis factors or cis elements (top) are DNA sequences recognized by transcription factors, or trans factors, or DNA binding proteins (bottom).

For some genes whose products are in continual use by the cell, gene expression is constant or constitutive. For other genes, expression is tightly regulated throughout the life of the cell. Because gene products often function together to bring about a specific cellular response, specific combinations of proteins in stoichiometric balance are crucial for cell differentiation and development. Protein availability and function are controlled at the levels of transcription, translation, and protein modification and stability. The most immediate and well-studied level of control of gene expression is transcription initiation. Molecular technology has led to an extensive study of transcription initiation, so a large amount of information on gene expression refers to this level of transcription.

Regulation of RNA Synthesis at Initiation

Two types of factors are responsible for regulation of RNA synthesis: **cis factors** and **trans factors** (transcription factors) (Fig. 2-8). Cis factors are DNA sequences that mark places on the DNA involved in the initiation and control of RNA synthesis. Trans factors are proteins that bind to the cis sequences and direct the assembly of transcription complexes at the proper gene. In order for transcription to occur, several proteins must assemble at the gene's transcription initiation site, including specific

and general transcription factors and the RNA polymerase complex.

An **operon** is a series of structural genes transcribed together on one mRNA and subsequently separated into individual proteins. In organisms with small genomes, such as bacteria and viruses, operons bring about coordinate expression of proteins required at the same time, for example, the enzymes of a metabolic pathway. The lactose operon (lac operon) contains three structural genes: *LacZ*, *LacY*, and *LacA*, which are all required for the metabolism of lactose. The *LacZ* gene product, β-galactosidase, hydrolyzes lactose into glucose and galactose. The *LacY* gene product, lactose permease, transports lactose into the

Historical Highlights

The production of particular proteins by bacteria growing in media containing specific substrates was observed early in the last century, a phenomenon termed **enzyme adaptation**, later called **induction**. Detailed analysis of the lactose operon in *E. coli* was the first description of an inducible gene expression at the molecular level. The effect of gene expression on phenotype was initially demonstrated by Monod and Cozen-Bazire in 1953 when they showed that synthesis of tryptophan in *Aerobacter* was inhibited by tryptophan.[62] Jacob and Monod subsequently introduced the concept of two types of genes, structural and regulatory, in the lactose operon in *E. coli*.[63]

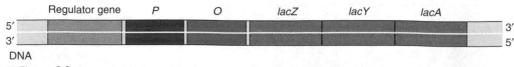
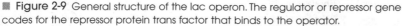

■ **Figure 2-9** General structure of the lac operon. The regulator or repressor gene codes for the repressor protein trans factor that binds to the operator.

cell. The *LacA* gene product, thiogalactoside transacetylase, transacetylates galactosides. The *LacI* gene that encodes a protein **repressor** along with the repressor's binding site in the DNA (the **operator**) just 5' to the start of the operon is responsible for the regulated expression of the operon. When *E. coli* is growing on glucose as a carbon source, the lactose-metabolizing enzymes are not required and this operon is minimally expressed. Within 2 to 3 minutes after shifting to a lactose-containing medium, the expression of these enzymes is increased a thousandfold.

Figure 2-9 shows a map of the lac operon. The three structural genes of the operon are preceded by the promoter, where RNA polymerase binds to the DNA to start transcription and the cis regulatory element, the operator. The sequences coding for the repressor protein are located just 5' to the operon. In the absence of lactose, the repressor protein binds to the operator sequence and prevents transcription of the operon. When lactose is present, it binds to the repressor protein

and changes its conformation and lowers its affinity to bind the operator sequence. This results in expression of the operon (Fig. 2-10). Jacob and Monod deduced these details through analysis of a series of mutants (changes in the DNA coding for the various components of the operon). Since their work, numerous regulatory systems have been described in prokaryotes and eukaryotes, all using the same basic idea of combinations of cis and trans factors.

Other operons are controlled in a similar manner by the binding of regulatory trans factors to cis sequences preceding the structural genes (Fig. 2-11). A different type of negative control is that found in the arg operon where a **corepressor** must bind to a repressor in order to turn off transcription (**enzyme repression**). Compare this with the inducer that prevents the repressor from binding the operator to turn on expression of the lac operon (**enzyme induction**). The mal operon is an example of positive control where an **activator** binds with RNA polymerase to turn on transcription.

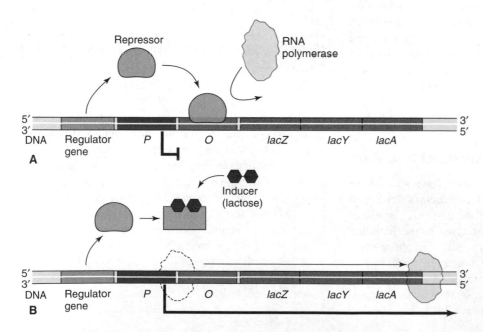

■ **Figure 2-10** Two states of the lac operon. (A) The repressor protein (R) binds to the operator cis element (O) preventing transcription of the operon from the promoter (P). (B) In the presence of the inducer lactose, the inducer binds to the repressor, changing its conformation, decreasing its affinity for the operator, allowing transcription to occur.

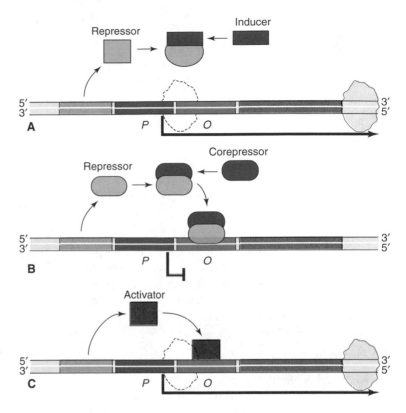

Figure 2-11 Modes of regulation in prokaryotes include induction as found in the lac operon (A), repression as found in the arg operon (B), and activation as in the mal operon (C).

Another mechanism of control in bacteria is **attenuation**. This type of regulation works through formation of stems and loops in the RNA transcript by intrastrand hydrogen bonding of complementary bases. These secondary structures allow or prevent transcription, for instance by respectively exposing or sequestering ribosome binding sites at the beginning of the transcript.

The general arrangement of cis factors in prokaryotes and eukaryotes is shown in Figure 2-12. These sequences are usually 4–20 bp in length. Some are inverted repeats with the capacity to form a cruciform structure in the DNA duplex recognizable by specific proteins. Prokaryotic regulatory sequences are usually found within close proximity of the gene. Eukaryotic genes have both proximal and

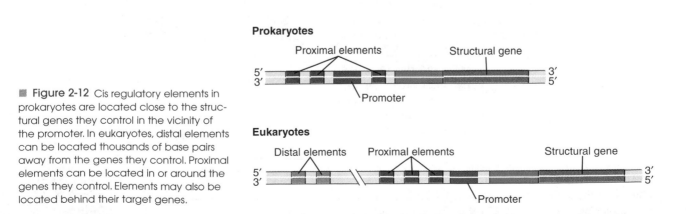

Figure 2-12 Cis regulatory elements in prokaryotes are located close to the structural genes they control in the vicinity of the promoter. In eukaryotes, distal elements can be located thousands of base pairs away from the genes they control. Proximal elements can be located in or around the genes they control. Elements may also be located behind their target genes.

Advanced Concepts

Unlike prokaryotes, eukaryotes do not have operons. Coordinately expressed genes can be scattered in several locations. Synchronous expression is brought about in eukaryotes by combinatorial control, that is, genes that are expressed in a similar pattern share similar cis elements so that they respond simultaneously to specific combinations of controlling trans factors.

distal regulatory elements. Distal eukaryotic elements can be located thousands of base pairs away from the genes they control. **Enhancers** and **silencers** are examples of distal regulatory elements that, respectively, stimulate or dampen expression of distant genes.

Epigenetics

Histone Modification

Gene activity (transcription) can be altered in ways other than by cis elements and transcription factors. Histone modification, DNA methylation, and gene silencing by double-stranded or antisense RNA regulate gene expression. These types of gene regulation are called **epigenetic regulation**. The term *epigenetics* reflects the idea that the phenotypic effects of these regulatory factors are heritable but not encoded in the DNA.

Chromatin is nuclear DNA that is compacted onto nucleosomes. A **nucleosome** is about 150 bases of DNA wrapped around a complex of 8 **histone** proteins, two each of H2A, H2B, H3, and H4. Histones not only are structural proteins but can also regulate access of trans factors and RNA polymerase to the DNA helix. Modification of histone proteins affects the activity of chromatin-associated proteins and transcription factors that increase or decrease gene expression. Through these protein interactions, chromatin can move between transcriptionally active and transcriptionally silent states. Different types of DNA modifications, including methylation, phosphorylation, ubiquitination, and acetylation, establish a complex system of control. Histone modifications create a docking surface that forms an environment for interaction with other chromatin binding factors and, ultimately, regulatory proteins (Fig. 2-13).[64] A collection of such

architectural and regulatory proteins assembled on an enhancer element has been termed an **enhanceosome**.[65]

The involvement of histone modification with gene expression has led to the study of aberrations in these modifications in disease states such as viral infections and neoplastic cells. Thus, analysis of histone states may be another target for diagnostic, prognostic, and therapeutic applications.

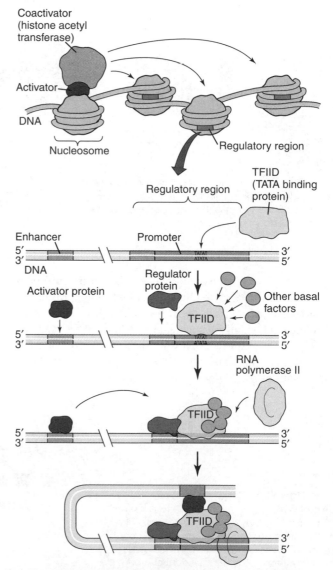

■ Figure 2-13 Interaction of transcription factors and nucleosome acetylation at the regulatory region of a gene (top) induce assembly of protein factors and RNA polymerase at the promoter (bottom).

DNA Modification

DNA methylation is another type of epigenetic regulation of gene expression in eukaryotes and prokaryotes. In vertebrates, methylation occurs in cytosine-guanine–rich sequences in the DNA (**CpG islands**) (Fig. 2-14). CpG islands were initially defined as regions >200 bp in length with an observed/expected ratio of the occurrence of CpG >0.6.[68] This definition may be modified to a more selective GC content to exclude unrelated regions of naturally high GC content.[69] CpG islands are found around the first exons, promoter regions, and sometimes toward the 3' ends of genes. Aberrant DNA methylation at these sites is a source of dysregulation of genes in disease states. For example, methylation of cytosine residues in the promoter regions of tumor suppressor genes is a mechanism of inactivation of these genes in cancer.[70] Methods to analyze promoter methylation have been developed.[71,72]

Methylation of DNA is the main mechanism of genomic **imprinting**, the gamete-specific silencing of genes.[73,74] Imprinting maintains the balanced expression of genes in growth and embryonic development by selective methylation of homologous genes. This controlled methylation occurs during gametogenesis and is different in male and female gametes. A convenient illustration of imprinting is the comparison of mules and hinnies. A mule (progeny of a female horse and male donkey) has a

---

Advanced Concepts

One theory holds that preexisting and gene-specific histone modifications constitute a **histone code** that extends the information potential of the genetic code.[66] Accordingly, **euchromatin**, which is transcriptionally active, has more acetylated histones and less methylated histones than transcriptionally silent **heterochromatin** made up of more condensed nucleosome fibers. Although methylated histones can activate transcription by recruiting histone acetylases, establishment of localized areas of histone methylation can also prevent transcription by recruiting proteins for DNA methylation and heterochromatin formation. This is one form of gene or transcriptional silencing.[67] Transcriptional silencing is responsible for inactivation of the human X chromosome in female embryo development and

position effects, the silencing of genes when placed in heterochromatic areas.

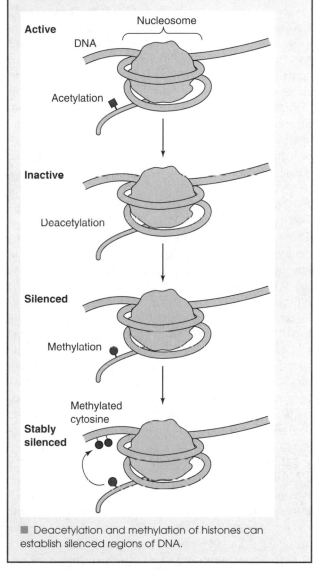

■ Deacetylation and methylation of histones can establish silenced regions of DNA.

...GGAGGAG<u>CG</u>C<u>GCG</u>G<u>CG</u>G<u>CG</u>GCCAGAGA

AAAG<u>C</u><u>CG</u>CAG<u>CG</u>G<u>CG</u><u>CG</u><u>CG</u><u>CG</u>CAC<u>CCGG</u>A

CAG<u>CCGG</u><u>CGG</u>AGG<u>CGGG</u>...

■ **Figure 2-14** CpG islands are sequences of DNA rich in the C-G dinucleotides. These structures have no specific sequence other than a higher-than-expected occurrence of CpG.

distinct phenotype from that of a hinny (progeny of a male horse and a female donkey). The difference is due to distinct imprinting of genes inherited through egg formation (oogenesis) versus those inherited through sperm formation (spermatogenesis). Genetic diseases in humans, Angelman's syndrome and Prader-Willi syndrome, are clinically distinct conditions that result from the same genetic defect on chromosome 15. The phenotypic differences depend on whether the genetic lesion involves the maternally or paternally inherited chromosome. Imprinting may be partly responsible for abnormal development and phenotypic characteristics of cloned animals as the process of cloning by nuclear transfer bypasses egg and sperm formation (gametogenesis).[75,76]

Regulation of Gene Expression by MicroRNA

There are thousands of microRNAs encoded among genes in higher eukaryotes.[77] These small RNAs regulate gene expression posttranscription by binding to the 3' end of mRNA and preventing its translation into protein (Fig. 2-15). MicroRNAs are transcribed as larger precursors (pre-miRNA), which are cleaved into hairpins by RNase III-like endonucleases called dicer and Drosha.[78] The hairpins are further digested into short, single-stranded RNA imperfectly complementary to the 3' end of the target gene. Hybridization between the micro-RNA and the mRNA prevents translation of the target RNA and eventually results in degradation of the mRNA.

Regulation of Gene Expression by RNAinterference

Another phenomenon that affects transcription is **RNA interference**, or RNAi. First discovered in the worm *Caenorhabditis elegans* in 1993, RNAi is not present in higher eukaryotes; however, it is a useful tool in the research laboratory used to selectively eliminate expression of specific genes. RNAi is mediated through siRNAs.[79] Like microRNA, the siRNAs and other proteins assemble into an enzyme complex, called the **RNA induced silencing complex (RISC)** (see Fig. 2-15). The RISC uses the associated siRNA to bind and degrade mRNA with sequences exactly complementary to the siRNA. Translation of specific genes can thus be inhibited. Alternatively, siRNAs may bind to specific sequences in already transcribed homologous RNA, targeting them for degradation into more siRNAs. Although the regulatory

mechanisms are similar, regulation by siRNA requires introduction of foreign RNA into the cell, while micro-RNAs are encoded in the cell's DNA.[80]

Advanced Concepts

siRNAs may also guide methylases to homologous sequences on the chromosome, either through direct interaction with the methylating enzymes or by hybridizing to specific sequences in the target genes, forming a bulge in the DNA molecule that attracts methylases. RNAi, however is not always required for DNA methylation.[81]

Advanced Concepts

RNA interference has been utilized as a method to specifically inactivate genes in the research laboratory. Preferable to gene deletions or "knock-out" methods that take months to inactivate a single gene, RNAi can specifically inactivate several genes in a few days.

Initially, this method did not work well in mammalian cells, due to a cellular response elicited by introduction of long dsRNAs that turns off multiple genes and promotes cell suicide. Studies with shorter dsRNAs, however, have been demonstrated to work in mammalian cell cultures.[32] This type of specific gene control in vitro may lead to control cell cultures or transcriptional states useful in the clinical laboratory setting as well as the research laboratory.

Advanced Concepts

Because of the high specificity of siRNAs, RNAi has also been proposed as a manner of gene and viral therapy.[82] Silencing has been targeted to growth-activating genes such as the vascular endothelial growth factor in tumor cells. Small interfering RNA silencing may also be aimed at HIV and influenza viruses. As with other gene therapy methods, stability and delivery of the therapeutic siRNAs are major challenges.

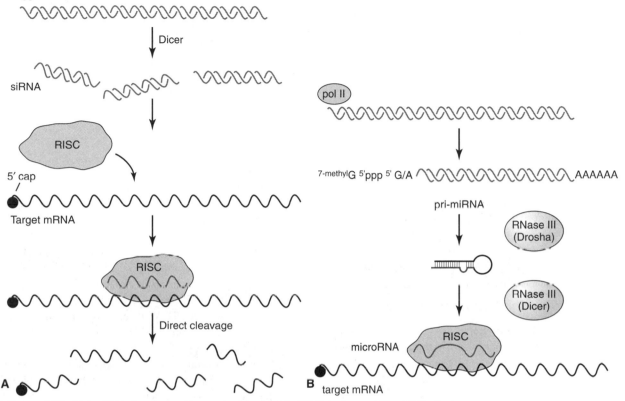

■ **Figure 2-15** (A) In siRNA silencing, a trigger double-stranded RNA is cleaved into siRNAs that become part of the RNA-Induced Silencing Complex (RISC). Led by the complementary siRNA sequences, RISC binds to the target RNA and begins RNA cleavage.[31] (B) In miRNA silencing; miRNA transcripts are transcribed from host genes, processed and joined to the RISC assembly.

Gene expression is the fundamental process for cell regulation, differentiation, and development. **Signal transduction** pathways that are the targets of several therapeutic strategies funnel internal and external signals to the nucleus where transcription factors bind to specific sequences in DNA and initiate or turn off transcription.

• **STUDY QUESTIONS** •

RNA Secondary Structure

1. Draw the secondary structure of the following RNA. The complementary sequences (inverted repeat) are underlined.

5'CAU<u>GUUCA</u>GCUCAUG<u>UGAAC</u>GCU 3'

2. Underline *two* inverted repeats in the following RNA.

5'CUGAACUUCAGUCAAGCAAAGAGUUUGCACU G 3'

RNA Processing

1. Name three processing steps undergone by messenger RNA.

2. What is the function of polyadenylate polymerase?

3. What is unusual about the phosphodiester bond formed between mRNA and its 5' cap?

4. The parts of the hnRNA that are translated into protein (open reading frames) are the _____.

5. The intervening sequences that interrupt protein coding sequences in hnRNA are _____.

Gene Expression

1. Proteins that bind to DNA to control gene expression are called _____ factors.

2. The binding sites on DNA for proteins that control gene expression are _____ factors.

3. How might a single mRNA produce more than one protein product?

4. The type of transcription producing RNA that is continually required and relatively abundant in the cell is called _____ transcription.

5. A set of structural genes transcribed together on one polycistronic mRNA is called an _____.

The Lac Operon

Using the depiction of the lac operon in Figures 2-9 and 2-10, indicate whether gene expression (transcription) would be on or off under the following conditions: (P = promoter; O = operator; R = repressor).

   a. P+ O+ R+, no inducer present – OFF
   b. P+ O+ R+, inducer present – ON
   c. P– O+ R+, no inducer present –
   d. P– O+ R+, inducer present –
   e. P+ O– R+, no inducer present –
   f. P+ O– R+, inducer present –
   g. P+ O+ R–, no inducer present –
   h. P+ O+ R–, inducer present –
   i. P– O– R+, no inducer present –
   j. P– O– R+, inducer present –
   k. P– O+ R–, no inducer present –
   l. P– O+ R–, inducer present –
   m. P+ O– R–, no inducer present –
   n. P+ O– R–, inducer present –
   o. P– O– R–, no inducer present –
   p. P– O– R–, inducer present –

Epigenetics

1. Indicate whether the following events would increase or decrease expression of a gene:
   a. Methylation of cytosine bases 5' to the gene
   b. Histone acetylation close to the gene
   c. siRNAs complementary to the gene transcript

2. How does the complementarity of siRNA to its target mRNA differ from that of miRNA?

3. What is imprinting in DNA?

4. What sequence structures in DNA, usually found 5' to structural genes, are frequent sites of DNA methylation?

5. What is the RISC?

References

1. Werner M, Thuriaux P, Soutourina J. Structure-function analysis of RNA polymerases I and III. *Current Opinion in Structural Biology* 2009;19: 740–745.
2. Lamond A, Earnshaw WC. Structure and function in the nucleus. *Science* 1998;280:547–553.
3. Tollervey D. Termination by torpedo. *Nature* 2004;432:456–457.
4. Epshtein V, Dutta D, Wade J, Nudler E. An allosteric mechanism of Rho-dependent transcription termination. *Nature* 2010;463:245–249.
5. Kuhn A, Bartsch I, Grummt I. Specific interaction of the murine transcription termination factor TTF I with class-I RNA polymerases. *Nature* 1990;344:559–562.
6. Weinberg RA, Penman S. Processing of 45S nucleolar RNA. *Journal of Molecular Biology* 1970;47: 169–178.
7. Yusupov M, Yusupova GZH, Baucom A, et al. Crystal structure of the ribosome at 5.5A resolution. *Science* 2001;292:883–896.
8. Ogle JM, Brodersen DE, Clemons WM Jr, et al. Recognition of cognate transfer RNA by the 30S ribosomal subunit. *Science* 2001;292:897–902.
9. Edmonds M, Caramela MG. The isolation and characterization of AMP-rich polynucleotide synthesized by Ehrlich ascites cells. *Journal of Biological Chemistry* 1969;244:1314–1324.
10. Tilghman SM, Tiemeier DC, Seidman JG, et al. Intervening sequence of DNA identified in the structural portion of a mouse β-globin gene. *Proceedings of the National Academy of Sciences* 1978;75:725–729.
11. White R, Hogness DS. R loop mapping of the 18S and 28S sequences in the long and short repeating units of *D. melanogaster* rDNA. *Cell* 1977;10:177–192.

12. Wickens M, Gonzalez TN. Knives, accomplices and RNA. *Science* 2004;306:1299–1300.

13. Paushkin S, Patel M, Furia BS, et al. Identification of a human endonuclease complex reveals a link between tRNA splicing and pre-mRNA 3'-end formation. *Cell* 2004;117:311–321.

14. Milcarek CR. The metabolism of a polyA minus mRNA fraction in HeLa cells. *Cell* 1974;3:1–10.

15. Perry RP, Kelly DE. Existence of methylated mRNA in mouse L cells. *Cell* 1974;1:37–42.

16. Both GW, Furuichi Y, Muthukrishman S, et al. Effect of 5+ terminal structure and base composition on polyribonucleotide binding to ribosomes. *Journal of Molecular Biology* 1975;104:637–658.

17. Lewin BM. Gene Expression 2: Eucaryotic Chromosomes, 2nd ed. New York: John Wiley & Sons, 1980.

18. Amara SG, Jonas V, Rosenfield MG, et al. Alternative RNA processing in calcitonin gene expression generates mRNA encoding different polypeptide products. *Nature* 1982;298:240–244.

19. Toro I, Thore S, Mayer C, et al. RNA binding in an Sm core domain: X-ray structure and functional analysis of an archaeal Sm protein complex. *EMBO Journal* 2001;20(9):2293–2303.

20. Mura C, Cascio D, Sawaya MR, et al. The crystal structure of a heptameric archaeal Sm protein: Implications for the eukaryotic snRNP core. *Proceedings of the National Academy of Sciences* 2001;98(10):5532–5537.

21. Liu Z, Luyten I, Bottomley MJ, et al. Structural basis for recognition of the intron branch site RNA by splicing factor 1. *Science* 2001;294:1098–1101.

22. Lehninger A. Principles of Biochemistry. New York, NY: Worth Publishers, 1982.

23. Holley RW. The Nucleotide Sequence of a Nucleic Acid. San Francisco: Freeman, 1968.

24. Lee R, Feinbaum RL, Ambros V. The *C. elegans* heterochronic gene lin-4 encodes small RNAs with antisense complementarity to lin-14. *Cell* 1993;75(5):843–854.

25. Reinhart B, Slack FJ, Basson M, et al. The 21-nucleotide let-7 RNA regulates developmental timing in *Caenorhabditis elegans*. *Nature* 2000;403(6772):901–906.

26. Wightman HI, Ruvkun G. Posttranscriptional regulation of the heterochronic gene lin-14 by lin-4 mediates temporal pattern formation in C. elegans. *Cell* 1993;75(5):855–862.

27. Lee RC, Ambros V. An extensive class of small RNAs in *Caenorhabditis elegans*. *Science* 2001;294:862–864.

28. Adams A. RNAi inches toward the clinic. *The Scientist* 2004;18(6):32–35.

29. Lagos-Quintana M, Rauhut R, Lendeckel W, et al. Identification of novel genes coding for small expressed RNAs. *Science* 2001;294:853–858.

30. Lau NC, Lim LP, Weinstein, EG, et al. An abundant class of tiny RNAs with probable regulatory roles in Caenorhabditis elegans. *Science* 2001;294: 858–862.

31. Tam W. The emergent role of microRNAs in molecular diagnostics of cancer. *Journal of Molecular Diagnostics* 2008;10(5):411–414.

32. Pfeffer ZM, Grasser FA, Chien M, et al. Identification of virus-encoded microRNAs. *Science* 2004;304:734–736.

33. Hamilton A, Baulcombe D. A species of small antisense RNA in posttranscriptional gene silencing in plants. *Science* 1999;286(5441):950–952.

34. Knight S, Bass BL. A role for the RNase III enzyme DCR-1 in RNA interference and germ line development in *Caenorhabditis elegans*. *Science* 2001;293(5538):2269–2271.

35. Fire A, Xu S, Montgomery MK, et al. Potent and specific genetic interference by double-stranded RNA in *Caenorhabditis elegans*. *Nature* 1998;391(6669):806–811.

36. Novina C, Sharp PA. The RNAi revolution. *Nature* 2004;430:161–164.

37. Sum E, Segara D, Duscio B, et al. Overexpression of LMO4 induces mammary hyperplasia, promotes cell invasion, and is a predictor of poor outcome in breast cancer. *Proceedings of the National Academy of Sciences of the United States of America* 2005;102(21):7659–7664.

38. Calderon A, Lavergne JA. RNA interference: A novel and physiologic mechanism of gene silencing with great therapeutic potential. *Puerto Rico Health Sciences Journal* 2005;24(1):27–33.

39. Ambros V, Lee RC, Lavanway A, et al. MicroRNAs and other tiny endogenous RNAs in *C. elegans*. *Current Biology* 2003;13:807–818.

40. Kuwabara T, Hsieh J, Nakashima K, et al. A small modulatory dsRNA specifies the fate of adult neural stem cells. *Cell* 2004;116:779–793.

41. Eliceiri G. Small nucleolar RNAs. *Cellular and Molecular Life Sciences* 1999;56(1–2):22–31.

42. Sunohara T, Jojima K, Yamamoto Y, et al. Nascent-peptide-mediated ribosome stalling at a stop codon induces mRNA cleavage resulting in nonstop mRNA that is recognized by tmRNA. *RNA* 2004; 10(3):378–386.

43. Adler B, Hajduk SL. Mechanisms and origins of RNA editing. *Current Opinion in Genetic Development* 1994;4:316–322.

44. Greeve J, Navaratnam N, Scott J. Characterization of the apolipoprotein B mRNA editing enzyme: no similarity to the proposed mechanism of RNA editing in kinetoplastid protozoa. *Nucleic Acids Research* 1991;19:3569–3576.

45. Travers A, Burgess RR. Cyclic reuse of the RNA polymerase sigma factor. *Nature* 1969;222:537–540.

46. Burgess R, Travers AA, Dunn JJ, et al. Factor-stimulating transcription by RNA polymerase. *Nature* 1969;221:43–47.

47. Roeder R, Rutter WJ. Specific nucleolar and nucleoplasmic RNA polymerases. *Proceedings of the National Academy of Sciences of the United States of America* 1970;65:675–682.

48. Jacob ST, Sajdel EM, Munro HN. Different responses of soluble whole nuclear RNA polymerase and soluble nucleolar RNA polymerase at divalent cations and to inhibition by α-amanitin. *Biochemical Biophysical Research Communications* 1970;38: 765–770.

49. Lindell TJ, Weinber F, Morris PW, et al. Specific inhibition of nuclear RNA polymerase by amanitin. *Science* 1970;170:447–448.

50. Lee Y, Kim M, Han J, et al. MicroRNA genes are transcribed by RNA polymerase II. *EMBO Journal* 2004;23(20):4051–4060.

51. Bird G, Zorio DA, Bentley DL. RNA polymerase II carboxy-terminal domain phosphorylation is required for cotranscriptional pre-mRNA splicing and 3'-end formation. *Molecular and Cellular Biology* 2004;24(20):8963–8969.

52. Gong X, Nedialkov YA, Burton ZF. Alpha-amanitin blocks translocation by human RNA polymerase II. *Journal of Biological Chemistry* 2004;279(26): 27422–27427.

53. Dalmay T, Hamilton A, Rudd S, et al. An RNA-dependent RNA polymerase gene in Arabidopsis is required for posttranscriptional gene silencing mediated by a transgene but not by a virus. *Cell* 2000;101(5):543–553.

54. Dickson K, Thompson SR, Gray NK, et al. Poly (A) polymerase and the regulation of cytoplasmic polyadenylation. *Journal of Biological Chemistry* 2001;276(45):41810–41816.

55. Ryan K, Calvo O, Manley JL. Evidence that polyadenylation factor CPSF-73 is the mRNA 3' processing endonuclease. *RNA* 2004;10(4): 565–573.

56. Dantonel J, Murthy KG, Manley JL, et al. Transcription factor TFIID recruits factor CPSF for formation of 3' end of mRNA. *Nature* 1997; 389(6649):399–402.

57. Harder J, Schroder J-M. RNase 7, a novel innate immune defense antimicrobial protein of healthy human skin. *Journal of Biological Chemistry* 2002;277:46779–46784.

58. Probst J, Brechtel S, Scheel B, et al. Characterization of the ribonuclease activity on the skin surface. *Genetic Vaccines and Therapy* 2006;4:4.

59. Cramer P, Bushnell DA, Kornberg R. Structural basis of transcription: RNA polymerase II at 2.8 angstrom resolution. *Science* 2001;292:1863–1876.

60. Gnatt AL, Cramer P, Fu J, et al. Structural basis of transcription: An RNA polymerase II elongation complex. *Science* 2001;292:1876–1881.

61. Linder P. The life of RNA with proteins. *Science* 2004;304:694–695.

62. Monod J, Cozen-Bizare G. L'effect d'inhibition specifique dans la biosynthese de la tryptophane-desmase chez *Aerobacter aerogenes*. *Comptes Rendus de l'Academie des Sciences* 1953;236: 530–532.

63. Jacob F, Monod J. Genetic regulatory mechanisms in the synthesis of proteins. *Journal of Molecular Biology* 1961;3:318–356.

64. Berger SL. The histone modification circus. *Science* 2001;292:64–65.

65. Munshi NT, Agalioti S, Lomvardas M, et al. Coordination of a transcriptional switch by HMGI(Y) acetylation. *Science* 2001;293:1133–1136.

66. Jenuwein T. Translating the histone code. *Science* 2001;293:1074–1079.

67. Bird A. Methylation talk between histones and DNA. *Science* 2001;294:2113–2115.

68. Gardiner-Garden M, Frommer M. CpG islands in vertebrate genomes. *Journal of Molecular Biology* 1987;196(2):261–282.

69. Jones D. The role of DNA methylation in mammalian epigenetics. *Science* 2001;293(5532):1068–1070.

70. Jones PA, Laird PW. Cancer epigenetics comes of age. *Nature Genetics* 1999;21:163–167.

71. Lehmann UB, Hasemeier R, Kreipe H. Quantitative analysis of promoter hypermethylation in laser-microdissected archival specimens. *Laboratory Investigation* 2001;81(4):635–637.

72. Gonzalgo ML, Bender CM, You EH, et al. Low frequency of p16/CDKN2A methylation in sporadic melanoma: Comparative approaches for methylation analysis of primary tumors. *Cancer Research* 1997;57:5336–5347.

73. Li E, Beard C, Forster AC, et al. DNA methylation, genomic imprinting, and mammalian development. *Cold Spring Harbor Symposium on Quantitative Biology* 1993;58:297–305.

74. Gold J, Pedersen RA. Mechanisms of genomic imprinting in mammals. *Current Topics in Developmental Biology* 1994;29:227–247.

75. Solter D. Lambing by nuclear transfer. *Nature* 1996;380(6569):24–25.

76. Yang L, Chavatte-Palmer P, Kubota C, et al. Expression of imprinted genes is aberrant in deceased newborn cloned calves and relatively normal in surviving adult clones. *Molecular Reproduction and Development* 2005;71(4):431–438.

77. Lee RC, Ambros V. An extensive class of small RNAs in *Caenorhabditis elegans*. *Science* 2001;294:862–864.

78. Lee Y, Ahn C, Han J, et al. The nuclear RNase III Drosha initiates microRNA processing. *Nature* 2003;425:415–419.

79. Matzke M, Kooter JM. RNA: guiding gene silencing. *Science* 2001;293:1080–1083.

80. Tuschl T, Weber K. Duplexes of 21-nucleotide RNAs mediate RNA interference in cultured mammalian cells. *Nature* 2001;411(6836):494–498.

81. Freitag M, Lee DW, Kothe GO, et al. DNA methylation is independent of RNA interference in *Neurospora*. *Science* 2004;304:1939.

82. Wall N, Shi Y. Small RNA: Can RNA interference be exploited for therapy? *Lancet* 2003;362:1401–1403.

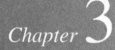

Chapter 3

Proteins and the Genetic Code

OBJECTIVES

- Describe the structure and chemical nature of the 20 amino acids.
- Show how the chemistry of the amino acids affects the chemical characteristics and functions of proteins.
- Define primary, secondary, tertiary, and quaternary structure of protein organization.
- Give the definition of a gene.
- Recount how the genetic code was solved.
- Describe how amino acids are polymerized into proteins, using RNA as a guide (translation).

Proteins are the products of transcription and translation of the nucleic acids. Even though nucleic acids are most often the focus of "molecular analysis," the ultimate effect of the information stored and delivered by the nucleic acid is manifested in proteins. In the medical laboratory, analysis of the amount and mutational status of specific proteins has long been performed in situ using immunohistochemistry, on live cells using flow cytometry and on isolated proteins by enzyme-linked immunosorbent assays, capillary electrophoresis, and Western blots. More recently, global protein analysis by mass spectrometry (proteomics) has been applied to clinical work on a research basis. Even if proteins are not being tested directly, they manifest the phenotype directed by the nucleic acid information. In order to interpret results of nucleic acid analysis accurately, therefore, it is important to understand the movement of genetic information from DNA to protein as dictated by the genetic code.

Amino Acids

Proteins are polymers of **amino acids**. Each amino acid has characteristic biochemical properties determined by the nature of its amino acid **side chain** (Fig. 3-1). Amino acids are grouped according to their polarity (tendency to interact with water at pH 7) as follows: **nonpolar**, uncharged **polar**, negatively charged polar, and positively charged polar (Table 3.1).

The properties of amino acids that make up a protein determine the shape and biochemical nature of the protein. A single protein can have separate **domains** with different properties. For example, transmembrane proteins have several stretches of hydrophobic amino acids positioned in the lipid membrane of the cell while they might also have hydrophilic or charged **extracellular** domains (Fig. 3-2).

Amino acids are synthesized in vivo by stereospecific enzymes so that naturally occurring proteins are made of amino acids of L-stereochemistry. The central asymmetric carbon atom of the amino acid is attached to a carboxyl group, an amino group, a hydrogen atom, and the side chain. Proline differs from the rest of the amino acids in that its side chain is cyclic, the amino group attached to the end carbon of the side chain making a five-carbon ring (see Fig. 3-1).

Amino acids are also classified by their biosynthetic origins or similar structures based on a common biosynthetic precursor (Table 3.2). Histidine has a unique synthetic pathway using metabolites common to purine nucleotide biosynthesis, which affords the connection of amino acid synthesis to nucleotide synthesis.

At pH 7, most of the carboxyl groups of the amino acids are ionized and the amino groups are not. The ionization can switch between the amino and carboxyl groups, making the amino acids **zwitterions** at physiological pH (Fig. 3-3). At certain pH levels, amino acids will become completely positively or negatively charged. These are the pK values for each amino acid. At the pH where an amino acid is neutral, its positive and negative charges are in balance. This is the pI value. Each amino acid will have its characteristic pI. The pI of a **peptide** or protein is determined by the ionization state (positive and negative charges) of the side chains of its constituent amino acids.

The amino and carboxyl terminal groups of the amino acids are joined in a carbon-carbon-nitrogen (–C–C–N–) substituted amide linkage (**peptide bond**) to form the protein backbone (Fig. 3-4). Two amino acids joined together by a peptide bond make a dipeptide. Peptides with additional units are tri-, tetra-, pentapeptides, and so forth, depending on how many units are attached to each other. At one end of the peptide will be an amino group (the **amino terminal**, or NH_2 end), and at the opposite terminus of the peptide will be a carboxyl group (the **carboxy terminal**, or COOH end). Like the 5' to 3' direction of nucleic acids, peptide chains grow from the amino to the carboxy terminus.

Proteins are **polypeptides** that can reach sizes of more than a thousand amino acids in length. The information stored in the sequence of nucleotides in DNA is transcribed and translated into an amino acid sequence that will ultimately bring about the genetically coded phenotype.

Proteins constitute the most abundant macromolecules in cells. The collection of proteins encoded in all of an organism's DNA is a **proteome**. The proteome of humans is larger than the genome (collection of all genes), possibly 10 times its size.[1] This is because a single gene can give rise to more than one protein through alternate splicing and other post-transcriptional/post-translational modifications.

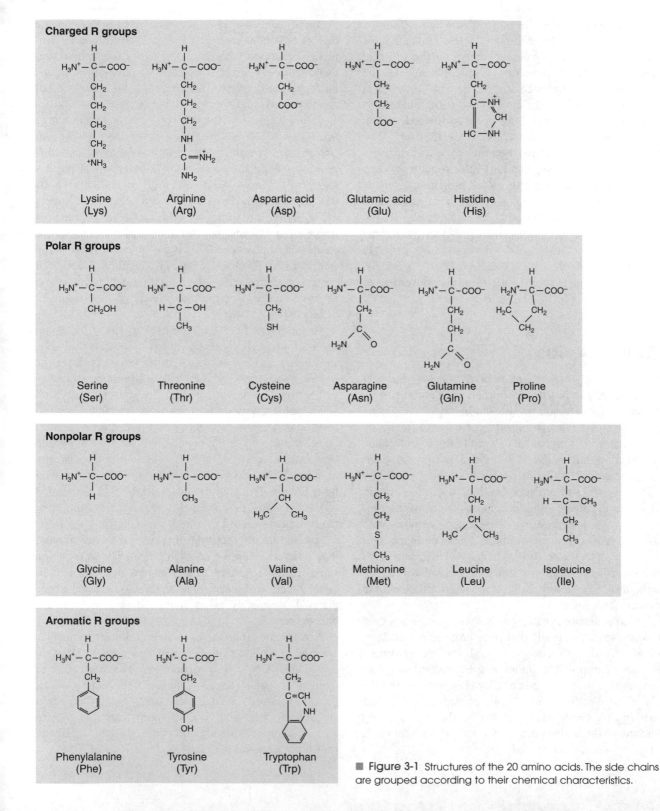

Figure 3-1 Structures of the 20 amino acids. The side chains are grouped according to their chemical characteristics.

Table 3.1 **Classification of Amino Acids Based on Polarity of Their Side Chains**

Classification	Amino Acid	Abbreviations
Nonpolar	Alanine	Ala, A
	Isoleucine	Ile, I
	Leucine	Leu, L
	Methionine	Met, M
	Phenylalanine	Phe, F
	Tryptophan	Trp, W
	Valine	Val, V
Polar	Asparagine	Asn, N
	Cysteine	Cys, C
	Glutamine	Gln, Q
	Glycine	Gly, G
	Proline	Pro, P
	Serine	Ser, S
	Threonine	Thr, T
	Tyrosine	Tyr, Y
Negatively charged (acidic)	Aspartic acid	Asp, D
	Glutamic acid	Glu, E
Positively charged (basic)	Arginine	Arg. R
	Histidine	His, H
	Lysine	Lys, K

Table 3.2 **Amino Acid Biosynthetic Groups**

Biosynthetic Group	Precursor	Amino Acids
α-Ketoglutarate group	α-Ketoglutarate	Gln, Q
		Glu, E
		Pro, P
		Arg. R
Pyruvate group	Pyruvate	Ala, A
		Val, V
		Leu, L
Oxalate group	Oxalacetic acid	Asp, D
		Asn, N
		Lys, Q
		Ile, I
		Thr, T
		Met, M
Serine group	3 Phosphoglycerate	Gly, G
		Ser, S
		Cys, C
Aromatic group	Chorismate	Phe, F
		Trp, W
		Tyr, Y
(Unique biosynthesis)		His, H

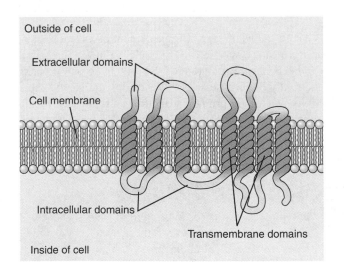

■ **Figure 3-2** Transmembrane proteins have hydrophobic transmembrane domains and hydrophilic domains exposed to the intracellular and extracellular spaces. The biochemical nature of these domains results from their distinct amino acid compositions.

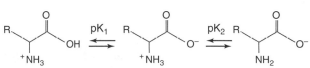

■ **Figure 3-3** An amino acid is positively charged at pK$_1$ and negatively charged at pK$_2$. At the pH where the positive and negative charges balance (pI), the molecule is neutral.

Advanced Concepts

An unusual 21st amino acid, **selenocysteine**, is a component of **selenoproteins**, such as glutathione peroxidase and formate dehydrogenase. There are 25 known mammalian selenoproteins. Selenocysteine is cysteine with the sulfur atom replaced by selenium.[2] Selenocysteine is coded by a predefined UGA codon that inserts selenocysteine instead of a termination signal.

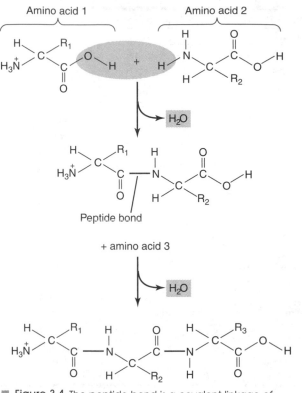

Figure 3-4 The peptide bond is a covalent linkage of the carboxyl C of one amino acid with the amino N of the next amino acid. One molecule of water is released in the reaction.

Historical Highlights

The primary sequence of proteins can be determined by a method first described in the Fred Sanger's report of the amino acid sequence of insulin.[3,4] This procedure was carried out in six steps. First, the protein was dissociated to amino acids. The dissociation products were separated by ion exchange chromatography in order to determine the type and amount of each amino acid. Second, the amino terminal and carboxy terminal amino acids were determined by labeling with 1-fluoro-2,4-dinitrobenzene and digestion with carboxypeptidase, respectively. The complete protein was then fragmented selectively at lysines and arginines with trypsin to 10–15 amino acid peptides. Fourth, Edmund degradation with phenylisothiocyanate and dilute acid labeled and removed the amino terminal residue. This was repeated on the same peptide until all the amino acids were identified. Fifth, after another selected cleavage of the original protein using cyanogen bromide, chymotrypsin, or pepsin and identification of the peptides by chromatography, the peptides were again sequenced using the Edmund degradation. Sixth, the complete amino acid sequence could be assembled by identification of overlapping regions.

The sequence of amino acids in a protein determines the nature and activity of that protein. This sequence is the **primary structure** of the protein and is read by convention from the amino terminal end to the carboxy terminal end. Minor changes in primary structure can alter the activity of proteins dramatically. The single amino acid substitution that produces hemoglobin S in sickle cell anemia is a well-known example. Replacement of a soluble glutamine residue with a hydrophobic valine at the sixth residue changes the nature of the protein so that it packs aberrantly in corpuscles and drastically alters cell shape. Minor changes in primary structure can have such drastic effects because the amino acids must often cooperate with one another to bring about protein structure and function.

Advanced Concepts

Even small peptides can have biological activity. Hormones such as insulin, glucagons, corticotropin, oxytocin, bradykinin, and thyrotropin are examples of peptides (9–40 amino acids long) with strong biological activity. Several antibiotics, such as penicillin and streptomycin, are also peptides.

Advanced Concepts

Protein sequence can be inferred from DNA sequence, although the degeneracy of the genetic code will result in several possible protein sequences for a given DNA sequence. Many databases on the frequency of codon usage in various organisms are available.[5-7] These can be used to predict the correct amino acid sequence.

Interactions between amino acid side chains fold a protein into predictable configurations. These include ordered beta or **beta-pleated sheets** and less-ordered **alpha helices**, or **random coils**. The alpha helix and beta sheet structures in proteins (Fig. 3-5) were first described by Linus Pauling and Robert Corey in 1951.[8–11] This level of organization is the **secondary structure** of the protein. Some proteins, especially structural proteins,

---

Advanced Concepts

Specialized secondary structures can identify functions of proteins. **Zinc finger** motifs are domains frequently found in proteins that bind to DNA. These structures consist of two beta sheets followed by an alpha helix with a stabilizing zinc atom. There are three types of zinc fingers, depending on the arrangement of cysteine residues in the protein sequence. Another example of specialized secondary structure is the **leucine zipper**, also found in transcription factors.[12] The conserved sequence has a leucine or other hydrophobic residue at each seventh position for approximately 30 amino acids arranged in an alpha helical conformation such that the leucine side chains radiate outwardly to facilitate association with other peptides of similar structure. Because other amino acids besides leucine can participate in this interaction, the term basic zipper, or bZip, has been used to describe this type of protein structure. Another similar structure found in transcriptional regulators is the helix loop helix,[13] consisting of basic amino acids that bind **consensus DNA** sequences (CANNTG) of target genes. This structure is sometimes confused with the helix turn helix. The helix turn helix is two alpha helices connected by a short sequence of amino acids, a structure that can easily fit into the major groove of DNA.

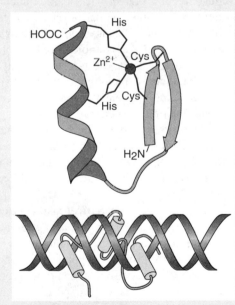

■ Zinc finger motif of the Sp1 protein, a eukaryotic transcription regulator. The side chains of histidine (H) and cysteine (C)—part of the zinc finger amino acid sequence, $C\text{-}X_{2\text{-}4}\text{-}C\text{-}X_3\text{-}F\text{-}X_5\text{-}L\text{-}X_2\text{-}H\text{-}X_3\text{-}H$ (~23 amino acids)—bind a Zn atom in the active protein. Sp1 binds DNA in the regulatory region of genes. Note: For single-letter amino acid code, see Figure 3-7. X in this consensus denotes any amino acid.

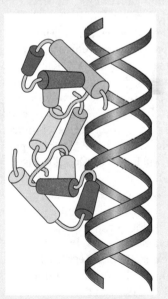

■ The lambda repressor, a transcription factor of the bacteriophage lambda, has a helix turn helix motif. One of each of the helices fits into the major groove of the DNA. Lambda repressor prevents transcription of genes necessary for active growth of the bacteriophage leading to host cell lysis.

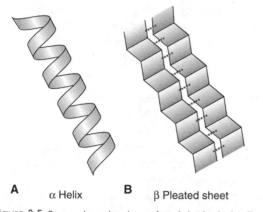

A   α Helix   **B**   β Pleated sheet

■ Figure 3-5 *Secondary structure of proteins includes the alpha helix (A) and the beta pleated sheet (B). The ribbon like structures in the pictures are composed of chains of amino acids hydrogen-bonded through their side chains.*

consist almost entirely of alpha helices or beta sheets. Globular proteins have varying amounts of alpha helix and beta sheets.

The secondary structures of proteins are further folded and arranged into a **tertiary structure**. Tertiary structure is also important for protein function. If a protein loses its tertiary structure, it is denatured. Mutations in DNA that substitute different amino acids in the primary structure can also alter tertiary structure. Denatured or improperly folded proteins are not functional. Proteins can also be denatured by heat (e.g., the albumin in egg white) or by conformations forced on innocuous peptides by infectious **prions**. Aggregations of prion-induced aberrantly folded proteins cause transmissible spongiform encephalopathies, such as Creutzfeldt-Jakob disease and bovine spongiform encephalitis (mad cow disease).

As previously mentioned, proteins often associate with other proteins in order to function. Two proteins bound together to function form a dimer, three form a trimer, four a tetramer, and so forth. Proteins that work together in this way are called **oligomers**, each component protein being a **monomer**. This is the **quaternary structure** of proteins. The combinatorial nature of protein function may account for the genetic complexity of higher organisms without a concurrent increase in gene number.

Proteins are classified according to function as enzymes and as transport, storage, motility, structural, defense, or regulatory proteins. Enzymes and transport, defense, and regulatory proteins are usually globular in nature, making them soluble and allowing them to diffuse freely across membranes. Structural and motility proteins are fibrous and insoluble.

In contrast to simple proteins that have no other components except amino acids, **conjugated proteins** do have components other than amino acids. The nonprotein component of a conjugated protein is the nonprotein **prosthetic group**. Examples of conjugated proteins are those covalently attached to lipids (**lipoproteins**), for example, low density lipoproteins; sugars (**glycoproteins**), for example, mucin in saliva; and metal atoms (**metalloproteins**), for example, ferritin. One of the most familiar examples of a conjugated protein is hemoglobin. Hemoglobin is a tetramer, having four Fe^{2+}-containing heme groups, one covalently attached to each monomer.

Genes and the Genetic Code

A **gene** is defined as the ordered sequence of nucleotides on a **chromosome** that encodes a specific functional product. A gene is the fundamental physical and functional unit of inheritance. The physical definition of a gene was complicated in early studies because of the methods used to define units of genetic inheritance. Genes were first studied by tracking mutations (changes in the order or sequence of nucleotides in the DNA) that took away their function. A gene was considered that part of a chromosome responsible for the function affected by mutation. Genes were not delineated well in terms of their physical size but were mapped relative to each other based on the frequency of recombination between them.

A gene contains not only **structural sequences** that code for an amino acid sequence but also **regulatory sequences** that are important for the regulated expression of the gene (Fig. 3-6). Cells expend a good deal of energy to coordinate protein synthesis so that the proper proteins are available at specific times and in specific amounts. Loss of this controlled expression will result in an abnormal phenotype, even though there may be no changes in the structural sequence of the gene. The failure to appreciate the importance of **proximal** and distal regulatory sequences was another source of confusion in early efforts to define a gene. Regulatory effects and the interaction between proteins still challenge interpretation of genetic analyses in the clinical laboratory.

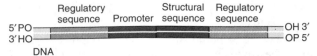

5′PO   OH 3′
3′HO   OP 5′
DNA

■ **Figure 3-6** A gene contains not only structural (coding) sequences but also sequences important for regulated transcription of the gene. These include the promoter, where RNA polymerase binds to begin transcription, and regulatory regions, where transcription factors and other regulatory factors bind to stimulate or inhibit transcription by RNA polymerase.

The Genetic Code

The nature of a gene was further clarified with the deciphering of the **genetic code** by Francis Crick, Marshall Nirenberg, Philip Leder, Gobind Khorana, and Sydney Brenner.[16–18] The genetic code is not information in itself but is a dictionary to translate the four-nucleotide sequence information in DNA to the 20–amino acid sequence information in proteins.

The triplet nature of the genetic code was surmised based on mathematical considerations. It was reasoned that the smallest set of 4 possible letters that would yield enough unique groups to denote 20 different amino acids was 3. A 1-nucleotide code could only account for $4^1 = 4$ different amino acids, whereas a 2-nucleotide code would yield $4^2 = 16$ different possibilities. A 3-nucleotide code would give $4^3 = 64$ different possibilities, enough to account for all 20 amino acids.

Historical Highlights

In the early 1960s, Seymour Benzer[14,15] used the T4 bacteriophage to investigate the gene more closely. By mixing phage with several different phenotypes, he could observe the restoration of normal phenotype or complementation of one mutant with another. Benzer could distinguish mutations that could **complement** each other, even though they affected the same phenotype and mapped to the same location in the phage DNA. He determined that these were mutations in different places within the same gene. He organized many mutants into a series of sites along the linear array of the phage chromosome so that he could structurally define the gene as a continuous linear span of genetic material.

Historical Highlights

The interesting history of the breaking of the genetic code began with a competitive scramble. A physicist and astronomer, George Gamow, organized a group of scientists to concentrate on the problem. They called themselves the RNA Tie Club. Each of the 20 members wore a tie emblazoned with a depiction of RNA and a pin depicting a different amino acid. The club members,—William Astbury, Oswald Avery, Sir William Laurence Bragg, Erwin Chargaff, Martha Chase, Robert Corey, Francis Crick, Max Delbruck, Jerry Donohue, Rosalind Franklin, Bruce Fraser, Sven Furgerg, Alfred Hershey, Linus Pauling, Peter Pauling, Max Perutz, J.T. Randall, Verner Schomaker, Alexander R. Todd, James Watson, and Maurice Wilkins—met regularly during the 1950s. They made some progress, including Crick's "adaptor" hypothesis (predicting tRNA) and Gamow's mathematical prediction of three nucleotides coding for one amino acid. Ultimately, however, they did not exclusively break the genetic code.

The next challenge was to decipher this triplet code and to prove its function. The simplest way to prove the code would have been to determine the order of nucleotides in a stretch of DNA coding for a protein and compare it with the order of amino acids in the protein. In the early 1960s, protein sequencing was possible, but only limited DNA sequencing was available. Marshall Nirenberg made the initial attempts at the code by using short synthetic pieces of RNA to support protein synthesis in a cell-free extract of *Escherichia coli*. In each of 20 tubes he mixed a different radioactive amino acid, cell lysate from *E. coli,* and an RNA template. In the first definitive experiment, the input template was a polymer of uracil, UUUUUUU.... If the input template supported synthesis of protein, the radioactive amino acids would be joined together and the radioactivity detected in a precipitable protein extract from the mixture. On May 27, 1961, Nirenberg measured radioactive protein levels from all but 1 of the 20 vials at around 70 counts/mg. The one vial, which contained the amino acid phenylalanine, yielded protein of 38,000 counts/mg.

After the first successful demonstration of this strategy, other templates were tested. Each synthetic nucleic acid incorporated different amino acids, based on the composition of bases in the RNA sequence. Codes for phenylalanine (UUU), proline (CCC), lysine (AAA), and glycine (GGG) were soon deduced from the translation of RNA synthesized from a single nucleotide population. More of the code was indirectly deduced using mixtures of nucleotides at different proportions. For instance, an RNA molecule synthesized from a 2:1 mixture of U and C polymerized mostly phenylalanine and leucine into protein. Similar tests with other nucleotide mixtures resulted in distinct amino acid incorporations. Although the nucleotide content of each RNA molecule in these tests was known, the exact order of nucleotides in the triplet was not known.

Nirenberg and Leder used another technique to get at the basic structure of the code. They observed binding of specific amino acids to RNA molecules containing three nucleotides (triplets) in ribosome-tRNA mixtures. By noting which triplet/amino acid combination resulted in binding of the amino acid to ribosomes, they were able to assign 50 of the 64 triplets to specific amino acids.

Meanwhile, Gobind Khorana had developed a system to synthesize longer RNA polymers of known nucleotide sequence. With polynucleotides of repeated sequence, he could predict and then observe the peptides that would come from that RNA. For example, a polymer consisting of two bases, such as . . . UCUCUCUCUCUCUC . . . , was expected to code for a peptide of two different amino acids, one coded for by UCU and one by CUC. This polymer yielded a peptide with the sequence . . . Ser-Leu-Ser-Leu . . . . This experiment did not indicate which triplet coded for which amino acid, but combined with the results from Nirenberg and Leder, the UCU was assigned to serine and CUC to leucine.

By 1965, all 64 triplets, or **codons**, were assigned to amino acids (Fig. 3-7). Once the code was confirmed, specific characteristics of it were apparent. The code is redundant, so that all but two amino acids (methionine and tryptophan) have more than one codon. Triplets coding for the same amino acid are similar, often differing in the third base of the triplet. Crick first referred to this as

Second position of codon

First position		U		C		A		G		Third position
U	UUU UUC	Phenylalanine	UCU UCC	Serine	UAU UAC	Tyrosine	UGU UGC	Cysteine	U C
	UUA UUG	Leucine	UCA UCG		UAA UAG	Ter (end) Ter (end)	UGA UGG	Ter (end) Tryptophan	A G
C	CUU CUC CUA CUG	Leucine	CCU CCC CCA CCG	Proline	CAU CAC	Histidine	CGU CGC CGA CGG	Arginine	U C A G
					CAA CAG	Glutamine			
A	AUU AUC AUA	Isoleucine	ACU ACC ACA ACG	Threonine	AAU AAC	Asparagine	AGU AGC	Serine	U C
	AUG	Methionine			AAA AAG	Lysine	AGA AGG	Arginine	A G
G	GUU GUC GUA GUG	Valine	GCU GCC GCA GCG	Alanine	GAU GAC	Aspartic acid	GGU GGC GGA GGG	Glycine	U C A G
					GAA GAG	Glutamic acid			

■ **Figure 3-7** The genetic code. Codons are read as the nucleotide in the left column, then the row at the top, and then the right column. Note how there are up to six codons for a single amino acid. Only methionine and tryptophan have a single codon. Note also the three termination codons (ter): TAA, TAG, and TGA.

wobble in the third position.[19] Wobble is also used to describe movement of the base in the third position of the triplet to form novel pairing between the carrier tRNA and the mRNA template during protein translation. Investigations have revealed that wobble may affect the severity of disease phenotype.[20]

All amino acids except leucine, serine, and arginine are selected by the first two letters of the genetic code. The first two letters, however, do not always specify unique amino acids. For example, CA begins the code for both histidine and glutamine. Three codons—UAG, UAA, and UGA—that terminate protein synthesis are termed **nonsense codons**. UAG, UAA, and UGA were named amber, ocher, and opal, respectively, when they were first defined in bacterial viruses.

The characteristics of the genetic code have consequences for molecular analysis. Mutations or changes in the DNA sequence will have different effects on phenotype, depending on the resultant changes in the amino acid sequence. Accordingly, mutations range from silent to drastic in terms of their effects on phenotype. This will be discussed in more detail in later chapters.

An interesting observation about the genetic code is that, with limited exceptions, the repertoire of amino acids is limited to 20 in all organisms, regardless of growing environments. Thermophilic and cryophilic organisms adapt to growth at 100°C and freezing temperatures, respectively, not by using structurally different amino acids, but by varying the combinations of the naturally occurring amino acids. Cells have strict control and editing systems to protect the genetic code and avoid incorporation of unnatural amino acids into proteins. Studies have shown that it is possible to manipulate the genetic code to incorporate modified amino acids.[21,22] This ability to introduce chemically or physically reactive sites into proteins in vivo has significant implications in biotechnology.

Advanced Concepts

The termination codon UGA also codes for selenocysteine. Selenoproteins have UGA codons in the middle of their coding regions. In the absence of selenium, protein synthesis stops prematurely in these genes.

Translation

Amino Acid Charging

After transcription of the sequence information in DNA to RNA, the transcribed sequence must be transferred into proteins. Through the genetic code, specific nucleic acid sequence is translated to amino acid sequence and, ultimately, to phenotype. As proposed in the adaptor hypothesis, there must be a molecular factor that can recognize both nucleic acid and protein sequence components. This factor is tRNA.

Protein synthesis starts with activation of the amino acids by covalent attachment to tRNA, or **tRNA charging**, a reaction catalyzed by 20 **aminoacyl tRNA synthetases**. The Mg^{++}-dependent **charging** reaction was first described by Hoagland and Zamecnik, who observed that amino acids incubated with ATP and the cytosol fraction of liver cells became attached to heat-soluble RNA (tRNA).[25] The reaction takes place in two steps. First, the amino acid is activated by addition of AMP:

amino acid + ATP → aminoacyl-AMP + PPi

Second, the activated amino acid is joined to the tRNA:

aminoacyl-AMP + tRNA → aminoacyl-tRNA + AMP

The product of the reaction is an ester bond between the 3' hydroxyl of the terminal adenine of the tRNA and the carboxyl group of the amino acid.

Advanced Concepts

According to evolutionary theory, the genetic code has evolved over millions of years of selection. An interesting analysis was done to compare the natural genetic code shared by all living organisms with millions of other possible triplet codes generated by computer (4 nucleotides coding for 20 amino acids).[23] The results showed that the natural code was significantly more resistant to damaging changes (mutations in the DNA sequence) compared with the other possible codes. The code is still undergoing "fine-tuning" through common mechanisms in prokaryotes and eukaryotes.[24]

Advanced Concepts

Once the amino acid is esterified to the tRNA, it makes no difference in specificity of its addition to the protein. The fidelity of translation is now determined by the **anticodon** (the three bases complementary to the amino acid codon) of the tRNA as an adaptor between mRNA and the growing protein. This association has been exploited by attaching amino acids synthetically to selected tRNAs. If amino acids are attached to tRNAs carrying anticodons to UAG, UAA, or UGA, the peptide chain will continue to grow instead of terminating at the stop codon. These tRNAs are called **suppressor tRNAs**, as they can suppress point mutations (single base-pair changes) that generate stop codons within a protein coding sequence.

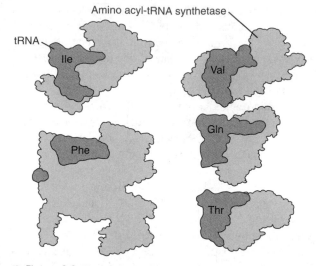

■ **Figure 3-8** Five amino acyl tRNA synthetases. Each enzyme is unique for a tRNA (shown in purple) and its matching amino acid. The specificity of these enzymes is key to the fidelity of translation.

There are 20 amino acid tRNA synthetases, one for each amino acid. Designated as class I and class II synthetases, these enzymes interact, respectively, with the minor or major groove of the tRNA acceptor arm. Both classes also recognize tRNAs by their anticodon sequences and amino acids by their side chains. Only the appropriate tRNA and amino acid will fit into its cognate synthetase (Fig. 3-8). An errant amino acid bound to the wrong synthetase will dissociate rapidly before any conformation changes and charging can occur. In another level of editing, mischarged aminoacylated tRNAs are hydrolyzed at the point of release from the enzyme. The fidelity of this system is such that mischarging is 10^3–10^6 less efficient than correct charging.[26]

Protein Synthesis

Translation takes place on **ribosomes**, ribonucleoprotein particles first observed by electron microscopy of animal cells. In the early 1950s, Zamecnik demonstrated that these particles were the site of protein synthesis in bacteria.[27] There are about 20,000 ribosomes in an *E. coli* cell, making up almost 25% of the cell's dry weight. Ribosomal structure is similar in prokaryotes and eukaryotes (see Fig. 2-3). In prokaryotes, 70S ribosomes are assembled from a 30S small subunit and a 50S large subunit, in association with mRNA and initiating factors. (S stands for sedimentation units in density gradient centrifugation, a method used to determine sizes of proteins and protein complexes.) The 30S subunit (1 million daltons) is composed of a 16S ribosomal RNA (rRNA) and 21 ribosomal proteins. The 50S subunit (1.8 million daltons) is composed of a 5S rRNA, a 23S rRNA, and 34 ribosomal proteins. Eukaryotic ribosomes are slightly larger (80S) and more complex, with a 40S small subunit (1.3 million daltons) and a 60S subunit (2.7 million daltons). The 40S subunit is made up of an 18S rRNA and about 30 ribosomal proteins. The 60S subunit contains a 5S rRNA, a 5.8S rRNA, a 28S rRNA, and about 40 ribosomal proteins.

Protein synthesis in the ribosome almost always starts with the amino acid methionine in eukaryotes and *N*-formylmethionine in bacteria, mitochondria, and chloroplasts. Initiating factors that participate in the formation of the ribosome complex differentiate the initiating methionyl tRNAs from those that add methionine internally to the protein.[28] In protein translation, the small ribosomal subunit first binds to initiation factor 3 (IF-3) and then to specific sequences near the 5' end of the mRNA, the **ribosomal binding site**. This guides the AUG codon (the "start" codon) to the proper place in the ribosomal subunit. Another initiation factor, IF-2 bound to GTP and the initiating tRNA^{Met} or tRNA^{fMet}, then joins the complex (Fig. 3-9). The large ribosomal

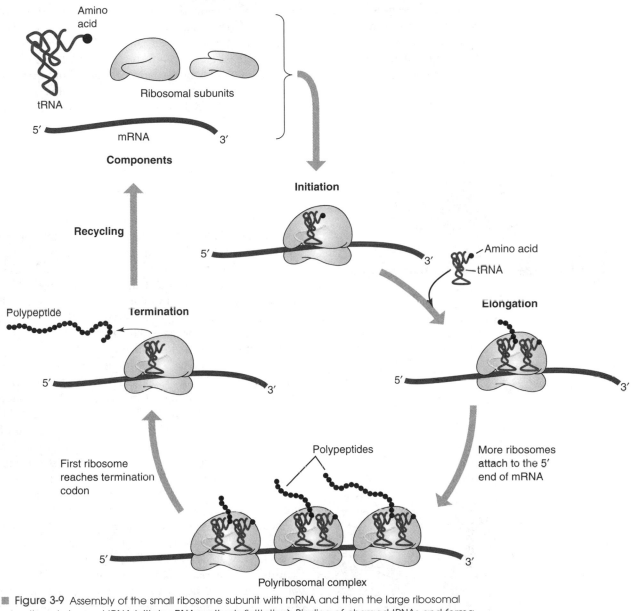

■ **Figure 3-9** Assembly of the small ribosome subunit with mRNA and then the large ribosomal subunit, and charged tRNA initiates RNA synthesis (initiation). Binding of charged tRNAs and formation of the peptide bond produce the growing polypeptide (elongation). Several ribosomes can simultaneously read a single mRNA (polyribosome complex). When the complex encounters a nonsense codon, protein synthesis stops (termination) and the components are recycled.

subunit then associates with the hydrolysis of GTP and release of GDP and phosphate, IF-2 and IF-3. The resulting functional 70S or 80S ribosome is the initiation complex. In this complex, the tRNA^{Met} or tRNA^{fMet} is situated in the peptidyl site (**P site**) of the functional ribosome. tRNA^{Met} or tRNA^{fMet} can only bind to the P site in the ribosome, which is formed in combination by both ribosomal subunits. In contrast, all other tRNAs bind to an adjacent site, the aminoacyl site (**A site**) of the ribosome.

Synthesis proceeds in the elongation step where the tRNA carrying the next amino acid binds to the A site of the ribosome in a complex with elongation factor Tu (EF-Tu) and GTP (Fig. 3-10). The fit of the incoming tRNA takes place by recognition and then proofreading of the codon-anticodon base pairing. Hydrolysis of GTP by EF-Tu occurs between these two steps.[29] The EF-Tu-GDP is released, and the EF-Tu-GTP is regenerated by another elongation factor, EF-Ts. Although these interactions ensure the accurate paring of the first two codon positions, the pairing at the third position is not as stringent, which might be related to the wobble in the genetic code.[30,31]

The first peptide bond is formed between the amino acids in the A and P sites by transfer of the *N*-formylmethionyl group of the first amino acid to the amino group of the second amino acid, generating a dipeptidyl-tRNA in the A site. This step is catalyzed by an enzymatic activity in the large subunit, **peptidyl transferase**. This activity might be mediated entirely through RNA, as no proteins are in the vicinity of the active site of the ribosome where the peptide bond formation occurs.[32] After formation of the peptide bond, the ribosome moves, shifting the dipeptidyl-tRNA from the A site to the P site with the release of the "empty" tRNA from a third position, the **E site**, of the ribosome. This movement (translocation) of tRNAs across a distance of 20 angstroms from the A to the P site and 28 angstroms from the P to the E site requires elongation factor EF-G. As the ribosomal complex moves along the mRNA, the growing peptide chain is always attached to the incoming amino acid. Two GTPs are hydrolyzed to GDP with the addition of each amino acid. This energy-dependent translocation occurs with shifting and rotation of ribosomal subunits (Fig. 3-11).[33]

During translation, the growing polypeptide begins to fold into its mature conformation. This process is assisted by molecular **chaperones**.[34] These specialized proteins bind to the large ribosomal subunit, forming a hydrophobic pocket that holds the emerging polypeptide (Fig. 3-12). Chaperones apparently protect the growing unfinished polypeptides until they can be safely folded into mature protein. In the absence of this activity, unfinished proteins might bind to each other and form nonfunctional aggregates. The DnaK protein of *E. coli* can also act as a chaperone by binding to the hydrophobic regions of the emerging polypeptide.[35]

Termination of the amino acid chain is signaled by one of the three nonsense, or termination, codons—UAA, UAG, or UGA—which are not charged with an amino acid. When the ribosome encounters a termination codon, termination, or **release factors** (R_1, R_2, and S in *E. coli*),

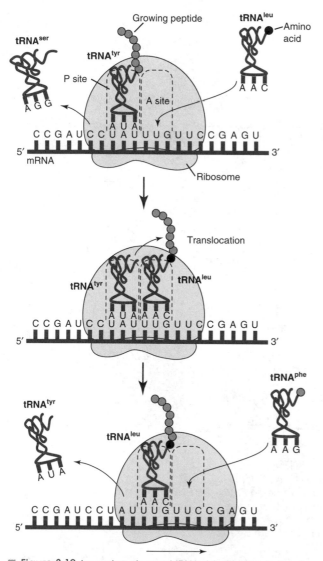

Figure 3-10 Incoming charged tRNAs bind to the A site of the ribosome, guided by matching codon-anticodon pairing. After formation of the peptide bond between the incoming amino acid and the growing peptide, the ribosome moves to the next codon in the mRNA, translocating the peptide to the P site and creating another A site for the next tRNA.

Advanced Concepts

In eukaryotes, accumulation of unfolded proteins in the endoplasmic reticulum elicits an unfolded protein response (**ER stress**), intended to correct the problem by cessation of protein synthesis or induction of more chaperones. If correction doesn't occur, ER stress will send the cell into a programmed death (apoptosis). ER stress has been found to be associated with a number of diseases, including diabetes, neurodegenerative disorders, cancer, and cardiovascular disease.[36,37]

causes hydrolysis of the finished polypeptide from the final tRNA, release of that tRNA from the ribosome, and dissociation of the large and small ribosomal subunits. In eukaryotes, termination codon–mediated binding of polypeptide chain release factors (eRF1 and eRF3) triggers hydrolysis of peptidyl-tRNA at the ribosomal peptidyl transferase center.[38,39] *E. coli* can synthesize a 300–400 amino acid protein in 10–20 seconds. Because the protein takes on its secondary structure as it is being synthesized, it already has its final conformation when it is released from the ribosome.

In bacteria, translation and transcription occur simultaneously. In nucleated cells, the majority of translation occurs in the cytoplasm. Several lines of evidence suggest, however, that translation might also occur in the nucleus. One line of evidence is that nuclei contain factors required for translation.[40,41] Furthermore, isolated nuclei can aminoacylate tRNAs and incorporate amino acids into proteins. Another support for nuclear translation is that **nonsense-mediated decay (NMD)**, degradation of messenger RNAs with premature termination codons, supposedly occurred in mammalian nuclei. Further investigations have shown, however, that NMD may not occur in the nuclei of lower eukaryotes.[42] As in prokaryotes, nuclear translation may require concurrent transcription.[43,44]

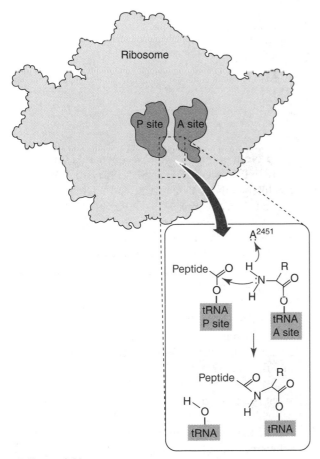

■ **Figure 3-11** Protein synthesis (translation) as it takes place in the ribosome. The peptide bond is formed in an area between the large and small subunits of the ribosome. The ribozyme theory holds that the ribosome is an enzyme that functions through RNA and not protein. The close proximity of only RNA to this site is evidence for the ribozyme theory.

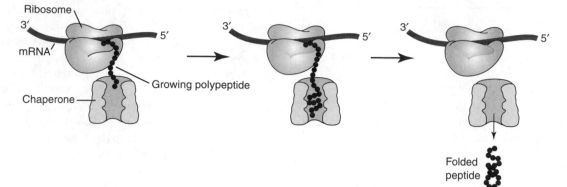

■ **Figure 3-12** Molecular chaperones catch the growing peptide as it emerges from the active site. The peptide goes through stages of holding (left), folding (center), and release (right). When the protein is completely synthesized and released from the ribosome, it should be in its folded state. This protects the nascent (growing) peptide from harmful interactions with other proteins in the cell before it has had an opportunity to form its protective and active tertiary structure.

• STUDY QUESTIONS •

1. Indicate whether the following peptides are hydrophilic or hydrophobic.
   a. MLWILAA
   b. VAIKVLIL
   c. CSKEGCPN
   d. SSIQKNET
   e. YAQKFQGRT
   f. AAPLIWWA
   g. SLKSSTGGQ

2. Is the following peptide positively or negatively charged at neutral pH?

   GWWMNKCHAGHLNGVYYQGGTY

3. Consider an RNA template made from a 2:1 mixture of C:A. What would be the three amino acids *most* frequently incorporated into protein?

4. What is the peptide sequence encoded in AUAUAUAUAUAUAUA ...?

5. Write the *anticodons* 5' to 3' of the following amino acids:
   a. L
   b. T
   c. M
   d. H
   e. R
   f. I

6. A protein contains the sequence LGEKKW-CLRVNPKGLDESKDYLSLKSKYLLL. What is the likely function of this protein? (Note: See Advanced Concepts box.)

7. A histone-like protein contains the sequence PKKGSKKAVTKVQKKDGKKRKRSRK. What characteristic of this sequence makes it likely to associate with DNA?

8. A procedure for digestion of DNA with a restriction enzyme includes a final incubation step of 5 minutes at 95°C. What is the likely purpose of this final step?

9. What is a ribozyme?

10. Name the nonprotein prosthetic groups for the following conjugated proteins:

    glycoprotein

    lipoprotein

    metalloprotein

References

1. Fields S. Proteomics in genomeland. *Science* 2001; 291:1221–1224.
2. Schomburg L, Schweizer U, Kahrle J. Selenium and selenoproteins in mammals: Extraordinary, essential, enigmatic. *Cellular and Molecular Life Science* 2004;61(16):1988–1995.
3. Sanger F, Tuppy H. The amino-acid sequence in the phenylalanyl chain of insulin. II: The investigation of peptides from enzymic hydrolysates. *Biochemical Journal* 1951;49(4):481–490.
4. Sanger F, Tuppy H. The amino-acid sequence in the phenylalanyl chain of insulin. I. The identification of lower peptides from partial hydrolysates. *Biochemical Journal* 1951;49(4):463–481.
5. Carbone F, Zinovyev A, Kepes F. Codon adaptation index as a measure of dominating codon bias. *Bioinformatics* 2003;19(16):2005–2015.
6. Ma J, Zhou T, Gu W, et al. Cluster analysis of the codon use frequency of MHC genes from different species. *Biosystems* 2002;65(2–3):199–207.
7. Van Den Bussche RA, Hansen EW. Characterization and phylogenetic utility of the mammalian protamine p1 gene. *Molecular and Phylogenetic Evolution* 2002;22(3):333–341.
8. Pauling L, Corey RB. The structure of proteins; two hydrogen-bonded helical configurations of the polypeptide chain. *Proceedings of the National Academy of Sciences* 1951;205(4):205–211.
9. Pauling L, Corey RB. The pleated sheet, a new layer configuration of polypeptide chains. *Proceedings of the National Academy of Sciences* 1951;37(5): 251–256.
10. Pauling L, Corey RB. The structure of synthetic polypeptides. *Proceedings of the National Academy of Sciences* 1951;37(5):241–250.
11. Pauling L, Corey RB. Atomic coordinates and structure factors for two helical configurations of polypeptide chains. *Proceedings of the National Academy of Sciences* 1951;37(5):235–240.
12. Landschulz W, Johnson PF, McKnight SL. The leucine zipper: A hypothetical structure common to a new class of DNA binding proteins. *Science* 1988;240(4860):1759–1764.
13. Ferre-D'Amare A, Prendergast GC, Ziff EB, et al. Recognition by Max of its cognate DNA through a dimeric b/HLH/Z domain. *Nature* 1993;363(6424): 38–45.
14. Benzer S. On the topography of genetic fine structure. *Proceedings of the National Academy of Sciences* 1961;47(3):403–415.
15. Benzer S. The fine structure of the gene. *Scientific American* 1962;206(1):70–84.
16. Crick F, Barnett, L, Brenner, S, et al. General nature of the genetic code for proteins. *Nature* 1961;192 (4809):1227–1232.
17. Nirenberg M, Leder, P, Bernfield, M, et al. RNA code words and protein synthesis, VII: On the general nature of the RNA code. *Proceedings of the National Academy of Sciences* 1965;53(5):1161–1168.
18. Jones D, Nishimura S, Khorana HG. Studies on polynucleotides, LVI: Further synthesis, in vitro, of copolypeptides containing two amino acids in alternating sequence dependent upon DNA-like polymers containing two nucleotides in alternating sequence. *Journal of Molecular Biology* 1966; 16(2):454–472.
19. Crick FHC. Codon-anticodon pairing: The wobble hypothesis. *Journal of Molecular Biology* 1966;19:548–555.
20. Kirino Y, Goto Y, Campos Y, et al. Specific correlation between the wobble modification deficiency in mutant tRNAs and the clinical features of a human mitochondrial disease. *Proceedings of the National Academy of Sciences* 2005;102(20): 7127–7132.
21. Wang L, Brock A, Herberich B et al. Expanding the genetic code of *Escherichia coli*. *Science* 2001;292: 498–500.
22. Doring V, Mootz HD, Nangle LA, et al. Enlarging the amino acid set of *Escherichia coli* by infiltration of the valine coding pathway. *Science* 2001;292: 501–504.
23. Vogel G. Tracking the history of the genetic code. *Science* 1998;281:329–331.
24. Grosjean H, de Crecy-Lagard V, Marck C. Deciphering synonymous codons in the three domains of life: Co-evolution with specific tRNA modification enzymes. *FEBS Letters* 2010;584: 252–264.
25. Hoagland MB, Keller EB, Zamecnik PC. Enzymatic carboxyl activation of amino acids. *Journal of Biological Chemistry* 1956;218:345–358.
26. Szymansk M, Deniziak M, Barciszewski J. The new aspects of aminoacyl-tRNA synthetases. *Acta Biochimica Polonica* 2000;47(3):821–834.

27. Zamecnik PC. An historical account of protein synthesis with current overtone: A personalized view. *Cold Spring Harbor Symposium on Quantitative Biology* 1969;34:1–16.
28. Kolitz S, Lorsch JR. Eukaryotic initiator tRNA: Finely tuned and ready for action. *FEBS Letters* 2010;584:396–404.
29. Ruusala T, Ehrenberg M, Kurland CG. Is there proofreading during polypeptide synthesis? *EMBO Journal* 1982;1(6):741–745.
30. Ogle JM, Brodersen DE, Clemons WM Jr, et al. Recognition of cognate transfer RNA by the 30S ribosomal subunit. *Science* 2001;292:897–902.
31. Agris P, Vendeix FA, Graham WD. tRNA's wobble decoding of the genome: 40 years of modification. *Journal of Molecular Biology* 2007;366:1–13.
32. Steitz T, Moore PB. RNA, the first macromolecular catalyst: The ribosome is a ribozyme. *Trends in Biochemical Sciences* 2003;28(8):411–418.
33. Yusupov M, Yusupova GZ, Baucom A, et al. Crystal structure of the ribosome at 5.5A resolution. *Science* 2001;292:883–896.
34. Horwich A. Sight at the end of the tunnel. *Nature* 2004;431:520–522.
35. Deuerling E, Schulze-Specking A, Tomoyasu, T, et al. Trigger factor and DnaK cooperate in folding of newly synthesized proteins. *Nature* 1999;400:693–696.
36. Civelek M, Manduchi E, Riley RJ, Stoeckert CJ, Davies PF. Chronic endoplasmic reticulum stress activates unfolded protein response in arterial endothelium in regions of susceptibility to atherosclerosis. *Circulation Research* 2009;105:453–461.
37. Austin R. The unfolded protein response in health and disease. *Antioxidants & Redox Signalling* 2009;11:2279–2287.
38. Zhouravleva G, Frolova L, Le Goff X, et al. Termination of translation in eukaryotes is governed by two interacting polypeptide chain release factors, eRF1 and eRF3. *EMBO Journal* 1995;14(16):4065–4072.
39. Frolova L, Merkulova TI, Kisselev LL. Translation termination in eukaryotes: Polypeptide release factor eRF1 is composed of functionally and structurally distinct domains. *RNA* 2000;6(3):381–390.
40. Gunasekera N, Lee SW, Kim S, et al. Nuclear localization of aminoacyl-tRNA synthetases using single-cell capillary electrophoresis laser-induced fluorescence analysis. *Analytical Chemistry* 2004;76(16):4741–4746.
41. Brogna S, Sato TA, Rosbash M. Ribosome components are associated with sites of transcription. *Molecular Cell* 2002;10(4):93–104.
42. Kuperwasser N, Brogna S, Dower K, et al. Nonsense-mediated decay does not occur within the yeast nucleus. *RNA* 2004;10(2):1907–1915.
43. Iborra FJ, Jackson DA, Cook PR. Coupled transcription and translation within nuclei of mammalian cells. *Science* 2001;293:1139–1142.
44. Sommer P, Nehrbass U. Quality control of messenger ribonucleoprotein particles in the nucleus and at the pore. *Current Opinions in Cell Biology* 2005;17(3):294–301.

Common Techniques in Molecular Biology

Chapter *4*

Nucleic Acid Extraction Methods

OUTLINE

OBJECTIVES

- Compare and contrast organic, inorganic, and solid-phase approaches for isolating cellular and mitochondrial DNA.
- Note the chemical conditions in which DNA precipitates and goes into solution.
- Compare and contrast organic and solid-phase approaches for isolating total RNA.
- Distinguish between the isolation of total RNA with that of messenger RNA.
- Describe the gel-based, spectrophotometric, and fluorometric methods used to determine the quantity and quality of DNA and RNA preparations.
- Calculate the concentration and yield of DNA and RNA from a given nucleic acid preparation.

The purpose of nucleic acid extraction is to release the nucleic acid from the cell for use in subsequent procedures. Ideally, the target nucleic acid should be free of contamination with protein, carbohydrate, lipids, or other nucleic acid, that is, DNA free of RNA or RNA free of DNA. The initial release of the cellular material is achieved by breaking the cell and nuclear membranes (cell lysis). Lysis must take place in conditions that will not damage the nucleic acid. Following lysis, the target material is purified, and then the concentration and purity of the sample can be determined.

Isolation of DNA

Although Miescher first isolated DNA from human cells in 1869,[1] the initial routine laboratory procedures for DNA isolation were developed from density gradient centrifugation strategies. Meselson and Stahl used such a method in 1958 to demonstrate semi-conservative replication of DNA.[2] Later procedures took advantage of solubility differences among chromosomal DNA, plasmids, and proteins in alkaline buffers. Large (>50 kbp) chromosomal DNA and proteins cannot renature properly when neutralized in acetate at low pH after alkaline treatment, forming large aggregates instead. As a result, they precipitate out of solution. The relatively small plasmids return to their supercoiled state and stay in solution. Alkaline lysis procedures were used extensively for extraction of 1–50 kb plasmid DNA from bacteria during the early days of recombinant DNA technology.

Preparing the Sample

Nucleic acid is routinely isolated from human, fungal, bacterial, and viral sources in the clinical laboratory

---

Advanced Concepts

In surveying the literature, especially early references, the starting material for DNA extraction had to be noted because that determined which extraction procedure was used. Extraction procedures were also modified to optimize the yield of specific products. A procedure designed to yield plasmid DNA does not efficiently isolate chromosomal DNA and vice versa.

(Table 4.1). The initial steps in nucleic acid isolation depend on the nature of the starting material.

Nucleated Cells in Suspension (Blood and Bone Marrow Aspirates)

Depending on the type of specimen sent for analysis, pretreatment may be necessary to make cells available from which the nucleic acid will be extracted. For instance,

Table 4.1 Yield of DNA from Different Specimen Sources[23-30]

Specimen	Expected Yield*
Specimens adequate for analysis without DNA amplification	
Blood[†] (1 mL, 3.5–10 × 10[6] WBCs/mL)	
Buffy coat[†] (1 mL whole blood)	50–200 µg
Bone marrow[†] (1 mL)	100–500 µg
Cultured cells (10[7] cells)	30–70 µg
Solid tissue[‡] (1 mg)	1–10 µg
Lavage fluids (10 mL)	2–250 µg
Mitochondria (10-mg tissue, 10[7] cells)	1–10 µg
Plasmid DNA, bacterial culture, (100-mL overnight culture)	350 µg–1 mg
Bacterial culture (0.5 mL, 0.7 absorbance units)	10–35 µg
Feces[§] (1 mg; bacteria, fungi)	2–228 µg
Specimens adequate for analysis with DNA amplification	
Serum, plasma, cerebrospinal fluid[‖] (0.5 mL)	0.3–3 µg
Dried blood (0.5–1-cm diameter spot)	0.04–0.7 µg
Saliva (1 mL)	5–15 µg
Buccal cells (1 mg)	1–10 µg
Bone, teeth (500 mg)	30–50 µg
Hair follicles[#]	0.1–0.2 µg
Fixed tissue[**] (5–10 × 10-micron sections; 10 mm[2])	6–50 µg
Feces[††] (animal cells, 1 mg)	2–100 pg

*Yields are based on optimal conditions. Assays will vary in yield and purity of sample DNA.

[†]DNA yield will vary with WBC count.

[‡]DNA yield will depend on type and condition of tissue.

[§]Different bacterial types and fungi will yield more or less DNA.

[‖]DNA yield will depend on degree of cellularity.

[¶]Dried blood yield from paper is less than from textiles.

[#]Mitochondrial DNA is attainable from hair shafts.

[**]Isolation of DNA from fixed tissue is affected by the type of fixative used and the age and the preliminary handling of the original specimen.

[††]Cells in fecal specimens are subjected to digestion and degradation.

white blood cells (WBCs) in blood or bone marrow specimens are removed from red blood cells (RBCs) and other blood components by either differential density gradient centrifugation or differential lysis. For differential density gradient centrifugation, whole blood or bone marrow mixed with isotonic saline is overlaid with Ficoll.

Ficoll is a highly branched sucrose polymer that does not penetrate biological membranes. Upon centrifugation, the mononuclear WBCs (the desired cells for isolation of nucleic acid) settle into a layer in the Ficoll gradient that is below the less dense plasma components and above the polymorphonuclear cells and RBCs. The layer containing the mononuclear cells is removed from the tube and washed by rounds of resuspension and centrifugation in saline before proceeding with the nucleic acid isolation procedure.

Another method used to isolate nucleated cells takes advantage of the differential osmotic fragility of RBCs and WBCs. Incubation of whole blood or bone marrow in hypotonic buffer or water will result in the lysis of the RBCs before the WBCs. The WBCs are then pelleted by centrifugation, leaving the empty RBC membranes (ghosts) and hemoglobin, respectively, in suspension and solution.

Tissue Samples

Fresh or frozen tissue samples must be dissociated before DNA isolation procedures can be started. Grinding the frozen tissue in liquid nitrogen, homogenizing the tissue, or simply mincing the tissue using a scalpel can disrupt whole tissue samples. Fixed, embedded tissue may be deparaffinized by soaking in xylene (a mixture of three isomers of dimethylbenzene). Less toxic xylene substitutes, such as Histosolve, Anatech Pro-Par, or ParaClear, are also often used for this purpose. After xylene treatment, the tissue is usually rehydrated by soaking it in decreasing concentrations of ethanol. Alternatively, fixed tissue may be used directly without dewaxing.

Depending on the fixative, DNA in fixed tissue may be broken and/or cross-linked to varying extents. Comparative studies have shown that buffered formalin is the least damaging among tested fixatives, with mercury-based fixatives, such as Bouin's and B-5, being the worst for DNA recovery (Table 4.2).[3,4] DNA quality will also depend on how the tissue was handled prior to fixation and the length of time tissue was in fixation. In general,

Table 4.2 **Tissue Fixatives Influencing Nucleic Acid Quality[4]**

Fixative	Relative Quality of Nucleic Acid	Average Fragment Size Range (kb)
10% buffered neutral formalin	Good	2.0–5.0
Acetone	Good	2.0–5.0
Zamboni's	Not as good	0.2–2.0
Clarke's	Not as good	0.8–1.0
Paraformaldehyde	Not as good	0.2–5.0
Metharcan	Not as good	0.7–1.5
Formalin-alcohol-acetic acid	Not as good	1.0–4.0
B-5	less desirable	<0.1
Carnoy's	less desirable	0.7–1.5
Zenker's	less desirable	0.7–1.5
Bouin's	less desirable	<0.1

DNA target products of 100 bp or less can consistently be obtained from fixed tissue. Extended digestion in proteinase K may yield longer fragments.

Microorganisms

Some bacteria and fungi have tough cell walls that must be broken to allow the release of nucleic acid. Several enzyme products (e.g., lyzozyme or zymolyase) that digest cell wall polymers are commercially available. Alternatively, cell walls can be broken mechanically by grinding or by vigorously mixing with glass beads. Gentler enzymatic methods are less likely to damage chromosomal DNA and thus are preferred for methods involving larger chromosomal targets as opposed to plasmid DNA. Treatment with detergent (1% sodium dodecyl sulfate) and strong base (0.2 M NaOH) in the presence of Tris base, ethylenediaminetetraacetic acid (EDTA), and glucose can also break bacterial cell walls.

Boiling in dilute sucrose, Triton X-100 detergent, Tris buffer, and EDTA after lysozyme treatment releases DNA that can be immediately precipitated with alcohol (see below). DNA extracted by boiling or alkaline (NaOH) procedures is denatured (single-stranded) and may not be suitable for methods such as restriction enzyme analysis that require double-stranded DNA.

Reagents such as PrepMan Ultra Sample Preparation Reagent (Applied Biosystems) can be used for isolation of DNA to be used in amplification procedures, such as polymerase **chain** reaction, from yeast, filamentous fungi, and gram positive bacteria. The advantage of these types of extraction is their speed and simplicity.

Organic Isolation Methods

After release of DNA from the cell, further purification requires removal of contaminating proteins, lipids, carbohydrates, and cell debris. This is accomplished using a combination of high salt, low pH, and an organic mixture of phenol and chloroform. The combination readily dissolves hydrophobic contaminants, such as lipids and **lipoproteins**, collects cell debris, and strips away most DNA-associated proteins (Fig. 4-1). Isolation of small amounts of DNA from challenging samples such as fungi can be facilitated by pretreatment with cetyltrimethylammonium bromide, a cationic detergent that efficiently separates DNA from polysaccharide contamination. To avoid RNA contamination, RNAse, an enzyme that degrades RNA, can be added at this point. Alternatively, RNAse may also be added to the resuspended DNA at the end of the procedure.

A biphasic emulsion forms when phenol and chloroform are added to the hydrophilic suspension of lysed cells (lysate). At the proper pH, centrifugation will settle the hydrophobic phase on the bottom, with the hydrophilic phase on top. Lipids and other hydrophobic components will dissolve in the lower hydrophobic phase. DNA will dissolve in the upper aqueous phase. Amphiphilic components, which have both hydrophobic and hydrophilic properties and cell debris, will collect as a white precipitate at the interface between the two layers.

The DNA in the upper phase is then precipitated by mixing with ethanol or isopropanol and salt (ammonium, potassium or sodium acetate, or lithium or sodium chloride). The ethyl or isopropyl alcohol is added to the upper phase solution at 2:1 or 1:1 ratios, respectively, and the DNA forms a solid precipitate.

Advanced Concepts

Both ethanol and isopropanol are used for molecular applications. The ethanol is one of the general-use formulas, reagent grade. Reagent-grade alcohol (90.25% ethanol, 4.75% methanol, 5% isopropanol) is denatured; that is, the ethanol is mixed with other components because pure 100% ethanol cannot be distilled. The isopropanol used is undenatured, or pure, as it is composed of 99% isopropanol and 1% water with no other components.

The choice of which alcohol to use depends on the starting material, the size and amount of DNA to be isolated, and the design of the method. Isopropanol is less volatile than ethanol and precipitates DNA at room temperature. Precipitation at room temperature reduces coprecipitation of salt. Also, compared with ethanol, less isopropanol is added for precipitation; therefore, isopropanol can be more practical for large-volume samples. For low concentrations of DNA, longer precipitation times at freezer temperatures may be required to maximize the amount of DNA that is recovered. An important consideration to precipitating the DNA at freezer temperatures is that the increased viscosity of the alcohol at low temperatures will require longer centrifugation times to pellet the DNA.

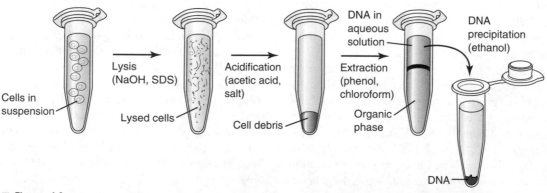

■ Figure 4-1 General scheme of organic DNA isolation.

Recovery of minimal amounts of DNA can be optimized using carrier molecules. In early studies, yeast RNA or glycogen was used to coprecipitate low concentrations of DNA.[5] More recently, glycogen or linear polyacrylamide have been used for this purpose. Glycogen is a biological material derived from mussels (e.g., *Mytilus edulis*). As a result, some preparations of glycogen may contain DNA.[6] Commercial preparations may be treated with DNase to avoid nucleic acid contamination. Commercial glycogen may also include a color indicator to aid in detecting small pellets. Generally, 10 to 20 micrograms of carrier is added per mL of isopropanol mixture before incubation and centrifugation.

The DNA precipitate is collected by centrifugation. Excess salt is removed by rinsing the pelleted nucleic acid in 70% ethanol, centrifuging and discarding the supernatant, and then dissolving the DNA pellet in rehydration buffer, usually 10 mM Tris, 1 mM EDTA (TE), or water.

Inorganic Isolation Methods

Safety concerns in the clinical laboratory make the use of caustic reagents such as phenol undesirable. Methods of DNA isolation that do not require phenol extraction have, therefore, been developed and are used in many laboratories. Initially, these methods did not provide the efficient recovery of clean DNA achieved with phenol extraction; however, newer methods have proven to produce high-quality DNA preparations in good yields.

Inorganic DNA extraction is sometimes called "**salting out**" (Fig. 4-2). It makes use of low pH and high salt conditions to selectively precipitate proteins, leaving the DNA in solution. The DNA can then be precipitated as described above using isopropanol, pelleted and resuspended in TE buffer or water.

Advanced Concepts

The presence of the chelating agent, EDTA, protects the DNA from damage by DNAses present in the environment of DNA preparations intended for long-term storage. EDTA is a component of TE buffer (10 mM Tris, 1 mM EDTA) and other resuspension buffers. The EDTA will also inhibit enzyme activity when the DNA is used in various procedures such as restriction enzyme digestion or polymerase chain reaction (PCR). One must be careful not to dilute the DNA too far so that large volumes (e.g., more than 10% of a reaction volume) of the DNA-EDTA solution are required for subsequent analysis methods. When DNA yield is low, as is the case with some clinical samples, it is better to dissolve it in water. More of this can be used in analysis procedures without adding excess amounts of EDTA. Because most of or the entire sample will be used for analysis, protection on storage is not a concern.

Advanced Concepts

Precipitation of the DNA excludes hydrophilic proteins, carbohydrates, and other residual contaminants still present after protein extraction. In addition, the concentration of the DNA can be controlled by adjusting the buffer or water volume used for resuspension of the pellet.

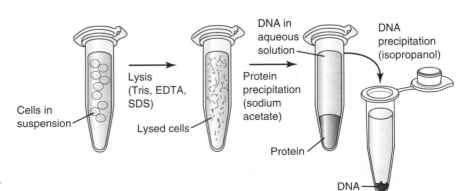

■ **Figure 4-2** Inorganic DNA isolation.

Solid-Phase Isolation

More rapid and comparably effective DNA extraction can be performed using solid matrices to bind and wash the DNA. Silica-based products were shown to effectively bind DNA in high salt conditions.[7] Many variations on this procedure were developed, including use of diatomaceous earth as a source of silica particles.[8] Modern systems can be purchased with solid matrices in the form of columns or beads. Columns come in various sizes, depending on the amount of DNA to be isolated. Columns used in the clinical laboratory are most often small "spin columns" that fit inside microcentrifuge tubes. These columns are commonly used to isolate viral and bacterial DNA from serum, plasma, or cerebrospinal fluid. They are also used routinely for isolation of cellular DNA in genetics and oncology. Preparation of samples for isolation of DNA on solid-phase media starts with cell lysis and release of nucleic acids, similar to organic and inorganic procedures (Fig. 4-3). Specific buffers are used to lyse bacterial, fungal, or animal cells. Buffer systems designed for specific applications (e.g., bacterial cell lysis or human cell lysis) are commercially available.

Advanced Concepts

Alkaline lysis can be used to specifically select for plasmid DNA because chromosomal DNA will not renature properly upon neutralization and form a precipitate. The denatured chromosomal DNA and protein can be removed by centrifugation before the supernatant containing plasmid DNA is applied to the column.

Advanced Concepts

Solid matrices conjugated to specific sequences of nucleic acid can also be used to select for DNA containing complementary sequences by hybridization. After removal of noncomplementary DNA, the bound complementary DNA can be eluted by heating the matrix or by breaking the hydrogen bonds chemically.

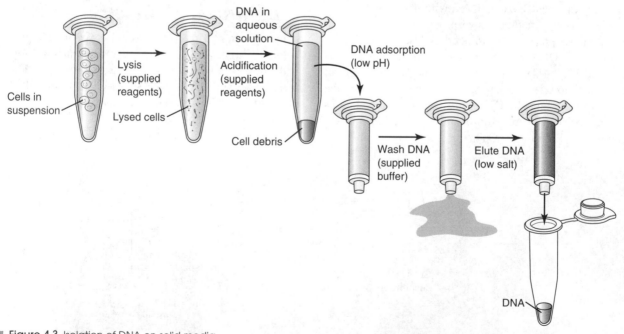

■ **Figure 4-3** Isolation of DNA on solid media.

For solid-phase separation, the cell lysate is applied to a column in high salt buffer, and the DNA in solution adsorbs to the solid matrix. Carrier RNA or DNA is applied with the DNA to enhance recovery, preventing irreversible binding of the small amount of target DNA. The carrier must be nucleic acid of more than 200 nucleotides in length in order to bind to the silica membrane. Other carriers used to enhance precipitation, such as glycogen and linear polyarcylamide, cannot be used in this application. After the immobilized DNA is washed with buffer, the DNA is eluted in a specific volume of water, TE, or other low salt buffer. The washing solutions and the eluant can be drawn through the column by gravity, vacuum, or centrifugal force. DNA absorbed to magnetic beads is washed by suspension of the beads in buffer and collection of the beads using a magnet applied to the outside of the tube while the buffer is aspirated or poured off. The DNA IQ system (Promega) uses a magnetic resin that holds a specific amount of DNA (100 ng). When the DNA is eluted in 100 μL, the DNA concentration is known (1 ng/μL) and ready for analysis.

Solid-phase isolation is the methodology employed for several robotic DNA isolation systems, such as Roche MagnaPure, Promega Maxwell, Qiagen BioRobot, and QIAcube, which use magnetized glass beads or membranes to bind DNA (Fig. 4-4). These systems are finding increased use in clinical laboratories for automated isolation of DNA from blood, tissue, bone marrow, plasma, and other body fluids. DNA isolated from specimens,

such as urine and amniotic fluid, has been reported to work better in polymerase chain reaction (PCR) applications, possibly due to removal of inhibitory substances found in these types of specimens by the prefiltering step. In most systems, a measured amount of sample—for example, 200–1000 μL of whole blood, 100 μL cell suspensions (10^6 to 10^7 cells), or 10–50 mg of tissue, in sample tubes—is placed into the instrument along with cartridges or racks of tubes containing the reagents used for isolation. Reagents are formulated in sets depending on the type and amount of starting material. The instrument is then programmed to lyse the cells and isolate and elute the DNA automatically.

Crude Lysis

Although high-quality DNA preparations are tantamount to successful procedures, there are circumstances that either preclude or prohibit extensive DNA purification. These include screening large numbers of samples by simple methods (e.g., electrophoresis with or without restriction enzyme digestion and some amplification procedures), isolation of DNA from limited amounts of starting material, and isolation of DNA from challenging samples such as fixed, paraffin-embedded tissues. In these cases, simple lysis of cellular material in the sample will yield sufficiently useful DNA for amplification procedures.

Proteolytic Lysis of Fixed Material

Simple screening methods are mostly used for research purposes in which large numbers of samples must be processed. In contrast, analysis of paraffin samples is frequently performed in the clinical laboratory. Fixed tissue is more conveniently accessed in the laboratory and may sometimes be the only source of patient material. Thin sections are usually used for analysis, although sectioning is not necessary with very small samples such as needle biopsies. Although paraffin-embedded specimens can be dewaxed with xylene or other agents and then rehydrated before nucleic acid isolation, the fixed tissue can be used without dewaxing. For some tests, such as somatic mutation analyses, a separate stained serial section can be examined microscopically to identify areas of the tissue comprising at least 40% tumor cells. The identifiable areas of tumor can then be isolated directly from the slide by simple scraping in buffer (microdissection)

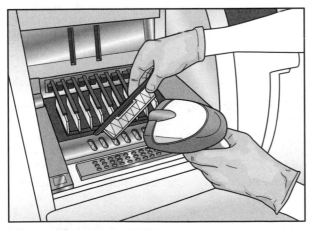

■ **Figure 4-4** Automated DNA isolation systems use cartridges containing lysis, adsorption, and elution agents and magnetic beads.

or laser capture (Fig. 4-5) and deposited into microcentrifuge tubes.

Before lysis, cells may be washed by suspension and centrifugation in saline or other isotonic buffer. Reagents used for cell lysis depend on the subsequent use of the DNA. For simple screens, cells can be lysed in detergents, such as SDS or Triton. For use in PCR amplification (see Chapter 7, "Nucleic Acid Amplification"), cells may be lysed in a mixture of Tris buffer and proteinase K. The proteinase K will digest proteins in the sample, lysing the cells and inactivating other enzymes. The released DNA can be used directly in the amplification reaction.

Extraction with Chelating Resin

Chelex is a cation-chelating resin that can be used for simple extraction of DNA.[9,10] A suspension of 10%

chelex resin beads is mixed with specimen, and the cells are lysed by boiling. After centrifugation of the suspension, DNA in the supernatant is cooled and may be further extracted with chloroform before use in amplification procedures. This method is most commonly used in forensic applications but may also be useful for purification of DNA from clinical samples and fixed, paraffin-embedded specimens.[11,12]

Other Rapid Extraction Methods

With the advent of PCR, new and faster methods for DNA isolation have been developed. The minimal sample requirements of amplification procedures allow for the use of material previously not utilizable for analysis. Rapid lysis methods (produced by Sigma, New England BioLabsor Epicentre Technologies) and DNA extraction/storage cards (produced by Whatman) provide sufficiently clean DNA that can be used for amplification.

Isolation of Mitochondrial DNA

There are two approaches to the isolation of mitochondrial DNA from eukaryotic cells. One method is to first isolate the mitochondria by centrifugation. After cell preparations are homogenized by grinding on ice, the homogenate is centrifuged at low speed (700–2600 × g) to pellet intact cells, nuclei, and cell debris. The mitochondria are pelleted from the supernatant in a second high-speed centrifugation (10,000–16,000 × g) and lysed with detergent. The lysate is treated with proteinase to remove protein contaminants. Mitochondrial DNA can then be precipitated with cold ethanol and resuspended in water or appropriate buffers for analysis. The second approach to mitochondrial DNA preparation is to isolate

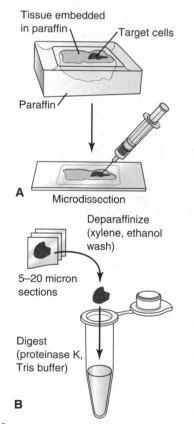

Figure 4-5 Crude extraction of DNA from fixed, paraffin-embedded tissue. Selected regions of tissue are scraped from slides (A) and extracted (B).

Advanced Concepts

When homogenizing cells for isolation of mitochondria, care must be taken not to over-grind the tissue and dissociate the mitochondrial membranes. Grinding in alkaline buffers with reducing agents such as β-mercaptoethanol will protect the mitochondria during the isolation process. A high-ionic-strength buffer can also be used to selectively lyse the nuclear membranes.

total DNA as described above. The preparation will contain mitochondrial DNA that can be analyzed within the total DNA background by hybridization or PCR.

Isolation of RNA

Working with RNA in the laboratory requires strict precautions to avoid sample RNA degradation. RNA is especially labile due to the ubiquitous presence of RNAses. These enzymes are small proteins that can renature, even after autoclaving, and regain activity. They remain active at a wide range of temperatures (down to −20°C and below). Unlike DNAses, RNAses must be eliminated or inactivated before isolation of RNA.

It is necessary to allocate a separate **RNAse-free (RNF)** area of the laboratory for storage of materials and specimen handling intended for RNA analysis. Gloves must always be worn in the RNF area. Disposables (tubes, tips, etc.) that come in contact with the RNA should be kept at this location and never be touched by ungloved hands. Articles designated DNAse-free/RNF by suppliers may be used directly from the package. Although reusable glassware is seldom used for RNA work, it can be rendered RNF. After cleaning, glassware must be baked for 4 to 6 hours at 400°C to inactivate the RNAses.

Total RNA

There are several types of RNA in prokaryotes and eukaryotes. (Refer to Chapter 2, "RNA," for a more detailed discussion of RNA type and structure.) The most abundant (80% to 90%) RNA in all cells is ribosomal RNA (rRNA). This RNA consists of two components, large and small, which are visualized by agarose gel electrophoresis (see Fig. 4-9). Depending on the cell type and conditions, the next most abundant RNA fraction (2.5% to 5%) is messenger RNA (mRNA). This mRNA may be detected as a faint background underlying the rRNA detected by agarose gel electrophoresis. Transfer RNA and small nuclear RNAs are also present in the total RNA sample.

Specimen Collection

RNA tests, especially those that involve gene expression, such as array analysis or quantitative reverse transcriptase PCR, are most accurate when the RNA is stabilized from further metabolism or degradation after collection.

Advanced Concepts

Several chemical methods have been developed to inactivate or eliminate RNAses. **Diethyl pyrocarbonate (DEPC)** can be added to water and buffers (except for Tris buffer) to inactivate RNAses permanently. DEPC converts primary and secondary amines to carbamic acid esters. It cross-links RNAse proteins through intermolecular covalent bonds, rendering them insoluble. Because of its effect on amine groups, DEPC will adversely affect Tris buffers. DEPC will also interact with polystyrene and polycarbonate and is not recommended for use on these types of materials.

Other RNAse inhibitors include vanandyl-ribonucleoside complexes, which bind the active sites of the RNAse enzymes, and macaloid clays, which absorb the RNAse proteins. Ribonuclease inhibitor proteins can be added directly to RNA preparations. These proteins form a stable noncovalent complex with the RNAses in solution. Some of these interactions require reducing conditions; therefore, dithiothreitol might be added in addition to the inhibitor.

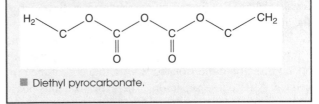

■ Diethyl pyrocarbonate.

Specialized collection tubes have been devised to stabilize RNA immediately upon blood draw (see Chapter 16, "Quality Assurance and Quality Control in the Molecular Laboratory"). In the laboratory, tissue or cell pellets can be stored and/or transported in preservative reagents such as RNAlater, (Qiagen).[13]

Extraction of Total RNA

Preparation of specimen material for RNA extraction differs in some respects from DNA extraction. Reticulocytes in blood and bone marrow samples are lysed by osmosis or separated from WBCs by centrifugation. When dissociating tissue, the sample should be kept frozen in liquid nitrogen or immersed in buffer that will inactivate **intracellular** RNAses. This is especially true for tissues such as pancreas that contain large amounts of innate RNAses. Bacterial and fungal RNA are also isolated by chemical lysis or by grinding in liquid nitrogen. Viral RNA can be isolated directly from serum, plasma, culture medium, or other cell-free fluids by means of specially formulated spin columns or beads. Cell-free material is used for these isolations, as most total RNA isolation methods cannot distinguish between RNA from microorganisms and those from host cells.

The cell lysis step for RNA isolation is performed in detergent or phenol in the presence of high salt (0.2 to 0.5 M NaCl) or RNAse inhibitors. Guanidine isothiocyanate (GITC) is a strong denaturant of RNAses and can be used instead of high salt buffers. Strong reducing agents such as 2-mercaptoethanol may also be added during this step.

Once the cells are lysed, proteins can be extracted by organic means (Fig. 4-6). Acid phenol:chloroform:isoamyl alcohol (25:24:1) solution efficiently extracts RNA. Chloroform enhances the extraction of the nucleic acid by denaturing proteins and promoting phase separation. Isoamyl alcohol prevents foaming. For RNA, the organic phase must be acidic (pH 4–5). The acidity of the organic phase is adjusted by overlaying it with buffer of the appropriate pH. In some isolation procedures, DNAse is added at the lysis step to eliminate contaminating DNA. Alternatively, RNAse-free DNAse also may be added directly to the isolated RNA at the end of the procedure. After phase separation, the upper aqueous phase containing the RNA is removed to a clean tube, and the RNA is precipitated by addition of two volumes of ethanol or one volume of isopropanol. Glycogen or

yeast-transfer RNA may be added at this step as a carrier to aid RNA pellet formation. The RNA precipitate is then washed in 70% ethanol and resuspended in RNF buffer or water.

Solid-phase separation of RNA begins with similar steps as described above for organic extraction. The strong denaturing buffer conditions must be adjusted before application of the lysate to the column (Fig. 4-7). In some procedures, ethanol is added at this point. Some systems provide a filter column to remove particulate material before application to the adsorption column. As with DNA columns, commercial reagents are supplied with the columns to optimize RNA adsorption and washing on the silica-based matrix.

After lysate is applied to the column in high salt chaotropic buffer, the adsorbed RNA is washed with the supplied buffers. DNAse may be added directly to the adsorbed RNA on the column to remove contaminating DNA. Washing solutions and the eluant are drawn through the column by gravity, vacuum, or centrifugal force. Small columns of silica-based material that fit inside **microfuge** tubes (spin columns) are widely used for routine nucleic acid isolation from all types of specimens. The eluted RNA is usually of sufficient concentration and purity for direct use in most applications. Automated systems like those shown in Figure 4-4 use magnetic beads or particles for RNA isolation as well. Special reagent sets are available for RNA or total nucleic acid (RNA and DNA) on these instruments.

Generally, 1 million eukaryotic cells or 10 to 50 mg of tissue will yield about 10 µg of RNA. The yield of RNA from biological fluids will depend on the concentration of microorganisms or other target molecules present in the specimen (Table 4.3).

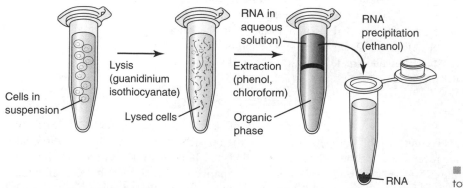

■ **Figure 4-6** Organic extraction of total RNA.

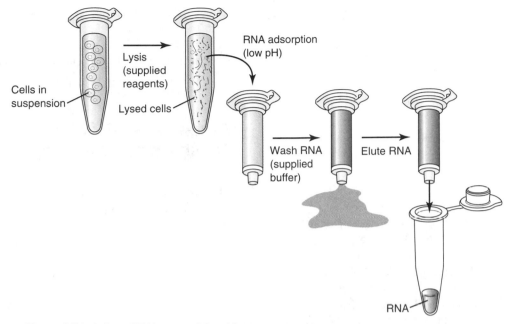

RNA adsorption
(low pH)

Cells in
suspension

Lysis
(supplied
reagents)

Lysed cells

Wash RNA
(supplied
buffer)

Elute RNA

RNA

■ **Figure 4-7** Isolation of RNA on a solid matrix

Table 4.3 **Yield of RNA From Various Specimen Sources[31-33]**

Specimen	Expected Yield*
Blood[†] (1 mL, 3.5–10 × 10^6 WBCs/mL)	1–10 µg
Buffy coat[†] (1 mL whole blood)	5–10 µg
Bone marrow[†] (1 mL)	50–200 µg
Cultured cells[‡] (10^7 cells)	50–150 µg
Buccal cells (1 mg)	1–10 µg
Solid tissue[§] (1 mg)	0.5–4 µg
Fixed tissue[||] (1 mm^3)	0.2–3 µg
Bacterial culture[¶] (0.5 mL, 0.7 absorbance units)	10–100 µg

*Specimen handling especially affects RNA yield. Isolation of polyA RNA will result in much lower yields. See text.

[†]RNA yield will depend on WBC count.

[‡]RNA yield will depend on type of cells and the conditions of cell culture.

[§]Liver, spleen, and heart tissues yield more RNA than brain, lung, ovary, kidney, or thymus tissues.

[||]Isolation of RNA from fixed tissue is especially affected by the type of fixative used and the age and the preliminary handling of the original specimen.

[¶]Different bacterial types and fungi will yield more or less RNA.

Proteolytic Lysis of Fixed Material

The quality of RNA from fixed, paraffin-embedded tissue will depend on the fixation process and handling of the specimen before fixation (Table 4.2).[14] Commercial reagent sets are available for extraction of RNA from fixed tissue specimens. These reagents are designed to provide lysis and incubation conditions that reverse formaldehye modification of RNA and efficiently release RNA from tissue sections while avoiding further RNA degradation. Specialized reagents or spin columns for removal of genomic DNA contamination are included in some systems. Automated isolation systems also have reagent kits and cartridges designed to isolate RNA from fixed tissue.

Isolation of polyA (messenger) RNA

As previously stated, approximately 80% to 90% of total RNA is rRNA. Often the RNA required for analysis is mRNA, accounting for only about 2.5% to 5% of the total RNA yield. The majority of mRNA consists of mRNA from highly expressed genes. Rare or single-copy mRNA is, therefore, a very minor part of the total RNA isolation. To enrich the yield of mRNA, especially rare

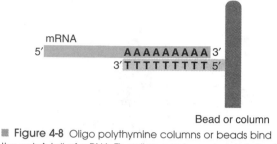

Figure 4-8 Oligo polythymine columns or beads bind the polyA tail of mRNA. The oligo can be poly uracil. Peptide nucleic acid dU or dT can also be used.

transcripts, protocols employing single-stranded oligomers of thymine or uracil immobilized on a matrix resin column or beads are used (Fig. 4-8). The polyT or polyU oligomers will bind the polyA tail found exclusively on mRNA. After washing away residual RNA, polyA RNA is eluted by washing the column with warmed, low salt buffer containing detergent to break the hydrogen bonds between the mRNA and the column. With this approach, approximately 30–40 ng of mRNA can be obtained from 1 μg of total RNA.

There are limitations to the isolation of polyA RNA using oligo dT or dU. The efficiency of polyA and polyU binding is variable. Secondary structure (intrastrand or interstrand hydrogen bonds) in the target sample may compete with binding to the capture oligomer. Also, mRNAs with short polyA tails may not bind efficiently or at all. AT-rich DNA fragments might bind to the column and not only compete with the desired mRNA target but also contaminate the final eluant. Potential digestion of the oligo-conjugated matrices precludes the use of DNase on the RNA before it is bound to the column.

Treatment of the eluant with RNase-free DNase is possible, but the DNase should be inactivated if the mRNA is to be used in procedures involving DNA components. Furthermore, rRNA may copurify with the polyA RNA. The final product, then, is enriched in polyA RNA but is not a pure polyA preparation.

Measurement of Nucleic Acid Quality and Quantity

Laboratory analysis of nucleic acids produces variable results, depending on the quality and quantity of input material. This is an important consideration in the medical laboratory, as test results must be accurately interpreted with respect to disease pathology. Consistent results require that run-to-run variation be minimized. Fortunately, measurement of the quality and quantity of DNA and RNA is straightforward.

Electrophoresis

DNA and RNA can be analyzed for quality by resolving an aliquot of the isolated sample on an agarose gel (Fig. 4-9; see Chapter 5, "Resolution and Detection of Nucleic Acids," for a more detailed discussion of electrophoresis). Fluorescent dyes such as **ethidium bromide** or SybrGreen I bind specifically to DNA and are used to visualize the sample preparation. Ethidium bromide or SybrGreen II are used to detect RNA. Less frequently, **silver stain** has been used to detect small amounts of DNA by visual inspection.

The appearance of DNA on agarose gels depends on the type of DNA isolated. A good preparation of plasmid

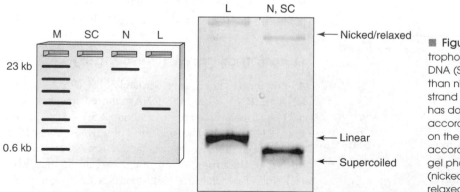

Figure 4-9 After agarose gel electrophoresis, compact supercoiled plasmid DNA (SC) will travel farther through the gel than nicked plasmid (N), which has single-strand breaks. Relaxed plasmid DNA (R) has double-strand breaks and will migrate according to its size, 23 kb in the drawing on the left. Linear (L) plasmids migrate according to the size of the plasmid. A gel photo shows a plasmid preparation. (nicked, N; supercoiled, SC; linear, L; relaxed, R; molecular weight markers, M).

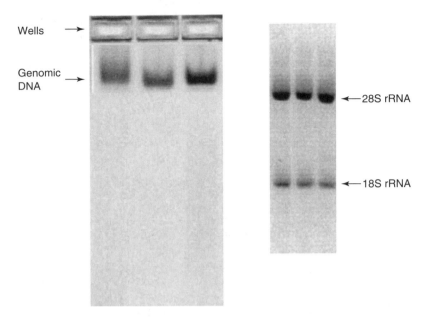

Wells

Genomic DNA

28S rRNA

18S rRNA

Figure 4-10 Intact ethidium bromide–stained human chromosomal DNA (left) and total RNA (right) after agarose gel electrophoresis. High-quality genomic DNA runs as a tight smear close to the loading wells. High-quality total RNA appears as two rRNA bands (shown with molecular weight markers, M).

DNA will yield a bright, moderate-**mobility** single **band** of supercoiled plasmid DNA with minor or no other bands that represent nicked or broken plasmid (see Fig. 4-9). High-molecular-weight chromosomal DNA should collect as a bright band with low mobility (near the top of the gel in Fig. 4-10). A high-quality preparation of RNA will yield two distinct bands of ribosomal RNA. The integrity of these bands is an indication of the integrity of the other RNA species present in the same sample. If these bands are degraded (smeared) or absent, the quality of the RNA in the sample is deemed unacceptable for use in molecular assays.

When fluorescent dyes are used, DNA and, less accurately, RNA can be quantified by comparison of the fluorescence intensity of the sample aliquot run on the gel with that of a known amount of control DNA or RNA loaded on the same gel. Densitometry of the band intensities gives the most accurate measurement of quantity. For some procedures, estimation of DNA or RNA quantity can be made by visual inspection.

Spectrophotometry

Nucleic acids absorb light at 260 nm through the adenine residues. Using the Beer-Lambert Law, concentration can be determined from the **absorptivity constants** (50 for double-stranded DNA, 40 for RNA). The relationship of concentration to absorbance is expressed as

$$A = \epsilon bc$$

where A = absorbance, ϵ = molar absorptivity (L/mol-cm), b = path length (cm), and c = concentration (mg/L). The absorbance at this wavelength is thus directly proportional to the concentration of the nucleic acid in the sample. Using the absorptivity as a conversion factor from optical density to concentration, one optical density unit (or absorbance unit) at 260 nm is equivalent to 50 mg/L (or 50 µg/mL) of double-stranded DNA and 40 µg/mL of RNA. To determine concentration, multiply the spectrophotometer reading in absorbance units by the appropriate conversion factor. Phenol absorbs ultraviolet light at 270 nm to 275 nm, close to the wavelength of maximum absorption by nucleic acids. This means that residual phenol from organic isolation procedures can increase 260 readings, so phenol contamination must be avoided when measuring concentration at 260 nm.

If the DNA or RNA preparation is of sufficient concentration to require dilution before spectrophotometry in order for the reading to fall within the linear reading range, the dilution factor must be included in the calculation of quantity. Multiply the absorbance reading by the conversion factor and the dilution factor to find the concentration of nucleic acid.

EXAMPLE 1. A DNA preparation diluted $1/100$ yields an absorbance reading of 0.200 at 260 nm. To obtain the concentration in µg/mL, multiply:

0.200 absorbance units $\times$ 50 µg/mL per absorbance unit $\times$ 100 = 1000 µg/mL

The yield of the sample is calculated using the volume of the preparation. If in the case illustrated above, the DNA was eluted or resuspended in a volume of 0.5 mL, the yield would be:

1000 µg/mL $\times$ 0.5 mL = 500 µg

EXAMPLE 2. An RNA preparation diluted $1/10$ yields an absorbance reading of 0.500 at 260 nm. The concentration is:

0.500 absorbance units $\times$ 40 µg/mL per absorbance unit $\times$ 10 = 200 µg/mL

The yield of the sample is calculated using the volume of the preparation. If in the case illustrated above, the DNA was eluted or resuspended in 0.2 mL, the yield would be:

200 µg/mL $\times$ 0.2 mL = 40 µg

Historical Highlights

The maximum absorption of light at 260 nm was one of the clues suggesting that DNA was the molecular matter of genetic material. In 1942, Lewis Stadler reported results on studies of the effect of wavelength of ultraviolet (uv) light on mutagenesis in corn plants.[15] He observed that the most mutagenic monochromatic light had a wavelength of 260 nm. Together with the data of Avery[16] and Hershey and Chase[17] (see Chapter 1, "DNA"), Stadler's observations further supported the notion that DNA is the carrier of genetic information.

Spectrophotometric measurements may also be used to estimate the purity of nucleic acid. Ideally, contamination can be detected by reading the concentration over a range of wavelengths. Graphing the absorbance reading as a function of wavelength produces a curve or spectrum that should peak at A_{260} nm for nucleic acid. Some spectrophotometers produce this graph automatically. Even with such automation, however, spectral analysis for each specimen sample is not practical for most routine medical laboratory work. In practice, nucleic acid solutions are read at 2 or 3 distinct wavelengths (Table 4.4). Absorbance over background at any wavelength other than the A_{260} maxima of the nucleic acid indicates contamination.

Routine nucleic acid isolation procedures produce reasonably pure DNA solutions free from particles, organic compounds, and phenol. Due to its abundance and close association with nucleic acid in the cell, the most likely contaminant in a nucleic acid preparation will be protein. Protein absorbs light at 280 nm through the aromatic tryptophan and tyrosine residues. Although this measurement is not highly accurate, general ranges indicate at least the presence of protein contaminants. The absorbance of the nucleic acid at 260 nm should be 1.6 to 2.00 times more than the absorbance at 280 nm. If the 260 nm/280 nm ratio is less than 1.6, the nucleic acid preparation may be contaminated with unacceptable amounts of protein and not of sufficient purity for use. Such a sample can be improved by column purification, reprecipitating the nucleic acid or repeating the protein removal step of the isolation procedure. It should be noted that low pH affects the 260 nm/280 nm ratio. Somewhat alkaline buffers (pH 7.5) are recommended for accurate determination of purity. RNA affords a somewhat higher 260 nm/280 nm ratio, 2.0 to 2.3. A DNA preparation with a ratio higher than 2.0 may be contaminated with RNA. Some procedures for DNA analysis are not affected by contaminating RNA, in

Wavelength (nm)	Contaminant
230	Organic compounds
270	Phenol
280	Protein
>330	Particulate matter

Table 4.4 **Common Contaminants and Their Wavelengths of Peak Absorbance**

which case the DNA is still suitable for use. If, however, RNA may interfere or react with DNA detection components, RNase should be used to remove the contaminating RNA. Because it is difficult to detect contaminating DNA in RNA preparations, RNA should be treated with RNase-free DNase where DNA contamination may interfere with subsequent applications.

Absorbance ratios do not necessarily predict successful amplification or hybridization reactions. Since the light is absorbed by single nitrogen base moieties, fragmented or degraded DNA will produce an A_{260} reading comparable to intact DNA. In this regard, fluorometry is considered by some to be a better method of quality assessment.

Historical Highlights

Estimation of protein contamination in nucleic acid is based on a method by Warburg and Christian designed to measure nucleic acid contamination in protein.[18] This method utilizes the natural light absorption at 280 nm of the aromatic amino acid side chains, tryptophan and tyrosine. Nucleic acids are common contaminants of protein preparations and naturally absorb light at 260 nm, where there is no interference by protein. In the Warburg-Christian method, the test material was read at 260 nm and 280 nm and then a nomograph was used to determine the relative amounts of protein and nucleic acid.

Advanced Concepts

Ultraviolet spectrophotometers dedicated to nucleic acid analysis can be programmed to calculate absorbance ratios and concentrations. The operator must enter the type of nucleic acid, the dilution factor, and the desired conversion factor. The instrument will automatically read the sample at the appropriate wavelengths and do the required calculations, giving a reading of concentration in μg/mL and a 260 nm/280 nm ratio.

Fluorometry

Fluorometry, or fluorescent spectroscopy, measures fluorescence related to DNA concentration in association with DNA-specific fluorescent dyes. Early methods used 3,5-diaminobenzoic acid 2HCl (DABA).[19] This dye combines with alpha methylene aldehydes (deoxyribose) to yield a fluorescent product. It is still used for the detection of nuclei and as a control for hybridization and spot integrity in microarray analyses.

More modern procedures use the DNA-specific dye **Hoechst 33258** {2-[2-(4-hydroxyphenyl)-(6-benzimidazol)]-6-(1-methyl-4-piperazyl)-benzimidazol/.3HCl}. This dye combines with adenine-thymine base pairs in the minor groove of the DNA double helix and is thus specific for intact double-stranded DNA. The binding specificity for A-T residues, however, complicates measurements of DNA that have unusually high or low GC content. A standard measurement is required to determine concentration by fluorometry, and this standard must have GC content similar to that of the samples being measured. Calf thymus DNA (GC content = 50%) is often used as a standard for specimens with unknown DNA GC content. Fluorometric determination of DNA concentration using Hoechst dye is very sensitive (down to 200 ng DNA/mL).

PicoGreen and OliGreen (Molecular Probes, Inc.) are other DNA-specific dyes that can be used for fluorometric quantification. Due to brighter fluorescence upon binding to double-stranded DNA, PicoGreen is more sensitive than Hoechst dye (detection down to 25 pg/mL concentrations). Like Hoechst dye, single-stranded DNA and RNA do not bind to PicoGreen. OliGreen is designed to bind to short pieces of single-stranded DNA (oligonucleotides). This dye will detect down to 100 pg/mL of single-stranded DNA. OliGreen will not fluoresce when bound to double-stranded DNA or RNA.

RNA may be measured in solution using SybrGreen II RNA gel stain.[20] Intensity of SyBrGreen II fluorescence is 20%–26% lower with polyadenylated RNA than with total RNA. The sensitivity of this dye is 2 ng/mL. SybrGreen II, however, is not specific to RNA and will bind and fluoresce with double-stranded DNA as well. Contaminating DNA must, therefore, be removed in order to get an accurate determination of RNA concentration.

Fluorometry measurements require **calibration** of the instrument with a known amount of standard before measurement of the sample. For methods using Hoechst dye, the dye, diluted to a working concentration of 1 µg/mL in water, is mixed with the sample (usually a dilution of the sample). Once the dye and sample solution are mixed, fluorescence must be read within 2 hours because the dye/sample complex is stable only for approximately this amount of time. The fluorescence is read in a quartz cuvette. A programmed fluorometer will read out a concentration based on the known standard calibration.

Absorption and fluorometry readings may not always agree. First, the two detection methods recognize different targets. Single nucleotides do not bind to fluorescent dyes, but they can absorb ultraviolet light and affect spectrometric readings. Furthermore, absorption measurements do not distinguish between DNA and RNA, so contaminating RNA may be factored into the DNA measurement. RNA does not enhance fluorescence of the fluorescent dyes and is thus invisible to fluorometric detection. In fact, specific detection of RNA in the presence of DNA in solution is not yet possible. Deciding which instrument to use is at the discretion of the laboratory. Most laboratories use spectrophotometry because the samples can be read directly without staining or mixing with dye. For methods that require accurate measurements of low amounts of DNA or RNA (in the range of 10–100 ng/mL), fluorometry may be preferred.

Microfluidics

Lab-on-a-chip technology has been applied to nucleic acid quantification and analysis. The Agilent 2100 Bioanalyzer is a microfluidics-based instrument used for this purpose. To make a measurement, the sample is applied to a multiwell chip that is placed into the Bioanalyzer. The sample then moves through microchannels across a detector. The instrument software generates images in electrophoerogram (peak) or gel (band) configurations. For RNA, a quantification estimate called the RNA Integrity Number is determined as a standard measure of RNA integrity. The presence of ribosomal impurities in mRNA preparations may also be calculated. This system is more automated than standard spectrophotometry or fluorometry, uses minimal volume of sample (as low as 1 µL), and can test multiple samples simultaneously. Microfluidics are useful for analysis of studies on small RNAs, such as microRNAs in eukaryotes[21] and gene expression in bacteria.[22]

• **STUDY QUESTIONS** •

DNA Quantity/Quality

1. Calculate the DNA concentration in µg/mL from the following information:
   a. Absorbance reading at 260 nm from a 1:100 dilution = 0.307
   b. Absorbance reading at 260 nm from a 1:50 dilution = 0.307
   c. Absorbance reading at 260 nm from a 1:100 dilution = 0.172
   d. Absorbance reading at 260 nm from a 1:100 dilution = 0.088

2. If the volume of the above DNA solutions was 0.5 mL, calculate the yield for (a)–(d).

3. Three DNA preparations have the following A_{260} and A_{280} readings:

Sample	OD_{260}	OD_{280}
(i) 1	0.419	0.230
(ii) 2	0.258	0.225
(iii) 3	0.398	0.174

For each sample, based on the A_{260}/A_{280} ratio, is each preparation suitable for further use? If not, what is contaminating the DNA?

4. After agarose gel electrophoresis, a 0.5 microgram aliquot of DNA isolated from a bacterial culture produced only a faint smear at the bottom of the gel lane. Is this an acceptable DNA sample?

5. Compare and contrast the measurement of DNA concentration by spectrophotometry with analysis by fluorometry with regard to staining requirements and accuracy.

RNA Quantity/Quality

1. Calculate the RNA concentration in µg/mL from the following information:
   a. Absorbance reading at 260 nm from a 1:100 dilution = 0.307

b. Absorbance reading at 260 nm from a 1:50 dilution = 0.307

c. Absorbance reading at 260 nm from a 1:100 dilution = 0.172

d. Absorbance reading at 260 nm from a 1:100 dilution = 0.088

2. If the volume of the above RNA solutions was 0.5 mL, calculate the yield for (a)–(d).

3. An RNA preparation has the following absorbance readings:

$A_{260} = 0.208$

$A_{280} = 0.096$

Is this RNA preparation satisfactory for use?

4. A blood sample was held at room temperature for 5 days before being processed for RNA isolation. Will this sample likely yield optimal RNA?

5. Name three factors that will affect yield of RNA from a paraffin-embedded tissue sample.

References

1. Mirsky AE. The discovery of DNA. *Scientific American* 1968;218(6):78–88.
2. Meselson M, Stahl FW. The replication of DNA in *Escherichia coli*. *Proceedings of the National Academy of Sciences* 1958;44:671–682.
3. Nagasaka T, Lai R, Chen Y-y, et al. The use of archival bone marrow specimens in detecting B-cell non-Hodgkin's lymphomas using polymerase chain reaction. *Leukemia and Lymphoma* 2000;36:347–352.
4. Greer C, Peterson SL, Kivat NB, Manos MM. PCR amplification from paraffin-embedded tissues. *American Journal of Clinical Pathology* 1991;95: 117–124.
5. Gallagher M, Burke WF Jr, Orzech K. Carrier RNA enhancement of recovery of DNA from dilute solutions. *Biochemical Biophysical Research Communications* 1987;144:271–276.
6. Bartram A, Poon C, Neufeld JD. Nucleic acid contamination of glycogen used in nucleic acid precipitation and assessment of linear polyacrylamide as an alternative co-precipitant. *BioTechniques* 2009;47:1019–1022.
7. Vogelstein GD. Preparative and analytical purification of DNA from agarose. *Proceedings of the National Academy of Sciences* 1979;76:615–619.
8. Carter MJ, Milton ID. An inexpensive and simple method for DNA purifications on silica particles. *Nucleic Acids Research* 1993;21(4):1044.
9. Walsh P, Metzger DA, Higuchi R. Chelex 100 as a medium for simple extraction of DNA for PCR-based typing from forensic material. *BioTechniques* 1991;10(4):506–513.
10. de Lamballerie X, Zandotti C, Vignoli C, et al. A one-step microbial DNA extraction method using "Chelex 100" suitable for gene amplification. *Research in Microbiology (Paris)* 1992;143(8):785–790.
11. de Lamballerie X, Chapel F, Vignoli C, et al. Improved current methods for amplification of DNA from routinely processed liver tissue by PCR. *Journal of Clinical Pathology* 1994;47:466–467.
12. Coombs N, Gough AC, Primrose JN. Optimisation of DNA and RNA extraction from archival formalin-fixed tissue. *Nucleic Acids Research* 1999;27(16):e12.
13. Yeh I, Martin MA, Robetorye RS, et al. Clinical validation of an array CGH test for HER2 status in breast cancer reveals that polysomy 17 is a rare event. *Modern Pathology* 2009;22:1169–1175.
14. Mizumo T, Nagamura H, Iwamoto KS, et al. RNA from decades-old archival tissue blocks for retrospective studies. *Diagnostic Molecular Pathology* 1998;7:202–208.
15. Stadler L, Uber FM. Genetic effects of ultraviolet radiation in maize. IV. Comparison of monochromatic radiations. *Genetics* 1942;27:84–118.
16. Avery O, MacLeod CM, McCarty M. Studies on the chemical nature of the substance inducing transformation of pneumococcal types. I. Induction of transformation by a DNA fraction isolated from pneumococcal type III. *Journal of Experimental Medicine* 1944;79:137–158.
17. Hershey AD, Chase M. Independent function of viral protein and nucleic acid in growth of bacteriophage. *Journal of General Physiology* 1952;26: 36–56.
18. Warburg O, Christian W. Isolierung und kristallisation des gärungsferments enolase. *Biochemische Zeitschrift* 1942;310:384–421.

19. Kissane J, Robins E. The fluorometric measurement of deoxyribonucleic acid in animal tissues with special reference to the central nervous system. *Journal of Biological Chemistry* 1958;233:184–188.

20. Schmidt D, Ernst JD. A fluorometric assay for the quantification of RNA in solution with nanogram sensitivity. *Analytical Biochemistry* 1995;232:144–146.

21. Becker C, Hammerle-Fickinger A, Riedmaier I, et al. mRNA and microRNA quality control for RT-qPCR analysis. *Methods.* 2010;50:237–243.

22. Jahn C, Charkowski AO, Willis DK. Evaluation of isolation methods and RNA integrity for bacterial RNA quantitation. *Journal of Microbiological Methods* 2008;75:318–324.

23. Aplenc R, Orudjev E, Swoyer J, et al. Differential bone marrow aspirate DNA yields from commercial extraction kits. *Leukemia* 2002;16(9):1865–1866.

24. Dani S, Gomes-Ruiz AC, Dani MAC. Evaluation of a method for high yield purification of largely intact mitochondrial DNA from human placentae. *Genetic and Molecular Research* 2003;2(2):178–184.

25. Leal-Klevezas D, Martínez-Vázquez IO, Cuevas-Hernández B, et al. Antifreeze solution improves DNA recovery by preserving the integrity of pathogen-infected blood and other tissues. *Clinical and Diagnostic Laboratory Immunology* 2000;7(6):945–946.

26. O'Rourke D, Hayes MG, Carlyle SW. Ancient DNA studies in physical anthropology. *Annual Review of Anthropology* 2000;29:217–242.

27. Shia S-R, Cotea RJ, Wub L, et al. DNA extraction from archival formalin-fixed, paraffin-embedded tissue sections based on the antigen retrieval principle: Heating under the influence of pH. *Journal of Histochemistry and Cytochemistry* 2002;50:1005–1011.

28. Cao W, Hashibe M, Rao J-Y, et al. Comparison of methods for DNA extraction from paraffin-embedded tissues and buccal cells. *Cancer Detection and Prevention* 2003;27:397–404.

29. Blomeke B, Bennett WP, Harris CC, et al. Serum, plasma and paraffin-embedded tissues as sources of DNA for studying cancer susceptibility genes. *Carcinogenesis* 1997;18:1271–1275.

30. McOrist A, Jackson M, Bird AR. A comparison of five methods of extraction of bacterial DNA from human faecal samples. *Journal of Microbiological Methods* 2002;50:131–139.

31. Barbaric D, Dalla-Pozza L, Byrne JA. A reliable method for total RNA extraction from frozen human bone marrow samples taken at diagnosis of acute leukaemia. *Journal of Clinical Pathology* 2002;55(11):865–867.

32. Byers R, Roebuck J, Sakhinia E, et al. PolyA PCR amplification of cDNA from RNA extracted from formalin-fixed paraffin-embedded tissue. *Diagnostic Molecular Pathology* 2004;13(3):144–150.

33. Medeiros M, Sharma VK, Ding R, et al. Optimization of RNA yield, purity, and mRNA copy number by treatment of urine cell pellets with RNA later. *Journal of Immunological Methods* 2003;279(1-2):135–142.

Chapter 5

Resolution and Detection of Nucleic Acids

OBJECTIVES

- Explain the principle and performance of electrophoresis as it applies to nucleic acids.

- Compare and contrast the agarose and polyacrylamide gel polymers commonly used to resolve nucleic acids, and state the utility of each polymer.

- Explain the principle and performance of capillary electrophoresis as it is applied to nucleic acid separation.

- Give an overview of buffers and buffer additives used in electrophoretic separation, including the constituents, purpose, and importance.

- Describe the general types of equipment used for electrophoresis and how samples are introduced for electrophoretic separation.

- Compare and contrast pulse field gel electrophoresis and regular electrophoresis techniques with regard to method and applications.

- Compare and contrast detection systems used in nucleic acid applications.

OBJECTIVES—cont'd

- Resolution and detection of nucleic acids are done in several ways. Gel and capillary electrophoresis are the most practical and frequently used methods. DNA can also be spotted and detected using specific hybridization probes, as will be described in Chapter 10, "DNA Sequencing."

Electrophoresis

Electrophoresis is the movement of molecules by an electric current. This can occur in solution, but it is practically done in a matrix to limit migration and contain the migrating material. Electrophoresis is routinely applied to the analysis of proteins and nucleic acids. Each phosphate group on a DNA polymer is ionized, making DNA a negatively charged molecule. Under an electric current, DNA will migrate toward the positive pole (**anode**). When DNA is applied to a macromolecular cage such as an **agarose** or **polyacrylamide gel**, its migration under the pull of the current is impeded, depending on the size of the DNA and the spaces in the gel. Because each nucleotide has one negative charge, the charge-to-mass ratio of molecules of different sizes will remain constant. DNA fragments will therefore migrate at speeds inversely related to their size. Electrophoresis is performed in tubes, slab gels, or capillaries. Slab gel electrophoresis has either a horizontal or vertical format (Fig. 5-1).

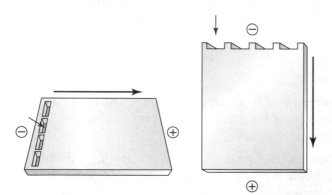

■ **Figure 5-1** Horizontal (left) and vertical (right) gel electrophoresis. In both formats, sample is introduced into the gel at the cathode end (small arrows) and migrates with the current toward the anode.

Advanced Concepts

Double-stranded DNA and RNA are analyzed by native gel electrophoresis. The relationship between size and speed of migration can be improved by separating single-stranded nucleic acids; however, both DNA and RNA favor the double-stranded state. Unpaired, or denatured, DNA and RNA must, therefore, be analyzed in conditions that prevent the hydrogen bonding between complementary sequences. These conditions are maintained through a combination of formamide mixed with the sample, urea mixed with the gel, and/or heat.

Historical Highlights

Arne Tiselius developed an electrophoresis apparatus while studying resolution of proteins and diffusion and adsorption in naturally occurring porous silicate particles. This "moving boundary" method required equipment over 5 meters long. By the early 1930s, his method was further refined.[1] In the early 1950s, granular starch was introduced as a matrix.[2] Oliver Smithies later found that if he heated about 15 grams of starch in 100 mL of his electrophoretic medium and allowed it to cool, he could make a gel matrix with resolving properties similar to a paper electrophoresis method he had previously devised. He used this gel to first separate serum proteins.[3] In 1956, Smithies and Poulik described resolution of 20 serum protein components using a two-dimensional electrophoresis system with paper in one dimension and starch in the other.[4]

Gel Systems

Gel matrices provide resistance to the movement of molecules under the force of the electric current. They prevent diffusion and reduce convection currents so that the separated molecules form a defined group, or "band." The gel can then serve as a support medium for analysis of the separated components. These matrices must be unaffected by electrophoresis, simple to prepare, and amenable to modification. Agarose and polyacrylamide are polymers that meet these criteria.

Agarose Gels

Agarose is a polysaccharide polymer extracted from seaweed. It is a component of agar used in bacterial culture dishes, which is comprised of agaropectin and agarose. Agarose is a linear polymer of agarobiose, which consists of 1,3-linked-β-D-galactopyranose and 1,4-linked 3, 6-anhydro-α-L-galactopyranose (Fig. 5-2).

Hydrated agarose gels in various concentrations, **buffers**, and sizes can be purchased ready for use. Alternatively, agarose is purchased and stored in the laboratory in powdered form. For use, powdered agarose is suspended in buffer, heated, and poured into a mold. The concentration of the agarose dictates the size of the spaces in the gel (100 to 300 nm). The size of DNA to be resolved is considered in determining the appropriate agarose concentration to use (Table 5.1). Small pieces of DNA (50–500 bp) are resolved on more concentrated agarose gels, for example, 2%–3% (Fig. 5-3). Larger fragments of DNA (2000–50,000) are best resolved in lower agarose concentrations, for example, 0.5%–1%. Agarose concentrations above 5% and below 0.5% are not practical. High-concentration agarose will impede migration, whereas very low concentrations produce a weak gel that is easily broken. Gel strength of any concentration of agarose will also decrease over time and with exposure to chaotropic agents such as urea.

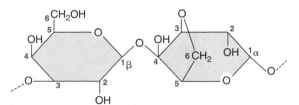

■ Figure 5-2 Agarobiose is the repeating unit of agarose.

Table 5.1 **Choice of Agarose Concentration for DNA Gels*[14]**

Agarose Concentration (%)	Separation Range (size in bp)
0.3	5000–60,000
0.6	1000–20,000
0.8	800–10,000
1.0	400–8000
1.2	300–7000
1.5	200–4000
2.0	100–3000

*The table shows the range of separation for linear double-stranded DNA molecules in TAE agarose gels with regular power sources. Note that these values may be affected if another running buffer is used and if voltage is over 5 V/cm.

Advanced Concepts

The physical characteristics of the agarose gel can be modified by altering its polymer length and helical parameters. Several types of agarose are thus available for specific applications. The resolving properties differ in these preparations as well as the gelling properties. Low-melting point agarose is often used for re-isolating resolved fragments from the gel. Other agarose types give better resolution of larger or smaller fragments. Modern agarose preparations are sufficiently pure to avoid problems such as **electroendosmosis**, a solvent flow toward one of the electrodes, usually the **cathode** (negative), in opposition to the DNA or RNA migration, which slows and distorts the migration of the samples, reducing resolution and smearing the bands.

Pulsed Field Gel Electrophoresis

Very large pieces (50,000–250,000+ bp) of DNA cannot be resolved efficiently by simple agarose electrophoresis. Even in the lowest concentrations of agarose, megabase fragments are too severely impeded for correct resolution (referred to as limiting mobility). Limiting mobility is reached when a DNA molecule is of such a size that it can move only lengthwise through successive pores of the gel.

For very large (megabasepair) DNA molecules, pulses of current applied to the gel in alternating dimensions

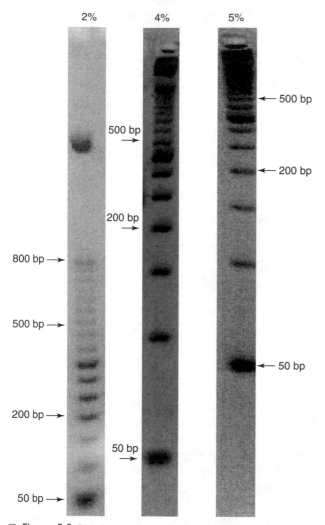

Figure 5-3 Resolution of double-stranded DNA fragments on 2%, 4%, and 5% agarose.

enhance migration. This process is called **pulsed field gel electrophoresis (PFGE)** (Fig. 5-4). The simplest approach to this method is **field inversion gel electrophoresis (FIGE)**.[5] FIGE works by alternating the positive and negative electrodes during electrophoresis. In this type of separation, the DNA goes periodically forward and backward. FIGE requires temperature control and a switching mechanism. Field inversion or reorientation to move very large molecules is performed in other configurations. Contour-clamped homogeneous electric field,[6] transverse alternating field electrophoresis,[7] and rotating gel electrophoresis[8,9] are examples of commonly used pulsed field or transverse angle reorientation electrophoresis methods.

Field inversion/reorientation systems require gel box, electrode, and gel configurations as well as appropriate electronic control to accommodate switching the electric fields during electrophoresis. Using various forms of PFGE, the large fragments are resolved, not only by sifting through the spaces in the polymer but also by their reorientation. PFGE methods require long separation times as the electrophoresis requires low voltage and the time necessary for the DNA molecules to realign themselves to move in a second dimension, usually an angle

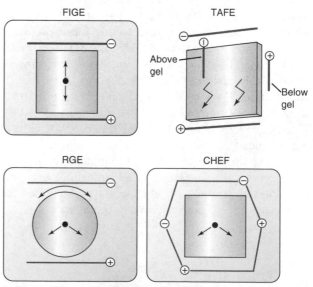

Figure 5-4 Field inversion gel electrophoresis (FIGE), contour-clamped homogeneous electric field (CHEF), transverse alternating field electrophoresis (TAFE), and rotating gel electrophoresis (RGE) are all examples of pulsed field gel configurations. Arrows indicate the migration path of the DNA.

Table 5.2 **Choice of Polyacrylamide Concentration for DNA Gels*[14]**

Acrylamide Concentration (%)	Separation Range (size in bp)
3.5	100–1000
5.0	80–500
8.0	60–400
12.0	40–200
20.0	10–100

*The indicated figures are referring to gels run in TBE buffer. Voltages over 8 V/cm may affect these values.

Advanced Concepts

FIGE is a special modification of PFGE in which the alternating currents are aligned 180° with respect to each other. The current pulses must be applied at different strengths and/or durations so that the DNA will make net progress in one dimension. The parameters for this type of separation must be matched to the DNA being separated so that both large and small fragments have time to reorient properly. For example, if timing is not sufficient for reorientation of the large fragments, small fragments will preferentially reorient and move backward and gradually lose distance with respect to the large molecules, which will continue forward progress on the next pulse cycle. Unlike PFGE that requires special equipment, FIGE can be performed in a regular gel apparatus; however, its upper resolution limit is 2 megabases compared with 5 megabases for PFGE.

apply current in alternating directions at specific times (called the switch interval) that are set by the operator. These parameters are based on the general size of the fragments to be analyzed; that is, a larger fragment will require a longer switch interval. PFGE is a slow migration method. Sample runs will take 24 hours or more.

Alternating field electrophoresis is used for applications that require the resolution of chromosome-sized fragments of DNA, such as in bacterial typing for epidemiological purposes. Enzymatic digestion of genomic DNA will yield a set of fragments that produce a band pattern specific to each type of organism. By comparing band patterns, the similarity of organisms isolated from various sources can be assessed. This information is especially useful in determining the epidemiology of infectious diseases, for example, identifying whether two biochemically identical isolates have a common source. This will be discussed in more detail in Chapter 12, "Detection and Identification of Microorganisms."

of 120° (180° for FIGE) from the original direction of migration.

The large molecules resolved by these methods must be protected from breakage and shearing. Therefore, specimens for PFGE analysis are immobilized in an agarose plug before cell lysis. Further purification and enzymatic digestion of the DNA are also performed while the DNA is immobilized in the agarose plug. After treatment, the plug is inserted directly into a space or well in the agarose gel for electrophoresis. PFGE instruments are designed to

Polyacrylamide Gels

Very small DNA fragments and single-stranded DNA are best resolved on **polyacrylamide** gels in **polyacrylamide gel electrophoresis** (**PAGE**). Acrylamide, in combination with the cross-linker methylene bisacrylamide (Fig. 5-5), polymerizes into a matrix that has consistent resolution characteristics (Fig. 5-6).

Polyacrylamide was originally applied mostly for protein separation, but it is now routinely applied to nucleic acid analysis. Polyacrylamide gels are used for sequencing nucleic acids, mutation analyses, nuclease protection assays, and other applications requiring high resolution of nucleic acids. Acrylamide is supplied to the laboratory

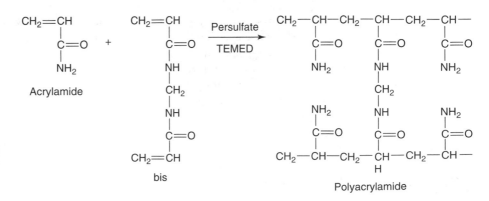

■ **Figure 5-5** The repeating unit of polyacrylamide is acrylamide; bis introduces branches into the polymer.

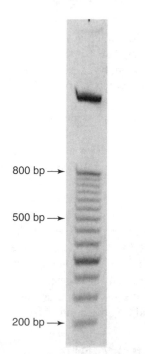

800 bp →

500 bp →

200 bp →

■ **Figure 5-6** Resolution of double-stranded DNA fragments on a 5%, 19:1 acrylamide:bis gel.

Advanced Concepts

Different cross-linkers affect the physical nature of the acrylamide mesh. Piperazine diacrylate can reduce the background staining that may occur when the gel is stained. *N,N*+-bisacrylylcystamine and *N,N*+-diallyltartardiamide enable gels to be solubilized to facilitate extraction of separated products.

---

in several forms. The powdered form is a dangerous neurotoxin and must be handled with care. Solutions of mixtures of acrylamide and bis-acrylamide are less hazardous and more convenient to use. Preformed gels are the most convenient, as the procedure for preparation of acrylamide gels is more difficult than that for agarose gels.

The composition of polyacrylamide gels is represented as the total percentage concentration (w/v) of monomer (acrylamide with cross-linker), T, and the percentage of monomer that is cross-linker, C. For example, a 6% 19:1

acrylamide:bis gel has a T value of 6% and a C value of 1/20, or 5%.

Unlike agarose gels that polymerize upon cooling, polymeration of polyacrylamide gels requires the use of a catalyst. The catalyst may be the nucleating agents **ammonium persulfate (APS)** plus *N,N,N+,N+-***tetramethylethylenediamine (TEMED)** or light activation. APS produces free oxygen radicals in the presence of TEMED to drive the polymerization mechanism. Free radicals can also be generated by a photochemical process using riboflavin plus TEMED. Excess oxygen inhibits the polymerization process. Therefore, deaeration, or the removal of air, of the gel solution is done before the addition of the nucleating agents.

Polyacrylamide gels for nucleic acid separation can be very thin, for example, 50 μm, making gel preparation difficult. Available systems are designed to facilitate the preparation of single and multiple gels. A more convenient, albeit more expensive, alternative is to use preformed polyacrylamide gels to avoid the hazards of working with acrylamide and the labor time involved in gel preparation. Use of preformed gels must be scheduled, keeping in mind the limited shelf life of the product.

The main advantage of polyacrylamide over agarose is the higher resolution capability of polyacrylamide for small fragments. A variation of 1 base pair in a 1-kb molecule (0.1% difference) can be detected in a polyacrylamide gel. Another advantage of polyacrylamide is that, unlike agarose, the components of polyacrylamide gels are synthetic; thus, there is not as much difference in batches obtained from different sources. Further, altering T and C in a polyacrylamide gel can change the pore size and, therefore, the sieving properties in a predictable and reproducible manner. Increasing T decreases the pore size proportionally. The minimum pore size (highest resolution for small molecules) occurs at a C value of 5%. Variation of C above or below 5% will increase pore size. Usually, C is set at 3.3% (29:1) for native and 5% (19:1) for standard DNA and RNA gels.

Capillary Electrophoresis

The widest application of **capillary electrophoresis** has been in the separation of such organic chemicals as pharmaceuticals and carbohydrates. It has also been applied to the separation of inorganic anions and metal ions. For these applications, it is an alternate method to high-performance liquid chromatography (HPLC). Capillary electrophoresis has the advantage of faster analytical runs and lower cost per run than HPLC. Increasingly, capillary electrophoresis is being used for the separation and analysis of nucleic acids.

In this type of electrophoresis, the analyte is resolved in a thin glass (fused silica) capillary that is 30–100 cm in length with an internal diameter of 25–100 μm. Fused silica is used as the capillary tube because it is the most transparent material allowing for the passage of fluorescent light. The fused silica is covered with a polyimide coating for protection, except for an uncoated window where the light is shone on the fragments as they pass a detection device, and has a negative charge along the walls of the capillary, generated by the dissociation of hydroxyl ions from the molecules of silicone. This establishes an electro-osmotic flow when a current is introduced along the length of the capillary. Under the force of the current, small and negatively charged molecules migrate faster than large and positively charged molecules (Fig. 5-7). Optimal separation requires the use of the proper buffer to ensure that the solute being separated is charged.

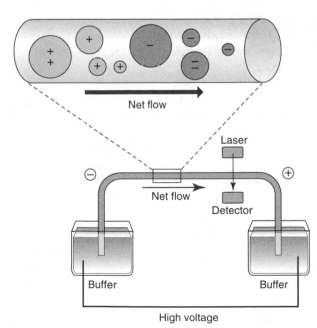

■ **Figure 5-7** Capillary electrophoresis separates particles by size (small, fast migration; large, slow migration) and charge (negative, fast migration; positive, slow migration).

Capillary electrophoresis was originally applied to molecules in solution. Separation was based on their size and charge (charge/mass ratio). Negatively charged molecules are completely ionized at high pH, whereas positively charged solutes are completely protonated in low pH buffers.

Nucleic acids do not separate well in solution. As the size or length of a nucleic acid increases (retarding migration), so does its negative charge (speeding migration), effectively confounding the charge/mass resolution. Introducing a polymer inside the capillary restores resolution by retarding nucleic acid migration according to its size more than its charge. It is important that the nucleic acid be completely denatured (single stranded) so that it will be separated according to its size, because secondary structure will affect the migration speed. Generally, picogram to nanogram quantities of fluorescently labeled, denatured nucleic acid in buffer containing formamide is introduced to the capillary, which is held at a denaturing temperature, usually 50°C to 60°C.

The sample is introduced into the capillary through electrokinetic, hydrostatic, or pneumatic injection. Electrokinetic injection is used for nucleic acid analysis. In this process, the platinum electrode close to the end of the capillary undergoes a transient high-positive charge to draw the sample into the end of the capillary. When the current is established, the injected nucleic acids migrate through the capillary. Capillary electrophoresis is analogous to gel electrophoresis with regard to the electrophoretic parameters for the resolution of nucleic acids. The capillary's small volume, as compared with that of a slab gel, can dissipate heat more efficiently during the electrophoresis process. More efficient heat dissipation allows the technologist to run the samples at higher charge per unit area, which means that the samples migrate faster, thereby decreasing the resolution (run) time.

Nucleic acid resolution by capillary electrophoresis is used extensively in forensic applications and parentage testing performed by analyzing short, tandem, repeat polymorphisms (see Chapter 11, "DNA Polymorphisms and Human Identification"). It has other applications in the clinical laboratory, such as clonality testing, microsatellite instability detection, and bone marrow engraftment analysis. Specially designed software can use differentially labeled molecular weight markers or allelic markers that, when run through the capillary with the sample, help to identify sample bands.

The capillary system has the advantages over traditional slab gel electrophoresis of increased sensitivity and immediate detection. With multiple color detection systems, standards, controls, and test samples are run through the capillary together, thereby eliminating the lane-to-lane variations that can occur across a gel. Although instrumentation for capillary electrophoresis is costly and detection requires fluorescent labeling of samples that can also be expensive, labor and run time are greatly decreased as compared with gel electrophoresis. In addition, analytical software programs automatically analyze results that are gathered by the detector in the capillary electrophoresis instrument.

Buffer Systems

The purpose of a buffer system is to carry the current and protect the samples during electrophoresis. This is accomplished through the electrochemical characteristics of the buffer components.

A buffer is a solution of a weak acid and its **conjugate** base. The pH of a buffered solution remains constant as the buffer molecules take up or release protons given off or absorbed by other solutes. The equilibrium between acid and base in a buffer is expressed as the dissociation constant, K_a:

$$K_a = \frac{[H^+][A^-]}{[HA]}$$

where $[H^+]$, $[A^-]$, and $[HA]$ represent the dissociated proton, dissociated base, and non-dissociated acid concentrations, respectively. K_a is most commonly expressed as its negative logarithm, pK_a, such that

$$pK_a = - \log K_a$$

A pK_a of 2 ($K_a = 10^{-2}$) favors the release of protons. A pK_a of 12 ($K_a = 10^{-12}$) favors the association of protons.

A given buffer maintains the pH of a solution near its pKa. The amount the pH of a buffer will differ from the pKa is expressed as the Henderson-Hasselbalch equation:

$$pH = pK_a + \log \frac{[\text{basic form}]}{[\text{acidic form}]}$$

If the acidic and basic forms of the buffer in solution are of equal concentration, $pH = pK_a$. If the acidic form predominates, the pH will be less than the pK_a; if the

basic form predominates, the pH will be greater than the pK_a.

The Henderson-Hasselbalch equation predicts that, in order to change the pH of a buffered solution by one point, either the acidic or basic form of the buffer must be brought to a concentration of 1/10 that of the other form. Therefore, addition of acid or base will barely affect the pH of a buffered solution as long as the acidic or basic forms of the buffer are not depleted.

Control of the pH of a gel by the buffer protects sample molecules from damage. Furthermore, the current through the gel is carried by buffer ions, preventing severe fluctuations in the pH of the gel. A buffer concentration must be high enough to provide sufficient acidic and basic forms to buffer its solution. Raising the buffer concentration, however, also increases the conductivity of the electrophoresis system, generating more heat at a given voltage. This can lessen gel stability and increase sample denaturation. High buffer concentrations must therefore be offset by low voltage.

In order for nucleic acids to migrate properly, the gel must be immersed in a buffer that conducts the electric

---

Advanced Concepts

The Henderson-Hasselbalch equation also predicts the concentration of the acidic or basic forms at a given pH. It can be used to calculate the state of ionization of a species in solution, that is, the predominance of acidic or basic forms. A buffer should be chosen that has a pK_a within a half point of the desired pH, which is about 8.0 for nucleic acids.

Advanced Concepts

The migration of buffer ions is not restricted by the gel matrix, so the speed of their movement under a current is governed strictly by the size of the ion and its charge (charge/mass ratio). Tris is a relatively large molecule, with a low charge-to-mass, and it moves through the current relatively slowly, even at high concentrations, giving increased buffering capacity.

current efficiently in relation to the buffering capacity. Ions with high-charge differences, +2, –2, +3, and so on, move through the gel more quickly; that is, they increase conductivity without increasing buffering capacity. This results in too much current passing through the gel as well as faster depletion of the buffer. Therefore, buffer components such as Tris base [2-amino-2-(hydroxymethyl)-1,3-propanediol] or borate are preferred because they remain partly uncharged at the desired pH and thus maintain constant pH without high conductivity. In addition to pKa, charge, and size, other buffer characteristics that might be taken into account when choosing a buffer include toxicity, interaction with other components, solubility, and ultraviolet absorption.

The Tris buffers, Tris borate EDTA (TBE; 0.089 M Tris-base, 0.089 M boric acid, 0.0020 M EDTA), Tris phosphate EDTA (TPE; 0.089 M Tris-base, 1.3% phosphoric acid, 0.0020 M EDTA), and Tris acetate EDTA (TAE; 0.04 M Tris-base, 0.005 M sodium acetate, 0.002 M EDTA) are most commonly used for electrophoresis of DNA. There are some advantages and disadvantages of both TBE and TAE that must be considered before one of these buffers is used for a particular application. TBE has a greater buffering capacity than TAE. Although the ion species in TAE are more easily exhausted during extended or high-voltage electrophoresis, DNA will migrate twice as fast in TAE than in TBE in a constant current. TBE is not recommended for some postelectrophoretic isolation procedures. When using any buffer, especially TBE and TPE, care must be taken that the gel does not overheat when run at high voltage in a closed container. Finally, stock solutions of TBE are prone to precipitation. This can result in differences in concentration between the buffer in the gel and the running buffer. Such a gradient will cause localized distortions in nucleic acid migration patterns, often causing a salt wave that is visible as a sharp horizontal band through the gel.

Buffer Additives

Buffer additives modify sample molecules in ways that affect their migration. Examples of these additives are formamide, urea, and various detergents. With regard to nucleic acids, **denaturing agents**, such as formamide or urea, break hydrogen bonds between complementary strands or within the same strand of DNA or RNA. The conformation or solubility of molecules can be standardized by the addition of one or both of these agents. Formamide and heat added to DNA and RNA break and block the hydrogen bonding sites, hindering complementary sequences from reannealing. As a result, the molecules become long, straight, unpaired chains. Urea and heat in the gel systems maintain this conformation such that intrachain hybridization (folding) of the nucleic acid molecules does not affect migration speeds, and separation occurs strictly according to the size or length of the molecule.

Electrophoresis of RNA requires different conditions imparted by different additives from those that are used with DNA. Because RNA is single-stranded and tends to fold to optimize internal homology, it must be completely denatured to prevent folding in order to accurately determine its size by migration in a gel system. The secondary structures formed in RNA are strong and more difficult to denature than DNA homologies. Denaturants used for RNA include methylmercuric hydroxide (MMH), which reacts with amino groups on the RNA to prevent base pairing between homologous nucleotides and with aldehydes (e.g., formaldehyde, glyoxal), which also disrupt base pairing. MMH is not used routinely because of its extreme toxicity.

Examples of RNA electrophoresis buffers are 10-mM sodium phosphate, pH 7, and MOPS buffer [20 mM 3-(N-morpholino) propanesulfonic acid, pH 7, 8 mM sodium acetate, 1 mM EDTA, pH 8]. The RNA sample is incubated in dimethyl sulfoxide, 1.1 M glyoxal (ethane 1.2 dione) and 0.01 M sodium phosphate, pH 7, to denature the RNA prior to loading the sample on the gel. Due to **pH drift** (decrease of pH at the cathode [–] and increase of the pH at the anode [+]) during the run, the buffer may have to be recirculated from the anode end of the bath to the cathode end (Fig. 5-8). This is accomplished by using a peristaltic pump or stopping the gel at intervals and transferring the buffer from the cathode to the anode ends.

Electrophoresis Equipment

Gel electrophoresis is performed in one of two conformations, horizontal or vertical. In general, agarose gels are run horizontally and polyacrylamide gels are run vertically.

Horizontal gels are run in acrylic containers called gel boxes or baths that are divided into two parts with a

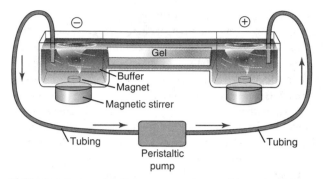

■ **Figure 5-8** A peristaltic pump can be used to recirculate buffer from the cathode to the anode end while running a **denaturing gel**.

platform in the middle on which the gel rests (Fig. 5-9). The electrodes in the gel compartments (platinum wires) are connected to a power supply by banana clips or connectors through the walls of the container. The gel in the box is submerged in electrophoresis buffer that fills both compartments and makes a continuous system through which the current flows. The thickness of the gel and the volume of the buffer affect the current, and, therefore, migration of the sample, so these parameters should be kept constant for consistent results. Because the gel is submerged throughout the loading and electrophoresis process, horizontal gels are sometimes referred to as **submarine gels**. Enclosed cassettes containing gel, buffer, electrodes, and detection do not require submersion in running buffer. The sample is loaded directly into the wells of these systems.

Once the sample is introduced into the gel, the electrodes are connected to the power source. The power supply will deliver voltage, setting up a current that will run through the gel buffer and the gel, carrying the charged sample through the gel matrix at a speed corresponding to the charge/mass ratio of the sample molecules.

Horizontal agarose gels are cast as square or rectangular slabs of varying size. Commercial gel boxes come with casting trays that mold the gel to the appropriate size for the gel box. The volume of the gel solution will determine the thickness of the gel. Agarose, supplied as a dry powder, is mixed at a certain percentage (w/v) with electrophoresis buffer and heated on a heat block or by microwave to dissolve and melt the agarose. The molten agarose is cooled to between 55°C and 65°C, and the appropriate volume is poured into the casting tray as dictated by the gel box manufacturer or application. A **comb** is then inserted into the top of the gel to create holes, or **wells**, in the gel into which the sample will be loaded. The size of the teeth in the comb will determine the capacity of the well for the sample, and the number of teeth in the comb will determine the number of wells that are available in the gel to receive the samples. The gel is then allowed to cool, during which time it will solidify. After the gel has polymerized, the comb is carefully removed and the gel is placed into the gel box and submerged in electrophoresis buffer.

Vertical gel boxes have separate chambers connected by the gel itself. Electrodes are attached to the upper and lower buffer chambers to set up the current that will run through the gel. The gel must be in place before filling

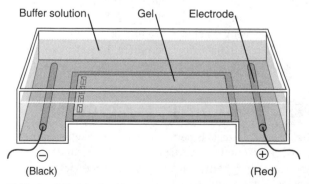

■ **Figure 5-9** A typical horizontal submarine gel system. A red connector is attached to the positive outlet on the power supply and a black to the negative port.

Advanced Concepts

Self-contained agarose gel systems have been developed to facilitate the electrophoresis process. They are manufactured in closed plastic cassettes containing buffer, gel, and stain. These are convenient for routine use, but restrict the gel configuration, that is, the number and size of wells, and so forth. Also, the percentage of agarose or acrylamide is limited to what is available from the manufacturer. Furthermore, the separated nucleic acids cannot easily be removed from these closed cassettes, limiting their analysis.

the upper chamber with buffer. Some systems have a conductive plate attached to the back of the gel to maintain constant temperature across the gel. Maintaining constant temperature is more of a problem with vertical gels because the outer edges of the gel cool more than the center, slowing migration in the outer lanes compared with lanes in the center of the gel. This is called "gel smiling" because similar-sized bands in the cooler outer lanes will be higher than comparable bands in the inside lanes. Vertical gel systems can range from large sequencing systems (35 cm × 26 cm) to minisystems (8 cm × 10 cm). Some minisystems accommodate two or more gels at a time (Fig. 5-10). Minisystems are used extensively for analyses that do not require single base-pair resolution. The larger systems are used for procedures requiring higher resolution. The gels are loaded from the top, below a layer of buffer in the upper chamber. Long, narrow, gel-loading pipette tips that deposit the sample neatly on the floor of the well increase band resolution and sample recovery.

Vertical gels are cast between glass plates that are separated by spacers. The spacers determine the thickness of the gel, ranging from 0.05 mm to 4 mm. The bottom of the gel is secured by tape or by a gasket in specially designed gel casting trays. After addition of polymerization agents, the liquid acrylamide is poured or forced between the glass plates with a pipet or a syringe. The comb is then placed on the top of the gel. During this process, it is important to prevent air from getting into the gel or beneath the comb. Bubbles will form discontinuities in the gel, and oxygen will inhibit the polymerization of the acrylamide. The comb is of a thickness equal to that of the spacers so that the gel will be the same thickness throughout.

As with horizontal gels, the number and size of the comb's teeth determine the number of wells in the gel and the sample volume that can be added to each well. Specialized combs, called **shark's-tooth combs**, are often used for sequencing gels (Fig. 5-11). These combs are placed upside down (teeth up, not in contact with

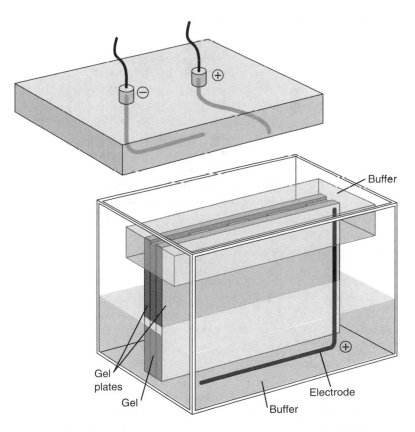

■ **Figure 5-10** A typical vertical gel apparatus. Polymerized gels are clamped into the gel insert (left) and placed in the gel bath (right). The positive electrode will be in contact with the bottom of the gel and the buffer, filling about a third of the gel bath. The negative electrode will be in contact with the top of the gel and a separate buffer compartment in the top of the insert.

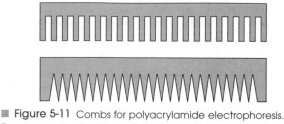

■ **Figure 5-11** Combs for polyacrylamide electrophoresis. Regular combs (top) have teeth that form the wells in the gel. Shark's-tooth combs (bottom) are placed onto the polymerized gel, and the sample is loaded between the teeth of the comb.

the gel) to form a trough on the gel during polymerization. After polymerization is complete, the comb is removed and placed tooth-side down on top of the gel for loading. With this configuration, the spaces *between* the comb teeth form the well walls, as opposed to the teeth themselves forming wells in the horizontal gels. The advantage to this arrangement is that the lanes are placed immediately adjacent to one another to facilitate lane-to-lane comparisons. When used, standard combs are removed before the gel is loaded, whereas the shark's-tooth combs are made so that the wells can be loaded while the comb is in place. When the standard combs are removed from the gel, care must be taken not to break or displace the "ears" that were formed by the spaces between the teeth in the comb that separate the gel wells.

Polyacrylamide gels can also be cast in tubes for isoelectric focusing or two-dimensional gel electrophoresis. The tubes containing the gels are placed in a chamber separated like those for vertical slab gels. The tubes are held in place by gaskets in the upper chamber. However, this gel configuration limits the number of samples, as only one sample can be run per gel.

Gel Loading

Prior to loading the sample containing isolated nucleic acid onto the gel, **tracking dye** and a density agent are added to the sample. The density agent (either Ficoll, sucrose, or glycerol) increases the density of the sample as compared with the electrophoresis buffer. When the sample solution is dispensed into the wells of the gel below the surface of the buffer, it sinks into the well instead of diffusing in the buffer. The tracking dyes are used to monitor the progress of the electrophoresis run. The dyes

migrate at specific speeds in a given gel concentration and usually run ahead of the smallest fragments of DNA (Table 5.3). They are not associated with the sample DNA, and thus they do not affect the its separation. The movement of the tracking dye is monitored, and when the dye approaches the end of the gel, or the desired distance, electrophoresis is terminated. Bromophenol blue is a tracking dye that is used for many applications, and xylene cyanol green is another of the chromophores used as tracking dyes for both agarose and polyacrylamide gels.

Detection Systems

The following are descriptions of the status of samples during and after electrophoresis performed using dyes that specifically associate with nucleic acid. The agents used most frequently for this application are fluorescent dyes and silver stain.

> ### Advanced Concepts
>
> A type of "bufferless" electrophoresis system supplies buffer in gel form or strips. These are laid next to the preformed gel on a platform that replaces the electrophoresis chamber. These systems can offer the additional advantage of precise temperature control during the run.

Table 5.3 **Tracking Dye Comigration***

Gel %	Bromophenol Blue (Nucleotides)	Xylene Cyanol (Nucleotides)
Agarose		
0.5–1.5	300–500	4000–5000
2.0–3.0	80–120	700–800
4.0–5.0	20–30	100–200
PAGE		
4	95	450
6	60	240
8	45	160
10	35	120
12	20	70
20	12	45

*Migration depends on buffer type (TAE, TBE, or TPE) and the formulation of agarose, acylamide, and bis.

Advanced Concepts

Gels in cassette systems and gel strip systems can be loaded without loading buffer because the wells are "dry," precluding the need for density gradients. These systems also have automatic shut-off at the end of the run, so tracking dye is usually not necessary, although some systems have a tracking dye built into the gel and/or buffer.

Nucleic Acid–Specific Dyes

Intercalating agents intercalate, or stack, between the nitrogen bases in double-stranded nucleic acid. Ethidium bromide [3,8-diamino-5-ethyl-6-phenylphenanthridinium bromide (EtBr)] is one of these agents and was the most widely used dye in early DNA and RNA analyses. It is carcinogenic and should be used with care, however. Under excitation with ultraviolet light at 300 nm, EtBr in DNA emits visible light at 590 nm. Therefore, DNA separated in agarose or acrylamide and exposed to EtBr will emit orange light when illuminated at 300 nm. After electrophoresis, the agarose or acrylamide gel is soaked in a solution of 0.1–1-mg/ml EtBr in running buffer (TAE, TBE, or TPE) or TE. Alternatively, dye is added directly to the gel before polymerization or to the running buffer. The latter two measures save time and allow visualization of the DNA during the run, however, dye added to the gel may form a bright front across the gel that could mask informative bands. Dye added to the running buffer produces more consistent staining, although more hazardous waste is generated by this method. Some enclosed gel systems contain EtBr inside a plastic-enclosed gel cassette, limiting exposure and limiting waste. After soaking or running in EtBr, the DNA illuminated with ultraviolet light will appear as orange bands in the gel. The image is captured with a Polaroid camera equipped with appropriate filters or by digital transfer to analytical software.

SyBr green (N',N'-dimethyl-N-[4-[(E)-(3-methyl-1,3-benzothiazol-2-ylidene)methyl]-1-phenylquinolin-1-ium-2-yl]-N-propylpropane-1,3-diamine) is one of a set of stains introduced in 1995 as another type of nucleic acid–specific dye system. The related dyes include SyBr green I used for double-stranded DNA staining; SyBr green II, for single-stranded DNA or RNA staining; and SyBr Gold, for both DNA and RNA staining. SyBr green I differs from EtBr in that it does not intercalate between bases; it sits in the minor groove of the double helix. SyBr green in association with DNA or RNA also emits light in the orange range (522 nm). In agarose gel electrophoresis, SyBr staining is 25–100 times more sensitive than EtBr (detection level: 60 pg of double-stranded DNA vs. 5 ng for EtBr). This is due, in part, to background fluorescence from EtBr in agarose. A 1X dilution of the manufacturer's 10,000X stock solution of SyBr green I in TAE, TBE, or TE is used in methods described for EtBr. SyBr green can also be added directly to the DNA sample before electrophoresis. DNA prestaining decreases the amount of dye required for DNA visualization but lowers the sensitivity of detection and may, at higher DNA concentrations, interfere with DNA migration through the gel.[10] Because SyBr green is not an intercalating agent, it is not as mutagenic and is therefore safer to use.[11]

Although SyBr green dyes have some advantages over EtBr, many laboratories continue to use the EtBr due to the requirement for special optical filters for detection of SyBr green. Scanning and photographic equipment optimized for EtBr would have to be modified for optimal detection of the SyBr stains. New instrumentation with more flexible detection systems allows utilization of the SyBr stains. SyBr green is the preferred dye for real-time PCR methods (see Chapter 7, "Nucleic Acid Amplification").

Silver Stain

Another sensitive staining system originally developed for protein visualization is silver stain. After electrophoresis, the sample is fixed with methanol and acetic acid. The gel is then impregnated with ammoniacal silver (silver diamine) solutions or silver nitrate in a weakly acid solution.[12] Interaction of silver ions with acidic or nucleophilic groups on the target results in crystallization or deposition of metallic silver under optimal pH conditions. The insoluble black silver salt precipitates upon introduction of formaldehyde in a weak acid solution, or alkaline solution for silver nitrate. Of the two procedures, silver diamine is best for thick gels, whereas silver nitrate is considered to be more stable.[13]

Silver staining avoids the hazards of the intercalators, but silver nitrate is itself also a biohazard and must be handled accordingly. In addition, silver staining is more complicated than simple fluorescent stains. Color development must be carefully watched in order to stop the reaction once the optimal signal is reached. Overdevelopment of the color reaction will result in high backgrounds and masking of results. The increased sensitivity of this staining procedure, however, makes up for its limitations. It is especially useful for protein analysis and for detection of limiting amounts of product.

• STUDY QUESTIONS •

1. You wish to perform an electrophoretic resolution of your restriction enzyme–digested DNA. The size of the expected fragments ranges from 100 to 500 bp. You discover two agarose gels polymerizing on the bench. One is 0.5% agarose; the other is 2% agarose. Which one might you use to resolve your fragments?

2. After completion of the electrophoresis of DNA fragments along with the proper molecular weight standard on an agarose gel, suppose (a) or (b) below was observed. What might be the explanations?
   a. The gel is blank (no bands, no molecular weight standard).
   b. Only the molecular weight standard is visible.

3. How does PFGE separate larger fragments more efficiently than standard electrophoresis?

4. A 6% solution of 19:1 acylamide is mixed, deaerated, and poured between glass plates for gel formation. After an hour, the solution is still liquid. What might be one explanation for the gel not polymerizing?

5. A gel separation of RNA yields aberrantly migrating bands and smears. Suggest two possible explanations for this observation.

6. Why does DNA not resolve well in solution (without a gel matrix)?

7. Why is SyBr green less toxic than EtBr?

8. What are the general components of loading buffer used for introducing DNA samples to submarine gels?

9. Name two dyes that are used to monitor migration of nucleic acid during electrophoresis.

10. When a DNA fragment is resolved by slab gel electrophoresis, a single sharp band is obtained. What is the equivalent observation had this fragment been fluorescently labeled and resolved by capillary electrophoresis?

References

1. Tiselius A. A new apparatus for electrophoretic analysis of colloidal mixtures. *Transactions of the Faraday Society* 1937;33:524.
2. Kunkel H, Slater RJ. Zone electrophoresis in a starch supporting medium. *Proceedings of the Society of Experimental Biology and Medicine* 1952;80:42–44.
3. Smithies O, Walker NF. Genetic control of some serum proteins in normal humans. *Nature* 1955;176:1265–1266.
4. Smithies O, Poulik MD. Two-dimensional electrophoresis of serum proteins. *Nature* 1956;177:1033.
5. Carle G, Frank M, Olson MV. Electrophoretic separation of large DNA molecules by periodic inversion of the electric field. *Science* 1986;232: 65–68.
6. Chu G, Vollrath D, Davis RW. Separation of large DNA molecules by contour-clamped homogeneous electric fields. *Science* 1986; 234:1582–1585.
7. Gardiner K, Laas W, Patterson DS. Fractionation of large mammalian DNA restriction fragments using vertical pulsed-field gradient gel electrophoresis. *Somatic Cell Molecular Genetics* 1986;12:185–195.
8. Southern E, Anand R, Brown WRA, et al. A model for the separation of large DNA molecules by crossed field gel electrophoresis. *Nucleic Acids Research* 1987;15:5925–5943.
9. Gemmill R. Pulsed field gel electrophoresis. In Chrambach A, Dunn MJ, Radola BJ, eds. Advances of Electrophoresis, vol. 4. Weinheim, Germany: VCH, 1991, pp. 1–48.
10. Miller S, Taillon-Miller P, Kwok P. Cost-effective staining of DNA with SyBr green in preparative

agarose gel electrophoresis. *BioTechniques* 1999; 7(1):34–36.

11. Singer V, Lawlor TE, Yue S. Comparison of SyBr green I nucleic acid gel stain mutagenicity and ethidium bromide mutagenicity in the salmonella/ mammalian microsome reverse mutation assay (Ames test). *Mutation Research* 1999;439(1):37–47.

12. Rabilloud T. A comparison between low background silver diamine and silver nitrate protein stains. *Electrophoresis* 1992;13(6):429–439.

13. Merrill C. Gel-staining techniques. *Methods in Enzymology* 1990;182:477–488.

14. Perbal B. A Practical Guide to Molecular Cloning, 2nd. ed. New York: John Wiley & Sons, 1988.

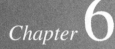

Chapter **6**

Analysis and Characterization of Nucleic Acids and Proteins

OUTLINE

RESTRICTION ENZYME MAPPING

HYBRIDIZATION TECHNOLOGIES
  Southern Blots
  Northern Blots
  Western Blots

PROBES
  DNA Probes
  RNA Probes
  Other Nucleic Acid Probe Types
  Protein Probes
  Probe Labeling
  Nucleic Acid Probe Design

HYBRIDIZATION CONDITIONS, STRINGENCY

DETECTION SYSTEMS

INTERPRETATION OF RESULTS

OBJECTIVES

- Describe how restriction enzyme sites are mapped on DNA.
- Construct a restriction enzyme map of a DNA plasmid or fragment.
- Diagram the Southern blot procedure.
- Explain depurination and denaturation of resolved DNA.
- Describe the procedure involved in blotting (transfer) DNA from a gel to a membrane.
- Discuss the purpose and structure of probes that are used for blotting procedures.
- Define hybridization, stringency, and melting temperature.
- Calculate the melting temperature of a given sequence of dsDNA.
- Compare and contrast radioactive and nonradioactive DNA detection methods.

OBJECTIVES—cont'd

• Compare and contrast dot and slot blotting methods.
• Describe microarray methodology.
• Discuss solution hybridization.

Restriction Enzyme Mapping

Clinical and forensic analyses require characterization of specific genes or genomic regions at the molecular level. Because of their sequence-specific activity (see Chapter 1), restriction endonucleases provide a convenient tool for molecular characterization of DNA (see Chapter 1, "DNA").

Restriction enzymes commonly used in the laboratory have four to six base-pair recognition sites, or binding/cutting sites, on the DNA. Any four to six base pair nucleotide sequence occurs at random in a sufficiently long stretch of DNA. Therefore, restriction sites will occur in all DNA molecules of sufficient length. Restriction site mapping, i.e., determining where in the DNA sequence a particular restriction enzyme recognition site is located, was developed using small circular bacterial plasmids. The resultant maps were used to identify and characterize naturally occurring plasmids and to engineer the construction of recombinant plasmids.

To make a restriction map, DNA is exposed to several restriction enzymes separately and then in different combinations. Take, for example, a linear fragment of DNA digested with the enzyme *Pst*I. After incubation with the enzyme, the resulting fragments are separated by gel electrophoresis. The gel image reveals four fragments, labeled A, B, C, and D, produced by *Pst*I (Fig. 6-1). From the number of fragments one can deduce the number of *Pst*I sites: three. The sizes of the fragments, as determined by comparison with known molecular-weight standards, indicate the distance between *Pst*I sites or from one *Pst*I site to the end of the fragment. Although *Pst*I analysis of this fragment yields a characteristic four-band restriction pattern, it does not indicate the order of the four restriction products in the original fragment.

To begin to determine the order of the restriction fragments, another enzyme is used, for example *Bam*HI. Cutting the same fragment with *Bam*HI yields two pieces, indicating one *Bam*HI site in this linear fragment (see Fig. 6-1). In this figure, observe that one restriction product (F) is much larger than the other (E). This means that the *Bam*HI site is close to one end of the fragment. When the fragment is cut simultaneously with *Pst*I and *Bam*HI, five products are produced, with *Pst*I product A cut into two pieces by *Bam*HI. This indicates that A is on one end of the DNA fragment. By measuring the number and length of products produced by other enzymes, the restriction sites can be placed in linear order along the DNA sequence. Figure 6-2 shows two possible maps based on the results of cutting the fragment with *Pst*I and *Bam*HI. With adequate enzymes and enzyme combinations, a detailed map of this fragment is generated.

Mapping of a circular plasmid is slightly different, as there are no free ends (Fig. 6-3). The example shown in the figure is a 4-kb pair circular plasmid with one *Bam*HI site and two *Xho*I sites. Cutting the plasmid with *Bam*HI will yield one fragment. The size of the fragment is the size of the plasmid. Two fragments released by *Xho*I indicate that there are two *Xho*I sites in the plasmid and that these sites are 1.2 and 2.8 kb pairs away from each other. As with linear mapping, cutting the plasmid with *Xho*I and *Bam*HI at the same time will start to order the sites with respect to one another on the plasmid. One possible arrangement is shown in Figure 6-3. As more enzymes are used, the map becomes more detailed.

Under the proper reaction conditions, restriction enzymes are highly specific for their recognition and cutting properties. Under nonstandard conditions, some restriction enzymes will bind to and cut sequences other than their defined recognition sequence. This altered specificity is called **star activity**. The propensity for star

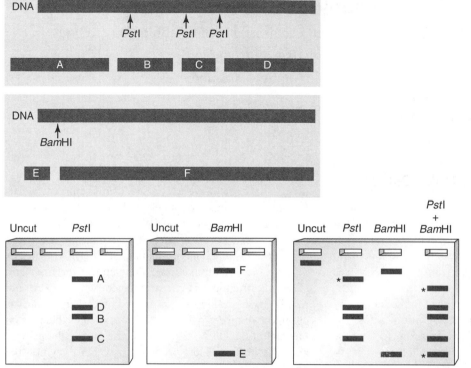

■ **Figure 6-1** Restriction mapping of a linear DNA fragment (top green bar). The fragment is first cut with the enzyme *Pst*I. Four fragments result, as determined by agarose gel electrophoresis, indicating that there are three *Pst*I sites in the linear fragment. The size of the pieces indicates the distance between the restriction sites. A second cut with *Bam*HI (bottom) yields two fragments, indicating one site. Since one *Bam*HI fragment (E) is very small, the *Bam*HI site must be near one end of the fragment. Cutting with both enzymes indicates that the *Bam*HI site is in the *Pst*I fragment A.

activity varies among enzymes.[1] Thus, the nature and degree of star activity depends on the enzyme and the reaction conditions.[2] Reaction conditions that induce star activity include suboptimal buffer, contamination with solvents or high concentrations of glycerol, prolonged reaction time, high concentration of enzymes, and divalent cation imbalance.

The pattern of fragments produced by restriction enzyme digestion of a DNA fragment or region can be

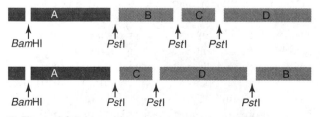

■ **Figure 6-2** Two possible maps inferred from the observations described in Figure 6-1. The *Bam*HI site positions fragment A at one end (or the other) of the map. Determination of the correct map requires information from additional enzyme cuts.

used to identify that DNA and to monitor certain changes in its size, structure, or sequence. Because of inherited or somatic differences in the nucleotide sequences in human DNA, the number or location of restriction sites for a given restriction enzyme are not the same in all individuals. The resulting differences in the size or number of restriction fragments are called **restriction fragment length polymorphisms (RFLPs)**. RFLPs were the basis of the first molecular-based human identification and mapping methods. RFLPs can also be used for the clinical analysis of structural changes in chromosomes associated with disease (translocations, deletions, insertions, and so forth).

Hybridization Technologies

Procedures performed in the clinical molecular laboratory are aimed at specific targets in genomic DNA. This requires visualization or detection of a particular gene or region of DNA in the backdrop of all other genes. There are several ways to find a target region of DNA. The first

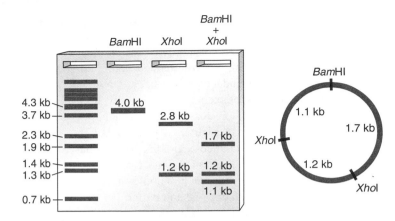

■ **Figure 6-3** Restriction mapping of a plasmid. After incubating plasmid DNA with restriction enzymes, agarose gel electrophoresis banding patterns indicate the number of restriction sites and the distance between them.

method for molecular analysis of specific DNA sites within a complex background without cloning that region was the Southern blot. Modifications of the Southern blot are applied to analysis of RNA, proteins, and lipids in order to study gene expression, regulation, and protein modifications (see Table 6.1).

Southern Blots

The **Southern blot** is named for Edwin Southern, who first reported the procedure.[3] In the Southern blot, DNA is isolated and cut with restriction enzymes. The fragments are separated by gel electrophoresis, denatured, and then transferred to a solid support such as **nitrocellulose**. In the final steps of the procedure, the DNA fragments are exposed to a labeled **probe** (complementary DNA or RNA) that is complementary to the region of interest. The signal of the probe is detected to indicate the presence or absence (lack of signal) of the sequence in

question. The original method entailed hybridization of a radioactively labeled probe to detect the DNA region to be analyzed. As long as there is a probe of known identity, this procedure can analyze any gene or gene region in the genome at the molecular level. The following sections will describe the parts of the Southern blot procedure in detail as well as discuss modifications of the procedure in order to analyze RNA and protein.

Restriction Enzyme Cutting and Resolution

The first step in the Southern blot procedure is digestion of test DNA with restriction enzymes. The choice of enzymes used will depend on the genetic locus and the application. For routine laboratory tests, restriction maps of the target DNA regions will have previously been determined, and the appropriate enzymes will be recommended. For other methods, such as typing of unknown organisms or cloning, several enzymes may be tested to find those that will be most informative.

Table 6.1 **Hybridization Technologies**

Hybridization Method	Target	Probe	Purpose
Southern blot	DNA	Nucleic acid	Gene structure
Northern blot	RNA	Nucleic acid	Transcript structure, processing, gene expression
Western blot	Protein	Protein	Protein processing, gene expression
Southwestern blot	Protein	DNA	DNA binding proteins, gene regulation
Eastern blot	Protein	Protein	Modification of Western blot using enzymatic detection (PathHunter™); also, detection of specific agriculturally important proteins[34]
Far-eastern blot[35,36]	Lipids	(None)	Transfer of HPLC-separated lipids to PVDF membranes for analysis by mass spectometry

Ten to 50 μg of genomic DNA are used for each restriction enzyme digestion for Southern analysis. More or less DNA may be required depending on the sensitivity of the detection system, the volume and configurations of wells, and the abundance of the target DNA. In the clinical laboratory, specimen availability may limit the amount of DNA available for testing. The DNA is mixed with the appropriate restriction enzyme and buffer. Restriction enzymes are supplied with 10X buffers that are diluted ¹/₁₀ into the final reaction volume. If more than one enzyme is to be used, each sample must be digested separately for each enzyme and buffer.

Digestion is carried out for an extended time (1 to 3 hours) to allow complete cutting of all sites in the DNA sample. High-specific-activity enzymes are also used to ensure complete cutting of every site. Incomplete cutting

will result in anomalous patterns, complicating interpretation of the Southern blot data. The fragments resulting from the restriction digestions are resolved by gel electrophoresis. The percentage and nature of the gel will depend on the size of the DNA region to be analyzed (see Chapter 5, Tables 5.1 and 5.2). As with all electrophoresis, a molecular-weight standard should be run with the test samples. Large fragments require longer runs at low voltage to get the best resolution. For example, 10,000 to 20,000 bp fragments are resolved in 0.7% agarose at 20 amperes for 16 hours.

After electrophoresis, it is important to observe the cut DNA. Figure 6-4A shows a 0.7% agarose gel stained with ethidium bromide and illuminated by ultraviolet (uv) light. Genomic DNA cut with restriction enzymes should produce a smear representing the billions of fragments of

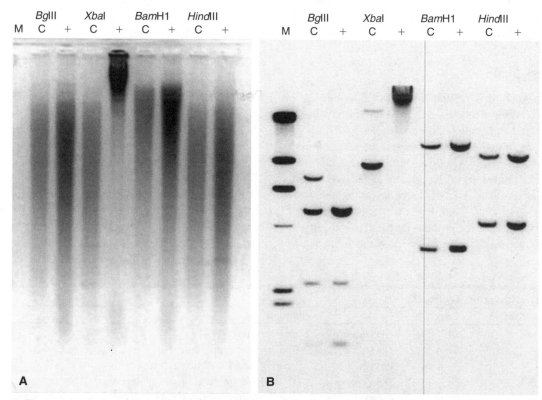

■ **Figure 6-4** (A) Genomic DNA fragments cut with restriction enzymes *Bgl*II, *Xba*I, *Bam*HI, and *Hind*III and separated by gel electrophoresis. (B) Autoradiogram of the fragments hybridized to a radioactive or chemiluminescent probe. Control lanes, 2, 4, 6, and 8, show the restriction pattern of DNA with a t(9;22) translocation. Test lanes 3, 5, 7, and 9 show the different restriction patterns that result from the normal or untranslocated DNA. Lane 1, molecular size marker.

all sizes released by digestion by the enzyme. The brightness of the DNA smears should be similar from lane to lane, ensuring that equal amounts of DNA were added to all lanes. A large aggregate of DNA near the top of the lane indicates that the restriction enzyme activity was incomplete. A smear located primarily in the lower region of the lane is a sign that the DNA is degraded. Uncut or degraded DNA will prevent accurate analysis. The DNA should digest if the restriction enzyme is active and the reaction mix is prepared correctly. Repeat of the restriction digest will be required if uncut DNA is present. If an impurity in the DNA results in resistance to restriction digestion or degradation of the DNA, re-isolation or further purification of the DNA will be required.

Preparation of Resolved DNA for Blotting (Transfer)

The goal of the Southern blot procedure is to analyze a specific region of the sample DNA. The restriction fragments containing the target sequence to be analyzed are obviously not distinguishable in the smear from other fragments that do not have the target sequence. Target fragments can be detected by hybridization with a complementary sequence of single-stranded DNA or RNA labeled with a detectable **marker**. To achieve optimal hydrogen bonding between the probe and its complementary sequence in the resolved sample DNA, the double-stranded DNA fragments in the gel must be separated into single strands (denatured) and transferred to a nitrocellulose membrane.

Depurination

Before moving the DNA fragments from the gel to the membrane for blotting, the double-stranded DNA fragments are denatured as the DNA remains in place in the gel. Although short fragments can be denatured directly as described below, larger fragments (>500 bp) are more efficiently denatured if they are depurinated before denaturation (Fig. 6-5). Therefore, for large fragments, the gel is first soaked in dilute hydrogen chloride (HCl) solution, a process that removes purine bases from the sugar-phosphate backbone. This will "loosen up" the larger fragments for more complete denaturation.

Denaturation

DNA is denatured by exposing it in the gel to the strong base sodium hydroxide (NaOH). NaOH promotes

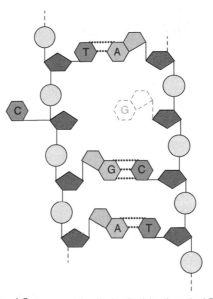

■ **Figure 6-5** An apurinic site in double-stranded DNA. Loss of the guanine (right) leaves an open site but does not break the sugar-phosphate backbone of the DNA.

breakage of the hydrogen bonds holding the DNA strands to one another. The resulting single strands are then available to hydrogen bond with the single-stranded probe. Further, the single-stranded DNA will bind more tightly than double-stranded DNA to the nitrocellulose membrane upon transfer.

Blotting (Transfer)

Before exposing the denatured sample DNA to the probe, the DNA is transferred, or blotted, to a solid substrate that will facilitate probe binding and signal detection. This substrate is usually nitrocellulose, nitrocellulose on an inert support, nylon or cellulose modified with a diethyl amino ethyl, or a carboxy methyl (CM) chemical group. Membranes of another type, polyvinyl difluoride (PVDF), are used for immobilizing proteins for probing with antibodies (western blots).

Membrane Types

Single-stranded DNA avidly binds to nitrocellulose membranes with a noncovalent, but irreversible, connection. The binding interaction is hydrophobic and electrostatic between the negatively charged DNA and the positive charges on the membrane. Nitrocellulose-based membranes bind 70–150 µg of nucleic acid per square centimeter. Membrane pore sizes (0.05 µm to 0.45µm) are suitable for DNA fragments from a few hundred bases up to those >20,000 bp in length.

Pure nitrocellulose has a high binding capacity for proteins as well as nucleic acids. It is the most versatile medium for molecular transfer applications. It is also compatible with different transfer buffers and detection systems. Nitrocellulose is not as sturdy as other media and becomes brittle with multiple reuses. Reinforced nitrocellulose is more appropriate for applications where multiple probings may be necessary. Mechanically stable membranes can be formulated with a net neutral charge to decrease non-specific binding. These membranes have a very high binding capacity (<400 µg/cm^2), which increases test sensitivity. A covalent attachment of nucleic acid to these membranes is achieved by exposure of the DNA on the membrane to ultraviolet light (uv) cross-linking.

Membranes with a positive charge more effectively bind small fragments of DNA. These membranes, however, are more likely to retain protein or other contaminants that will contribute to background noise after the membrane is probed.

Before transfer of the sample, membranes are moistened by floating them on the surface of the transfer buffer. Any dry spots (areas where the membrane does not properly hydrate) will remain white while the rest of the membrane darkens with buffer. If the membrane does

not hydrate evenly, dry spots will inhibit binding of the sample.

Transfer Methods

Transfer is performed in several ways. The goal of all methods is to move the DNA from the gel to a membrane substrate for probing. The membrane must be equilibrated in the transfer buffer before coming into contact with the DNA in the gel. Membranes should be handled carefully, preferably with powder-free gloves. Folding or creasing the membrane should also be avoided.

The original method developed by Southern used capillary transfer (Fig. 6-6). For capillary transfer, the gel is placed on top of a reservoir of buffer, which can be a shallow container or filter papers soaked in high salt

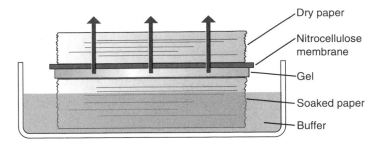

■ **Figure 6-6** Capillary transfer. Driven by capillary movement of buffer from the soaked paper to the dry paper, denatured DNA moves from the gel to the membrane.

Advanced Concepts

Capillary transfer is simple and relatively inexpensive, as no instruments are required. The transfer, however, can be less than optimal, especially with large gels. Bubbles, crystals, or other particles between the membrane and the gel can cause loss of information or staining artifacts. The procedure is also slow, taking from a few hours to overnight for large fragments.

buffer, for example, 10X saline sodium citrate (10X SSC: 1.5 M NaCl, 0.15 M Na citrate) or commercially available transfer buffers. The nitrocellulose membrane is placed directly on the gel, and dry absorbent filter paper or paper towels are stacked on top of the membrane. The buffer will move by capillary action from the lower reservoir to the dry material on top of the gel. The movement of the buffer transversely through the gel will carry the denatured DNA out of the gel. When the DNA contacts the nitrocellulose membrane, the DNA will bind to it.

A second method, called **electrophoretic transfer**, uses electric current to move the DNA from the gel to the membrane (Fig. 6-7). This system utilizes electrodes attached to membranes above (**anode**) and below (**cathode**) the gel. The current carries the DNA transversely from the gel to the membrane. Electrophoretic transfer is performed in a "tank" or by a "semidry" approach. In the tank method, the electrodes transfer current through the membrane through electrophoresis buffer, as shown in Figure 6-7. In the semidry method, the electrodes contact the gel-membrane sandwich directly, requiring only enough buffer to soak the gel and membrane. The tank electrophoretic transfer is preferred for large proteins resolved on acrylamide gels, whereas the semidry method is frequently used for small proteins.

Vacuum transfer is a third method of DNA blotting (Fig. 6-8). This blotting technique uses suction to move the DNA from the gel to the membrane in a recirculating buffer. Like electrophoretic transfer, this method transfers the DNA more rapidly than capillary transfer—in 2 to 3 hours rather than overnight. Also, it avoids discontinuous transfer due to air trapped between the membrane and the gel. One disadvantage of the second and third

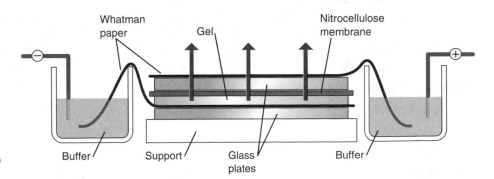

■ **Figure 6-7** Electrophoretic transfer. This system uses electric current to mobilize the DNA from the gel to the membrane.

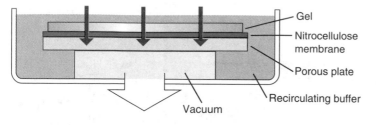

Figure 6-8 Vacuum transfer. This system uses suction to move the DNA out of the gel and onto the membrane.

methods is the expense and maintenance of the electrophoresis and vacuum equipment.

After transfer, the cut, denatured DNA is avidly bound to the membrane. The DNA can be permanently immobilized to the membrane by baking in a vacuum oven (80°C, 30–60 minutes) or by uv cross-linking, that is, covalently attaching the DNA to the nitrocellulose using UV light energy. Baking or cross-linking covalently attaches the DNA to the membrane and prevents the DNA fragments from washing away or moving on the membrane during extended procedures or when sequential probings are to be done.

Following immobilization of the DNA, a **prehybridization** step is required to prevent the probe from binding to nonspecific sites on the membrane surface, which will cause high background noise. Prehybridization involves incubating the membrane in the same buffer in which the probe will subsequently be introduced or in a specially formulated prehybridization buffer. At this point, the buffer does not contain probe. Prehybridization buffer consists of such blocking agents as Denhardt solution (Ficoll, polyvinyl pyrrolidane, bovine serum albumin) and salmon sperm DNA. Sodium dodecyl sulfate (SDS, 0.01%) may also be included, along with formamide, the latter especially for RNA probes. The membrane is exposed to the prehybridization buffer at the optimal hybridization temperature for 30 minutes to several hours, depending on the specific protocol. At this stage the sample is ready for hybridization with the probe, which will allow visualization of the specific gene or region of interest.

Northern Blots

The **northern blot** is a modification of the Southern blot technique and was designed to investigate RNA structure and quantity. Although most northern analyses are performed to investigate levels of gene expression (transcription from DNA) and stability, the analyses are also used to investigate RNA structural abnormalities resulting from aberrations in synthesis or processing, such as **alternative splicing**. Splicing abnormalities are responsible for a number of diseases, such as beta-thalassemias and familial isolated growth hormone deficiency. Analysis of RNA structure and quantity indirectly reveals mutations in the regulatory or splicing signals in DNA.

An RNase-free environment must always be maintained for RNA preparation. After isolation and quantification of RNA, the samples (up to approximately 30 μg total RNA or 0.5–3.0 μg polyA RNA, depending on the relative abundance of the transcript under study) are applied directly to agarose gels. Agarose concentrations of 0.8%–1.5% are usually employed. Polyacrylamide gels may also be used, especially for smaller transcripts—for instance, for analysis of viral gene expression.[4] Gel electrophoresis of RNA must be carried out under denaturing conditions for accurate transcript size assessment (see Chapter 5, "Resolution and Detection of Nucleic Acids"). Complete denaturation is also required for efficient transfer of the RNA from the gel to the membrane, as with the transfer of DNA in the Southern blot. Because the denaturation is maintained during electrophoresis, a separate denaturation step is not required for northern blots. After electrophoresis, representative lanes can be cut from the gel, soaked in ammonium acetate to remove the denaturant, and stained with acridine orange or ethidium bromide to assess quality and equivalent sample loading (see Chapter 4, "Nucleic Acid Extraction Methods").

Denaturant such as formaldehyde must be removed from the gel before transfer because it inhibits binding of the RNA to nitrocellulose. This is accomplished by rinsing the gel in deionized water. RNA is transferred in 10X or 20X SSC or 10X SSPE (1.8 M NaCl, 0.1 M sodium phosphate, pH 7.7, 10 mM EDTA) to nitrocellulose as described above for DNA. 20X SSC should be used for small transcripts (500 bases or less). The blotting procedure for RNA in the northern blot is performed in 20X

SSC, similar to the procedure for DNA transfer in the Southern blot. Prehybridization and hybridization in formamide/SSC/SDS prehybridization/hybridization buffers are performed also as with Southern blot. If the RNA has been denatured in glyoxal, the membrane must be soaked in warm Tris buffer (65°C) to remove any residual denaturant immediately before prehybridization.

Western Blots

Another modification of the Southern blot is the **western blot**.[5] The immobilized target for a western blot is protein. There are many variations on western blots. Generally, serum, cell lysate, or extract is separated on SDS-polyacrylamide gels (SDS-PAGE) or isoelectric focusing gels (IEF). The former resolves proteins according to molecular weight, and the latter according to charge. Dithiothreitol or 2-mercaptoethanol may also be used to separate proteins into subunits. Polyacrylamide concentrations vary from 5% to 20%. Depending on the complexity of the protein and the quantity of the target protein, 1–50 μg of protein is loaded per well. Before loading, the sample is treated with denaturant, such as mixing 1:1 with 0.04 M Tris HCl, pH 6.8, 0.1% SDS. The accuracy and sensitivity of the separation can be enhanced by using a combination of IEF gels followed by SDS-PAGE or by using two-dimensional gel electrophoresis. Prestained molecular-weight standards are run with the samples to orient the membrane after transfer and to approximate the sizes of the proteins after probing. Standards ranging from 11,700 d (cytochrome C) to 205,000 d (myosin) are commercially available.

The gel system used may affect subsequent probing of proteins with antibodies. Specifically, denaturing gels could affect **epitopes** (antigenic sites on the protein) such that they will not bind with the labeled antibodies. Gel pretreatment with mild buffers such as 20% glycerol in 50 mM Tris-HCl, pH 7.4, can renature proteins before transfer.[6]

After electrophoresis, proteins are blotted to membranes by capillary or electrophoretic transfer. Nitrocellulose has high affinity for proteins and is easily treated with detergent (0.1% Tween 20 in 0.05 M Tris and 0.15 M sodium chloride, pH 7.6) to prevent binding of the **primary antibody** probe to the membrane itself (**blocking**) before hybridization. Binding of proteins to nitrocellulose is probably hydrophobic, as nonionic detergents can remove proteins from the membrane. Other membrane types used for protein blotting are PVDF and **anion** (DEAE) or cation (CM) exchange cellulose.

Probes

The probe for Southern and northern blots is a single-stranded fragment of nucleic acid attached to a signal-producing moiety. The purpose of the probe is to identify one or more sequences of interest within a large amount of nucleic acid. The probe therefore should hybridize

---

Advanced Concepts

Some protocols call for destaining of the RNA gel in sodium phosphate buffer (acridine orange) or 200 mM sodium acetate, pH 4.0 (ethidium bromide), before transfer. The latter destaining method may interfere with the movement of RNA from the gel during transfer. If formaldehyde has been used as a denaturant during electrophoresis, the gel must be rinsed and held in deionized water. Rinsing is not necessary if the formaldehyde concentration is less than 0.4 M.

Advanced Concepts

The western blot method is used to confirm enzyme-linked immunoassay results for human immunodeficiency virus (HIV) and hepatitis C virus among other organisms. In this procedure, known HIV proteins are separated by electrophoresis and transferred and bound to a nitrocellulose membrane. The patient's serum is overlaid on the membrane, and antibodies with specificity to HIV proteins bind to their corresponding protein antigens. Unbound patient antibodies are washed off, and binding of antibodies is detected by adding a labeled antihuman immunoglobulin antibody. If HIV antibodies are present in the patient's serum, they can be detected with antihuman antibody probes appearing as a dark band on the blot corresponding to the specific HIV protein to which the antibody is specific.

specifically with the target DNA or RNA that is to be analyzed. The probe can be RNA, denatured DNA, or other modified nucleic acids. **Peptide nucleic acids (PNAs)** and **locked nucleic acids** have also been used as probes. These structures contain normal nitrogen bases that can hybridize with complementary DNA or RNA, but the bases are connected by backbones different from the natural phosphodiester backbone of DNA and RNA. These modified nucleic acids are resistant to nuclease degradation and, because of a reduced negative charge on their backbone, can hybridize more readily to target DNA or RNA.

Probes for western blots are specific binding proteins or antibodies. A labeled **secondary antibody** directed against the primary binding protein is then used for the visualization of the protein band of interest.

DNA Probes

DNA probes are created in several ways. In early methods, a fragment of the gene to be analyzed was cloned on a bacterial plasmid and then isolated by restriction enzyme digestion and gel purification. The fragment, after labeling (see below) and denaturation, was then used in Southern or northern blot procedures.

Other sources of DNA probes include the isolation of a sequence of interest from viral genomes and in vitro organic synthesis of a piece of nucleic acid of a predetermined sequence. The latter is used only for short, oligomeric probes. Probes may also be synthesized using the polymerase chain reaction (PCR) (see Chapter 7, "Nucleic Acid Amplification") to generate large amounts of specific DNA sequences.

The length of the probe will, in part, determine the specificity of the hybridization reaction. Probe lengths range from tens to thousands of base pairs. In analysis of the entire genome in a Southern blot, longer probes are more specific for a DNA region because they must match a longer sequence on the target. Shorter probes are not usually used in Southern blots because short sequences are more likely to be found in multiple locations in the genome, resulting in high background binding to sequences not related to the target region of interest. Short probes are more appropriate for mutational analysis as they are sensitive to single-base mismatches (see Chapter 8, "Chromosomal Structure and Chromosomal Mutations").

The probe is constructed so that it has a complementary sequence to the targeted gene. In order to bind to the probe, then, the target nucleic acid has to contain the sequence of interest. Properly prepared and stored DNA probes are relatively stable. Double-stranded DNA probes must be denatured before use. This is usually accomplished by heating the probe (e.g., 95°C, 10–15 min) in hybridization solution or treating with 50% formamide/2X SSC at a lower temperature for a shorter time (e.g., 75°C, 5–6 min)

RNA Probes

RNA probes are often made by transcription from a synthetic DNA template in vitro. These probes are similar to DNA probes with equal or greater binding affinity to complementary sequences. Because RNA and DNA form a stronger helix than DNA/DNA, the RNA probes may offer more sensitivity than DNA probes in the Southern blot.

RNA probes can be synthesized directly from a plasmid template or from template DNA produced by PCR (see Chapter 7). Predesigned systems commercially available for this purpose include plasmid vector DNA, such as pGEM (Promega) or pBluescript (Stratagene), containing a binding site for RNA polymerase (promoter) and a cloning site for the sequences of interest, and a DNA-dependent RNA polymerase from *Salmonella* bacteriophage SP6 or *E. coli* bacteriophage T3 or T7. DNA sequences complementary to the RNA transcript to be analyzed are cloned into the plasmid vector using restriction enzymes. The recombinant vector containing the gene of interest is then linearized, and the RNA probe is transcribed in vitro from the promoter. The normal transcript can be used for Southern blots. For northern blots, the antisense transcript (complementary to the normal transcript on the blot) is generated by placing the fragment backwards so that the promoter starts at the end of the gene. RNA probes are labeled by incorporating a radioactive or modified nucleotide during the in vitro transcription process.

Either coding or complementary RNA will hybridize to a double-stranded DNA target. RNA probes for northern blots must be designed so that the probe is complementary to the target sequence. A probe of identical sequence to the target RNA (coding sequence) will not hybridize. Labeling during synthesis provides RNA probes with a high specific activity (signal to micrograms of probe) that increases the sensitivity of the probe. To avoid background noise, some protocols include digestion of nonhybridized RNA, using a specific RNase such as RNase A, after hybridization is complete.

RNA probes are generally less stable than DNA probes and cannot be stored for long periods. Synthesis of an RNA probe by transcription from a stored template is relatively simple and is easily performed within a few days of use. The DNA template can be removed from the probe by treatment with RNase-free DNase. Although RNA is already single-stranded, denaturation before use is recommended in order to eliminate secondary structure internal to the RNA molecule.

Other Nucleic Acid Probe Types

Peptide nucleic acid and locked nucleic acid probes (Figs. 6-9 and 6-10) are synthesized using chemical methods.[7–10] These modified nucleic acids have the advantage of being resistant to nucleases that degrade DNA and RNA by breaking the phosphodiester backbone. Further, the negative charge of the phosphodiester backbones of DNA and RNA counteract hydrogen bonding between the bases of the probe and target sequences. Structures such as PNA that do not have a negative charge hybridize more efficiently.

Protein Probes

Western blot protein probes are antibodies that bind specifically to the immobilized target protein. Polyclonal or monoclonal antibodies can be used for this purpose. **Polyclonal antibodies** are products of a generalized response to a specific antigen, usually a peptide or protein. Small molecules (**haptens**) attached to protein carriers, carbohydrates, nucleic acids, and even to whole cells and tissue extracts can be used to generate an antibody response. Adjuvants, such as Freund's adjuvant, enhance the antibody titer by slowing the degradation of the protein and lengthening the time the immune system is exposed to the stimulating antigen. Specific immunoglobulins are subsequently isolated from sera by affinity chromatography.

Polyclonal antibodies are comprised of a mixture of immunoglobulins directed at more than one epitope (molecular structure) on the antigen. **Monoclonal antibodies** are more difficult to produce. Kohler and Milstein first demonstrated that spleen cells from immunized mice could be fused with mouse myeloma cells to form hybrid cells (**hybridomas**) that could grow in culture and secrete antibodies.[11] By cloning the hybridomas (growing small cultures from single cells), preparations of specific antibodies could be produced continuously. The clones could then be screened for antibodies that best react with the target antigen. The monoclonal antibodies are isolated from cell culture fluid; higher titers of antibodies are obtained by inoculating the antibody-producing hybridoma into mice and collecting the peritoneal fluid. The monoclonal antibody is then isolated by chromatography.

Polyclonal antibodies are useful for immunoprecipitation methods and for western blots. With their greater specificity, monoclonal antibodies can be used for almost

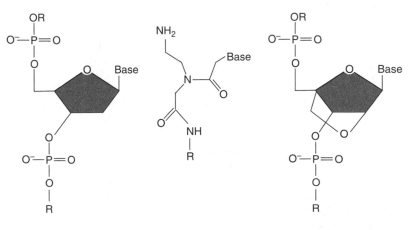

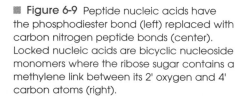

■ **Figure 6-9** Peptide nucleic acids have the phosphodiester bond (left) replaced with carbon nitrogen peptide bonds (center). Locked nucleic acids are bicyclic nucleoside monomers where the ribose sugar contains a methylene link between its 2' oxygen and 4' carbon atoms (right).

Advanced Concepts

Alternative nucleic acids are not only useful in the laboratory, they are also potentially valuable in the clinic. Several structures have been proposed for use in antisense gene therapy (Fig. 6-10). Introduction of sequences complementary to messenger RNA of a gene (antisense sequences) will prevent translation of that mRNA and expression of that gene. If this could be achieved in whole organisms, selected aberrantly expressed genes or even viral genes could be turned off. One drawback of this technology is the degradation of natural RNA and DNA by intracellular nucleases. The nuclease-resistant structures are more stable and available to hybridize to the target mRNA.

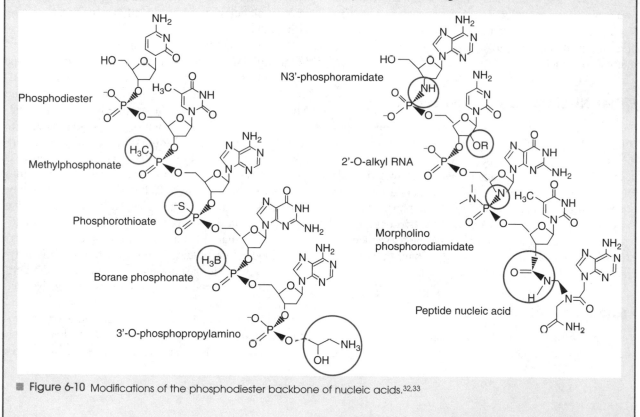

■ **Figure 6-10** Modifications of the phosphodiester backbone of nucleic acids.[32,33]

any procedure. In western blot technology, polyclonal antibodies can give a more robust signal, especially if the target epitopes are partially lost during electrophoresis and transfer. Monoclonal antibodies are more specific and may give less background noise; however, if the targeted epitope is lost, these antibodies do not bind and no signal is generated. Dilution of primary antibody can range from 1/100 to 1/100,000, depending on the sensitivity of the detection system.

Probe Labeling

In order to visualize the probe bound to target fragments on a membrane, the probe must be labeled and generate a detectable signal. In the past, classical Southern analysis methods called for radioactive labeling with ^{32}P. This labeling was achieved by introduction of nucleotides containing radioactive phosphorus to the probe. Today, many medical laboratories now use nonradioactive labeling to avoid the hazard and expense of working with radiation. Nonradioactive labeling methods are based on indirect detection of a tagged nucleotide incorporated in or added to the probe. The two most commonly used nonradioactive tags are **biotin** and **digoxygenin** (Fig. 6-11), either of which can be attached covalently to a nucleotide triphosphate, usually UTP or CTP.

There are three basic methods that are used to label a DNA probe: end labeling, nick translation, and random priming. In **end labeling**, labeled nucleotides are added to the end of the probe using terminal transferase or T4 polynucleotide kinase. In **nick translation**, the labeled nucleotides are incorporated into single-stranded breaks, or nicks, that are substrates for nucleotide addition by DNA polymerase. The polymerase uses the intact complementary strand for a template and displaces the previously hybridized strand as it extends the nick. **Random priming** generates new single-stranded versions of the probe with the incorporation of the labeled nucleotides. The synthesis of these new strands is primed by oligomers of random sequences that are 6 to 10 bases in length. These short sequences will, at some frequency, complement sequences in the denatured probe and prime synthesis of copies of the probe sequences with incorporated labeled nucleotides.

RNA probes are transcribed from cloned DNA or amplified DNA. These probes are labeled during their synthesis with radioactive, biotinylated, or digoxygenin-tagged nucleotides. Unlike double-stranded complementary DNA probes and targets that contain both strands of the complementary sequences, RNA probes are single-stranded with only one strand of the complementary sequence represented.

Nucleic Acid Probe Design

The most critical parts of any hybridization procedure are the design and optimal hybridization of the probe, both of which determine the specificity of the results. With nucleic acids, the more optimal the hybridization conditions for a probe/target interaction, the more specific the probe. Longer probes (500–5000 bp) offer greater specificity with decreased background noise, as they are less affected by point mutations or polymorphisms within the target sequence or within the probe itself. Long probes, however, may be difficult or expensive to synthesize.

Shorter probes (<500 bp) are less specific than longer ones in Southern blotting applications. A short sequence has a higher chance of being repeated randomly in unrelated regions of the genome. Short probes are ideal, however, for mutation analysis, as their binding affinity is sensitive to single base-pair changes within a target binding sequence.

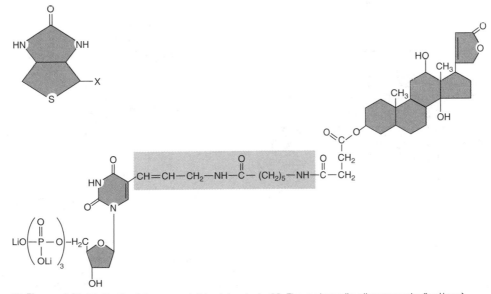

■ **Figure 6-11** Biotin (top) has a variable side chain (X). The polycyclic digoxygenin (bottom) is shown covalently attached to UTP (dig-11-UTP). This molecule can be covalently attached or incorporated into DNA or RNA to make a labeled probe.

Advanced Concepts

Protein probes used in western blot applications may be labeled with ^{35}S for radioactive detection. For nonradioactive detection, western protein probes can be covalently bound to an enzyme, usually horseradish peroxidase (HRP) or alkaline phosphatase. When exposed to a light- or color-generating substrate, the enzyme will produce a detectable signal on the membrane or on an autoradiogram. Unconjugated antibodies can be detected after binding with a conjugated secondary antibody to the primary probe, such as mouse antihuman or rabbit antimouse antibodies (Fig. 6-12). The secondary antibodies will recognize any primary antibody by targeting the FC region.

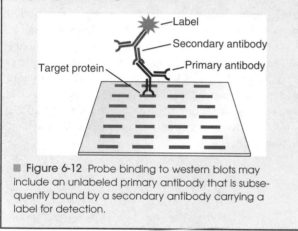

■ **Figure 6-12** Probe binding to western blots may include an unlabeled primary antibody that is subsequently bound by a secondary antibody carrying a label for detection.

The sequence of the probe can affect its binding performance as well. A sequence with numerous internal complementary sequences will fold and hybridize with itself, which will compete with hybridization to the intended target. The probe folding or secondary structure is especially strong in sequences with high GC content, decreasing the binding efficiency to the target sequence and, therefore, the test sensitivity.

Hybridization Conditions, Stringency

Southern blot and northern blot probing conditions must be empirically optimized for each nucleic acid target.

Stringency is the combination of conditions under which the target is exposed to the probe. Conditions of high stringency are more demanding of probe/target complementarity and length. Low stringency conditions are more forgiving. If conditions of stringency are set too high, the probe will not bind to its target. If conditions are set too low, the probe will bind unrelated targets, complicating interpretation of the final results.

Several factors affect stringency. These include temperature of hybridization, salt concentration of the hybridization buffer, and the concentration of denaturant such as formamide in the buffer. The length and nature of the probe sequence can also influence the level of stringency. A long probe or one with a higher percentage of G and C bases will bind under more stringent conditions than a short probe or one with greater numbers of A and T bases will bind. The ideal hybridization conditions are estimated from calculation of the **melting temperature**, or T_m, of the probe sequence. The T_m is a way to express the amount of energy required to separate the hybridized strands of a given sequence (Fig. 6-13). At the T_m, half of the sequence is double-stranded and half is single-stranded. The T_m for a double-stranded DNA sequence in solution is calculated by the following formula:

$$T_m = 81.5°C + 16.6 \log M + 0.41 \,(\% \, G + C)$$
$$- \,0.61 \,(\% \text{ formamide}) - (600/n)$$

where M = sodium concentration in mol/L and n = number of base pairs in the shortest duplex.

RNA:RNA hybrids are more stable than DNA:DNA hybrids due to less constraint by the RNA phosphodiester backbone. DNA:RNA hybrids have intermediate affinity.

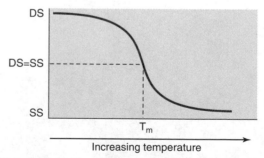

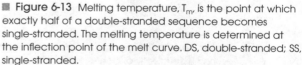

■ **Figure 6-13** Melting temperature, T_m, is the point at which exactly half of a double-stranded sequence becomes single-stranded. The melting temperature is determined at the inflection point of the melt curve. DS, double-stranded; SS, single-stranded.

The formulae for RNA:RNA or DNA:RNA hybrids, therefore, are slightly different from the formula for a DNA:DNA helix. The melting temperature will also be different if PNA or other alternative nucleic acids are used as probes.[12]

The T_m is also a function of the extent of complementarity between the sequence of the probe and that of the target sequence. For each 1% difference in sequence, the T_m decreases 1.5°C. Furthermore, since the T_m of RNA probes is higher, RNA:DNA hybrids increase T_m by 10°–15°C. RNA:RNA hybrids increase T_m by 20°–25°C.

The T_m for short probes (14–20 bases) can be calculated by a simpler formula:

$$T_m = 4°C \times \text{number of GC pairs} + 2°C \\ \times \text{number of AT pairs}$$

The hybridization temperature of oligonucleotide probes is about 5°C below the melting temperature.

The effect of sequence complexity on hybridization efficiency can be illustrated by the **C_0t value**. **Sequence complexity** is the length of unique (nonrepetitive) nucleotide sequences. After denaturation, complex sequences require more time to reassociate than simple sequences, such as polyA:polyU. C_0t is an expression of the sequence complexity (Fig. 6-14). C_0t is equal to the initial DNA concentration (C_0) times the time required to reanneal it (t). **$C_0t_{1/2}$** is the time required for half of a double-stranded sequence to anneal under a given set of conditions.

Advanced Concepts

C_0t was used to demonstrate that mammalian DNA consisted of sequences of varying complexity. Britten and Kohne[13] used *Escherichia coli* and calf thymus DNA to demonstrate this complexity. When they measured reassociation of *E. coli* DNA vs. time, a sigmoid curve was observed, as expected for DNA molecules with equal complexity. In comparison, the calf DNA reassociation was multifaceted and spanned several orders of magnitude (see Fig. 6-14). The spread of the curve results from the mixture of slowly renaturing unique sequences and rapidly renaturing repeated sequences (satellite DNA).

T_m and C_0t values can provide a starting point for optimizing stringency conditions for Southern or northern blot analysis. Hybridization at a temperature 25°C below the T_m for 1–3 $C_0t_{1/2}$ is considered optimal for a double-stranded DNA probe. Final conditions must be established empirically, especially for short probes. Stringency conditions for routine analyses, once established, will be used for all subsequent assays. In the event a component of the procedure is altered, new conditions may have to be established.

Hybridizations are generally performed in hybridization bags or in glass cylinders. Within limits, the sensitivity of the analysis increases with increased probe concentration. Because the probe is the limiting reagent, it is practical to keep the volume of the hybridization solution low. The recommended volume of hybridization buffer is approximately 10 mL/100 cm^2 of membrane surface area.

Formamide in the hybridization buffer effectively lowers the optimal hybridization temperature. This is especially useful for RNA probes and targets that, because of secondary structure, are more difficult to denature and tend to have a higher renaturation (hybridization) temperature. Incubation of the hybridization system in sealed bags in a water bath or in capped glass cylinders in rotary ovens maintains the entire membrane surface area at a constant temperature.

Short probes (<20 bases) can hybridize in 1 to 2 hours. In contrast, longer probes require much longer hybridization times. For Southern and northern blots with probes

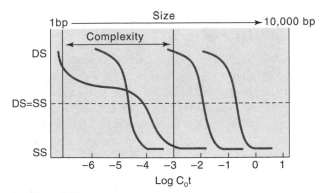

■ Figure 6-14 Reannealing of single-stranded (SS) DNA to double-stranded (DS) DNA vs. time at a constant concentration yields a sigmoid curve. The complexity of the DNA sequence will widen the sigmoid curve. Increasing the length of the double-stranded DNA will shift the curve to the right.

Advanced Concepts

The nature of the probe label will affect hybridization conditions. Unlike ^{32}P labeling, the bulky nonradioactive labels (see Fig. 6-12) disturb the hybridization of the DNA chain. The temperature of hybridization with these types of probes will be lower than that used for radioactively labeled probes.

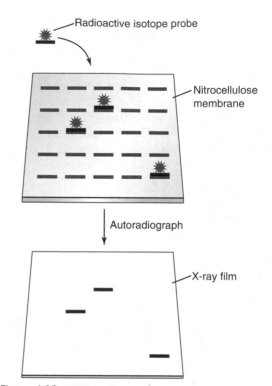

Figure 6-15 A DNA or RNA probe labeled with radioactive phosphorous atoms (^{32}P or ^{33}P) hybridized to target (homologous) sequences on a nitrocellulose membrane. The fragments to which the probe is bound can be detected by exposing autoradiography film to the membrane.

>1000 bases in length, incubation is carried out for 16 hours or more. Raising the probe concentration can increase the hybridization rates. Also, inert polymers, such as dextran sulfate, polyethylene glycol, or polyacrylic acid, accelerate the hybridization rates for probes longer than 250 bases.

Detection Systems

This chapter has so far addressed the transfer of gel-separated DNA, RNA, or protein to a solid membrane support and hybridization or binding of a specific probe to the target sequence of interest. The next step is to detect whether the probe has bound to the immobilized target and, if it has bound, the relative location of the binding. The original ^{32}P-labeled probes offered the advantages of simple and sensitive detection. After hybridization, unbound probe is washed off and the blot is exposed to light-sensitive film to detect the fragments that are hybridized to the radioactive probe (Fig. 6-15). Wash conditions must be formulated so that only completely hybridized probe remains on the blot. Typically, wash conditions are more stringent than those used for hybridization.

Nonradioactive detection systems require a more involved detection procedure. For most nonradioactive systems, the probe is labeled with a nucleotide covalently attached to either digoxygenin or biotin. The labeled nucleotide is incorporated into the nucleotide chain of the probe by in vitro transcription, nick translation, primer extension, or addition by terminal transferase. After a digoxygenin- or biotin-labeled probe is hybridized with the blot with sample(s) containing the target sequence of interest, unbound probe is washed away. Then, antidigoxygenin antibody or streptavidin, respectively,

Advanced Concepts

Optimization may not completely eliminate all non-specific binding of the probe. This will result in extra bands in control lanes or cross-hybridizations. At a given level of stringency, any increase to eliminate cross-hybridization will lower the binding to the intended sequences. It becomes a matter of balancing the optimal probe signal with the least amount of nontarget binding. Cross-hybridizations are usually recognizable as bands of the same size in multiple runs. It is important to take cross-hybridization bands into account in the final interpretation of the assay results.

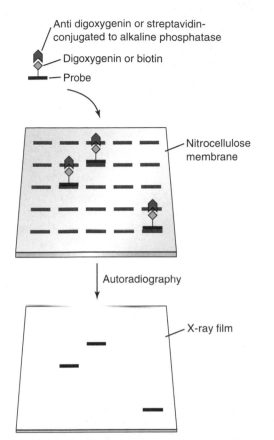

Anti digoxygenin or streptavidin-conjugated to alkaline phosphatase

Digoxygenin or biotin

Probe

Nitrocellulose membrane

Autoradiography

X-ray film

■ **Figure 6-16** Indirect nonradioactive detection. The probe is covalently attached to digoxygenin or biotin. After hybridization, the probe is bound by antibodies to digoxygenin or streptavidin conjugated to alkaline phosphatase (AP). This complex is exposed to color or light-producing substrates of AP, producing color on the membrane or light detected with autoradiography film.

conjugated to alkaline phosphatase (AP conjugate, Fig. 6-16) is added to the reaction mix to bind to the digoxigenin- or biotin-labeled probe:target complex. HRP conjugates may also be used in this procedure.

Advanced Concepts

In addition to CSPD and CDP-star (Roche Diagnostics Corp.), there are several substrates for chemiluminescent detection that are 1–2 dioxetane derivatives such as 3-(2'-spiroadamantane)-4-methoxy-4-(3'-phosphoryloxy) phenyl-1,2-dioxetane (AMPPD; Tropix, Inc.). Dephosphorylation of these compounds by the alkaline phosphatase conjugate bound to the probe on the membrane results in a light-emitting product (see Fig. 6-17).[14] Other luminescent molecules include acridinium ester and acridinium (*N*-sulfonyl) carboxamide labels, isoluminol, and electrochemiluminescent ruthenium trisbipyridyl labels.

The substrate used most often for chromogenic detection is a mixture of Nitroblue tetrazolium (NBT) and 5-bromo-4-chloro-3-indolyl phosphate (BCIP). Upon dephosphorylation of BCIP by **alkaline phosphatase**, it is oxidized by NBT to give a dark blue indigo dye as an oxidation product. BCIP is reduced in the process and also yields a blue product (see Fig. 6-18).

After the binding of the conjugate, and the washing away of unbound conjugate, the membrane is bathed in a solution of substrate that, when dephosphorylated by AP or oxidized by HRP, produces a signal. Substrates frequently used are dioxetane or tetrazolium dye derivatives, which generate chemiluminescent (Fig. 6-17) or color (Fig. 6-18) signals, respectively (see Table 6.2).

As with radioactive detection, the chemiluminescent signal produced by the action of the enzyme on dioxetane develops in the dark by autoradiography. The release of light by phosphorylation of dioxetane occurs at the

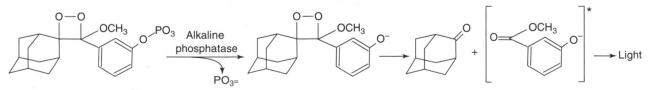

■ **Figure 6-17** Light is emitted from 1-2 dioxetane substrates after dephosphorylation by alkaline phosphatase to an unstable structure. This structure releases an excited anion that emits light.

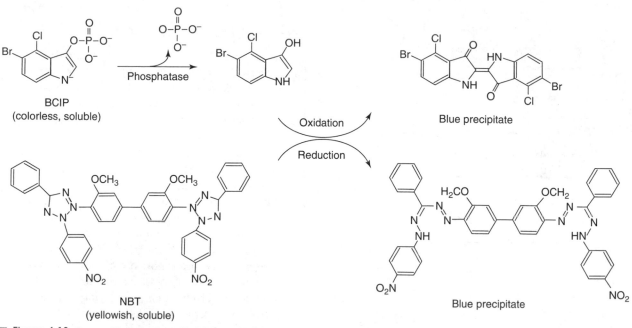

■ **Figure 6-18** Generation of color with BCIP and NBT. Alkaline phosphatase dephosphorylates BCIP, which then reduces NBT, making an insoluble blue precipitate.

location on the membrane where the probe is bound and darkens the light-sensitive film. Chemiluminescent detection is often stronger and develops faster than radioactive detection. A disadvantage of chemiluminescent detection is that it is harder to control and sometimes produces non-specific signals. New substrates have been designed to minimize these drawbacks. Unlike radioactive detection, in which testing the membrane with a Geiger counter can give an indication of how "hot" the bands are and consequently how long to expose the membrane to the film, chemiluminescent detection may require developing films at different intervals to determine the optimum exposure time.

Table 6.2 **Nonradioactive Detection Systems**

Type of Detection	Enzyme	Reagent	Reaction Product
Chromogenic	HRP	4-chloro-1-naphthol (4CN)	Purple precipitate
	HRP	3,3'-diaminobenzidine	Dark brown precipitate
	HRP	3,3',5,5',-tetramethylbenzidine	Dark purple stain
	Alkaline phosphatase	5-bromo-4-chloro-3-indolyl phosphate/nitroblue tetrazolium	Dark blue stain
Chemiluminescent	HRP	Luminol/H_2O_2/p-iodophenol	Blue light
	Alkaline phosphatase	1–2 dioxetane derivatives	Light
	Alkaline phosphatase	Disodium 3-(4-methoxyspiro {1,2-dioxetane-3,2'-(5'-chloro) tricyclo[3.3.1.1^{3,7}]decan} 4-yl)-1-phenyl phosphate and derivatives (CSPD, CDP-Star)	Light

For chromogenic detection, color is produced when the enzyme interacts with a derivative of a tetrazolium dye and is detected directly on the membrane. The advantage of this type of detection is that the color can be observed as it develops and the reaction stopped at a time when there is an optimum signal-to-background ratio. In general, chromogenic detection is not as sensitive as chemiluminescent detection and can also result in background noise, especially with probes labeled by random priming.

The key to a successful blotting method is a high **signal-to-noise ratio**. Ideally, the probe and detection systems should yield a specific and robust signal. High specific signal, however, may be accompanied by background noise. Blocking agents are used with nonradioactive detection systems to avoid nonspecific binding of conjugate to the membrane; however, blocking cannot be so strong that it interferes with specific binding of the conjugate to the probe. Therefore, specificity of detection may be sacrificed to get a stronger signal. Conversely, sensitivity may be sacrificed to generate a more specific signal.

Interpretation of Results

When a specific probe binds to its target immobilized on a membrane, the binding is detected as described in the previous section, with the end result being the visualization of a "band" on the membrane or film. A band is seen as a line running across the width of the lane.

Analysis of bands, that is, presence or absence or location in the lane, produced by Southern blot can be straightforward or complex, depending on the sample and the design of the procedure. Figure 6-19 is a depiction of a Southern blot result. The bands shown can be visualized either on a membrane or on an autoradiographic film, depending on the type of detection system. If a gene locus has a known restriction pattern, for instance, in lane 1, then samples can be tested to compare their restriction patterns. In Figure 6-19, the sample in lane 3 has the identical pattern; that is, both lanes have the same number of bands and the bands are all in the same location on the autoradiogram and are likely to be very similar if not identical in sequence to the sample in lane 1. Southern blot cannot detect tiny deletions or insertions of nucleotides or single nucleotide differences unless they affect a restriction enzyme site. For some assays, cross-hybridization may confuse results. These

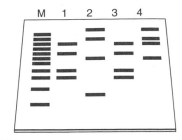

Figure 6-19 Example of a Southern blot result. The first lane (M) contains molecular-weight markers. Restriction digests of a genetic region can be compared to determine differences in structure. Two samples with the same pattern (for example, lanes 1 and 3) can be considered genetically similar.

artifacts can be identified by their presence in every lane at a constant size.

Northern (or western) blots are usually used for analysis of gene expression, although they can also be used to analyze transcript size, transcript processing, and protein modification. For these analyses, especially when estimating expression, it is important to include an internal control to correct for errors in isolation, gel loading, and transfer of samples. The amount of expression is then determined relative to the internal control (Fig. 6-20). In the example shown, the target transcript or protein product (top bands in all lanes, indicated by the arrow) is expressed in increasing amounts, left to right. The internal standardized control (lower bands in all lanes) assures that a sample has low expression of target transcript

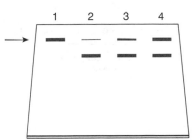

Figure 6-20 Example of a northern or western blot result. Lane 1 contains a positive control transcript or protein (arrow) to verify the probe specificity and target size. Molecular-weight markers can also be used to estimate size as in Southern analysis. The amount of gene product (expression level) is determined by the intensity of the signal from the test samples relative to a control gene product (lower band in lanes 2–4). The control transcript is used to correct for any differences in isolation or loading from sample to sample.

or protein product and that the low signal is not due to technical difficulties.

Array-Based Hybridization

Dot/Slot Blots

There are many variations on hybridization configurations. In cases where the determination of the size of the target is not required, DNA and RNA can be more quickly analyzed using dot blots or slot blots. These procedures are applied to expression, mutation, and amplification/deletion analyses.

For dot or slot blots, the target DNA or RNA is deposited directly on the membrane by means of various devices, some with vacuum systems. A pipet can be used for procedures testing only a few samples. For **dot blots**, the target is deposited in a circle or dot. For **slot blots**, the target is deposited in an oblong bar (Fig. 6-21). Slot blots are more accurate for quantitation by densitometry scanning because they eliminate the error that may arise from scanning through a circular target. Dot blots are useful for multiple qualitative analyses where many targets are being compared, such as in mutational screening.

Dot and slot blots are performed most efficiently on less complex samples, such as PCR products or selected mRNA preparations. Without gel resolution of the target fragments, it is important that the probe hybridization conditions be optimized because cross-hybridizations cannot be definitively distinguished from true target identification.

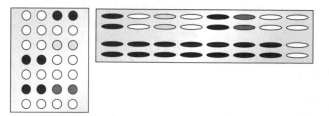

■ Figure 6-21 Example configuration of a dot blot (left) and a slot blot (right). The target is spotted in duplicate, side by side, on the dot blot. The last two rows of spots contain positive, sensitivity, and negative control followed by a blank with no target. The top two rows of the slot blot gel on the left represent four samples spotted in duplicate, with positive, sensitivity, and negative control followed by a blank with no target in the last four samples on the right. The bottom two rows represent a loading or normalization control that is often useful in expression studies to confirm that equal amounts of DNA or RNA were spotted for each test sample.

A negative control (DNA of equal complexity but without the targeted sequence) serves as the baseline for interpretation of these assays. When performing expression analysis by slot or dot blots, it is also important to include an amplification or normalization control, as shown on the slot blot in Figure 6-21. This allows correction for loading or sample differences. This control can also be analyzed on a separate, duplicate membrane to avoid cross-reactions between the test and control probes.

Genomic Array Technology

Array technology is a type of hybridization analysis allowing simultaneous study of large numbers of targets (or samples). Arrays are applied to gene (DNA) amplification or deletion on comparative genome hybridization arrays and to gene expression (RNA or protein) analysis on expression arrays. There are several approaches to array technology, including **macroarrays**, microarrays, high-density oligonucleotide arrays, and **microelectronic arrays**.

Macroarrays

In contrast to northern and Southern blots, dot (and slot) blots offer the ability to test and analyze larger numbers of samples at the same time. These methodologies are limited, however, by the area of the substrate material, nitrocellulose membranes, and the volume of hybridization solution required to provide enough probe to produce an adequate signal for interpretation. In addition, although up to several hundred test samples can be analyzed simultaneously on a dot blot, those samples can be tested for only one gene or gene product.

A variation of this technique is the **reverse dot blot**, in which many different probes are immobilized on the membrane and the test sample is labeled for hybridization with the immobilized probes. In this configuration, the terminology can be confusing. Immobilized probe is now effectively the target, and the labeled specimen DNA, RNA, or protein is actually the probe(s). Regardless of the designation, the general idea is that a known sequence is immobilized at a known location on the blot and the amount of sample that hybridizes to it is determined by the signal from the labeled sample.

Macroarrays are reverse dot blots of up to several thousand targets on nitrocellulose membranes. Radioactive or chemiluminescent signals are typically used to detect hybridization of a labeled sample to the target probes on the membrane. Macroarrays are created by spotting multiple probes onto nitrocellulose membranes. The hybridization of labeled sample material is read by eye or with a phosphorimager (a quantitative imaging device that uses storage **phosphor** technology instead of x-ray film). Analysis involves comparison of signal intensity from test and control samples spotted on duplicate membranes.

Although macroarrays greatly increase the capacity to assess numerous targets, this system is still limited by the area of the membrane and the specimen requirements. As the target number increases, the volume of sample material required increases. This limits the utility of this method for small amounts of test material, especially as might be encountered with clinical specimens.

Microarrays

In 1987, treated glass instead of nitrocellulose or nylon membranes for the production of arrays was introduced, increasing the versatility of array applications. With improved spotting technology and the ability to deposit very small target spots on glass substrates, the macroarray evolved into the **microarray**. Tens of thousands of targets can be screened simultaneously in a very small area by miniaturizing the deposition of droplets (Fig. 6-22). Automated depositing systems (arrayers) can place more than 80,000 spots on a glass substrate the size of a microscope slide. The completion of the rough draft of the human genome sequence revealed that the human genome may consist of fewer than 30,000 genes. Thus, even with spotting representative sequences of each gene in triplicate, simultaneous screening of the entire human genome on a single chip is within the scope of array technology.

Advanced Concepts

The first automated arrayer was described in 1995 by Patrick Brown at Stanford University.[15] This and later versions of automated arrayers used pen-type contact to place a dot of probe material onto the substrate. Modifications of this technology include the incorporation of ink-jet printing systems to deposit specific targets at designated positions using thermal, solenoid, or piezoelectric expulsion of target material (see Fig. 6-22).

The larger nitrocellulose membrane of the macroarray, then, is replaced by a glass microscope slide of the microarray. The slide carrying the array of targets is sometimes referred to as a chip (Fig. 6-23). This chip has led to some confusion of microarray technology with lab-on-a-chip technology. Lab-on-a-chip is a system of channels and reservoirs etched into glass or other material where chemical reactions can take place. It has no relationship to microarray chips in this regard.

Array targets immobilized on the glass slide are usually DNA—either cDNAs, PCR products, or oligomers—however, targets can be DNA, RNA, or protein. Targets are spotted in triplicate and spaced across the chip to avoid any geographic artifacts that may occur from uneven hybridization or other technical problems. Test samples are usually cDNA-generated from sample RNA but can, as well, be genomic DNA, RNA, or protein.

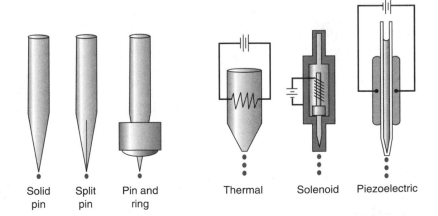

■ Figure 6-22 Pen-type (left) and ink-jet (right) technologies used to spot arrays.

Solid pin   Split pin   Pin and ring   Thermal   Solenoid   Piezoelectric

Advanced Concepts

The study of the entire genome or sets of related genes is the field of **genomics**. Knowing the combinatorial and interrelated functions of gene products, observing the behavior of sets of genes or genomes is a more accurate method for analyzing biological states or responses. The complete set of transcripts encoded by a genome is the **transcriptome**, and the set of encoded proteins is the **proteome**. One gene can encode multiple transcripts so that the transcriptome is more complex than the genome. One transcript can give rise to more than one protein, making the proteome even more complex. Stanley Fields[16] predicted that the proteome is likely to be 10 times more complex than the genome. The study of entire sets of proteins, or **proteomics**, is facilitated by array technology using antigen/antibody or receptor/ligand binding in the array format and mass spectrometry.

Another method used to deposit targets on chips is DNA synthesis directly on the glass or silicon support.[17] This technique uses sequence information to design oligonucleotides and to selectively mask, activate, and covalently attach nucleotides at designated positions on the chip. Proprietary photolithography techniques (Affymetrix) allow for highly efficient synthesis of short oligomers (10–25 bases long) on high-density arrays (Fig. 6-24). These oligomers are then probed with labeled fragments of the test sequences. Using this technology, hundreds of thousands of targets can be applied to chips. These types of arrays are called **high-density oligonucleotide arrays** and are used for mutation analysis, single nucleotide polymorphism analysis, and sequencing.

Sample preparation for array analysis requires fluorescent labeling of the test sample, as microarrays and other high-density arrays are read by automated fluorescent detection systems. The most frequent labeling method used for RNA is synthesis of cDNA or RNA copies with incorporation of labeled nucleotides. For DNA, random priming or nick translation is used. Several alternative methods have also been developed.[18]

For gene expression analyses, target probes immobilized on the chips are hybridized with labeled mRNA from treated cells or different cell types to assess the expression activity of the genes represented on the chip. Arrays used for this application are classified as **expression arrays**.[19] Expression arrays measure transcript or protein production relative to a reference control isolated from untreated or normal specimens (Fig. 6-25).[20]

In contrast, **comparative genome hybridization** (array CGH) is designed to test DNA. This method is used to screen the genome or specific genomic loci for deletions and amplifications.[21] In this method, genomic

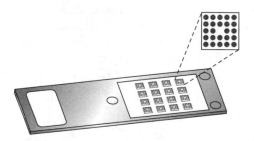

■ **Figure 6-23** Microarray, or DNA chip, is a glass slide carrying 384 spots. Arrays are sometimes supplied with fluorescent nucleotides for use in labeling the test samples and software for identification of the spots on the array by the array reader.

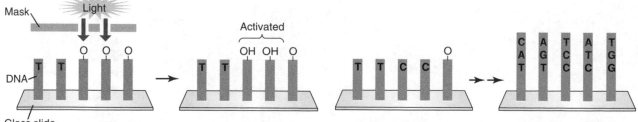

■ **Figure 6-24** Photolithographic target synthesis. A mask (left) allows light activation of the chip. When a nucleotide is added, only the activated spots will covalently attach it (center). The process is repeated until the desired sequences are generated at each position on the chip (right).

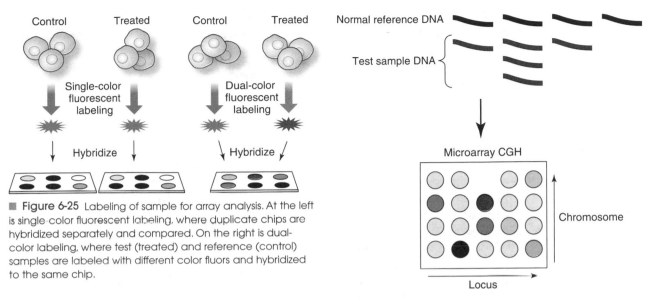

■ **Figure 6-25** Labeling of sample for array analysis. At the left is single-color fluorescent labeling, where duplicate chips are hybridized separately and compared. On the right is dual-color labeling, where test (treated) and reference (control) samples are labeled with different color fluors and hybridized to the same chip.

■ **Figure 6-26** Comparative genomic hybridization. Reference and test DNA are labeled with different fluors, represented here as black and green, respectively. After hybridization, excess green label indicates amplification of the test sample locus. Excess black label indicates deletion of the test sample locus. Neutral or gray indicates equal test and reference DNA.

DNA is isolated, fragmented, and labeled for hybridization on the chip (Fig. 6-26), which is analogous to the cytogenetic technique done on metaphase chromosomes (see Chapter 8, "Chromosomal Structure and Chromosomal Mutations"). Array CGH can provide higher resolution and more defined genetic information than traditional cytogenetic analysis, but it is limited to the analysis of loci represented on the chip. Genomic arrays can be performed on fixed tissue and limiting samples. Methods have been developed to globally amplify genomic DNA to enhance CGH analysis (see Chapter 7, "Nucleic Acid Amplification").[22,23]

Reading microarrays requires a fluorescent reader and analysis software. After correction for background noise and normalization with standards, the software averages signal intensity from duplicate or triplicate sample data. The results are reported as a relative amount of the reference and test signals. Depending on the program, variances of more than 2–3 standard deviations from 1 (test = reference) are considered an indication of significant increases (test/reference > 1) or decreases (test:reference < 1) in the test sample.

Several limitations of the array technology initially restrained the use of microarrays in the clinical laboratory. The lack of established standards and controls for optimal binding prevented the calibration of arrays from one laboratory to another, and not enough data had been accumulated to determine the degree of nonspecific

binding and cross-hybridization that might occur among and within a given set of sequences on an array. For instance, how much variation would result from comparing two normal samples together multiple times? Background noise can also affect the interpretation of array results. Furthermore, passive hybridization of thousands of different sequences results in different binding affinities under the same stringency conditions unless immobilized sequences are carefully designed to have similar melting temperatures. For mutation analysis, the length of the immobilized probe is limited due to the use of a single hybridization condition for all sequences. For gene expression applications, only relative, rather than absolute, quantitation is possible.

These and other concerns have been addressed to improve the reliability and consistency of array analysis. Baseline measurements, universal standards, and recommended controls are being established. Advances in microelectronics and microfluidics have also been applied to array design and manufacture.[24,25]

Arrays are seeing increased use in clinical laboratories due to improvements in price, applications, and availability of instrumentation. Premade chips increase opportunities for medical applications, from targeted pathway analysis to genomewide studies. Minimal sample requirements and comprehensive analysis with relatively small investments in time and labor are attractive features of array technology.

Bead Array Technology

Analysis of multiple targets in a single specimen is the key advantage of array technology. In microarrays, the probes are immobilized on a solid support. The probes may also be immobilized on beads, allowing hybridization of the targets in the bead suspension (Luminex Corp.). In this way, multiple suspensions can be tested simultaneously, for example, in each well of a 96-well plate, increasing the number of sample arrays that can be tested at one time. In order to distinguish specific probes carried on different beads, the beads are color-coded with a fluorescent dye. The sample is then labeled with a different dye so that the combination of the target and bead fluorescent signals indicates the presence or absence of a specific target. This technology can be used for protein as well as nucleic acid targets. Clinical tests using Luminex systems are available for infectious diseases and tissue typing (see Chapter 12, "Detection and Identification of Microorganisms," and Chapter 15, "DNA-Based Tissue Typing").

Solution Hybridization

In **solution hybridization**, neither the probe nor the target is immobilized. Probes and targets bind in solution, followed by resolution of the bound products. With the increasing interest in short interfering RNAs (siRNAs) and microRNAs (miRNAs), which are conveniently analyzed by this type of hybridization analysis, solution methods may come into more frequent use.

Solution hybridization has been used to measure mRNA expression, especially when there are low amounts of target RNA. One version of the method is called **RNase protection**, or S1 mapping, for the S1 single-strand–specific nuclease. In S1 mapping, the labeled probe is hybridized to the target sample in solution. After digestion of excess probe by a single-strand–specific nuclease, the resulting labeled, double-stranded fragments are resolved by polyacrylamide gel electrophoresis

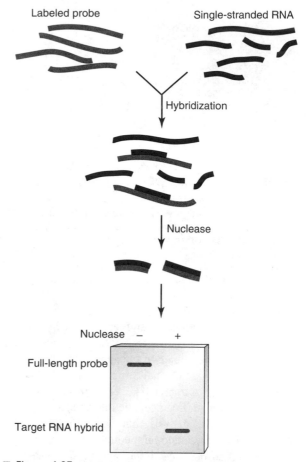

■ **Figure 6-27** Solution hybridization. Target RNAs are hybridized to a labeled RNA or DNA carrying the complementary sequence to the target. After digestion by a single strand-specific nuclease, only the target:probe double-stranded hybrid remains. The hybrid can be visualized by the label on the probe after electrophoresis.

(Fig. 6-27). S1 mapping is useful for determining the start point or termination point of transcripts.[26,27] This procedure is more sensitive than northern blotting because no target can be lost during electrophoresis and blotting. It is more applicable to RNA expression analysis due to limited sensitivity with double-stranded DNA targets.

In several variations of this type of analysis, DNA probe:RNA target hybrids are detected by capture on a solid support or beads rather than by electrophoresis.[28,29] For these "sandwich"-type assays, two probes are used, both of which hybridize to the target RNA. One probe, the capture probe, is biotinylated and will bind specifically to streptavidin immobilized on a plate or on magnetic beads. The other probe, called the detection probe, is detected by a monoclonal antibody directed against RNA:DNA hybrids or a covalently attached digoxygenin molecule used to generate a chromogenic or chemiluminescent signal (see "Detection Systems").

Solution hybridization can also be applied to the analysis of protein-protein interactions and to nucleic acid–binding proteins using a **gel mobility shift assay**.[30,31] After mixing the labeled DNA or protein with the test material, such as a cell lysate, a change in mobility, usually a shift to slower migration, indicates binding of a component in the test material to the probe protein or nucleic acid (Fig. 6-28). This assay has been used extensively to identify trans factors that bind to cis acting elements that control gene regulation. Solution hybridization can also be used to detect sequence changes in DNA or mutational analysis. These applications will be discussed in Chapter 9, "Gene Mutations."

Hybridization methods offer the advantage of direct analysis of nucleic acids at the sequence level without cloning of target sequences. The significance of hybridization methodology to clinical applications is the direct discovery of molecular genetic information from routine specimen types. A wide variety of modifications of the basic blotting methods have been and will be developed for clinical and research applications. Although amplification methods, specifically the polymerase chain reaction, have replaced many blotting procedures, a number of hybridization methods are still used in routine clinical analysis.

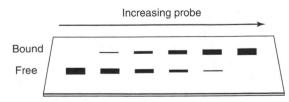

Increasing probe

Bound

Free

■ **Figure 6-28** Gel mobility shift assay showing protein-protein or protein-DNA interaction. The labeled test substrate is mixed with the probe in solution and then analyzed on a polyacrylamide gel. If the test protein binds the probe protein or DNA, the protein will shift up in the gel assay.

• STUDY QUESTIONS •

1. Calculate the melting temperature of the following DNA fragments using the sequences only:
   a. AGTCTGGGACGGCGCGGCAATCGCA
      TCAGACCCTGCCGCGCCGTTAGCGT
   b. TCAAAAATCGAATATTTGCTTATCTA
      AGTTTTTAGCTTATAAACGAATAGAT
   c. AGCTAAGCATCGAATTGGCCATCGTGTG
      TCGATTCGTAGCTTAACCGGTAGCACAC
   d. CATCGCGATCTGCAATTACGACGATAA
      GTAGCGCTAGACGTTAATGCTGCTATT

2. What is the purpose of denaturation of double-stranded target DNA after electrophoresis and prior to transfer in Southern blot?

3. Name two ways to permanently bind nucleic acid to nitrocellulose following transfer.

4. If a probe for Southern blot was dissolved in a hybridization buffer that contains 50% formamide, is the stringency of hybridization higher or lower than if there were no formamide?

5. If a high concentration of NaCl were added to a hybridization solution, how would the stringency be affected?

6. Does an increase in temperature from 65°C to 75°C during hybridization raise or lower stringency?

7. At the end of the Southern blot procedure, what would the autoradiogram show if the stringency was too high?

8. A northern blot is performed on an RNA transcript with the sequence GUAGGUATGUAUUUGGGCGC-GAACGCAAAA. The probe sequence is GUAG-GUATGUAUUUGGGCGCG. Will this probe hybridize to the target transcript?

9. In an array CGH experiment, three test samples were hybridized to three microarray chips. Each chip was spotted with eight gene probes (Genes A–H). Below

are results of this assay expressed as the ratio of test DNA to reference DNA. Are any of the eight genes consistently deleted or amplified in the test samples? If so, which ones?

Gene	Sample 1	Sample 2	Sample 3
A	1.06	0.99	1.01
B	0.45	0.55	0.43
C	1.01	1.05	1.06
D	0.98	1.00	0.97
E	1.55	1.47	1.62
F	0.98	1.06	1.01
G	1.00	0.99	0.99
H	1.08	1.09	0.90

10. What are two differences between CGH arrays and expression arrays?

References

1. Wei H, Therrien C, Blanchard A, Guan S, Zhu Z. The Fidelity Index provides a systematic quantitation of star activity of DNA restriction endonucleases. *Nucleic Acids Research* 2008;36:e50.
2. Robinson C, Sligar SG. Heterogeneity in molecular recognition by restriction endonucleases: Osmotic and hydrostatic pressure effects on BamHI, Pvu II, and EcoRV specificity. *Proceedings of the National Academy of Sciences* 1995;92:3444–3448.
3. Southern E. Detection of specific sequences among DNA fragments separated by gel electrophoresis. *Journal of Molecular Biology* 1975; 98:503–517.
4. Murthy S, Kamine J, Desrosiers RC. Viral-encoded small RNAs in herpes virus saimiri–induced tumors. *EMBO Journal* 1986;5(7):1625–1632.
5. Bowen B, Steinberg J, Laemmli UK, et al. The detection of DNA-binding proteins by protein blotting. *Nucleic Acids Research* 1980;8(1):1–20.
6. Dunn D. Effects of the modification of transfer buffer composition and the renaturation of proteins in gels on the recognition of proteins on western blots by monoclonal antibodies. *Analytical Biochemistry* 1986;157(1):144–153.
7. Koshkin AA, Nielson P, Rajwanshi VK, et al. Synthesis of the adenine, cytosine, guanine, 5-methlycysteine, thymine and uracil bicyclonucleoside monomers, oligomerisation, and unprecedented nucleic acid recognition. *Tetrahedron* 1998;54:3607–3630.
8. Singh SK, Koshkin AA, Wengel J. LNA (locked nucleic acids): Synthesis and high-affinity nucleic acid recognition. *Chemical Communications* 1998;4:455-456.
9. Buchardt O, Berg RH, Nielsen PE. Peptide nucleic acids and their potential applications in biotechnology. *Trends in Biotechnology* 1993;11(9):384–386.
10. Egholm M, Christensen L, Behrens C, et al. PNA hybridizes to complementary oligonucleotides obeying the Watson-Crick hydrogen-bonding rules. *Nature* 1993;365(6446):566–568.
11. Kohler G, Milstein C. Continuous cultures of fused cells secreting antibody of predefined specificity. *Nature* 1975;256:495–497.
12. Giesen U, Kleider W, Berding C, Geiger A, Orum H, Nielsen PE. A formula for thermal stability (T_m) prediction of PNA/DNA complexes. *Nucleic Acids Research* 1998;21:5004–5006.
13. Britten RJ. Repeated sequences in DNA. *Science.* 1968;161:529–540.
14. McCapra F. The chemiluminescence of organic compounds. *Quarterly Review of the Chemical Society* 1966; 20:485–510.
15. Schena M, Shalon D, Davis RW, et al. Quantitative monitoring of gene expression patterns with a complementary DNA microarray. *Science.* 1995;270:467–470.
16. Fields S. Proteomics: Proteomics in genomeland. *Science* 2001;291(5507):1221–1224.
17. Lipschultz RJ, Fodor TR, Gingeras DJ, et al. High-density synthetic oligonucleotide arrays. *Nature Genetics* 1999;21:20–24.
18. Richter A, Schwager C, Hentz S, et al. Comparison of fluorescent tag DNA labeling methods used for expression analysis by DNA microarrays. *BioTechniques* 2002;33(3):620–630.
19. Freeman W, Robertson DJ, Vrana KE. Fundamentals of DNA hybridization arrays for gene expression analysis. *BioTechniques* 2000;29(5):1042–1055.
20. Campbell MA. Department of Biology, DNA Microarray Methodology—Flash Animation. Davidson, NC: Davidson College, 28036. http://www.bio.davidson.edu/Courses/genomics/chip/chip.html 2001.
21. Oostlander A, Meijer GA, Ylstra B. Microarray-based comparative genomic hybridization and its applications in human genetics. *Clinical Genetics* 2004;66(6):488–495.

22. Huang Q, Schantz SP, Pulivarthi HR, et al. Improving degenerate oligonucleotide primed PCR comparative genomic hybridization for analysis of DNA copy number changes in tumors. *Genes, Chromosomes and Cancer* 2000;28:395–403.

23. Wang G, Maher E, Brennan C, et al. DNA amplification method tolerant to sample degradation. *Genome Research* 2004;14(11):2357–2366.

24. Edman CF, Raymond DK, Wu E, et al. Electric field–directed nucleic acid hybridization on microchips. *Nucleic Acids Research* 1997;25(24):4907–4914.

25. Sosnowski RG, Tu E, Butler WF, et al. Rapid determination of single base mismatch mutations in DNA hybrids by direct electric field control. *Proceedings of the National Academy of Sciences* 1997;94:1119–1123.

26. Squires C, Krainer A, Barry G, et al. Nucleotide sequence at the end of the gene for the RNA polymerase beta' subunit (rpoC). *Nucleic Acids Research* 1981;9(24):6827–6840.

27. Zahn K, Inui M, Yukawa H. Characterization of a separate small domain derived from the 5' end of 23S rRNA of an alpha-proteobacterium. *Nucleic Acids Research* 1999;27(21):4241–4250.

28. Rautio J, Barken KB, Lahdenperä J, et al. Sandwich hybridisation assay for quantitative detection of yeast RNAs in crude cell lysates. *Microbial Cell Factories* 2003;2:4–13.

29. Casebolt D, Stephenson CB. Monoclonal antibody solution hybridization assay for detection of mouse hepatitis virus infection. *Journal of Clinical Microbiology* 1992;30(3):608–612.

30. Malloy P. Electrophoretic mobility shift assays. *Methods in Molecular Biology* 2000; 130:235–246.

31. Park S, Raines RT. Fluorescence gel retardation assay to detect protein-protein interactions. *Methods in Molecular Biology* 2004;261:155–160.

32. Wickstrom E. DNA combination therapy to stop tumor growth. *Cancer Journal* 1998;4(suppl 1):S43.

33. Smith JB. Preclinical antisense DNA therapy of cancer in mice. *Methods in Enzymology* 1999;314:537–580.

34. Tanaka H, Fukuda N, Shoyama Y. Eastern blotting and immunoaffinity concentration using monoclonal antibody for ginseng saponins in the field of traditional chinese medicines. *Journal of Agricultural and Food Chemistry* 2007;55:3783–3787.

35. Taki T, Gonzalez TV, Goto-Inoue N, Hayasaka T, Setou M. TLC blot (far-eastern blot) and its applications. *Methods in Molecular Biology* 2009;536:545–556.

36. Ishikawa D, Taki T. Thin-layer chromatography blotting using polyvinylidene difluoride membrane (far-eastern blotting) and its applications. *Methods in Enzymology* 2000;312:145–157.

Chapter 7

Nucleic Acid Amplification

OBJECTIVES

- Compare and contrast among the following in vitro assays for amplifying **nucleic acids**: polymerase chain reaction (PCR), branched DNA amplification, ligase chain reaction, transcription-mediated amplification, and **Qβ replicase** with regard to type of target nucleic acid, principle, major elements of the procedure, type of amplicon produced, major enzyme(s) employed, and applications.

- Describe examples of modifications that have been developed for PCR.

- Discuss how amplicons are detected for each of the amplification methods.

- Design forward and reverse primers for a PCR, given the target sequence.

- Differentiate between target amplification and signal amplification.

Early analyses of nucleic acids were limited by the availability of material for analysis. Generating enough copies of a single gene required propagation of millions of cells in culture or isolation of large amounts of genomic DNA. If a gene had been cloned, many copies could be generated on bacterial plasmids, but this preparation was laborious, and some sequences were resistant to propagation in this manner.

The ability to amplify a specific DNA sequence opened the possibility of analyzing at the nucleotide level virtually any piece of DNA in nature. The first specific amplification method of any type was the **polymerase chain reaction (PCR)**. Other amplification methods have been developed based on making modifications to PCR. The methods that have been developed to amplify nucleic acids can be divided into three groups, based on whether the **target** nucleic acid itself, a probe specific for the target sequence, or the signal used to detect the target nucleic acid is amplified. These methods are discussed in this chapter.

Target Amplification

The **amplification** of nucleic acids by **target amplification** involves making copies of a target sequence to such a level (in the millions of copies) that they can be detected in vitro. This is analogous to growing cells in culture and allowing the cells to replicate their nucleic acid as well as themselves so that, for example, they can be visualized on an agar plate. Waiting for cells to replicate to detectable levels can take days to weeks or months, whereas replicating the nucleic acid in vitro only takes hours to days. PCR is the first and prototypical method for amplifying target nucleic acid.

Polymerase Chain Reaction

Kary Mullis visualized the idea of amplifying DNA in vitro in 1983 while driving one night on a California highway.[1,2] In the process of working through a mutation detection method, Mullis came upon a way to double his test target, a short region of double-stranded DNA, giving him 2^1, or 2, copies. If he repeated the process, the target would double again, giving 2^2, or 4, copies. After N doublings, he would have 2^N copies of his target. If $N = 30$ or 40, there would be millions of copies.

What Mullis had envisioned was the polymerase chain reaction (PCR). Over the next months in the laboratory, he synthesized short oligonucleotides (primers) complementary to sequences flanking a region of the human nerve growth factor and tried to amplify the region from human DNA, but the experiment did not work. Not sure of the nucleotide sequence information he had on the human gene, he tried a more defined target. The first successful amplification was a short fragment of the *Escherichia coli* plasmid, pBR322. The first paper describing a practical application, the amplification of beta-globin and analysis for diagnosis of patients with sickle cell anemia, was published 2 years later.[3] He called the method a "polymerase-catalyzed chain reaction" because DNA polymerase was the enzyme he used to drive the replication of DNA, and once it started the replication continued in a chain reaction. The name was quickly shortened to PCR. Since PCR was first performed, it has become increasingly user-friendly, more automated, and more amenable to use in a clinical laboratory, with infinite possible applications.

Basic PCR Procedure

When the cell replicates its DNA it requires the existing double-stranded DNA that serves as the **template** to give the order of the nucleotide bases, the deoxyribonucleotide bases themselves in the form of **deoxynucleotide triphosphates (dNTP)**—dATP, dGTP, dCTP, dTTP; DNA polymerase to catalyze the addition of nucleotides to the growing **strand**; and a primer (synthesized by primase in vivo) to which DNA polymerase adds subsequent bases (refer to Chapter 1, "DNA," for a detailed explanation).

PCR essentially duplicates the in vivo replication of DNA in vitro, using the same components (Table 7.1) to replicate DNA, with the same end result: one copy of double-stranded DNA becoming two copies (Fig. 7-1). In less than 2 hours, PCR can produce millions of copies, called **amplicons**, of DNA in contrast to days for a cell to produce the same number of copies in vivo. The real advantage of the PCR is the ability to amplify specific targets. Just as the Southern blot first allowed analysis of specific regions in a complex background, PCR presents the opportunity to amplify and effectively **clone** the target sequences. The amplified target, then, can be subjected to innumerable analytical procedures.

Table 7.1 **Components of a Typical PCR Reaction**

Component	Purpose
0.25 mM each primer (oligodeoxynucleotides)	Directs DNA synthesis to the desired region
0.2 mM each dATP, dCTP, dGTP, dTTP	Building blocks that extend the primers
50 mM KCl	Monovalent cation (salt), for optimal hybridization of primers to template
10 mM Tris, pH 8.4	Buffer to maintain optimal pH for the enzyme reaction
1.5 mM $MgCl_2$	Divalent cation, required by the enzyme
2.5 units polymerase	The polymerase enzyme that extends the primers (adds dNTPs)
10^2–10^5 copies of template	Sample DNA that is being tested

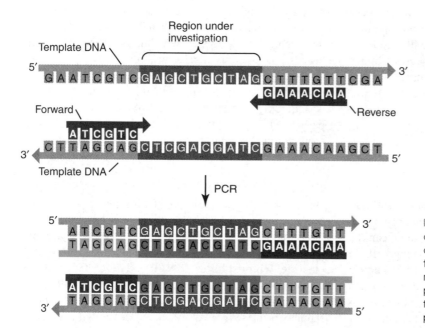

■ **Figure 7-1** The components and result of a PCR. Oligodeoxynucleotides (primers) are designed to hybridize to sequences flanking the DNA region under investigation. The polymerase extends the forward and reverse primers making many copies of the region flanked by the primer sequences, the PCR product.

The components of the PCR—DNA template, short oligonucleotide primers, nucleotides, polymerase, and buffers—are subjected to an **amplification program,** which consists of a specified number of **cycles** that are divided into steps during which the samples are held at particular temperatures for designated times. Table 7.2 shows the steps of a common three-step PCR cycle.

PCR starts with one double-stranded DNA target. In the first step (**denaturation**), the double-stranded DNA is denatured into two single strands (Fig. 7-2). This is accomplished by heating the sample at 94°C to 96°C for several seconds to several minutes, depending on the template. The initial denaturation step is lengthened for genomic or other large DNA template fragments. Subsequent denaturations can be shorter.

Historical Highlights

Kary Mullis was working at Cetus Corporation, where he synthesized short, single-stranded DNA molecules, or oligodeoxynucleotides (oligos), used by other laboratories. Mullis also tinkered with the oligos he made. One night, as he drove through the mountains of northern California, Mullis thought about a method he had designed to detect mutations in DNA. His scheme was to add radioactive dideoxynucleotides—ddATP, ddCTP, ddGTP, ddTTP—to four separate DNA synthesis reactions containing oligos, the test DNA template, and polymerase. In each reaction, the complementary oligo would hybridize to the template, and the polymerase would extend the oligo with the dideoxynucleotide, but only the dideoxynucleotide that was complementary to the next nucleotide in the template. He could then determine in which of the four tubes the oligo was extended with a radioactive ddNTP by gel electrophoresis.

He thought he might improve the method by using a double-stranded template and priming synthesis on both strands, instead of one at a time. Because the results of the synthesis reaction would be affected by contaminating deoxynucleotides (dNTPs) in the reagent mix, Mullis considered running a preliminary reaction without the ddNTPs to use up any dNTPs present. He would then heat the reaction to denature the dNTP-extended oligos and add an excess of unextended oligos and the ddNTPs. As he further considered the modification to his method, he realized that if the extension of an oligo in the preliminary reaction crossed the point where the other oligo was bound on the opposite strand, he would make a new copy of the region between the oligos. He considered the new copy and additional advantage, as it would improve the sensitivity of this method by doubling the target. Then, he thought, what if he did it again? The target would double again. If he added dNTPs intentionally he could do it over and over again.

In his own words: "I stopped the car at mile marker 46,7 on Highway 128. In the glove compartment I found some paper and a pen. I confirmed that two to the tenth power was about a thousand and that two to the twentieth power was about a million and that two to the thirtieth power was around a billion, close to the number of base pairs in the human genome. Once I had cycled this reaction thirty times I would be able to [copy] the sequence of a sample with an immense signal and almost no background."[4]

The next and most critical step for the specificity of the PCR is the **annealing** step. In the second step of the PCR cycle, the two oligonucleotide primers that will prime the synthesis of DNA anneal (hybridize) to complementary

Table 7.2 **Elements of a PCR Cycle**

Step	Temperature (°C)	Time (sec)
Denaturation	90–96	20–60
Annealing	50–70	20–90
Extension	68–75	10–60

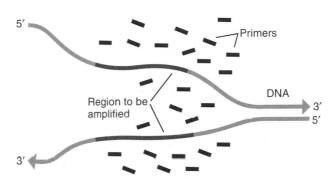

■ Figure 7-2 Denaturation of the DNA target. The region to be amplified is shown in dark green. The primers (black) are present in vast excess.

sequences on the template (Fig. 7-3). The primers dictate the part of the template that will be amplified; in other words, the primers determine the specificity of the amplification. It is important that the annealing temperature be optimized with the primers and reaction conditions. Annealing temperatures will range 50°C to 70°C and are usually established empirically. A starting point can be determined using the T_m of the primer sequences

Historical Highlights

Mullis's original method, using ddNTPs and oligos to detect mutations, is still in use today. Fluorescent polarization–template-directed dye terminator incorporation (described in Chapter 9, "Gene Mutations") uses fluorescently labeled ddNTPs to distinguish which ddNTP is added to the oligo. Another extension/termination assay, Homogeneous MassExtend, is a similar method, using mass spectrometry to analyze the extension products. Both of these methods were used in the Human Haplotype Mapping (HapMap) Project (see Chapter 11, "DNA Polymorphisms and Human Identification").

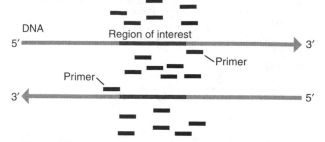

■ Figure 7-3 In the second step of the PCR cycle, annealing, the primers hybridize to their complementary sequences on each strand of the denatured template. The primers are designed to hybridize to the sequences flanking the region of interest.

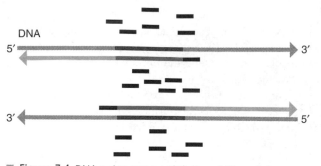

■ Figure 7-4 DNA polymerase catalyzes addition of deoxynucleotide triphosphates (dNTPs) to the primers, using the sample DNA as the template. This completes one PCR cycle. Note how in the original template there was one copy of the green region. Now, after one cycle, there are two copies.

(see Chapter 6, "Analysis and Characterization of Nucleic Acids and Proteins," for a discussion of stringency and hybridization). Reaction conditions, salt concentration, mismatches, template condition, and secondary structure will all affect the real T_m of the primers in the reaction.

The third and last step of the PCR cycle is the primer extension step (Fig. 7-4). This is where DNA synthesis

occurs. In this step, the polymerase synthesizes a copy of the template DNA by adding nucleotides to the hybridized primers. DNA polymerase catalyzes the formation of the phosphodiester bond between an incoming dNTP determined by hydrogen bonding to the template (A:T or G:C) and the base at the 3' end of the primer. In this way, DNA polymerase replicates the template DNA by simultaneously extending the primers on both strands of the template. This step occurs at the optimal temperature of the enzyme, 68°C to 72°C.

At the end of the three steps, or one cycle (denaturation, primer annealing, and primer extension), one copy of double-stranded DNA has been replicated into two copies. Returning to the denaturing temperature starts the second cycle (Fig. 7-5), with the end result being a doubling in the number of double-stranded DNA molecules again. At the end of the PCR program, millions of copies of the original region defined by the primer sequences will have been generated. Following is a more detailed discussion of each of the components of PCR.

Historical Highlights

As Kary Mullis realized early on, the key to the brilliance of PCR is that primers can be designed to target specific sequences: "I drove on down the road. In about a mile it occurred to me that the oligonucleotides could be placed at some arbitrary distance from each other, not just flanking a base pair and that I could make an arbitrarily large number of copies of any sequence I chose and what's more, most of the copies after a few cycles would be the same size. That size would be up to me. They would look like restriction fragments on a gel. I stopped the car again. Dear Thor!, I exclaimed. I had solved the most annoying problems in DNA chemistry in a single lightning bolt. Abundance and distinction. With two oligonucleotides, DNA polymerase, and the four nucleoside triphosphates I could make as much of a DNA sequence as I wanted and I could make it on a fragment of a specific size that I could distinguish easily."[4]

Advanced Concepts

In some cases, the annealing temperature is close enough to the extension temperature that the reaction can proceed with only two temperature changes. This is two-step PCR, as opposed to three-step PCR that requires a different temperature for all three steps.

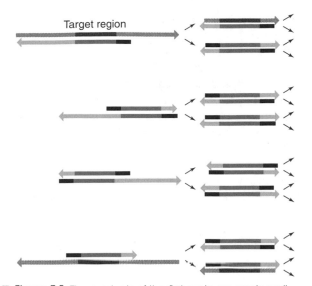

Target region

■ **Figure 7-5** The products of the first cycle are again replicated in the second PCR cycle, yielding four copies of the target region. At each cycle the number of copies of the target region doubles. In an ideal PCR, the PCR product (amplicon) is composed of $2N$ copies of the target region where N = number of PCR cycles.

Components of PCR

The PCR is a method of in vitro DNA synthesis. Therefore, to perform PCR, all of the components necessary for the replication of DNA in vivo are combined in optimal concentrations for replication of DNA to occur in vitro. This includes the template to be copied, primers to prime synthesis of the template, nucleotides, polymerase enzyme, and buffer components including monovalent and divalent cations to provide optimal conditions for accurate and efficient replication.

Primers

The primers are the critical component of the PCR because they determine the specificity of the PCR. Primers are analogous to the probes in blotting and hybridization procedures (see Chapter 6). Primers are chemically manufactured on a DNA synthesizer.

Primers are designed to contain sequences complementary to sites flanking the region to be analyzed. Primer design is therefore a critical aspect of the PCR. Primers are single-stranded DNA fragments, usually 20 to 30 bases in length. The forward primer hybridizes to the target DNA sequence on the opposite strand just 5'

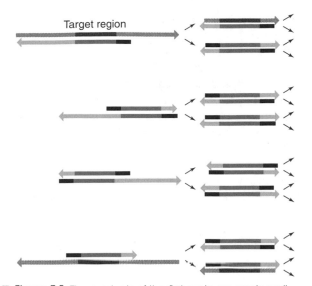

Target region

■ **Figure 7-5** The products of the first cycle are again replicated in the second PCR cycle, yielding four copies of the target region. At each cycle the number of copies of the target region doubles. In an ideal PCR, the PCR product (amplicon) is composed of $2N$ copies of the target region where N = number of PCR cycles.

optimally at the same annealing temperature. T_m can be adjusted by increasing the length of the primers or by placing the primers in areas with more or fewer Gs and Cs in the template.

The nature of the primer structure determines the accuracy of binding to its complementary sequence and not to other sequences. Just as cross-hybridization can occur with blot hybridization, aberrant primer binding, or **mispriming**, can occur in PCR. A fragment synthesized as a result of mispriming will carry the primer sequence and become a target for subsequent rounds of amplification (Fig. 7-6). Eventually, misprimed products will take components away from the intended reaction. The resulting misprimed products may also interfere with proper interpretation of results or with subsequent procedures, such as sequencing (see Chapter 10, "DNA Sequencing") or mutation analysis (see Chapter 9).

Secondary structure (internal folding and hybridization within DNA strands) may also interfere with PCR. Primer sequences that have internal homologies, especially at the 3' end, or homologies with the other member of the primer pair may not work as well in the PCR. An artifact often observed in the PCR is the occurrence of **primer dimers**, which are PCR products that are just double the size of the primers. They result from the binding of primers onto each other through short (2- to 3-base) homologies at their 3' ends and the copying of each primer sequence (Fig. 7-7). The

resulting doublet is then a very efficient target for subsequent amplification.

The entire primer sequence does not have to bind to the template to prime synthesis; however, the 3' nucleotide position is critical for extension of the primer. The polymerase will not form a phosphodiester bond if the 3' end of the primer is not hydrogen-bonded to the template. This characteristic of primer binding has been exploited to modify the PCR procedure for mutation analysis of the template (see Chapter 9). There is no such strict requirement for complementarity on the 5' end of the primer. Noncomplementary extensions or tails can be added to the 5' end of the primer sequences to introduce useful additions to the final PCR product, such as restriction enzyme sites, promoters, or binding sites for other primers. These **tailed primers** are designed to add or alter sequences to one or both ends of the PCR product (Fig. 7-8).

DNA Template

In a clinical sample, depending on the application, the template may be derived from the patient's genomic or mitochondrial DNA or from **viruses**, bacteria, fungi, or parasites that might be infecting the patient. Genomic DNA will have only one or two copies per cell equivalent of single-copy genes to serve as amplification targets. With robust PCR reagents and conditions, nanogram amounts of genomic DNA are sufficient for consistent results. For routine clinical analysis, 100 ng to 1 µg of

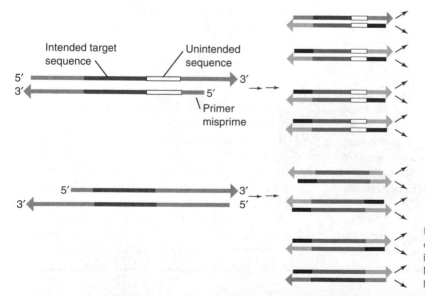

■ Figure 7-6 Mispriming of one primer creates an unintended product that could interfere with subsequent interpretation. Mispriming can also occur in regions unrelated to the intended target sequence.

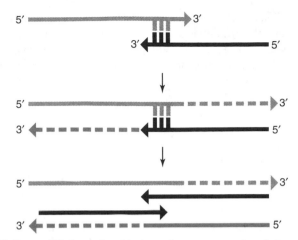

■ **Figure 7-7** Formation of primer dimers occurs when there are three or more complementary bases at the 3' end of the primers. With the primers in excess, these will hybridized during the annealing step (vertical lines) and the primers will be extended by the polymerase (dotted line) using the opposite primer as the template. The resulting product, denatured in the next cycle, will compete for primers with the intended template.

DNA is usually used. Lesser amounts are required for more defined template preparations, such as cloned target DNA or product from a previous amplification.

The best templates are in good condition, free of contaminating proteins, and without nicks or breaks that can stop DNA synthesis or cause misincorporation of nucleotide bases. Templates with high GC content and secondary structure may prove more difficult to optimize

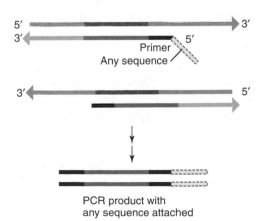

■ **Figure 7-8** Sequences unrelated to the template can be added to the 5' end of the primer. After PCR, the sequence will be on the end of the PCR product. These tailed primers can add useful sequences to one, as shown, or both ends of the PCR product.

Advanced Concepts

Reagent systems have been designed to facilitate amplification of targets with high GC content. These systems incorporate an analog of dGTP, called **deaza dGTP**, to destabilize secondary structure formed by G:C base pairing. Deaza dGTP interferes with EtBr staining in gels and is best used in procedures with other types of detection such as autoradiography.

for amplification. The DNA region affected in Fragile X syndrome, 5' to the *FMR*-1 gene, is an example of such a GC-rich target.

Deoxyribonucleotide Bases

Nucleotide triphosphates are the building blocks of DNA. An equimolar mixture of the four deoxynucleotide-triphosphates (dNTPs)—adenine, thymine, guanine, and cytosine—is added to the synthesis reaction in concentrations sufficient to support the exponential increase of copies of the template. Standard procedures require 0.1 to 0.5 mM concentrations of each nucleotide. Substituted or labeled nucleotides such as deaza dGTP may be included in the reaction for special applications. These nucleotides will require empirical optimization for best results.

Advanced Concepts

The concentration and purity of dNTP preparations affect the efficiency of the PCR reaction. A single solution containing a mixture of all four nucleotides is most convenient and lowers pipetting errors compared to four separate nucleotide solutions. The four dNTP working concentrations should be higher than the estimated K_m of each dNTP (10 to 15 mM, the concentration of substrate at half maximal enzyme velocity). Higher concentrations (at least 10 to 100 mM) are recommended for storage, as storing dNTPS in lower concentrations results in hydrolysis to dNDP and dNMP. Nucleotide di- and monophosphates can also result from poor manufacturing conditions or **contamination** with heavy metals. These molecules will inhibit the PCR reaction.

DNA Polymerase

Automation of the PCR procedure was greatly facilitated by the discovery of the thermostable enzyme *Taq* **polymerase**. When Kary Mullis first performed PCR, he used the DNA polymerase isolated from *E. coli*. Every time the sample was denatured, however, the high temperature inactivated the enzyme. Thus, after each round of denaturation, additional *E. coli* DNA polymerase had to be added to the tube. This was labor-intensive and provided additional opportunities for the introduction of contaminants into the reaction tube. The *Taq* polymerase was isolated from the thermophilic bacterium *Thermus aquaticus*.

Using an enzyme derived from a thermophilic bacterium meant that the DNA polymerase could be added once at the beginning of the procedure and would maintain its activity throughout the heating and cooling cycles. Other enzymes, such as *Tth* **polymerase**, from *Thermus thermophilus*, were subsequently exploited for laboratory use. *Tth* polymerase also has reverse transcriptase activity, so it can be used in **reverse-transcriptase PCR (RT-PCR**, see the section "Reverse Transcriptase

PCR" later in this chapter) in which the starting material is an RNA template. The addition of proofreading enzymes, for example, Vent polymerase, allows *Taq* or *Tth* polymerase to generate large products over 30,000 bases in length.

Cloning of the genes coding for these polymerases has led to modified versions of the polymerase enzymes, such as the **Stoffel fragment** lacking the N-terminal 289 amino acids of *Taq* polymerase and its inherent 3' to 5' exonuclease activity.[7] The half-life of the Stoffel fragment at high temperatures is about twice that of *Taq* polymerase, and it has a broader range of optimal $MgCl_2$ concentrations (2 to 10 mM) than *Taq*. This enzyme is recommended for allele-specific PCR and for amplification of regions with high GC content. Further modified versions of the *Taq* enzymes retaining 3' to 5' exonuclease, but not 5' to 3' exonuclease activity, are used where high **fidelity** (accurate copying of the template) is important. Other variants of *Taq* polymerase, ThermoSequenase and T7 Sequenase, efficiently incorporate dideoxy **NTPs** for application to chain termination sequencing (see Chapter 10). Hemo KlenTaq™ (New England BioLabs) is a truncated version of *Taq* polymerase with mutations rendering it resistant to inhibitors present in whole blood, a characteristic applicable to clinical analysis.

Despite its thermal stability, the *Taq* polymerase enzyme is still subject to loss of activity under adverse conditions. For example, although mixing is important for buffers and other solutions, especially after thawing, vigorous agitation of the polymerase enzymes is not recommended. This can result in mechanical shearing, altering secondary and tertiary structures of complex enzymes like the polymerases and causing irreversible denaturation. Most of the enzymes used in molecular biology have complex tertiary structure (with multiple subunits) and will lose enzyme activity upon vigorous mixing. In contrast, tiny proteins like RNAse can renature and are therefore resistant to this type of treatment.

PCR Buffer

PCR buffers provide the optimal conditions for enzyme activity. Potassium chloride (20 to 100 mM), ammonium sulfate (15 to 30 mM), or other sources of monovalent cations are important buffer components. These salts affect the denaturing and annealing temperatures of the DNA and the enzyme activity. An increase in salt concentration makes longer DNA products denature more slowly than shorter DNA products during the amplification process, so shorter molecules will be amplified preferentially. The influence of buffer/salt conditions varies with different primers and templates.

Divalent cations, provided by magnesium chloride, also affect primer annealing and are very important for enzyme activity. Magnesium requirements will vary depending on other components of the reaction mix; for example, each NTP will take up one magnesium atom. Furthermore, the presence of ethylenediaminetetraacetic acid (EDTA) or other chelators will lower the amount of magnesium available for the enzyme. Too few Mg^{2+} ions lower enzyme efficiency, resulting in a low yield of PCR product. Overly high Mg^{2+} concentrations promote misincorporation and thus increase the yield of nonspecific products. Lower Mg^{2+} concentrations are desirable when fidelity of the PCR is critical. The recommended range of $MgCl_2$ concentration is 1 to 4 mM, in standard reaction conditions. If the DNA samples contain EDTA or other chelators, the $MgCl_2$ concentration in the reaction mixture should be adjusted accordingly. Tris buffer and accessory buffer components are also important for optimal enzyme activity and accurate amplification of the intended product; 10 mM Tris-HCl maintains the proper pH of the buffer, usually between pH 8 and pH 9.5. As with other PCR components, the optimal conditions are established empirically.

Accessory components are sometimes used to optimize reactions. Bovine serum albumin (10 to 100 µg/mL) binds inhibitors and stabilizes the enzyme. Dithiothreitol (0.01 mM) provides reducing conditions that may enhance enzyme activity. Formamide (1% to 10%) added to the reaction mixture will lower the denaturing temperature of DNA with high secondary structure, thereby increasing the availability for primer binding. Chaotropic agents such as triton X-100, glycerol, and dimethyl sulfoxide added at concentrations of 1% to 10% may also reduce secondary structure to allow polymerase extension through difficult areas. These agents contribute to the stability of the enzyme as well.

Enzymes are usually supplied with buffers optimized by the manufacturer. Commercial PCR buffer enhancers of proprietary composition may also be purchased to optimize difficult reactions. Often, the buffer and its ingredients are mixed with the nucleotide bases and stored as aliquots of a **master mix**. The enzyme, target, and primers are then added when necessary. Dedicated master mixes will also include the primers, so only the target sequences must be added.

Thermal Cyclers

The first PCRs were performed using multiple water baths or heat blocks set at the required temperatures for each of the steps of the PCR cycle. The tubes were manually moved from one temperature to another. In addition, before the discovery of thermostable enzymes, new enzyme had to be added after each denaturation step, further slowing the procedure and increasing the chance of error and contamination.

Automation of this tedious process was greatly facilitated by the availability of the heat-stable enzymes. To accomplish the PCR, then, an instrument must only manage temperature according to a scheduled amplification program. **Thermal cyclers**, or **thermocyclers**, were thus designed to rapidly and automatically ramp (change) to the required incubation temperatures, holding at each one for designated periods.

Early versions of thermal cyclers were designed as heater/coolers with programmable memory to record the appropriate reaction conditions. Compared with modern models, the memory available for recording the reaction conditions and sample was limited. Wax or oil (vapor barriers) had to be added to the reactions to prevent condensation of the sample on the tops of the tubes during the temperature changes. The layer of wax or oil made subsequent sample handling more difficult. Later, thermal cycler models were designed with heated lids that eliminated the requirement for vapor barriers.

The several versions of thermal cyclers available differ in heating and/or refrigeration systems as well as the programmable software within the units. Some hold samples in open chambers for air heating and cooling; others hold samples in blocks designed to accommodate 0.2-mL tubes, usually in a 96-well format. Some models have interchangeable blocks to accommodate amplification in different sizes and numbers of tubes or in situ amplification of nucleic acid targets in tissue on slides. A cycler may run more than one block independently so that different PCR programs can be performed simultaneously. **Rapid PCR** systems work with small sample volumes in chambers that can be heated and cooled quickly by changing the air temperature surrounding the samples. **Real-time PCR** systems are equipped with fluorescent detectors to measure PCR product as the reaction proceeds. PCR can also be performed in a microchip device in which 1- to 2-µL samples are forced through tiny channels etched in a glass chip, passing through temperature zones as the chip rests on a specially adapted heat block.[8]

For routine PCR, an appropriate amount of DNA that has been isolated from a test specimen is mixed with the other PCR components, either separately or as a master mix. The final volume of the reaction mix varies from 1 to 50 µL for most PCR. Most thermal cyclers take thin-walled tubes, tube strips, or 96-well plates with 0.2-mL volume capacity. Preparation of the specimen for PCR is often referred to as **pre-PCR** work. To avoid contamination (see below), it is recommended that the pre-PCR work be performed in a designated area that is clean and free of amplified products. The sample tubes are then loaded into the thermal cycler. The computer is programmed with the temperatures and times for each step of the PCR cycle, the number of cycles to be completed (usually 30 to 50), the conditions for ramping from step to step, and the temperature at which to hold the tubes once all of the cycles are complete. Since the PCR products are stable at the holding temperature, the technologist does not have to retrieve the samples from the thermal cycler immediately after the PCR program is concluded.

After PCR, a variety of methods are used to analyze the product. Most commonly, the PCR product is analyzed by gel or capillary electrophoresis. Depending on the application, the size, presence, or intensity of PCR products is observed after electrophoresis. An example of the results from a PCR run is shown in Figure 7-9.

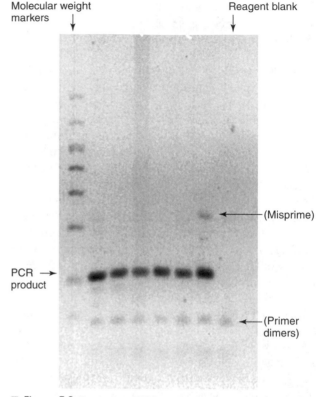

Figure 7-9 Example of PCR products after resolution on an agarose gel and staining with ethidium bromide. Molecular weight markers in the first gel lane are used to estimate the size of the PCR product. The intended product is 125 bp. Artifactual primer dimers and misprimed products are also present. Absence of products in the last gel lane (reagent blank) confirms that there is no contamination in the master mix.

Controls for PCR

As with any diagnostic assay, running the correct controls during every PCR run is essential for maintaining and ensuring the accuracy of the assay. Positive controls ensure that the enzyme is active, the buffer is optimal, the primers are priming the right sequences, and the thermal cycler is cycling appropriately. A negative **control** without DNA (also called a **contamination control** or **reagent blank**) ensures that the reaction mix is not contaminated with template DNA or amplified products from a previous run. A negative control with DNA that lacks the target sequence (**negative template control**) ensures that the primers are not annealing to nontarget sequences of DNA. In some applications of PCR, an internal **amplification control** is included that contains a second set of primers and an unrelated target added to the reaction mix. This control demonstrates that the reaction is working even if the test sample is not amplified. Amplification controls are performed preferably in the same tube with the test reaction, although it is acceptable to perform the amplification control in a duplicate reaction mix if the control cannot easily be distinguished from the target product in the same reaction. This type of control is most important when PCR results are reported as positive or negative, "negative" meaning that the target sequences are not present. The amplification control is critical to distinguish between a true negative for the sample and an amplification failure (false-negative).

Control of PCR Contamination

Contamination is a significant concern in methods that involve target amplification by PCR. The nature of the amplification procedure is such that, theoretically, a single molecule will give rise to product. This is of great concern in the medical or forensic laboratory where results may be interpreted based on the presence, absence, size, or amount of a PCR product. With modern reagent systems designed for robust amplification of challenging specimens, such as paraffin-embedded tissues or samples with low cell numbers, the balance between aggressive amplification of the intended target and avoidance of a contaminating template is delicate. For this reason, contamination control is of utmost importance in designing a PCR procedure and laboratory setup.

Although genomic DNA (e.g., from hair, skin, or ambient microorganisms) is a source of spurious PCR targets, the major cause of contamination is the presence of PCR products from previous amplifications. Unlike the relatively large and scarce genomic DNA, the small, highly concentrated PCR product DNA can aerosol when tubes are uncapped and when the amplified DNA is pipetted. This PCR product is a perfect template for primer binding and amplification in a subsequent PCR using the same primers. Contamination control procedures, therefore, are mainly directed toward eliminating PCR product from the setup reaction.

Contamination is controlled both physically and chemically. Physically, the best way to avoid PCR carryover is to separate the pre-PCR areas from the post-PCR analysis areas. Positive airflow, air locks, and more extensive measures are taken by high-throughput laboratories that process large numbers of samples and test for a limited number of amplification targets. Most laboratories can separate these areas by assigning separate rooms or using isolation cabinets. Equipment, including laboratory gowns and gloves, and reagents should be dedicated to either pre- or **post-PCR**. Gloves should be changed if contaminated areas are touched before proceeding with PCR setup. Items can flow from the pre- to the post-PCR area but not in the opposite direction without decontamination.

Ultraviolet (uv) light has been used to decontaminate and maintain pre-PCR areas.[9] Ultraviolet light catalyzes single- and double-strand breaks in the DNA that will then interfere with replication. Isolation cabinets are equipped with uv light sources that are turned on for about 20 minutes after the box has been used. The effectiveness of uv light may be increased by the addition of **psoralens** to amplification products after analysis. Psoralens intercalate between the bases of double-stranded DNA, and in the presence of long-wave uv light they covalently attach to the thymidines, uracils, and cytidines in the DNA chain. The bulky adducts of the psoralens prevent denaturation and amplification of the treated DNA.

The efficiency of uv light treatment for decontamination depends on the wavelength, energy, and distance of the light source. The technologist must avoid skin or eye exposure to uv light, and uv light will also damage Plexiglas and some plastics, so laboratory equipment, including pipets, may be affected by extended exposure. Although convenient, uv treatment may not be the most effective decontaminant for every procedure.[10-12] For example, the using overhead uv room lights for decontamination is not very efficient for surface DNA decontamination due to the hazardous high intensity (4000 microWatt-seconds/cm^2) required to damage DNA at the distances the light has to travel from the ceiling to the bench surface. A widely used method for decontamination and preparation of the workspace is 10% bleach (7 mM sodium hypochlorite). Frequently wiping bench tops, hoods, or any surface that comes in contact with specimen material with dilute bleach or alcohol removes most DNA contamination. As a practice in forensic work, before handling evidence or items that come in contact with evidence, gloves are wiped with bleach and allowed to air-dry.

A frequently used chemical method of contamination control is the dUTP-UNG system, which involves substitution of dUTP for dTTP in the PCR reagent master mix, resulting in incorporation of dUTP instead of dTTP into the PCR product. Although some polymerase enzymes may be more or less efficient in incorporating the nucleotide, the dUTP does not affect the PCR product in most applications. At the beginning of each PCR, the enzyme uracil-*N*-glycosylase (UNG) is added to the reaction mix. This enzyme will degrade any nucleic acid containing uracil, such as contaminating PCR product from previous reactions. A short incubation period is added to the beginning of the PCR amplification program, usually at 50°C for 2 to 15 minutes to allow the UNG enzyme to function. The initial denaturation step in the PCR cycle will degrade the UNG before synthesis of the new products. Note that this system will not work with some types of PCR, such as nested PCR (discussed below), because a second round of amplification requires the presence of the first-round product. The dUTP-UNG system is used routinely in real-time PCR procedures in which contamination control is more important because the contaminant will not be distinguishable from the desired amplicon by gel electrophoresis.

Wipe tests are performed in some laboratories as a routine check or to confirm successful decontamination. Filter paper is wiped on any exposed or touched surfaces in the pre-PCR setup, extraction, and amplification areas. The paper is then placed in robust PCR buffer with appropriate primers and subjected to amplification. Any production of amplicon indicates the presence of contamination.

Prevention of Mispriming

As shown in Figure 7-9, PCR products are analyzed for size and purity by electrophoresis. The amplicon size should agree with the size determined by the primer placement. For instance, if two 20-b primers were designed to hybridize to sequences flanking a 100-bp target, the amplicon should be 140 bp in size. Much larger or smaller amplicons are due to mispriming, primer dimers, or other artifacts of the reaction. For some procedures, these artifacts do not affect interpretation of results and can be ignored as long as they do not compromise the efficiency of the reaction. For other purposes, however, extraneous PCR products must be avoided or removed.

Misprimes are initially averted by good primer design and optimal amplification conditions. Even under the

best conditions, however, misprimes can occur during preparation of the reaction mix. This is because *Taq* polymerase has some activity at room temperature. While mixes are prepared and transported to the thermal cycler, the primers and template are in contact at 22°C to 25°C, a condition of very low stringency. (See Chapter 6, "Analysis and Characterization of Nucleic Acids and Proteins," for a discussion of stringency.) Under these conditions, the primers can bind sequences other than their exact complements in the target, and the low-level activity of *Taq* will extend them. These misprimed products, then, are already present before the amplification program begins. **Hot-start PCR** can be used to prevent this type of mispriming.

Hot-start PCR can be performed in three different ways. In one approach, the reaction mixes are prepared on ice and placed in the thermal cycler after it has been prewarmed to the denaturation temperature. A second way to perform hot-start PCR is to use a wax barrier. A bead of wax is placed in each reaction tube containing all components of the reaction mix except enzyme and template. The tubes are heated to 100°C to melt the wax and then cooled to room temperature. The melted wax will float to the top of the reaction mix and congeal into a physical barrier as it cools. The remainder of the reaction mix containing template and enzyme is then added on top of the wax barrier. When the tubes are placed in the thermal cycler, the wax will melt at the denaturation temperature, and the primers and template will first come in contact at the proper annealing temperature. The wax also serves as an evaporation barrier as the reaction proceeds. After amplification, however, the wax barrier must be punctured to gain access to the PCR products.

The third and most frequently used hot-start method uses sequestered enzymes, such as AmpliTaq Gold (Applied Biosystems), Platinum *Taq* (Invitrogen), Jump-Start *Taq* (Sigma), HotStarTaq (Qiagen), and numerous others. These enzymes are supplied in inactive form, sequestered and inactivated by monoclonal antibodies or by other proprietary methods. The enzyme will not extend the primers until it is activated by heat in the first denaturation step of the PCR program, thereby preventing any primer extension during preparation of the reagent mix.

A method called **touchdown PCR** is a modification of the PCR program that is also used to enhance amplification of the desired PCR product. In this method, the PCR

Advanced Concepts

In addition to breaking the sugar-phosphate backbone of DNA, uv light also stimulates covalent attachment of adjacent pyrimidines in the DNA chain, forming **pyrimidine dimers**. These boxy structures are the source of mutations in DNA in some diseases caused by sun exposure. DNA repair systems remove these structures in vivo. Loss of these repair systems is manifested in diseases such as xeroderma pigmentosum, Cockayne syndrome, and trichothiodystrophy.[13]

program begins with annealing temperatures higher than the optimal target primer binding temperature. The annealing temperature is decreased by 1°C every cycle or every other cycle until the optimal annealing temperature is reached. Subsequent cycles are carried out at the optimal temperature. Any difference in the annealing temperature will translate into an exponential advantage for correct versus mismatched primer binding.[14]

PCR Product Cleanup

Sequence limitations in primer design or reaction conditions may not completely prevent primer dimers or other extraneous products. These unintended amplicons are unacceptable for analytical procedures that demand pure product, such as sequencing or some mutation analyses (see Chapters 9 and 10). A direct way to obtain clean PCR product is to resolve the amplification products by gel electrophoresis and then cut out pieces of the gel containing desired bands and elute the PCR product. Agarose gel slices can be digested with enzymes, such as β-agarase (New England BioLabs), or by incubation with iodine, releasing the product DNA (Fig. 7-10).

Residual components of the reaction mix, such as leftover primers and unused nucleotides, also interfere with some post-PCR applications. Moreover, the buffers used for PCR may not be compatible with post-PCR procedures. Amplicons free of PCR components are most frequently and conveniently prepared using **spin columns** (Fig. 7-11) or silica beads. The DNA binds to the column

and the rest of the reaction components are rinsed away by centrifugation. The DNA can then be eluted from the column. Even though columns or beads provide better recovery than gel elution, they may not completely remove residual primers or misprimed products.

Addition of shrimp alkaline phosphatase (SAP) in combination with exonuclease I (ExoI) is an enzymatic method for removing nucleotides and primers from PCR products prior to sequencing or mutational analyses. During a 15-minute incubation at 37°C, SAP dephosphorylates nucleotides, and ExoI degrades primers. The enzymes must then be removed by extraction or inactivated by heating at 80°C for 15 minutes. This method is convenient, as it is performed in the same tube as the PCR. It does not, however, remove other buffer components.

In some post-PCR methods, such a small amount of PCR product is added to the next reaction that residual components of the amplification are of no consequence, so no further cleanup of the PCR product is required. The choice of cleanup procedure or whether cleanup is necessary at all will depend on the application.

PCR Modifications

PCR has been adapted for various applications, several of which are used in the medical laboratory. Among the large and increasing number of PCR modifications are the following methods that might be encountered in the clinical molecular laboratory. These methods are capable of detecting multiple targets in a single run (multiplex PCR) using RNA templates (reverse transcriptase PCR) or such amplified products as templates (nested PCR) and quantitating starting template (quantitative PCR, or real-time PCR).

Multiplex PCR

More than one primer pair can be added to a PCR so that multiple amplifications are primed simultaneously, resulting in the formation of multiple products. **Multiplex PCR** is especially useful in typing or identification analyses. Individual organisms, from viruses to humans, can be identified or typed by observing a set of several PCR products at once. Pathogen typing and forensic identification kits contain multiple sets of primers that amplify polymorphic DNA regions. The pattern of product sizes will be specific for a given type or individual.

Multiple organisms have been the target of multiplex PCR in clinical microbiology laboratories.[15–17] One

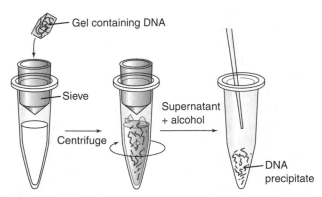

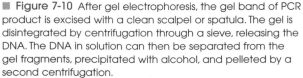

■ **Figure 7-10** After gel electrophoresis, the gel band of PCR product is excised with a clean scalpel or spatula. The gel is disintegrated by centrifugation through a sieve, releasing the DNA. The DNA in solution can then be separated from the gel fragments, precipitated with alcohol, and pelleted by a second centrifugation.

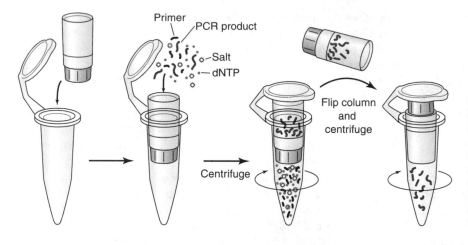

■ **Figure 7-11** PCR product cleanup in spin columns (left) removes residual components in the PCR mix. Amplicon DNA binds to a silica matrix in the column while the buffer components flow through during centrifugation. The column is then inverted, and the DNA is eluted by another centrifugation in low salt (Tris-EDTA) buffer.

respiratory sample, for example, can be used to test for the presence of more than one respiratory virus.[18] Organisms that cause sexually transmitted diseases can be targeted using multiplex PCR and one genital swab.[19] In a slightly different approach to testing for multiple targets, one set of primers can detect an infectious organism and a second set can then detect the presence of a gene that makes that organism resistant to a particular antimicrobial agent. This test has been performed for methicillin-resistant *Staphylococcus aureus* and the results published.[20]

Multiplex PCR reagents and conditions require more complex optimization. Often, target sequences will not amplify with the same efficiency and primers may interfere with each other in binding to the target sequences. The conditions for the PCR must be adjusted for the optimal amplification of all products in the reaction, but this may not be possible in all cases. Multiplexing primers is useful, not only to detect multiple targets but also to confirm accurate detection of a single target. Internal amplification controls are often multiplexed with test reactions that are interpreted by the presence or absence of product. The control primers and targets must be chosen so that they do not interfere or compete with the amplification of the test region. Internal amplification controls are the ideal for positive/negative qualitative PCR tests.

Sequence-Specific PCR

The strict requirement for complementarity of the 3' end of primers can be used to identify single base changes in the target DNA. By designing the forward or reverse primer to end with a 3' base complementary to the mutant sequence, the presence of the base change is detected by successful amplification. (Also see Chapter 9.) Although this method is used frequently in the medical laboratory to detect base changes in patient DNA, its high sensitivity risks detection of mutations at very low levels that may not be clinically significant.[21] Sequence-specific PCR is the basis for human leukocyte antigen allele analysis in tissue typing. (See Chapter 15, "DNA-Based Tissue Typing.")

Reverse Transcriptase PCR

If the starting material for a procedure is RNA, the RNA may first be converted to double-stranded DNA, which is a better template for amplification than single-stranded RNA. The conversion is accomplished through the action of reverse transcriptase (RT), an enzyme isolated from RNA viruses. This enzyme first copies the RNA single strand into a RNA:DNA **hybrid** strand and then uses a hairpin formation on the end of the newly synthesized DNA strand to prime synthesis of the complementary DNA strand, replacing the original RNA in the hybrid. The resulting double-stranded DNA is called **cDNA,** for copy or **complementary DNA**.

Like other DNA polymerases, reverse transcriptase requires priming. Specific primers—oligo dT primers or random hexamers—are most often used to prime the synthesis of the initial DNA strand. The yield of cDNA will be relatively low using this approach but highly specific for the target of interest. The specific primers will prime cDNA synthesis only from transcripts complementary to the primer sequences. Oligo dT primers are 18-base-long single-stranded polyT sequences that will prime cDNA synthesis only from messenger RNA with polyA tails. The yield of cDNA will be higher with oligo dT primers than with target-specific primers but potentially all mRNA could be included in the specimen. The highest yield of cDNA is achieved with random hexamers or decamers. These are 6- or 10-base-long single-stranded oligonucleotides of random sequences. The 6 or 10 bases will match and hybridize to random sites in the target RNA with some frequency, priming DNA synthesis. Random priming will generate cDNA from all RNA (and DNA) in the specimen.

RT PCR is used to measure RNA expression profiles, to detect rRNA, to analyze gene regions interrupted by long introns, and to detect microorganisms with RNA genomes. For gene expression analysis, the amount of cDNA reflects the amount of transcript in the preparation. In other applications, genes that are interrupted by long introns can be made more available for consistent amplification using cDNA versions lacking the interrupting sequences. cDNA is often used for sequencing because the sequence of the coding region can be determined without long stretches of introns that might complicate the analysis. The detection of RNA viruses such as *Coronavirus*, which is responsible for severe acute respiratory syndrome (SARS), can be accomplished using RT PCR.[22]

Originally, RT PCR was performed in two steps: cDNA synthesis and then PCR. *Tth* DNA polymerase, which has RT activity, and proprietary mixtures of RT and sequestered (hot-start) DNA polymerase are components of one-step RT PCR procedures.[23] These methods are more convenient than the two-step procedure, as RNA is added directly to the PCR. The amplification program is modified to include an initial incubation of 45°C to 50°C for 30 to 60 minutes, during which RT makes cDNA from RNA in the sample. The RT activity will then be inactivated in the first denaturation step of the PCR procedure.

Although RT PCR is a widely used and important adjunct to molecular analysis, it is subject to the vulnerabilities of RNA degradation. As with other procedures that target RNA, specimen handling is important for accurate results. Methods have been described for the RT PCR amplification of challenging specimens, such as paraffin-embedded tissues; however, fixed specimens are difficult to analyze consistently.[24]

Nested PCR

The increased sensitivity that PCR offers is very useful in clinical applications because clinical specimens are often limited in quantity and quality. The low level of target and the presence of interfering sequences can prevent a regular PCR from working with the reliability required for clinical applications. **Nested PCR** is a modification that increases the sensitivity and specificity of the reaction.[25-28]

In nested PCR, two pairs of primers are used to amplify a single target in two separate PCR runs. The second pair of primers, designed to bind slightly inside of the binding sites of the first pair, will amplify the product of the first PCR in a second round of amplification. The second amplification will specifically increase the amount of the intended product. In **semi-nested PCR**, one of the second-round primers is the same as the first-round primer (Fig. 7-12).

Several variations of nested and semi nested PCR have been devised. For example, as shown in Figure 7-12, the first-round primers can have 5' sequences added (5' tails) complementary to sequences used for second-round primers. This tailed primer method is valuable for multiplex procedures in which multiple first-round primers may differ in their binding efficiencies. With the tailed primers, sequences complementary to a single set of second-round primers are added to all of the first-round products. In the second round, then, all products will be amplified with the same primers and with equal efficiency. Although this tailed primer procedure increases sensitivity in multiplex reactions, it does not increase specificity.

Real-Time (Quantitative) PCR

Standard PCR procedures will indicate if a particular target sequence is present in a clinical sample. For some situations, though, the clinician is also interested in how much of the target sequence is present. There are several approaches to estimating the amount of starting template via PCR. The nature of amplification, however, makes calculating direct quantities of starting material complex. Strategies for quantifying starting material by quantifying the end products of PCRs have utilized specialized internal controls, that is, known quantities of starting material that are coamplified with the test template. These types of assays suffer, however, from primer incompatibilities and inconsistent results. Another approach is

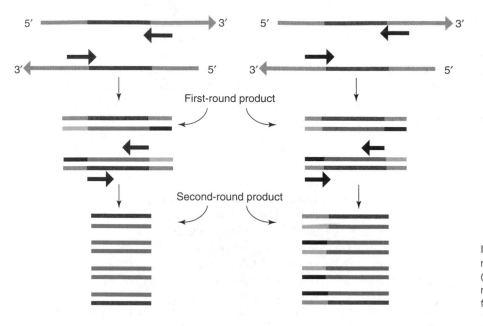

5' ———————→ 3'   5' ———————→ 3'
←   ←
→   →
3' ←——————— 5'   3' ←——————— 5'

First-round product

Second-round product

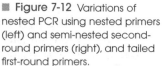

■ **Figure 7-12** Variations of
nested PCR using nested primers
(left) and semi-nested second-
round primers (right), and tailed
first-round primers.

adding competitor templates at several known levels to assess the amount of test material by preferential amplification over a known amount of competitor.[29] These assays are also at times unreliable and inconsistent when test and internal control templates differ by more than 10-fold. They are most accurate with a 1:1 ratio of test and internal control, requiring analysis of multiple dilutions of controls for optimal results.

A very useful modification of the PCR process is **real-time** or **quantitative PCR** (**qPCR**).[30,31] This method was initially performed by adding ethidium bromide (EtBr) to a regular PCR. Because EtBr intercalates into double-stranded DNA and fluoresces, it can be used to monitor the accumulation of PCR products during the PCR in real time, that is, as it is made. The advantage of this method over standard PCR is the ability to determine the amount of starting template accurately. These quantitative measurements are performed with the ease and rapidity of standard PCR without tedious addition of competitor templates or multiple internal controls. A growing number of clinically significant parameters, such as copy numbers of diseased human genes, **viral load**, tumor load, and the effects of treatment, are measured easily with this method.[32–34]

The rationale for qPCR is illustrated in Figure 7-13. If the target copy number in a PCR were graphed versus the number of PCR cycles (denaturation, annealing,

extension), the results would be an exponential curve where the number of target copies = 2^N, N being the number of PCR cycles. If the copy number is measured by detectable fluorescence as shown in the figure, the curve looks similar to a bacterial growth curve, with a lag phase, an exponential (log) phase, a linear phase, and a stationary phase.

In contrast to real-time PCR, analysis of PCR product by the standard method occurs at the end of the PCR stationary phase (**endpoint analysis**). The exhaustion of reaction components and competition between PCR product and primers during the annealing step slow the PCR product accumulation after the exponential phase of growth until it finally plateaus. In the endpoint analysis, products of widely different amounts of starting template are tested at the plateau where they are all the same (observe the ends of the amplification curves shown in Fig. 7-13A). Using the fluorescent signal to detect the growing target copy number during the amplification process, analysis in real-time PCR is performed in the exponential phase of growth. Since the length of the lag phase is inversely proportional to the amount of starting template, fluorescence will reach exponential growth in early cycles when a lot of target is present; when less target is present, fluorescence will not reach exponential growth until later cycles. With 10-fold dilutions of known positive standards, a relationship can be established between the starting target copy or cell number and the cycle number at which fluorescence crosses a threshold amount of fluorescence.

The PCR cycle at which sample fluorescence crosses the threshold is the **threshold cycle**, or **C_T**. Plotting the target copy number of the diluted standards against C_T for each standard generates the graph shown in Figure 7-13B. Once this relationship is established, the starting amount of an unknown specimen can be determined by the cycle number at which the unknown crosses the fluorescence threshold.

The first approach to real-time PCR utilizing the dye EtBr, which is specific to double-stranded DNA. Dye is still used for routine qPCR, except that EtBr has been replaced by **SYBR green**, another dye specific to double-stranded DNA. The advantage of SYBR green is its specificity and robust fluorescence comparable to that of EtBr but with less toxicity. These dyes bind and fluoresce

Advanced Concepts

The optimal threshold level is based on the background or baseline fluorescence and the peak fluorescence in the reaction. Instrument software is designed to set this level automatically. Alternatively, the threshold may be determined and set manually.

specifically in the double-stranded DNA product of the PCR (Fig. 7-14).

The use of nonspecific dyes to measure accumulation of product requires a clean PCR free of mispriming and primer dimers, because these artifactual products will also generate fluorescence. More specific systems, examples of which are described below, have been devised that

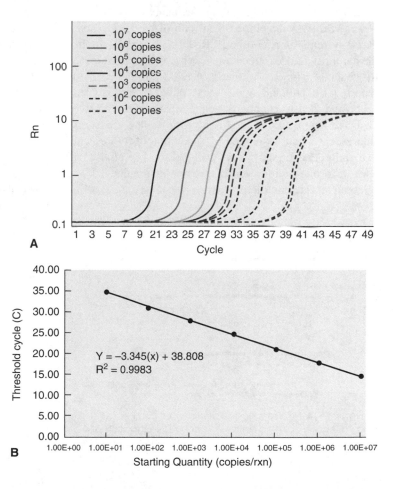

■ Figure 7-13 A plot of the accumulation of PCR product over 50 cycles of PCR. (A) is a sigmoid curve. The generation of fluorescence occurs earlier with more starting template (solid lines) than with less (dotted lines). The cycle number at which fluorescence increases over a set amount, or fluorescence threshold, is inversely proportional to the amount of starting material (B).

$Y = -3.345(x) + 38.808$
$R^2 = 0.9983$

Advanced Concepts

Fluorescence versus C_T is an inverse relationship. The more starting material, the fewer cycles are necessary to reach the fluorescence threshold. Samples that differ by a factor of 2 in the original concentration of target are expected to be 1 cycle apart, with the more dilute sample having a C_T 1 cycle higher than the more concentrated sample. Samples that differ by a factor of 10 (as in a 10-fold dilution series) would be 3.3 cycles apart. The slope of a standard curve made with 10-fold dilutions, therefore, should be –3.3.

Advanced Concepts

EtBR is a planar molecule that intercalates between the planar nucleotides in the DNA molecule. In doing so, it interferes with DNA metabolism and replication in vivo and is a mutagen. In contrast, SYBR green binds to the minor groove of the double helix without disturbing the nucleotide bases and thus does not upset DNA metabolism to the extent that EtBr does.

utilize probes designed to generate fluorescence. The probes increase specificity by only yielding fluorescence when they hybridize to the target sequences.

TaqMan was developed from one of the first probe-based systems for real-time PCR.[35] This method exploits the natural 5' to 3' exonuclease activity of *Taq* polymerase to generate signal. An early version of the method reported by Holland et al. used radioactively labeled probe and measured activity by the release of radioactive cleavage fragments.[36] The TaqMan procedure measures fluorescent signal generated by separation of fluorescent dye and quencher, a system developed by Lee et al. that uses a probe composed of a single-stranded DNA oligonucleotide complementary to a specific sequence in

the targeted region of the PCR template.[37] Note that this probe is present in the reaction mix in addition to the specific primers used to prime the DNA synthesis reaction. The probe is chemically modified at its 3' end so that it cannot be extended by the polymerase. The single-stranded DNA TaqMan probe is covalently attached to a fluorescent dye on the 5' end and another dye or nonfluorescent molecule that pulls fluorescent energy from the 5' dye (**quencher**) on the 3' end (Fig. 7-15).

As the polymerase proceeds to synthesize DNA guided by the template to which the probe is hybridized, the natural exonuclease activity of *Taq* polymerase will degrade the probe into single and oligonucleotides, thereby

Advanced Concepts

The 5' end of a Taqman probe is labeled with one of a number of dyes with different "colors," or peak wavelengths, of fluorescence, for example, FAM (6-carboxyfluorescein), TET (6-tetrachlorofluorescein), HEX (6-hexachlorofluorescein), JOE (4', 5'-dichloro-2', 7'-dimethoxy-fluorescein), Cy3, Cy5 (indodicarbocyanine), and so forth. The probe is covalently bound at the 3' end with a quencher, such as DABCYL (4-dimethylaminophenylazobenzoic acid) or TAMRA (5(6)-carboxytetramethylrhodamine), or nonfluorescent quenchers, such as BHQ1, BHQ2 (Black Hole Quenchers), and Eclipse. In the TaqMan system, the quencher prevents fluorescence from the 5' dye until they are separated during the synthesis reaction.

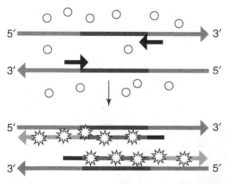

■ **Figure 7-14** Non-sequence–specific dyes, such as EtBr and SYBR green, bind to double-stranded DNA products of the PCR. As more copies of the target sequence accumulate, the fluorescence increases.

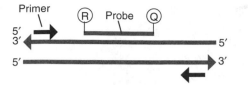

■ Figure 7-15 A TaqMan probe hybridizes to the target sequences between the primer binding sites. The probe is covalently attached to a fluorescent reporter dye (R) at the 5' end and a quencher (Q) at the 3' end.

removing the labeled nucleotide from the vicinity of the quencher and allowing it to fluoresce (Fig. 7-16). Excess probe is present so that with every doubling of the target sequences more probe binds and is digested and more fluorescence is generated. The TaqMan procedure has been applied to quantitative determinations in oncology[38] and microbiology.[39] Probe design, like primer design, is important for a successful qPCR amplification.[40,41]

Another probe-based detection system, **Molecular Beacons**, measures the accumulation of product at the annealing step in the PCR cycle. The signal from Molecular Beacons is detectable only when the probes are bound to the template *before* displacement by the polymerase. Here the probe is chemically modified so that it is not degraded during the extension step. Molecular beacons are designed with a specific binding sequence of approximately 25 bases flanked by a short, approximately 5-base-long inverted repeat that will form a stem and loop structure when the probe is not bound to the template. There is a reporter fluorophor (dye) at the 5' end of the oligomer and a quencher at the 3' end. Until specific product is present, the probe will form a hairpin structure that brings the fluorophore in proximity with the quencher (Fig. 7-17). Fluorescence will occur on binding of the probe to denatured template during the annealing step (Fig. 7-18). When the primers are extended in the PCR, displacement of the probe by *Taq* will restore the hairpin (nonfluorescent) structure. Excess probe in the reaction mix will assure binding to the increasing amount of target. The amount of fluorescence, therefore, will be directly proportional to the amount of template available for binding and inversely proportional to the C_T.

Scorpion-type primers are a variation of Molecular Beacons.[42,43] In contrast to free-labeled probes, the PCR product will be covalently bound to the dye. In this system, target-specific primers are tailed at the 5' end with a sequence complementary to part of the internal primer sequence, a quencher, a stem-loop structure, and a 5' fluorophore (Fig. 7-19). The fluorophore and the quencher are positioned so that they are juxtaposed when the hairpin in the primer is intact. After polymerization,

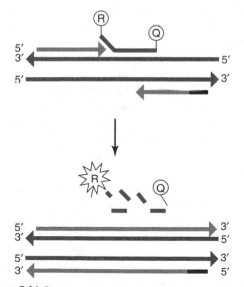

■ Figure 7-16 Taqman signal fluorescence is generated when *Taq* polymerase extends the primers and digests the probe and releases the reporter from the vicinity of the quencher.

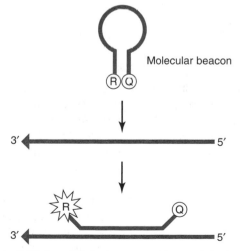

■ Figure 7-17 A molecular beacon probe contains target specific sequences and a short inverted repeat that hybridizes into a hairpin structure. The 5' end of the probe has a reporter dye (R), and the 3' end has a quencher dye (Q).

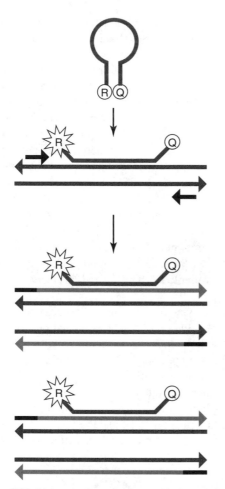

■ **Figure 7-18** Molecular beacons bound to target sequences fluoresce. Fluorescence doubles with every doubling of target sequences.

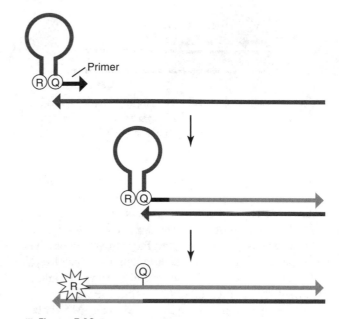

■ **Figure 7-19** Scorpion primer/probes are primers tailed with molecular beacon-type sequences. After extension of the primer/probe, the target-specific sequences fold over to hybridize with the newly synthesized target sequences, separating the reporter (R) from the quencher (P).

the secondary structure of the primer is overcome by hybridization of the primer sequence with the target sequence, removing the fluorophore from the quencher. This intramolecular system generates signal faster than the intermolecular Molecular Beacon strategy and may be preferred for methods requiring fast cycling conditions.[44]

Another frequently used system, **fluorescent resonance energy transfer** (**FRET**), utilizes two specific probes, one with a 3' fluorophore (acceptor) and the other with a 5' catalyst for the fluorescence (donor), that bind to adjacent targets.[45] Examples of frequently used donor-acceptor pairs are fluorescein-rhodamine, fluorescein-(2 aminopurine), and fluorescein-Cy5. When the donor and acceptor are brought within 1 to 10 nm (1 to 5 bases) through specific DNA binding, excitation energy is transferred from the donor to the acceptor (Fig. 7-20). The acceptor then loses the energy in the form of heat or fluorescence emission called sensitized emission. As with the molecular beacons, the more template available for binding of the probes, the more fluorescence will be generated. FRET probes are used in the medical laboratory for viral detection and quantitation and for amplification and detection of genetic diseases.[46-49]

Real-time PCR lends itself to several variations of technique, as exemplified above. These techniques can be further modified, for example, using FRET probes with different sequences to distinguish types of organisms or to detect mutations. Refer to Chapter 9 for a description of methods using fluorescent probes and melt curves to detect gene mutations. Methods can be combined, for example, using an intercalating dye (acridine orange) as the donor and a probe with a single receptor dye (rhodamine).[50] As with standard PCR, a large and growing number of such methods have been devised for a variety of applications.

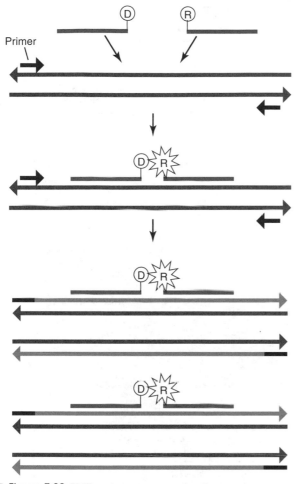

Primer

■ **Figure 7-20** FRET probes are separate oligomers, one covalently attached to a donor fluor (D) and one to an acceptor or reporter fluor (R). The acceptor/reporter will fluoresce only when both probes are bound next to one another on the target sequences. As more target accumulates, more probes bind and more fluorescence is emitted.

Advanced Concepts

Internal controls are often used with qPCR assays to detect false-negative results in the event of amplification failure. (See Chapter 16, "Quality Assurance and Quality Control in the Molecular Laboratory.") Ideally, these controls should be RNA for RNA expression assays and plasmid for DNA copy number analyses.

Transcription-Based Amplification Systems

In transcription-based amplification systems (TAS), RNA is the usual target instead of DNA. A DNA copy is synthesized from the target RNA, and then transcription of the DNA produces millions of copies of RNA. There are a number of commercial variations of this process: **transcription-mediated amplification (TMA)** (Gen-Probe), **nucleic acid sequence–based amplification (NASBA)** (Organon-Teknika), and **self-sustaining sequence replication (3SR)** (Baxter Diagnostics).

Kwoh and colleagues developed the first TAS in 1989.[51] TAS differs from other nucleic acid amplification procedures in that RNA is the target as well as the primary product. In the original method of TAS, a primer complementary to sequences in the target RNA that also has the binding site for RNA polymerase at one end is added to a sample of target RNA. The primer anneals, and reverse transcriptase makes a DNA copy of the target RNA. Heat is used to denature the DNA-RNA hybrid, and a second primer binds to the cDNA and is extended by reverse transcriptase, producing double-stranded DNA. RNA polymerase derived from the bacteriophage T7 then transcribes the cDNA, producing hundreds to thousands of copies of RNA. The transcribed RNA can then serve as target RNA to which the primers bind and synthesize more cDNA.

The original TAS procedure as described above had the disadvantage that a heating step was required to denature the intermediate RNA-DNA hybrid product. The heat also denatured the enzymes so that fresh enzyme had to be added after each denaturation step. The process was simplified with the addition of RNase H derived from *E. coli* (Fig. 7-21). RNase H degrades the RNA from the intermediate hybrid, eliminating the heating step. Thus, after synthesis of the DNA copy by reverse transcriptase, the RNA strand is degraded by RNase H. Binding of the second primer and extension of the primer, producing double-stranded DNA by reverse transcriptase, is followed by transcription of the cDNA with T7 RNA polymerase (Fig. 7-22).

This modified procedure has been marketed as TMA, NASBA, or 3SR, depending on the manufacturer. An additional modification and simplification of the procedure came about with the discovery that the reverse transcriptase derived from avian myeloblastosis virus (AMV) has inherent RNase H activity. Thus, TAS can be run with

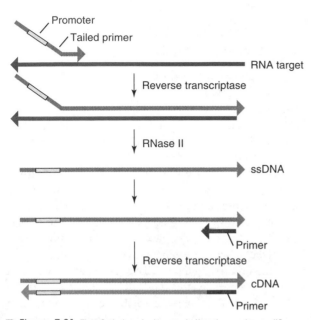

Figure 7-21 The first step in transcription-based amplification is the production of a complementary double-stranded DNA copy of the RNA target (A). Synthesis is performed by reverse transcriptase, which extends a primer that is tailed with an RNA polymerase binding site (promoter) sequence (purple). The RNA/DNA hybrid (B) is digested with RNase H, leaving the single-stranded DNA (C), which is converted to a double strand with a complementary primer (D). The DNA product (E) will have a promoter sequence at one end.

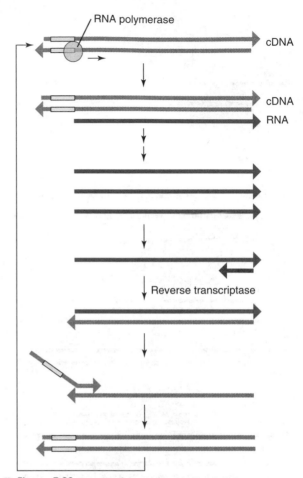

Figure 7-22 The cDNA produced in the first step serves as a template for RNA polymerase (A). Many copies of RNA are synthesized (B, C), which are primed by a complementary primer (D) for synthesis of another RNA/DNA hybrid (E). After RNase H degrades the RNA strand, the primer tailed with the promoter sequences synthesizes another template (F), cycling back into the system as (A).

only two enzymes, AMV reverse transcriptase and T7 RNA polymerase.

TAS has some advantages over PCR and other amplification procedures. First, in contrast to PCR and the ligase chain reaction (LCR, discussed below), TAS is an isothermal process, negating the requirement for thermal cycling to drive the reactions. Second, targeting RNA allows for the direct detection of RNA viruses, for example, hepatitis C virus[52,53] and human immunodeficiency virus.[54,55] Even targeting the RNA of organisms with DNA genomes, such as *Mycobacterium tuberculosis*, is more sensitive than targeting the DNA, because each bacterium, for example, has multiple copies of RNA, whereas it has only one copy of DNA.[56]

The NASBA procedure, with slight modifications, can also be performed on a DNA target.[57] For DNA, the sample is heated to denature the DNA, and the first primer anneals and is extended by reverse transcriptase (which in addition to having RNA-dependent DNA polymerase

activity also has DNA-dependent DNA polymerase activity). The sample is heated again to denature the double strands, and the second primer binds and is extended. The DNA product has also incorporated the T7 RNA polymerase binding site, as occurs when RNA is the target. Thus, T7 RNA polymerase transcribes the newly replicated DNA into hundreds to thousands of RNA copies.[58]

Detection of *M. tuberculosis* in smear-positive respiratory samples, *Chlamydia trachomatis* in genital specimens, and HIV and cytomegalovirus (CMV) quantitation in blood are a few of the current applications for TAS.

Arbitrarily Primed PCR

In **arbitrarily primed PCR**, also known as **randomly amplified polymorphic DNA** or random amplification of polymorphic DNA (RAPD), short primers (10 to 15 bases) with random sequences are used to amplify arbitrary regions in genomic DNA under low stringency conditions.[59,60] With this method, PCR products are generated without knowing the sequence of the target or targeting a specific gene. In contrast to standard PCR where only one or a few known products are generated, it is possible with this method to obtain multiple products depending how many times a short sequence appears in the genome (Fig. 7-23). Arbitrarily primed PCR has been used primarily in the epidemiological typing of microorganisms.[61] Similar band patterns obtained from performing PCR with the same arbitrary primers indicate that two organisms are the same or similar. (See Chapter 12, "Detection and Identification of Microorganisms.") The disadvantage of this method, however, is that the stringency is low enough that the reproducibility between runs is not very good, such that two organisms that had the same PCR product pattern on one day could have two different patterns and look like two different organisms when amplified on another day.

Whole Genome Amplification

In addition to amplification of single genes or transcripts, methods have been devised to amplify all regions of input DNA, or whole genomes. Whole genome amplification (WGA) methods are designed to survey all genes or transcripts of an organism for purposes of typing of microorganisms or screening for particular genetic lesions. Genomic amplification differs from standard amplification methods in that the primers used are not complementary to specific genetic regions, rather, replication initiates at random sites throughout the input nucleic acid (Fig. 7-24).[62]

In addition to typing, genomic amplification provides the ability to generate a lot of information from a very small amount of starting material. In biological samples especially, the target nucleic acid is not always clean, accessible, or in optimal condition for complex analyses, such as sequencing or microarray methods. Analyses that involve multiple targets demand enough starting material to accurately test each one. The following methods are approaches to genomic amplification applied to typing of microorganisms and generation of multiple genomic copies for genetic studies.

WGA can be performed using degenerative primers that prime random synthesis throughout the target genome or by nick translation.

Degenerative primers are synthetic single-stranded DNA sequences that vary with some frequency at each position where N = A T G or C. In primer extension preamplification (PEP), this variation occurs throughout the primer: N_{15-16}. In degenerative oligonucleotide primer (DOP) amplification, the variable sequences are flanked by a highly repeated sequence in DNA: $CCGACTCGAGN_6ATGTGG$. Tagged-PCR, T-PCR primers have a 5' sequence complementary to repetitive DNA followed by a random sequence of variable length: $CTCACTCTCAN_X$.

Alternatively, whole genome amplification can be achieved by introducing single-strand breaks or nicks in the

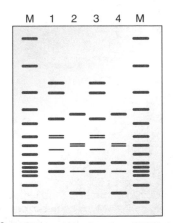

■ Figure 7-23 RAPD or arbitrarily primed PCR yields many products per PCR reaction. The band pattern produced by these fragments reflects the nature of the DNA template. M: Molecular weight markers. Lanes 1 and 3 are products from very similar templates, which are different from those in lanes 2 and 4.

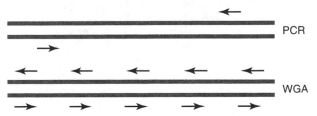

■ Figure 7-24 In contrast to PCR, the object of whole genome amplification (WGA) is to copy all regions of a genomic template. The primers may be of random sequence or directed to highly repeated sequences in the genome.

genomic DNA and amplification primed by short random sequences (hexamers) or the 3' ends of the breaks.[63] This process is called **multiple displacement amplification**, as the extension requires removal or denaturation of double-stranded DNA as extension proceeds. Amplification is performed using Phi29 DNA polymerase, a highly processive enzyme—one that can displace and copy thousands of bases without losing contact with the template.

WGA has multiple applications, including **comparative genomic arrays**,[64] detection of single nucleotide polymorphisms,[65] and analysis of minimal starting material, such as DNA in plasma,[66] single cell analysis,[67] and ancient DNA samples.[68]

Emulsion PCR

Emulsion PCR is designed to simultaneously amplify thousands of specific templates in a single reaction tube.[69] It was developed to amplify genomic libraries more efficiently. In this method, the ends of fragmented template DNA are ligated to universal primer sequences and, along with the other components of the PCR reaction (buffer, polymerase enzyme, forward and reverse primers, dNTPs), are added to an oil surfactant mixture (Span 80, Tween 80, Triton X-100, and mineral oil) (Fig. 7-25). With stirring, an emulsion is formed with

1 to 10 billion droplets, each of which can contain a single template in a tiny volume of reaction buffer. When the emulsion is subjected to an amplification program, the droplets will act as single reaction chambers producing many copies of a specific sequence. After amplification, the emulsion is broken. The pooled products are used for a variety of genomic study applications, such as array studies, haplotyping, or detection of rare mutations.

Solid phase emulsion PCR was developed for next-generation sequencing (Chapter 10) and other high-throughput technologies that have driven the development of equally high-throughput PCR technologies. In this method, templates ligated to a universal primer sequence are mixed with bead-immobilized primers and other reaction components in the water-in-oil emulsion (Fig. 7-26). Aqueous droplets in the oil contain a single

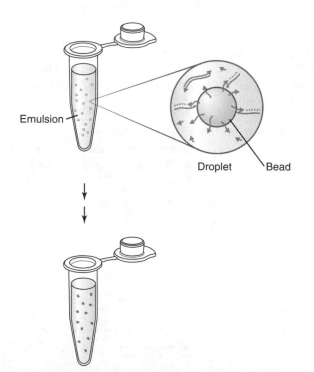

■ **Figure 7-26** For solid phase ePCR, the template is prepared as described in Figure 7-25. Many copies of one primer are covalently attached to a microsphere (bead). In the emulsion droplets, a single template will be copied into immobilized products on the beads. After the PCR reaction, the emulsion is broken, the beads are released, and the complementary strands are washed away, leaving many copies of immobilized single strands on each bead.

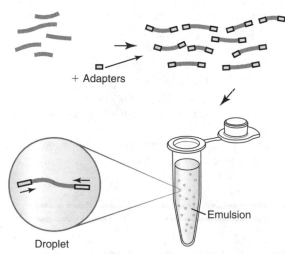

■ **Figure 7-25** Whole genome DNA is fragmented and the fragments are ligated to adapters that are complementary to forward and reverse PCR primers. The adapted templates, primers, and other PCR reagents in aqueous solution form an emulsion with oil such that each aqueous droplet in the emulsion contains a single template. Each of thousands of oil droplets then serve as reaction chambers for unique products.

template and a single bead coupled to multiple copies of the primer sequence. When the emulsion is broken, the PCR products are denatured, washing away the complementary strand and leaving the single-stranded sequencing templates attached to the beads. These templates can then be subjected to massive parallel (next-generation) sequencing technologies.

Surface Amplification (Bridge PCR)

Surface amplification is an isothermal, genomic PCR method used in high-throughput sequencing technologies. In this method, forward and reverse primers are immobilized on a solid support in a flow cell (Fig. 7-27). Fragmented or preamplified template is denatured and those single strands complementary to the immobilized primers will anneal under nondenaturing buffer conditions. Extension of the immobilized primer occurs at 60°C. Denaturing conditions are then introduced by

addition of formamide to the reaction mixture. After the template and reaction components are removed by washing, annealing conditions are reestablished chemically, allowing the attached copy of the template to anneal to the immobilized reverse primer. The reverse primer is extended, forming a bridge between the two immobilized primers. The process is repeated for 35 cycles, producing approximately 1000 copies of the template sequence. The double-stranded bridges are then denatured, resulting in a localized clone of single-stranded complementary molecules. To avoid re-annealing, a cleavable site located on one primer (either forward or reverse) allows removal of one of the complements (Fig. 7-27). For DNA sequence applications, the remaining strand is chemically blocked at the free 3' end using terminal DNA transferase and a dideoxynucleotide molecule that cannot be extended. Sequencing primer is then annealed to the template for sequencing. (See Chapter 10.)

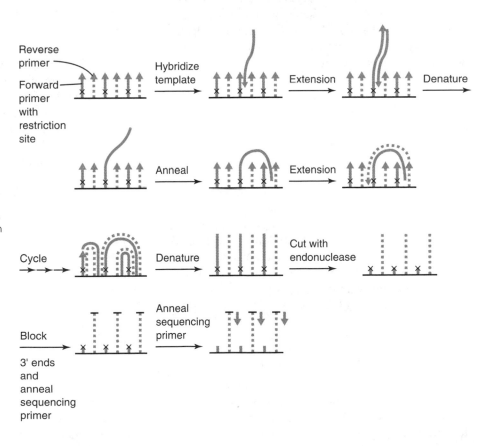

■ **Figure 7-27** Bridge PCR produces immobilized single-stranded products from immobilized forward and reverse primers. One primer is designed to contain a single-strand endonuclease recognition site. After amplification, the PCR products form bridges from the forward to the reverse primers so that upon denaturation, the single strands are also immobilized. Endonuclease digestion will remove one complement of single strands so that the remaining population of immobilized single strands is identical. The strands are then subjected to further analysis such as sequencing.

Probe Amplification

In **probe amplification** procedures, the number of target nucleic acid sequences in a sample is not changed. Rather, synthetic probes that are specific to the target sequences bind to the target where the probes themselves are amplified. There are three major procedures that involve the amplification of probe sequences: ligase chain reaction (LCR), **strand displacement amplification (SDA),** and Qβ replicase.

Ligase Chain Reaction

LCR is a method for amplifying synthetic primers/probes complementary to target nucleic acid. Similar to PCR, the entire target sequence must be known in order to prepare the oligonucleotide primers for LCR. In PCR, there is a distance between the primers of hundreds to thousands of bases that is part of the amplified sequence. In LCR, by contrast, the primers bind immediately adjacent to each other. Instead of DNA polymerase synthesizing complementary DNA by extending the primers as occurs in PCR, DNA ligase is used in LCR to ligate the adjacent primers together. The ligated primers can then serve as a template for the annealing and ligation of additional primers. Because the product of LCR is ligated primer, LCR is a method of probe amplification rather than target amplification as the copy number of target molecules does not change.

LCR requires a thermal cycler to change the temperature to drive the different reactions. In LCR the reaction is heated to denature the template. When the temperature is cooled, the primers anneal if the complementary sequence is present, and a thermostable ligase joins the two primers (Fig. 7-28). Even a 1-base-pair mismatch at the ligation point will prevent ligation of the primers. Thus, LCR can be used to detect point mutations in a target sequence. The DNA mutation that occurs in the beta globulin of patients with sickle cell disease, as compared with normal beta globulin, was one of the first applications of LCR.[70]

Strand Displacement Amplification

SDA differs from most of the previously described amplification methods in that SDA is an isothermal amplification process; that is, after an initial denaturation step, the reaction proceeds at one temperature.[71] In SDA

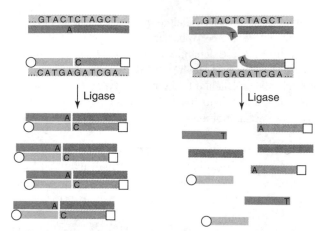

■ **Figure 7-28** Ligase chain reaction generates a signal by repeated ligation of probes complementary to specific sequences in the test DNA. One complementary oligomer is covalently attached to biotin for immobilization (square), and one has a signal-producing molecule (circle). The two oligomers will be ligated together only if the sequence of the target is complementary (left). The oligomers captured on a solid substrate by streptavidin will generate a signal. If the sequence of the target is not complementary (right), the captured probe will not yield a signal.

the major amplification products are the probes. There are two stages to the SDA process. In the first stage (target generation), the target DNA is denatured by heating to 95°C. At each end of the target sequence, two primers bind close to each other, an outer and an inner primer (Fig. 7-29). The inner primers have a 5' tail containing a recognition sequence for a restriction enzyme. Exonuclease-deficient DNA polymerase derived from *E. coli* DNA polymerase I extends all of the primers, incorporating a modified nucleotide, 2'-deoxyadenosine 5'-O-(1-thiotriphosphate) (dATPaS) included in the nucleotide mix. As the outer primers are extended, they displace the products formed by the extension of the inner primers. A second set of outer and inner primers then bind to the displaced inner primer products, and DNA polymerase extends the complementary primers, producing four double-stranded products (probes). These probes are the target DNA for the next stage of the process.

The second stage of the reaction is the exponential probe amplification phase using a restriction endonuclease enzyme, *Hinc*II (Fig. 7-30). When the restriction enzyme is added to the double-stranded probe DNA, only one strand of the probe will be cut due to the

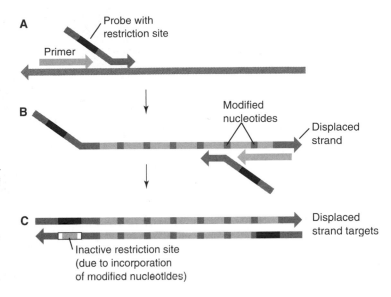

A Probe with restriction site

Primer

B Modified nucleotides

Displaced strand

C Displaced strand targets

Inactive restriction site (due to incorporation of modified nucleotides)

■ **Figure 7-29** The first stage of SDA is the denaturation of the double-stranded target and annealing of primers and probes tailed with sequences including a restriction enzyme site (A; only one strand of the initial target is shown). A second reaction (B) copies the probe, incorporating dATPαS and thereby inactivating the restriction site on the copied strand (C). This species is the target for amplification in the second stage of the reaction.

dATPαS introduced in the extension reaction. This forms a nick in the DNA that is extended by DNA polymerase, simultaneously displacing the opposite strands. The nicking and extension forms single-stranded probes and regenerates the restriction site. The nicking/extension reaction can repeat on the initial probe as well as the probes generated in the reaction. With the enzyme nicking reaction, strand displacement does not require denaturation of the double-stranded probes. Thus, the iterative process takes place at about 52°C without temperature cycling.

The SDA process was first widely applied to detection of *M. tuberculosis*.[72] Methods using fluorescence polarization to detect the amplified target have been designed to test for *M. tuberculosis*[73] and *C. trachomatis*.[74] Addition of a fluorogenic probe to the reaction produces a fluorescent signal that corresponds to the amount of amplified target. This is the basis for the BDProbeTecET test for *M. tuberculosis*,[75] *C. trachomatis*, and *Neisseria gonorrhoeae*.[76]

Advanced Concepts

For SDA of RNA or other single-stranded targets, the initial heat denaturation step is not necessary. The inner primer tailed with the restriction site is annealed to the 3' end of the target, forming a double-stranded probe that will enter the iterative restriction/strand displacement reactions.

Qβ Replicase

Qβ replicase is another method for amplifying probes that have specificity for a target sequence. The method is named for the major enzyme that is used to amplify probe sequences. Qβ replicase is an RNA-dependent RNA polymerase from the bacteriophage Qβ.[77] The target nucleic acid in this assay can be either DNA (which must first be denatured) or RNA.

The target nucleic acid is added to a well containing reporter probes, which are RNA molecules that have specificity for the target sequence and also contain a promoter sequence that is recognized by the Qβ replicase. The reporter probes are allowed to hybridize to the template. The template with bound probes is immobilized using polyG capture probes (Fig. 7-31, capture probe A) and paramagnetic beads covalently attached to polyC sequences. With a magnet applied to the outside of the wells, the unbound reporter molecules are washed away. The template-probe complexes are released from the polyC magnetic bead by denaturation and hybridized to a polyA capture probe (capture probe B). The complex is then hybridized to a polyT paramagnetic bead. After a series of washes to remove unbound reporter probe, the template-probe complex is again released from the magnetic bead.

For the amplification step, the probe-bound template is mixed with the Qβ replicase, which replicates the probe molecules. This replication is very efficient; it generates 10^6–10^9 RNA molecules (probes) in less than 15 minutes.

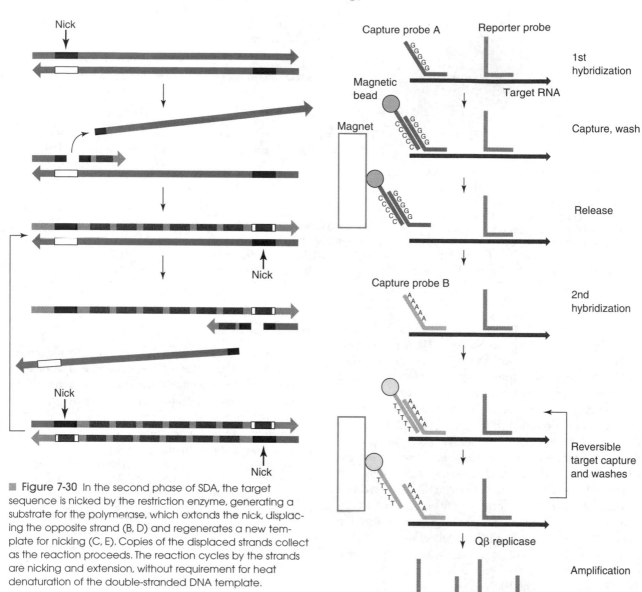

■ **Figure 7-30** In the second phase of SDA, the target sequence is nicked by the restriction enzyme, generating a substrate for the polymerase, which extends the nick, displacing the opposite strand (B, D) and regenerates a new template for nicking (C, E). Copies of the displaced strands collect as the reaction proceeds. The reaction cycles by the strands are nicking and extension, without requirement for heat denaturation of the double-stranded DNA template.

■ **Figure 7-31** The Qβ replicase method proceeds through a series of binding and washing steps.[77,78] Probe bound to the purified template is then amplified by Qβ replicase. The resulting RNA can be detected by fluorometry using propidium iodide as a fluorescent label of the synthesized probe or by chromogenic methods.

Because so many RNA molecules are produced, product detection can be achieved by colorimetric as well as real-time fluorogenic methods. Qβ replicase has been used primarily to amplify the nucleic acid associated with infectious organisms, particularly mycobacteria,[78,79] *Chlamydia*,[80] HIV,[81] and CMV[82].

Signal Amplification

In **signal amplification** procedures, there is no change in the number of target or probe sequences; instead, large amounts of signal are bound to the target sequences that are present in the sample. Signal amplification procedures are inherently better at quantifying the amount of target sequences present in the clinical sample. Several signal amplification methods are available commercially.

Branched DNA Amplification

In **branched DNA (bDNA) amplification**, a series of short oligomer probes are used to capture the target nucleic acid. Additional extender probes bind to the target nucleic acid and then to multiple reporter molecules,[83] loading the target nucleic acid with signal.

For the bDNA signal amplification procedure, target nucleic acid released from the cells is denatured (if DNA is the target; this method also works with RNA). The target nucleic acid binds to capture probes that are fixed to the plate well (Fig. 7-32). Extender or preamplifier probes then bind to the captured target. The extender probes have sequences that are complementary to sequences in the target molecules as well as to sequences in amplifier probes.

In the first-generation assay, the extender probes bind to a bDNA amplifier probe, which in turn binds multiple alkaline phosphatase-labeled nucleotides. Eight multimers or amplifiers, each with 15 branches, bind to each extender probe bound to the target. In the second- and third-generation assays, the extender probes bind preamplifiers, which in turn bind 14 to 15 amplifiers each

with the capacity to bind multiple alkaline phosphatase–labeled oligonucleotides (Fig. 7-33). Dioxetane is added as the substrate for the **alkaline phosphatase**, and chemiluminescence is measured in a luminometer. This system has a detection limit of about 50 target mol/mL.[84]

There are several advantages to the bDNA method. First, in the bDNA assay there is less risk of carryover contamination resulting in a positive test than in PCR.[85] Second, multiple capture and extender probes can be incorporated that detect slightly different target sequences, as occurs with different isolates of hepatitis C virus and HIV. By incorporating different probes that recognize slightly different sequences, multiple genotypes of the same virus can still be detected by the same basic system. Finally, the requirement for probes to bind multiple sequences in the same target increases the specificity of the system. It is highly unlikely that all of the required probes would bind nonspecifically to an unrelated target and produce a signal. The bDNA signal amplification assay has been applied to the qualitative and quantitative

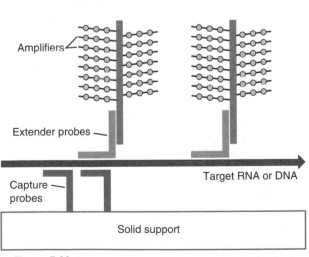

■ Figure 7-32 Branched DNA signal amplification of a single target. The target is captured or immobilized to a solid support by capture probes, after which extender probes and blocking probes create a stable cruciform structure with the amplifiers. Each amplifier has hybridization sites for 8–14 branches, which in turn bind substrate molecules for alkaline phosphatase.

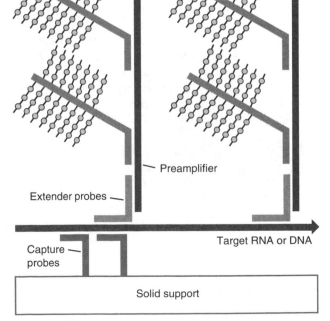

■ Figure 7-33 Second-generation bDNA assays use extender probes that bind multiple amplifiers, increasing the signal intensity and improving limits of detection.

detection of hepatitis B virus, hepatitis C virus, and HIV-1.[84,85] It is the basis of the VERSANT HIV-1 3.0, HCV 3.0, and HBV assays (Siemens).[86–89] By replacing the plate support with beads, the assay has been combined with the Luminex xMAP bead array technology to provide a multiplex system (QuantiGene Plex 2.0®, Affymetrix) that can detect 100 different targets in a single sample.

Hybrid Capture Assays

Digene Diagnostics has marketed the **hybrid capture** assays primarily for the detection and molecular characterization of human papilloma virus in genitourinary specimens.[90,91] It is also available for the detection of hepatitis B virus[92,93] and CMV.[94,95] For these assays, target DNA released from cells is bound to single-stranded RNA probes (Fig. 7-34). The DNA-RNA hybrid has a unique structure that is recognized by antibodies. Antibodies bound to the surface of a microtiter well capture the DNA-RNA hybrids. Double-stranded DNA or single-stranded RNA will not bind to these antibodies. Captured hybrids are detected by the binding of alkaline phosphatase–conjugated antibodies to the DNA-RNA hybrid antibodies in a typical sandwich assay. The substrate for the alkaline phosphatase is added, and chemiluminescence is measured. The sensitivity of this assay for human papilloma virus has been reported to be about 1000 copies of viral DNA.[96] The hybrid capture assay is considered a signal amplification assay because the amount of target DNA is not amplified; rather, the DNA is isolated bound to RNA and is recognized by multiple antibodies to the target/probe hybrid molecule.

Cleavage-Based Amplification

Cleavage-based amplification detects target nucleic acids by using a series of probes that bind to the target and overlap. Cleavase is a bacterial enzyme that recognizes overlapping sequences of DNA and makes a cut (cleaves) in the overlapping piece. In vivo, this activity is most likely important in repairing DNA. This method is the basis of the Invader system (Third Wave Technologies). Applications for this form of amplification include DNA polymorphisms, such as factor V Leiden mutation detection,[97,98] and infectious diseases, such as HCV and HPV genotyping.[99,100]

To start the amplification, the target nucleic acid is mixed with invader and signal probes (Fig. 7-35). The invader probe and the signal probes bind at the target, with the 5' end of the signal probe overlapping with the invader probe. Cleavase recognizes this overlap and cleaves the signal probe, which can act as an invader probe in the next step of the reaction. In the second step, a FRET probe is added that has sequences complementary to the cleaved signal probe. The 5' end of the FRET probe has a reporter molecule that is located in proximity to a quencher molecule. As a result, the intact FRET probe does not produce a signal. The signal probe (now an invader probe) binds to the FRET probe, producing an overlapping region that is recognized by Cleavase. When Cleavase cuts the FRET probe in the overlapping region, it releases the reporter molecule from the quencher, resulting in the production of signal. The amount of signal can be quantified and related directly to the amount of target molecules in the sample.

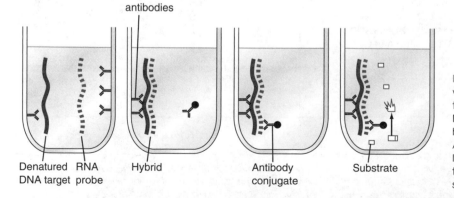

Capture antibodies

Denatured DNA target | RNA probe | Hybrid | Antibody conjugate | Substrate

■ **Figure 7-34** Hybrid capture starts with hybridization of the RNA probe to the denatured DNA target. The RNA-DNA hybrid is then bound by hybrid-specific immobilized antibodies. A secondary antibody bound to alkaline phosphatase generates signal in the presence of a chemiluminescent substrate (right).

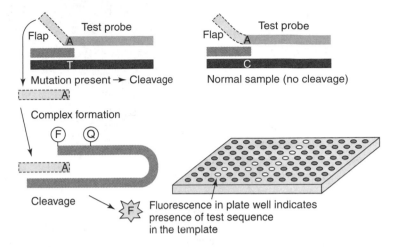

■ Figure 7-35 Invader assays exploit the substrate requirements of the Cleavase enzyme. A cleavable substrate is formed by the hybridization of two probes and template (top left). This structure will not form if the probe does not match the template (top right). If the proper substrate is formed, the enzyme removes part of one probe and that fragment forms another cleavable complex with the fluorescently labeled reporter probe (bottom left). Repeated binding and cleavage amplifies the signal. In a plate format, only those wells with template complementary to the test probe will produce fluorescent signal.

Cycling Probe

In the **cycling probe** method of amplification, target sequences are detected using a synthetic probe consisting of sequences of DNA and RNA arranged in a DNA-RNA-DNA sandwich sequence carrying a reporter dye at one end and a quencher dye at the other. The probe binds to the target nucleic acid (Fig. 7-36). RNase H cleaves the RNA from the middle of the probe. The loss of the RNA sequences lowers the hybridization temperature of the

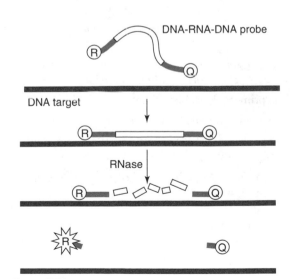

■ Figure 7-36 Cycling probe produces fluorescence only when the RNA probe binds to the DNA template. The RNA-DNA hybrid formed by the probe bound to the template is a substrate for RNase H, which digests the RNA probe and releases the reporter dye (R) from the vicinity of the quencher (Q).

probe and the DNA portions of the probes leave the template. When the probe is released, the reporter and quencher dye are separated, allowing fluorescence to escape from the reporter. The template remains available for additional probe hybridization. Since the cyclic denaturation of the probe depends on the digestion of the RNA portion, the method is isothermal. The amount of fluorescence from the **reporter dye** (produced when the target is present) is measured as an indication of the presence of target molecules. Alternatively, the presence of chimeric probes that remain when target sequences are not present can also be measured. This method has been used to detect genes associated with antimicrobial resistance in bacteria, such as methicillin resistance (***mecA***) in *Staphylococcus aureus* and vancomycin resistance (*vanA* and *vanB*) in *Enterococcus*.[101–103]

• STUDY QUESTIONS •

1. A master mix of all components (except template) necessary for PCR contains what basic ingredients?

2. The final concentration of *Taq* polymerase is to be 0.01 units/μL in a 50-μL PCR. If the enzyme is supplied as 5 units/μL, how much enzyme would you add to the reaction?
   a. 1 μL
   b. 1 μL of a 1:10 dilution of *Taq*
   c. 5 μL of a 1:10 dilution of *Taq*
   d. 2 μL

3. Primer dimers result from:
   a. High primer concentrations
   b. Low primer concentrations
   c. High GC content in the primer sequences
   d. 3' complementarity in the primer sequences

4. Which control is run to detect contamination?
   a. Negative control
   b. Positive control
   c. Molecular weight marker
   d. Reagent blank

5. Nonspecific extra PCR products can result from:
   a. Mispriming
   b. High annealing temperatures
   c. High agarose gel concentrations
   d. Omission of $MgCl_2$ from the PCR

6. Using which of the following is an appropriate way to avoid PCR contamination?
   a. High-fidelity polymerase
   b. Hot-start PCR
   c. A separate area for PCR setup
   d. Fewer PCR cycles

7. How many copies of a target are made after 30 cycles of PCR?
   a. 2×30
   b. 2^{30}
   c. 30^2
   d. 30/2

8. What are the three steps of a standard PCR cycle?

9. Which of the following is a method for purifying a PCR product?
   a. Treat with uracil N glycosylase
   b. Add divalent cations
   c. Put the reaction mix through a spin column
   d. Add DEPC

10. In contrast to standard PCR, real-time PCR is:
    a. Quantitative
    b. Qualitative
    c. Labor-intensive
    d. Sensitive

11. In real-time PCR, fluorescence is *not* generated by which of the following?
    a. FRET probes
    b. TaqMan probes
    c. SYBR green
    d. *Tth* polymerase

12. Prepare a table that compares PCR, LCR, bDNA, TMA, Qβ Replicase, and Hybrid Capture with regard to the type of amplification, target nucleic acid, type of amplicon, and major enzyme(s) for each.

13. Examine the following sequence. (The complementary strand is not shown.) You are devising a test to detect a mutation at the underlined position.

5' TATTTAGTTA TGGCCTATAC ACTATTTGTG
AGCAAAGGTG ATCGTTTTCT GTTTGAGATT
TTTATCTCTT GATTCTTCAA AAGCATTCTG
AGAAGGTGAG ATAAGCCCTG AGTCTCAGCT
ACCTAAGAAA AACCTGGATG TCACTGGCCA
CTGAGGAGC TTTGTTTCAAC CAAGTCATGT
GCATTTCCAC GTCAACAGAA TTGTTTATTG
TGACAGTT**A**T ATCTGTTGTC CCTTTGACCT
TGTTTCTTGA AGGTTTCCTC GTCCCTGGGC
AATTCCGCAT TTAATTCATG GTATTCAGGA
TTACATGCAT GTTTGGTTA AACCCATGAGA
TTCATTCAGT TAAAAATCCA GATGGCGAAT 3'

Design one set of primers (forward and reverse) to generate an amplicon containing the underlined base.

The primers should be 20 bases long.

The amplicon must be 100 to 150 bp in size.

The primers must have similar melting temperatures (T_m), +/- 2°C.

The primers should have no homology in the last three 3' bases.

a. Write the primer sequences 5'→ 3' as you would if you were to order them from the DNA synthesis facility.

b. Write the T_m for each primer that you have designed.

14. How does nested PCR differ from multiplex PCR?

15. What replaces heat denaturation in strand displacement amplification?

References

1. Mullis K. The unusual origin of the polymerase chain reaction. *Scientific American* 1990;262:56–61, 64–65.
2. Mullis K, Faloona FA. Specific synthesis of DNA *in vitro* via a polymerase-catalyzed chain reaction. *Methods in Enzymology* 1987;155:335–350.
3. Saiki R, Scharf S, Faloona F, et al. Enzymatic amplification of beta-globin genomic sequences and restriction site analysis for diagnosis of sickle cell anemia. *Science* 1985;230:1350–1354.
4. Mullis K. The polymerase chain reaction. *The Nobel Prize in Chemistry* 1993.
5. Guyer R, Koshland DE. The molecule of the year. *Science* 1989;246:1543–1546.
6. Saiki R, Scharf S, Faloona F, et al. Enzymatic amplification of beta-globin genomic sequences and restriction site analysis for diagnosis of sickle cell anemia. *Science* 1985;230:1350–1354.
7. Lawyer F, Stoffel S, Saiki RK, et al. Isolation, characterization, and expression in *Escherichia coli* of the DNA polymerase gene from *Thermus aquaticus. Journal of Biological Chemistry* 1989;264(11): 6427–6437.
8. Obeid P, Christopoulos TK, Crabtree HJ, et al. Microfabricated device for DNA and RNA amplification by continuous-flow polymerase chain reaction and reverse transcription-polymerase chain reaction with cycle number selection. *Analytical Chemistry* 2003;75(2):288–295.
9. Cone R, Fairfax MR. Protocol for ultraviolet irradiation of surfaces to reduce PCR contamination. *Genome Research* 1993;3:S15–S17.
10. Klaschik S, Lehmann LE, Raadts A, et al. Comparison of different decontamination methods for reagents to detect low concentrations of bacterial 16S DNA by real-time-PCR. *Molecular Biotechnology* 2002;22(3):231–242.
11. Meier A, Persing DH, Finken M, et al. Elimination of contaminating DNA within polymerase chain reaction reagents: Implications for a general approach to detection of uncultured pathogens. *Journal of Clinical Microbiology* 1993;31(3):646–652.
12. Fox J, Ait-Khaled M, Webster A, et al. Eliminating PCR contamination: Is UV irradiation the answer? *Journal of Virological Methods* 1991;33(3): 375–382.

13. Cleaver J, Crowley E. UV damage, DNA repair and skin carcinogenesis. *Frontiers in Bioscience* 2002;7:1024–1043.
14. Korbie DJ, Mattick JS. Touchdown PCR for increased specificity and sensitivity in PCR amplification. *Nature Protocols* 2008;3:1452–1456.
15. Waltenbury D, Leduc LG, Ferroni GD. The use of RAPD genomic fingerprinting to study relatedness in strains of *Acidithiobacillus ferrooxidans. Journal of Microbiological Methods* 2005;62(1):103–112.
16. Tzanakaki G, Tsopanomichalou M, Kesanopoulos K, et al. Simultaneous single-tube PCR assay for the detection of *Neisseria meningitidis, Haemophilus influenzae* type b and *Streptococcus pneumoniae. Clinical Microbiology and Infection* 2005;11(5): 386–390.
17. Nguyen T, Le Van P, Le Huy C, et al. Detection and characterization of diarrheagenic *Escherichia coli* from young children in Hanoi, Vietnam. *Journal of Clinical Microbiology* 2005;43(2):755–760.
18. Bellau-Pujol S, Vabret A, Legrand L, et al. Development of three multiplex RT-PCR assays for the detection of 12 respiratory RNA viruses. *Journal of Virological Methods* 2005;126(1–2):53–63.
19. Gaydos C, Crotchfelt KA, Shah N, et al. Evaluation of dry and wet transported intravaginal swabs in detection of *Chlamydia trachomatis* and *Neisseria gonorrhoeae* infections in female soldiers by PCR. *Journal of Clinical Microbiology* 2002;40(3):758–761.
20. Geha D, Uhl JR, Gustaferro CA, et al. Multiplex PCR for identification of methicillin-resistant staphylococci in the clinical laboratory. *Journal of Clinical Microbiology* 1994;32:1768–1772.
21. Jones D, Kamel-Reid S, Bahler D, et al. Laboratory practice guidelines for detecting and reporting BCR-ABL drug resistance mutations in chronic myelogenous leukemia and acute lymphoblastic leukemia. *Journal of Molecular Diagnostics* 2009;11:4–16.
22. Hui R, Zeng F, Chan CMF, et al. Reverse transcriptase PCR diagnostic assay for the coronavirus associated with severe acute respiratory syndrome. *Journal of Clinical Microbiology* 2004;42(5): 1994–1999.
23. Casabianca A, Orlandi C, Fraternale A, et al. A new one-step RT-PCR method for virus quantitation in murine AIDS. *Journal of Virological Methods* 2003;110(1):81–90.

24. Koopmans M, Monroe SS, Coffield LM, et al. Optimization of extraction and PCR amplification of RNA extracts from paraffin-embedded tissue in different fixatives. *Journal of Virological Methods* 1993;43(2):189–204.

25. Poggio G, Rodriguez C, Cisterna D, et al. Nested PCR for rapid detection of mumps virus in cerebrospinal fluid from patients with neurological diseases. *Journal of Clinical Microbiology* 2000;38(1):274–278.

26. Nakao M, Janssen JW, Flohr T, et al. Rapid and reliable quantification of minimal residual disease in acute lymphoblastic leukemia using rearranged immunoglobulin and T-cell receptor loci by light cycler technology. *Cancer Research* 2000;60(12):3281–3289.

27. Gibbons C, Awad-El-Kariem FM. Nested PCR for the detection of *Cryptosporidium parvum*. *Parasitology Today* 1999;15(8):345.

28. Knox C, Timms P. Comparison of PCR, nested PCR, and random amplified polymorphic DNA PCR for detection and typing of *Ureaplasma urealyticum* in specimens from pregnant women. *Journal of Clinical Microbiology* 1998;36(10):3032–3039.

29. Pinti M, Nasi M, Moretti L, et al. Quantitation of CD95 and CD95L mRNA expression in chronic and acute HIV-1 infection by competitive RT-PCR. *Annals of the New York Academy of Sciences* 2000;926:46–51.

30. Higuchi R, Dollinger G, Walsh PS, et al. Simultaneous amplification and detection of specific DNA sequences. *Biotechnology* 1992;10:413–417.

31. Higuchi R, Fockler C, Dollinger G, et al. Kinetic PCR: Real-time monitoring of DNA amplification reactions. *Biotechnology* 1993;11:1026–1030.

32. Sherman K, Rouster SD, Horn PS. Comparison of methodologies for quantification of hepatitis C virus (HCV) RNA in patients coinfected with HCV and human immunodeficiency virus. *Clinical Infectious Diseases* 2002;35(4):482–487.

33. Raab M, Cremer FW, Breitkreutz IN, et al. Molecular monitoring of tumour load kinetics predicts disease progression after non-myeloablative allogeneic stem cell transplantation in multiple myeloma. *Annals of Oncology* 2005;16(4):611–617.

34. Murthy S, Magliocco AM, Demetrick DJ. Copy number analysis of c-erb-B2 (HER-2/neu) and topoisomerase II alpha genes in breast carcinoma by quantitative real-time polymerase chain reaction using hybridization probes and fluorescence *in situ* hybridization. *Archives of Pathology & Laboratory Medicine* 2005;129(1):39–46.

35. Morris T, Robertson B, Gallagher M. Rapid reverse transcription-PCR detection of hepatitis C virus RNA in serum by using the TaqMan fluorogenic detection system. *Journal of Clinical Microbiology* 1996;34(12):2933–2936.

36. Holland P, Abramson RD, Watson R, Gelfand DH: Detection of specific polymerase chain reaction product by utilizing the 5' to 3' exonuclease activity of Thermus aquaticus DNA polymerase. *Proceedings of the National Academy of Sciences* 1991;88:7276–7280.

37. Lee LG, Connell CR, Bloch W. Allelic discrimination by nick-translation PCR with fluorogenic probes. *Nucleic Acids Research* 1993;21:3761–3766.

38. Branford S, Hughes TP, Rudzki Z. Monitoring chronic leukemia therapy by real-time quantitative PCR in blood is a reliable alternative to bone marrow cytogenetics. *British Journal of Haematology* 1999;107:587–599.

39. Kleiber J, Walter T, Haberhausen G, et al. Performance characteristics of a quantitative homogeneous TaqMan RT-PCR test for HCV RNA. *Journal of Molecular Diagnostics* 2000;2(3):158–166.

40. Rudert WA, Braun ER, Faas SJ, et al. Double-labeled fluorescent probes for 5' nuclease assays: Purification and performance evaluation. *BioTechniques* 1997;22:1140–1145.

41. Livak KJ, Flood SJ, Marmaro J, et al. Oligonucleotides with fluorescent dyes at opposite ends provide a quenched probe system useful for detecting PCR product and nucleic acid hybridization. *PCR Methods and Applications* 1995;4:357–362.

42. Whitcombe D, Theaker J, Guy SP, et al. Detection of PCR products using self-probing amplicons and fluorescence. *Nature Biotechnology* 1999;17:804–807.

43. Nazarenko IA, Bhatnagar SK, Hohman RJ. A closed tube format for amplification and detection of DNA based on energy transfer. *Nucleic Acids Research* 1997;25:2516–2521.

44. Thelwell NS, Millington S, Solinas A, et al. Mode of action and application of Scorpion primers to mutation detection. *Nucleic Acids Research* 2000;28: 3752–3761.

45. Didenko VV. DNA probes using fluorescence resonance energy transfer (FRET): Designs and applications. *BioTechniques* 2001;31(5):1106–1121.

46. Menard A, Dachet F, Prouzet-Mauleon V, et al. Development of a real-time fluorescence resonance energy transfer PCR to identify the main pathogenic *Campylobacter* spp. *Clinical Microbiology and Infection* 2005;11(4):281–287.

47. Aliyu S, Aliyu MH, Salihu HM, et al. Rapid detection and quantitation of hepatitis B virus DNA by real-time PCR using a new fluorescent (FRET) detection system. *Journal of Clinical Virology* 2004;30(2):191–195.

48. Neoh S, Brisco MJ, Firgaira FA, et al. Rapid detection of the factor V Leiden (1691 G > A) and haemochromatosis (845 G > A) mutation by fluorescence resonance energy transfer (FRET) and real-time PCR. *Journal of Clinical Pathology* 1999;52(10):766–769.

49. Gundry CN, Bernard PS, Hermann MG, et al. Rapid F508del and F508C assay using fluorescent hybridization probes. *Genetic Testing* 1999;3: 365–370.

50. Cardullo RA, Agarwal S, Flores C, et al. Nucleic acid hybridization by nonradioactive fluorescence resonance energy transfer. *Proceedings of the National Academy of Sciences* 1988;85:8790–8794.

51. Kwoh D, Davis GR, Whitfield KM, et al. Transcription-based amplification system and detection of amplified human immunodeficiency virus type 1 with a bead-based sandwich hybridization format. *Proceedings of the National Academy of Sciences* 1989;86(4):1173–1777.

52. Gorrin G, Friesenhahn M, Lin P, et al. Performance evaluation of the VERSANT HCV RNA qualitative assay by using transcription-mediated amplification. *Journal of Clinical Microbiology* 2003;41(1):310–317.

53. Allain J. Genomic screening for blood-borne viruses in transfusion settings. *Clinical and Laboratory Haematology* 2000;22(1):1–10.

54. Kimura T, Rokuhara A, Sakamoto Y, et al. Sensitive enzyme immunoassay for hepatitis B virus core-related antigens and their correlation to virus load. *Journal of Clinical Microbiology* 2002;40(2): 439–445.

55. Kievits T, van Gemen B, van Strijp D, et al. NASBA isothermal enzymatic *in vitro* nucleic acid amplification optimized for the diagnosis of HIV-1 infection. *Journal of Virological Methods* 1991;35(3):273–286.

56. van der Vliet G, Schukkink RA, van Gemen B, et al. Nucleic acid sequence-based amplification (NASBA) for the identification of mycobacteria. *Journal of General Microbiology* 1993;139(10): 2423–2429.

57. Deiman B, van Aarle P, Sillekens P. Characteristics and applications of nucleic acid sequence-based amplification (NASBA). *Molecular Biotechnology* 2002;20(2):163–180.

58. Romano J, van Gemen B, Kievits T. NASBA: A novel, isothermal detection technology for qualitative and quantitative HIV-1 RNA measurements. *Clinical Laboratory Medicine* 1996;16(1):89–103.

59. Welsh J, McClelland M. Fingerprinting genomes using PCR with arbitrary primers. *Nucleic Acids Research* 1990;18(24):7213–7218.

60. Perucho M, Welsh J, Peinado MA, et al. Fingerprinting of DNA and RNA by arbitrarily primed polymerase chain reaction: Applications in cancer research. *Methods in Enzymology* 1995;254: 275–290.

61. Kluytmans J, Berg H, Steegh P, et al. Outbreak of *Staphylococcus schleiferi* wound infections: Strain characterization by randomly amplified polymorphic DNA analysis, PCR ribotyping, conventional ribotyping, and pulsed-field gel electrophoresis. *Journal of Clinical Microbiology* 1998;36(8): 2214–2219.

62. Hawkins T, Detter JC, Richardson PM. Whole genome amplification—applications and advances. *Current Opinion in Biotechnology* 2002;13(1): 65–67.

63. Dean F, Hoson S, Fang L, et al. Comprehensive human genome amplification using multiple displacement amplification. *Proceedings of the National Academy of Sciences* 92002;9:5261–5266.

64. Huang Q, Schantz SP, Pulivarthi HR, Mo J, McCormick SA, Chaganti RSK. Improving

degenerate oligonucleotide primed PCR-comparative genomic hybridization for analysis of DNA copy number changes in tumors. *Genes, Chromosomes and Cancer* 2000;28:395–403.

65. Struan F, Grant A, Steinlight S, et al. SNP genotyping on a genome-wide amplified DOP-PCR template. *Nucleic Acids Research* 2002;30:e125.

66. Li J, Harris L, Mamon H, et al Whole genome amplification of plasma-circulating DNA enables expanded screening for allelic imbalance in plasma. *Journal of Molecular Diagnostics* 2006;8:22–30.

67. Klein C, Schmidt-Kittler O, Schardt JA, Pantel K, Speicher MR, Riethmuller G. Comparative genomic hybridization, loss of heterozygosity, and DNA sequence analysis of single cells. *Proceedings of the National Academy of Sciences* 1999;96:4494–4499.

68. Pusch C, Nicholson GJ, Bachmann L, Scholz M. Degenerative oligonucleotide-primed preamplification of ancient DNA allows the retrieval of authentic DNA sequences. *Analytical Biochemistry* 1999;279:118–122.

69. Williams R, Peisajovich SG, Miller OJ, Magdassi S, Tawfik DSS, Griffiths AD. Amplification of complex gene libraries by emulsion PCR. *Nature* 2008;3:545–550.

70. Barany F. The ligase chain reaction in a PCR world. *PCR Methods and Applications* 1991;1(1):5–16.

71. Walker G, Little MC, Nadeau JG, et al. Isothermal *in vitro* amplification of DNA by a restriction enzyme/DNA polymerase system. *Proceedings of the National Academy of Sciences* 1992;89(1):392–396.

72. Ichiyama S, Ito Y, Sugiura F, et al. Diagnostic value of the strand displacement amplification method compared to those of Roche Amplicor PCR and culture for detecting mycobacteria in sputum samples. *Journal of Clinical Microbiology* 1997;35(12):3802–3805.

73. Walker G, Linn CP. Detection of *Mycobacterium tuberculosis* DNA with thermophilic strand displacement amplification and fluorescence polarization. *Clinical Chemistry* 1996;42(10):1604–1608.

74. Spears P, Linn CP, Woodard DL, et al. Simultaneous strand displacement amplification and fluorescence polarization detection of *Chlamydia trachomatis* DNA. *Analytical Biochemistry* 1997;247(1):130–137.

75. Pfyffer G, Funke-Kissling P, Rundler E, et al. Performance characteristics of the BD ProbeTec system for direct detection of *Mycobacterium tuberculosis* complex in respiratory specimens. *Journal of Clinical Microbiology* 1999;37(1):137–140.

76. Little M, Andrews J, Moore R, et al. Strand displacement amplification and homogeneous real-time detection incorporated in a second-generation DNA probe system, BD ProbeTec ET. *Clinical Chemistry* 1999;45(6):777–784.

77. Blumenthal T, Carmichael GG. RNA replication: Function and structure of Qbeta-replicase. *Annual Review of Biochemistry* 1979;48:525–548.

78. Shah J, Liu J, Buxton D, et al. Detection of *Mycobacterium tuberculosis* directly from spiked human sputum by Q-beta replicase–amplified assay. *Journal of Clinical Microbiology* 1995;33:322–328.

79. Shah J, Liu J, Buxton D, et al. Q-beta replicase–amplified assay for detection of *Mycobacterium tuberculosis* directly from clinical specimens. *Journal of Clinical Microbiology* 1995;33(6):1435–1441.

80. Stefano J, Genovese L, An Q, et al. Rapid and sensitive detection of *Chlamydia trachomatis* using a ligatable binary RNA probe and Q beta replicase. *Molecular and Cellular Probes* 1997;11(6):407–426.

81. Lomeli H, Tyagi S, Pritchard CG, et al. Quantitative assays based on the use of replicatable hybridization probes. *Clinical Chemistry* 1989;35(9):1826–1831.

82. Fox R, Dotan I, Compton T, et al. Use of DNA amplification methods for clinical diagnosis in autoimmune diseases. *Journal of Clinical Laboratory Analysis* 1989;3(6):378–387.

83. Horn T, Chang CA, Urdea MS. Chemical synthesis and characterization of branched oligodeoxyribonucleotides (bDNA) for use as signal amplifiers in nucleic acid quantification assays. *Nucleic Acids Research* 1997;25(23):4842–4849.

84. Kern D, Collins M, Fultz T, et al. An enhanced-sensitivity branched-DNA assay for quantification of human immunodeficiency virus type 1 RNA in plasma. *Journal of Clinical Microbiology* 1996;34(12):3196–3202.

85. Lisby G. Application of nucleic acid amplification in clinical microbiology. *Methods in Molecular Biology* 1998;92:1–29.

86. Konnick E, Williams SM, Ashwood ER, et al. Evaluation of the COBAS hepatitis C virus (HCV) TaqMan analyte-specific reagent assay and

comparison to the COBAS Amplicor HCV Monitor V2.0 and Versant HCV bDNA 3.0 assays. *Journal of Clinical Microbiology* 2005;43(5):2133–2140.

87. Elbeik T, Markowitz N, Nassos P, et al. Simultaneous runs of the Bayer Versant HIV-1 version 3.0 and HCV bDNA version 3.0 quantitative assays on the System 340 platform provide reliable quantitation and improved work flow. *Journal of Clinical Microbiology* 2004;42(7):3120–3127.

88. Gleaves C, Welle J, Campbell M, et al. Multicenter evaluation of the Bayer Versant HIV-1 RNA 3.0 assay: Analytical and clinical performance. *Journal of Clinical Virology* 2002; 25(2):205–216.

89. Yao J, Beld MG, Oon LL, et al. Multicenter evaluation of the Versant hepatitis B virus DNA 3.0 assay. *Journal of Clinical Microbiology* 2004;42(2): 800–806.

90. Clavel C, Masure M, Levert M, et al. Human papillomavirus detection by the hybrid capture II assay: A reliable test to select women with normal cervical smears at risk for developing cervical lesions. *Diagnostic Molecular Pathology* 2000;9(3):145–150.

91. Farthing A, Masterson P, Mason WP, et al. Human papillomavirus detection by hybrid capture and its possible clinical use. *Journal of Clinical Pathology* 1994;47(7):649–652.

92. Barlet V, Cohard M, Thelu MA, et al. Quantitative detection of hepatitis B virus DNA in serum using chemiluminescence: Comparison with radioactive solution hybridization assay. *Journal of Virological Methods* 1994;49(2):141–151.

93. Poljak M, Marin IJ, Seme K, et al. Second-generation hybrid capture test and Amplicor monitor test generate highly correlated hepatitis B virus DNA levels. *Journal of Virological Methods* 2001;97(1-2): 165–169.

94. Caliendo A, Yen-Lieberman B, Baptista J, et al. Comparison of molecular tests for detection and quantification of cell-associated cytomegalovirus DNA. *Journal of Clinical Microbiology* 2003;41(8): 3509–3513.

95. Hebart H, Gamer D, Loeffler J, et al. Evaluation of Murex CMV DNA hybrid capture assay for detection and quantitation of cytomegalovirus infection in patients following allogeneic stem cell transplantation. *Journal of Clinical Microbiology* 1998;36(5): 1333–1337.

96. Schiffman M, Kiviat NB, Burk RD, et al. Accuracy and interlaboratory reliability of human papillomavirus DNA testing by hybrid capture. *Journal of Clinical Microbiology* 1995;33(3):545–550.

97. Hessner MJ, Budish MA, Friedman KD. Genotyping of factor V G1691A (Leiden) without the use of PCR by invasive cleavage of oligonucleotide probes. *Clinical Chemistry* 2000;46:1051–1056.

98. Ledford M, Friedman KD, Hessner MJ, et al. A multi-site study for detection of the factor V (Leiden) mutation from genomic DNA using a homogeneous invader microtiter plate fluorescence resonance energy transfer (FRET) assay. *Journal of Molecular Diagnostics* 2000;2:97–104.

99. Germer J, Majewski DW, Yung B, Mitchell PS, Yao JD. Evaluation of the invader assay for genotyping hepatitis C virus. *Journal of Clinical Microbiology* 2006;44:318–323.

100. Schutzbank T, Jarvis C, Kahmann N, Lopez K, Weimer M, Yount A. Detection of high-risk papillomavirus DNA with commercial invader-technology-based analyte-specific reagents following automated extraction of DNA from cervical brushings in ThinPrep media. *Journal of Clinical Microbiology* 2007;45:4067–4069.

101. Cloney L, Marlowe C, Wong A, et al. Rapid detection of *mecA* in methicillin resistant *Staphylococcus aureus* using cycling probe technology. *Molecular and Cellular Probes*. 1999;13(3):191–197.

102. Modrusan Z, Marlowe C, Wheeler D, et al. Detection of vancomycin-resistant genes *vanA* and *vanB* by cycling probe technology. *Molecular and Cellular Probes* 1999;13(3):223–231.

103. Merlino J, Rose B, Harbour C. Rapid detection of non-multidrug-resistant and multidrug-resistant methicillin-resistant Staphylococcus aureus using cycling probe technology for the mecA gene. *European Journal of Clinical Microbiology and Infectious Disease* 2003;22:322–323.

Chapter **8**

Chromosomal Structure and Chromosomal Mutations

OBJECTIVES

- Define mutations and polymorphisms.
- Distinguish the three types of DNA mutations: genome, chromosomal, and gene.
- Describe chromosomal compaction and the proteins involved in chromatin structure.
- Diagram a human chromosome, and label the centromere, q arm, p arm, and telomere.
- Illustrate the different types of structural mutations that occur in chromosomes.
- State the karyotype of a normal male and female.
- Identify the chromosomal abnormality in a given karyotype.
- Compare and contrast **interphase** and metaphase FISH analyses.
- Distinguish between the effects of balanced and unbalanced translocations on an individual and the individual's offspring.

The **human genome** is all of the genes found in a single individual. The human genome consists of 2.9 billion nucleotide base pairs of DNA organized into 23 chromosomes. As **diploid** organisms, humans inherit a **haploid** set of all their genes (23 chromosomes) from each parent, so that humans have two copies of every gene (except for some on the X and Y chromosomes). Each chromosome is a double helix of DNA, ranging from 246 million nucleotide base pairs in length in chromosome 1 (the largest) to 47 million nucleotide base pairs in chromosome 22 (the smallest; Table 8.1). Genetic information is carried on the chromosomes in the form of the order, or **sequence,** of nucleotides in the DNA helix. A **phenotype** is a trait or group of traits resulting from transcription and translation of these genes. The **genotype** is the DNA nucleotide sequence responsible for a phenotype.

Table 8.1 **Sizes of Human Chromosomes in Base Pairs**

Chromosome	Millions of Base Pairs
1	246
2	244
3	199
4	192
5	181
6	171
7	158
8	146
9	136
10	135
11	134
12	132
13	113
14	100
15	90
16	82
17	76
18	64
19	64
20	47
21	47
22	49
X	154
Y	57

Genotypic analysis is performed to confirm or predict phenotype. In the laboratory, some changes in chromosome structure and changes in chromosome number can be observed microscopically. Mutations at the nucleotide sequence level are detected using biochemical or molecular methods. Alterations of the DNA sequence may affect not only the phenotype of an individual but the progeny of that individual as well. The latter, heritable changes are the basis for prediction of the phenotype in the next generation. The probability of inheritance of a phenotypic trait can be estimated using the logical methods of Mendel's laws of genetics and statistics.

A transmissible (inheritable) change in the DNA sequence is a mutation or polymorphism. Although these terms are sometimes used interchangeably, they do have slightly different meanings based on population genetics. A DNA sequence change that is present in a relatively small proportion of a population is a **mutation**. The term **variant** may also be used, particularly to describe inherited sequence alterations, thus reserving the term *mutation* for somatic changes, for example, changes found only in tumor tissue. A change in the DNA sequence that is present in at least 1% to 2% of a population is a **polymorphism**. Both mutations and polymorphisms may or may not produce phenotypic differences.

Polymorphisms are casually considered mutations that do not severely affect phenotype; this is generally true, as any negative effect on survival and reproduction limits the persistence of a genotype in a population. Some polymorphisms are maintained in a population through a balance of positive and negative phenotype. The classic example is sickle cell anemia, a condition caused by a single-base substitution in the gene that codes for hemoglobin. The alteration is regarded as a mutation, but it is really a **balanced polymorphism**. In addition to causing abnormal red blood cells, the genetic alteration results in resistance to infection by *Plasmodium falciparum*, that is, resistance to malaria. The beneficial trait provides a survival and reproductive advantage that maintains the polymorphism in a relatively large proportion of the population. Examples of benign polymorphisms with no selective advantage are the ABO blood groups and the major histocompatibility complex (see Chapter 15, "DNA-Based Tissue Typing") and polymorphisms used for human identification and paternity testing (see Chapter 10, "DNA Sequencing").

DNA mutations can affect a single nucleotide or millions of nucleotides, even whole chromosomes, and thus can be classified into three categories: gene, chromosome, and genome mutations. **Gene mutations** affect single genes and are often, but not always, small changes in the DNA sequence. **Chromosome mutations** affect the structures of entire chromosomes. These changes require movement of large chromosomal regions (hundreds of thousands to millions of base pairs) either within the same chromosome or to another chromosome.

Genome mutations are changes in the number of chromosomes. A cell or cell population with a normal complement of chromosomes is **euploid**. Genome mutations result in cells that are **aneuploid**. Aneuploidy is usually (but not always) observed as increased numbers of chromosomes, because the loss of whole chromosomes is not compatible with survival. A single copy of each chromosome (23 in humans) is a **haploid** complement. Humans are normally **diploid**, with two copies of each chromosome. Aneuploidy can result when there are more than two copies of a single chromosome or when there are multiple copies of one or more chromosomes. Down syndrome is an example of a disease resulting from aneuploidy, where there are three copies, or **triploidy**, of chromosome 21.

Detection of mutations in the laboratory ranges from direct visualization of genome and chromosomal mutations under the microscope to indirect molecular methods to detect single-base changes. Methods used for detection of genome and chromosomal mutations are discussed in this chapter. Methods to detect gene mutations are described in Chapter 9, "Gene Mutations."

Chromosomal Structure and Analysis

Chromosomal Compaction and Histones

An important concept in the understanding of chromosomes is that chromosome behavior is dependent on chromosome structure as well as DNA sequence.[1] Genes with identical DNA sequences will behave differently, depending on their chromosomal location or the surrounding nucleotide sequence. It is a well-known phenomenon that a gene inserted or moved into a different chromosomal location may be expressed (transcribed and

translated) differently than it was in its original position. This is called **position effect**. Furthermore, certain functional features in chromosomes such as the **centromere** (where the chromosome attaches to the spindle apparatus for proper segregation during cell division) are not defined by specific DNA sequences.[2]

A eukaryotic chromosome is a double helix of DNA. A cell nucleus contains 4 cm of double helix, which must be compacted, both to fit into the cell nucleus and for accurate segregation in **mitosis**. An extended DNA double helix undergoes an 8000-fold **compaction** to make a metaphase chromosome (Fig. 8-1).[5] The winding of DNA onto **histones**, the most abundant proteins in the cell, is the first step. There are five histones: H1, H2a, H2b, H3, and H4. Approximately 160 to 180 bp of DNA is wrapped around a set of eight histone proteins (two each of H2a, H2b, H3, and H4) to form a **nucleosome**. Nucleosomes are visible by electron microscopy as 100-Å beadlike structures that are separated by short strands of a free double helix or linker region (Fig. 8-2).

Advanced Concepts

The structure of metaphase chromosomes is maintained by more than just histones. Metaphase chromatin is one-third DNA, one-third histones, and one-third nonhistone proteins. Nonhistone protein complexes, termed condensin I and condensin II, are apparently required for maintenance of mitotic chromosome structure.[3]

Historical Highlights

Before 1943, histones were thought to contain genetic information. Their function was later determined to be structural. It is now known that in addition to their structural role, histones control access to and expression of DNA. Modification of histones, through acetylation, methylation, phosphorylation, or ubiquitination, alters DNA access and plays a role in other cellular functions, such as recombination, replication, and gene expression.[4]

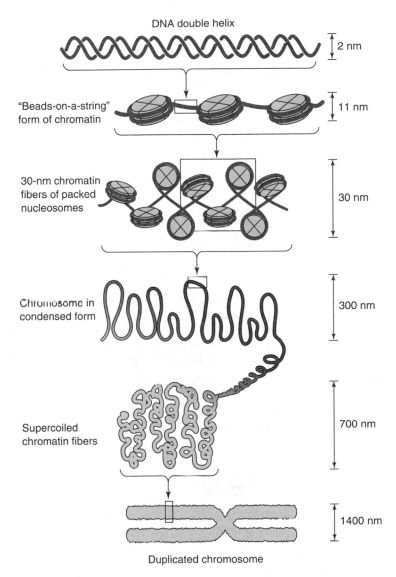

DNA double helix

2 nm

"Beads-on-a-string" form of chromatin

11 nm

30-nm chromatin fibers of packed nucleosomes

30 nm

Chromosome in condensed form

300 nm

Supercoiled chromatin fibers

700 nm

1400 nm

Duplicated chromosome

■ Figure 8-1 DNA compaction into metaphase chromosomes. (From Alberts B. Molecular Biology of the Cell, 4th ed, New York: Garland Science, 2002.)

DNA is wrapped around histones in such a way as to form a "bead-on-a-string" arrangement that comprises the 10-nm or 10-micron fiber.

In the interphase nucleus, the 10-micron fiber is further coiled around histone H1 into a thicker and shorter 30-nm or 30-micron fiber. The 30-nm interphase fibers represent the "resting state" of DNA. The fibers are locally relaxed into 10-nm fibers for DNA metabolism as required during the cell cycle. When the DNA is relaxed into 10-micron fibers for transcription or replication, the placement of nucleosomes along the double helix can be detected using nucleases (e.g., Mung bean nuclease, or DNase I). These enzymes cut the double helix in the **linker region**, the part of the double helix that is exposed between the histones.

The interphase fibers are looped onto protein scaffolds to form 300-nm fibers before entry into the M phase of the cell cycle (mitosis) and the looped fibers are wound into 700-nm solenoid coils.[6] The 700-nm coils are compacted into the 1400-nm fibers that can be seen

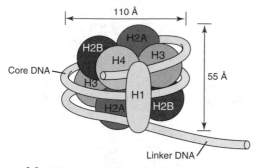

■ **Figure 8-2** DNA wrapped around eight histone proteins (two each of histone 2A, 2B, 3, and 4) forms a nucleosome. A further association with histone H1 coils the nucleosomal DNA into a 30-nm fiber.

in metaphase nuclei and as **karyotypes** in laboratory testing.

In the 30-nm interphase chromatin fiber, the internucleosomal DNA is associated with histone H1 and the beaded structure is wound into a solenoid coil. Loss of this level of organization is the first classic indicator of **apoptosis**, or programmed cell death. The 30-nm fibers are uncoiled, and the exposed linker DNA between the nucleosomes becomes susceptible to digestion by intracellular nucleases. The DNA wrapped into the nucleosomes remains intact so that DNA isolated from

---

Advanced Concepts

Members of a family of proteins called SMC proteins control chromosome condensation in eukaryotes and other aspects of chromosome behavior, including chromosome segregation in prokaryotes. Two of the SMC proteins, XCAP-C and XCAP-E, first isolated from frog eggs,[7] are integral parts of the condensin complex, a protein scaffold structure that can be isolated from both mitotic and interphase cells. This complex in the presence of topoisomerase can wrap DNA around itself in an ATP-driven reaction. SMC family proteins also play a role in the repair of chromosomal breaks.[8] Although the exact role of the SMC proteins in chromosome condensation and decondensation is not yet completely defined, this ability to change chromosome architecture is a significant feature of DNA metabolism.[9]

---

apoptotic cells contains "ladders," or multiples of discreet multiples of approximately 180 bp. These ladders can be resolved by agarose gel electrophoresis (Fig. 8-3). Chromosome topology (state of compaction of the DNA double helix) affects gene activity, for instance, in X chromosome inactivation in females. More highly compacted DNA is less available for RNA transcription. The more highly compacted state of DNA is closed chromatin, or **heterochromatin** (in contrast to open chromatin, or **euchromatin**). Maintenance of heterochromatin throughout interphase may require special proteins called condensin proteins or condensin-like protein complexes (**nonhistone proteins**).

Chromosome Morphology

Mitotic chromosomes have been distinguished historically by their relative size and centromere placement. As previously stated, the centromere is the site of attachment of the chromosome to the spindle apparatus. The connection is made between microtubules of the spindle and a protein complex called the **kinetochore** that assembles at the centromere sequences (Fig. 8-4). At the nucleotide level, the centromere is composed of a set of highly repetitive **alpha satellite** sequences.[10] These repetitive sequences interfere with chromosome compaction so that microscopically the centromere appears as a constriction in the metaphase chromosome. Chromosomes are **metacentric**, **sub-metacentric**, **acrocentric**, or **telocentric**, depending on the placement of the centromere (Fig. 8-5).

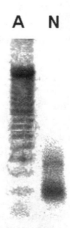

■ **Figure 8-3** Apoptotic DNA (A) is characterized by the ladder seen on gel electrophoresis. This is in contrast to degraded DNA from necrotic cells (N).

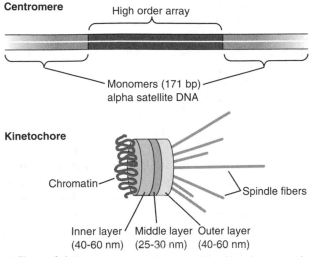

Figure 8-4 The centromere (top) consists of tandem repeats of 171 base-pair sequences flanking sets of single repeat units, or monomers repeated in groups in a higher-order array. The kinetochore (bottom) is a protein structure that connects the centromeres to the spindle apparatus.

The placement of the centromere divides the chromosome into arms. Metacentric chromosome arms are approximately equal in length, while one arm is longer than the other in sub-metacentric chromosomes. One arm is extremely small or missing in acrocentric or telocentric chromosomes, respectively.

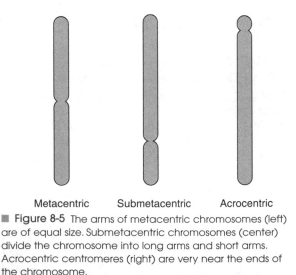

Figure 8-5 The arms of metacentric chromosomes (left) are of equal size. Submetacentric chromosomes (center) divide the chromosome into long arms and short arms. Acrocentric centromeres (right) are very near the ends of the chromosome.

Advanced Concepts

Some plants and insects have **holocentric** chromosomes. During cell division, these chromosomes associate with kinetochores along their entire length.

There are no telocentric human chromosomes. Human chromosomes are acrocentric or submetacentric and so have long and short arms (Table 8.2). The long arm of a chromosome is designated **q**, and the short arm is designated **p**. Acrocentric chromosomes have a long arm length/short arm length ratio of from 3:1 to 10:1. Chromosomes 13 to 15, 21, and 22 are acrocentric.

Visualizing Chromosomes

Conventional cytological stains, such as Feulgen, Wright, and hematoxylin, have been used to visualize chromosomes. An advance in the recognition of individual chromosomes was the discovery that fluorescent stains and chemical dyes can react with specific chromosome regions. This region-specific staining forms reproducible patterns where portions of the chromosome accept or reject the stain. For cytogenetic analysis, this allows unequivocal identification of every chromosome and the direct detection of some chromosomal abnormalities. Underlying the region-specific staining is the implication that the reproducible staining patterns occur

Table 8.2 **Classification of Chromosomes by Size and Centromere Position**

Group	Chromosomes	Description
A	1, 2	Large metacentric
	3	Large submetacentric
B	4, 5	Large submetacentric
C	6–12, X	Medium-sized submetacentric
D	13–15	Medium-sized acrocentric with satellites
E	16	Short metacentric
	17, 18	Short submetacentric
F	19, 20	Short metacentric
G	21, 22	Short acrocentric with satellites
	Y	Short acrocentric

as a result of defined regional ultrastructures of the mitotic chromosomes.

When chromosomes are stained with the fluorescent dyes quinacrine and quinacrine mustard, the resulting fluorescence pattern visualized after staining is called **Q banding** (Fig. 8-6). This method was first demonstrated in 1970 by Caspersson, Zech, and Johansson.[11] The results of this work confirmed that each human chromosome could be identified by its characteristic banding pattern. Q banding gives a particularly intense staining of the human Y chromosome and thus may also be used to distinguish the Y chromosome in interphase nuclei. Because Q banding requires a fluorescent microscope, it is not as widely used as other stains that are detectable by light microscopy.

The chemical dye Giemsa stains in patterns, or **G bands**, similar to those seen in Q banding. The appearance of G banding differs, depending on the treatment of the chromosomes before staining.[12] Mild treatment (2 × standard saline citrate for 60 minutes at 60°C) yields the region-specific banding pattern comparable to that seen with fluorescent dyes. Use of trypsin or other proteolytic agents to extract or denature proteins before Giemsa staining was found to map structural aberrations more clearly and is the most commonly used staining method for analyzing chromosomes.[13,14] G bands are also produced by Feulgen staining after treatment with DNase I.[15] The number of visualized bands can be increased from about 300 to 500 per chromosome by staining chromosomes before they reach maximal metaphase condensation. This is called **high-resolution banding**.

Harsher treatment of chromosomes (87°C for 10 minutes, then cooling to 70°C) before Giemsa staining will produce a pattern opposite to the G banding pattern called **R banding**.[16] R bands can also be visualized after staining with acridine orange.[17]

Alkali treatment of chromosomes results in centromere staining, or **C banding**.[18] Centromere staining is absent in G band patterns. C bands may be associated with heterochromatin, the "quiet," or poorly transcribed, sequences along the chromosomes that are also present around centromeres. In contrast, euchromatin, which is relatively rich in gene activity, may not be stained as much as heterochromatin in C banding.

Nucleolar organizing region (NOR) staining is another region-specific staining approach. Chromosomes treated with silver nitrate will stain specifically at the constricted regions, or stalks, on the acrocentric chromosomes.

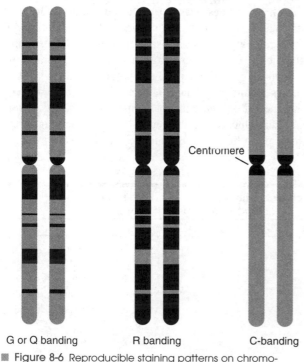

Centromere

G or Q banding   R banding   C-banding

■ **Figure 8-6** Reproducible staining patterns on chromosomes are used for identification and site location. Heterochromatin stains darkly by G or Q banding (left); euchromatin stains darkly by R banding (center); C banding stains centromeres (right).

Advanced Concepts

The correlation between heterochromatin and staining may also hold for noncentromeric G and Q bands. This association is complicated, however, because a variety of procedures and stains produce identical banding patterns. The correlation of staining with heterochromatin is contradicted by observations of the X chromosome. Although one X chromosome is inactive and replicates later than the active X in females, both X chromosomes stain with equal pattern and intensity. Staining differences, therefore, must be due to other factors. Possible explanations for differential interactions with dye include differences in DNA compaction, sequences, and DNA-associated nonhistone proteins.

Staining of chromosomes with **4',6-diamidino-2-phenylindole (DAPI)** was first described in 1976 as a way to detect mycoplasmal contamination in cell cultures.[19] DAPI binds to the surface grooves of double-stranded DNA and fluoresces blue under ultraviolet light (353-nm wavelength). DAPI is used to visualize chromosomes as well as whole nuclei.

Chromosome banding facilitates detection of small deletions, insertions, inversions, and other abnormalities and the identification of distinct chromosomal locations. For this purpose, the reproducible G-banding pattern has been ordered into regions, comprising bands and sub-bands. For example, in Figure 8-7 a site on the long arm (q) of chromosome 17 is located in region 1, band 1, sub-band 2, or 17q11.2.

Detection of Genome and Chromosomal Mutations

Karyotyping

Genome mutations, or aneuploidy, can be detected by indirect methods, such as flow cytometry and more directly by karyotyping. A **karyotype** is the complete set of chromosomes in a cell. Karyotyping is the direct observation of metaphase chromosome structure by arranging metaphase chromosomes according to size. It requires collecting living cells and growing them in culture in the laboratory for 48 to 72 hours. Cell division is stimulated by addition of a **mitogen**, usually phytohemagglutinin. Dividing cells are then arrested in metaphase with colcemid, an inhibitor of microtubule (mitotic spindle) formation. The chromosomes in dividing cells that arrest in metaphase will yield a **chromosome spread** when the cell nuclei are disrupted with hypotonic saline. The

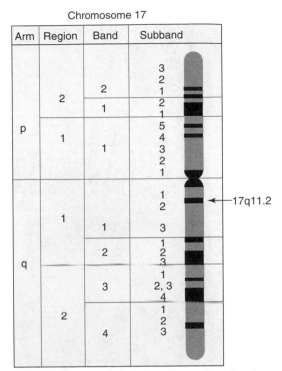

Chromosome 17

Arm	Region	Band	Subband
p	2	2	3 2 1
		1	2 1
	1	1	5 4 3 2 1
q	1	1	1 2 3
		2	1 2 3
		3	1 2, 3 4
	2	4	1 2 3

←—17q11.2

■ **Figure 8-7** Identification of chromosomal location by G-band patterns. Locations are designated by the chromosome number 17 in this example, the arm q, the region 1, the band 1, and the sub-band 2.

23 pairs of chromosomes can then be assembled into an organized display, or karyotype, according to their size and centromere placement (Fig. 8-8). Aneuploidy may be observed affecting several chromosomes[22] (Fig. 8-9) or a single chromosome (Fig. 8-10).

Karyotyping will also detect chromosomal mutations such as **translocations**, which are the exchange of genetic material between chromosomes. Translocations can be of several types. In **reciprocal translocations**, parts of two chromosomes exchange; that is, each chromosome breaks and the broken chromosomes reassociate or recombine with one another. When this type of translocation does not result in gain or loss of chromosomal material, it is **balanced** (Figs. 8-11 and 8-12). Balanced translocations may occur, therefore, without phenotypic effects. Balanced translocations in germ cells (cells that give rise to eggs or sperm) can, however, become **unbalanced** by not assorting properly during meiosis; as a result, they affect the phenotype of offspring. A **robertsonian** translocation involves the movement of most of

Advanced Concepts

Chromosomes can be prestained with the DNA-binding oligopeptide distamycin A to enhance chromosomal distinctions.[20,21] DAPI/distamycin A staining is useful in identifying pericentromeric breakpoints in chromosomal rearrangements and other rearrangements or chromosomes that are too small for standard banding techniques.

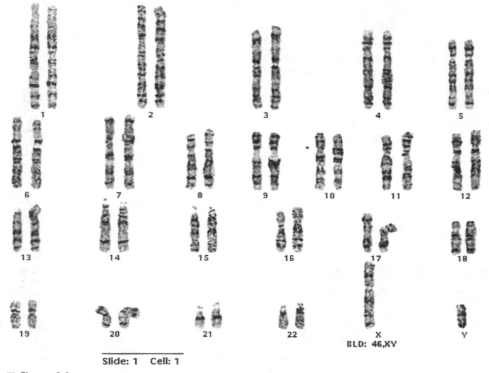

■ **Figure 8-8** A normal male karyotype. There are 22 sets of autosomes, one inherited from each parent, and one pair of sex chromosomes, XY. This karyotype is designated 46, XY.

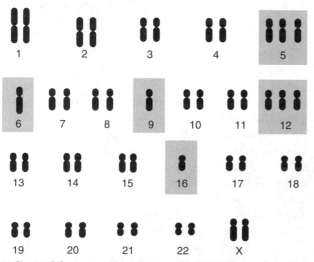

■ **Figure 8-9** Aneuploidy involving multiple chromosomes. Chromosomes 5 and 12 are triploid; chromosomes 6, 9, and 16 are monoploid.

one entire chromosome to the centromere of another chromosome (Fig. 8-13). This type of translocation may also become unbalanced during reproduction, resulting in a net gain or loss of chromosomal material in the offspring.

Other types of chromosome mutations that are visible by karyotyping are shown in Figure 8-14. A **deletion** is a loss of chromosomal material. Large deletions covering millions of base pairs can be detected using karyotyping; smaller **microdeletions** are not always easily seen using this technique. An **insertion** is a gain of chromosomal material. The inserted sequences arise from duplication of particular regions within the affected chromosome or from fragments of other chromosomes. As with deletions, insertions cause altered banding patterns and a change in the size of the chromosomes. **Inversions** result from excision, flipping, and reconnecting chromosomal material within the same chromosome. **Pericentric inversions** include the centromere in the inverted region,

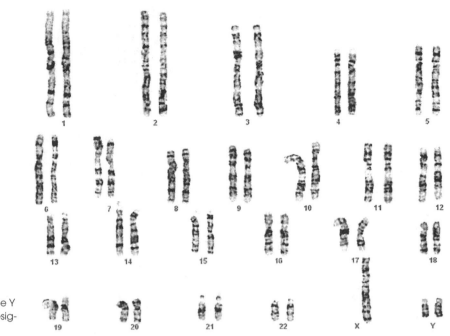

■ **Figure 8-10** Aneuploidy involving the Y chromosome (XYY syndrome). This is designated 47, XYY.

Historical Highlights

The first chromosome mutations were visualized in the 1960s in leukemia cells. Peter Nowell and David Hungerford observed an abnormally small chromosome 22 in leukemia cells, which they labeled the "Philadelphia" chromosome. A few years later, Janet Rowley, using chromosome banding, noted that tumor cells not only lost genetic material, they exchanged it. In 1972 she first described the translocation between chromosomes 8 and 21, t(8;21) in patients with acute myeloblastic leukemia. In that same year, she demonstrated that the Philadelphia chromosome was the result of a reciprocal exchange between chromosome 9 and chromosome 22.[23] She went on to identify additional reciprocal translocations in other diseases: the t(14;18) translocation in follicular lymphoma and the t(15;17) translocation in acute promyelocytic leukemia. This was the first evidence that cancer had a genetic basis.

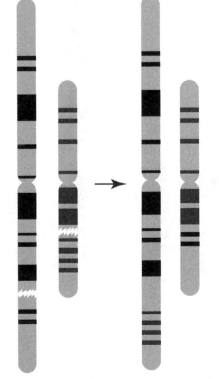

■ **Figure 8-11** A balanced reciprocal translocation.

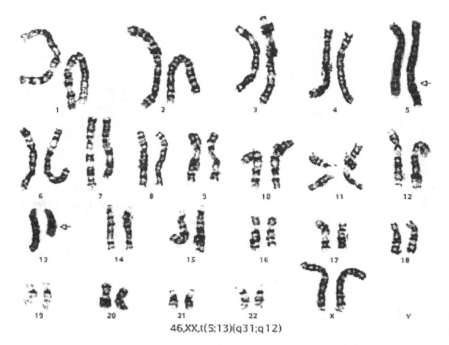

46,XX,t(5;13)(q31;q12)

■ **Figure 8-12** A karyotype showing a balanced reciprocal translocation between chromosomes 5 and 13. This is designated 46, XX,t(5;13).

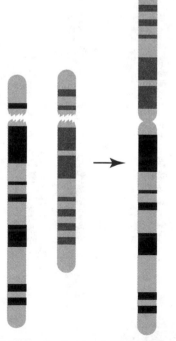

■ **Figure 8-13** A robertsonian translocation.

whereas **paracentric inversions** involve sequences within one arm of the chromosome. An **isochromosome** is a metacentric chromosome that results from transverse splitting of the centromere during cell division. Transverse splitting causes two long arms or two short arms to separate into daughter cells instead of normal chromosomes with one long arm and one short arm. The arms of an isochromosome are, therefore, equal in length and genetically identical. A **ring chromosome** results from deletion of genetic regions from both ends of the chromosome and a joining of the ends to form a ring. A **derivative chromosome** is an abnormal chromosome consisting of translocated or otherwise rearranged parts from two or more unidentified chromosomes joined to a normal chromosome.

Results of karyotyping analyses are expressed as the number of chromosomes per nucleus (normal is 46), the type of sex chromosomes (normal is XX or XY), followed by any genetic abnormalities observed. A normal karyotype is 46, XX in a female or 46, XY in a male. A karotype showing 46,XX,del(7)(q13) denotes a deletion in the long arm q of chromosome 7 at region 1, band 3. A karotype showing 46,XY,t(5;17)(p13.3;p13) denotes a translocation between the short arms of chromosomes

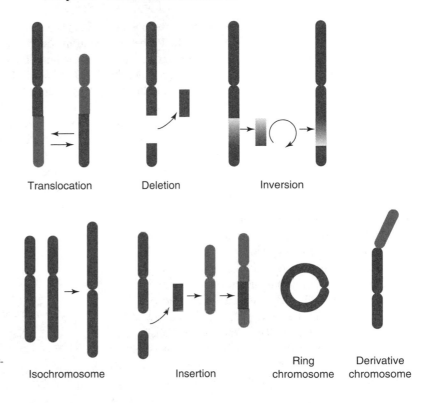

Translocation   Deletion   Inversion

Isochromosome   Insertion   Ring chromosome   Derivative chromosome

■ **Figure 8-14** Chromosome mutations involving alterations in chromosome structure.

5 and 17 and region 1, band 3, sub-band 3, and region 1, band 3, respectively. A karotype showing 47,XX+21 is the karyotype of a female with Down syndrome resulting from an extra chromosome 21. Klinefelter syndrome is caused by an extra X chromosome in males, for example, 47,XXY. Table 8.3 lists some of the terms used in expressing karyotypes.

Fluorescence In Situ Hybridization

Interphase FISH

Fluorescence in situ hybridization (FISH) is a method widely used to detect protein and RNA as well as DNA structures in place in the cell, or in situ. FISH offers a more rapid assay with higher resolution and flexibility than karyotyping.[24] Interphase FISH does not require culturing of cells, and metaphase FISH allows detection of much smaller regional abnormalities than are visible by karyotyping. Since growing cells in culture is not required, **interphase FISH** methods are used commonly to study prenatal samples, tumors, and hematological malignancies, not all of which are conveniently brought into metaphase in culture.

For FISH cytogenetic analysis, fixed cells are exposed to a probe. The probe is a 60- to 200-kb fragment of DNA attached covalently to a fluorescent molecule. The probe will hybridize, or bind, to its complementary sequences in the cellular DNA. In interphase FISH, the bound probe

Table 8.3 **A List of Descriptive Abbreviations**

Abbreviation	Indication
+	gain
−	loss
del	deletion
der	derivative chromosome
dup	duplication
ins	insertion
inv	inversion
i, iso	isochromosome
mat	maternal origin
pat	paternal origin
r	ring chromosome
t	translocation
tel	telomere (end of chromosome arm)

is visualized under a fluorescent microscope as a point of fluorescent light in the nucleus of the cell. Probes are designed to be complementary to a particular chromosome or chromosomal locus so that the image under the microscope will correlate with the state of that chromosome or locus. For example, a probe to any unique region on chromosome 22 should yield an image of two signals per nucleus, reflecting the two copies of chromosome 22 in the somatic cell nucleus (Fig. 8-15). A deletion or duplication of the DNA that is hybridized to the probe will result in a nucleus with only one signal or more than two signals, respectively. Multiple probes spanning large regions are used to detect regional deletions.[25,26]

Translocations or other rearrangements are detected using probes of different "colors" (or signals) complementary to regions on each chromosome taking part in the translocation. A normal nucleus will have two of each of the probe signals. A translocated chromosome will combine the two probe signals, resulting in a loss of one of each signal in the nucleus. Analysis of translocation signals is sometimes complicated by false signals that result from two chromosomes landing close to one another in the nucleus, such that the bound probes give a signal similar to that exhibited by a translocation. These false signals maybe distinguished from true translocations by the size of the fluorescent image, but this distinction requires a trained eye. Accounting for false-positive signals as background noise limits the sensitivity of this assay.

The sensitivity of interphase FISH analysis for detection of translocations is increased through the use of dual color probes, or **dual fusion probes**. These probes are mixtures of two single probes, each labeled with a different fluorescent dye. They are designed to bind to regions spanning the breakpoint of both translocation partners.

A translocation will be observed as a signal from both the translocation junction and the reciprocal of the translocation junction, for example, t(9;22) and t(22;9) (Fig. 8-16). Dual color **break-apart probes**, 0.6 to 1.5 Mb, are another approach to decrease background signals as well as to identify translocation events where one chromosome can recombine with multiple potential partners. These probes are designed to bind to the intact chromosome flanking the translocation breakpoint. When a translocation occurs, the two probes separate (Fig. 8-17). Sometimes called tri-FISH, break-apart probes are not the same as tricolor probes (see below).

Centromeric probes (CEN probes) are designed to hybridize to highly repetitive alpha satellite sequences surrounding centromeres. These probes detect aneuploidy

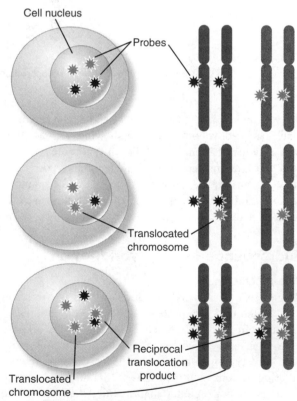

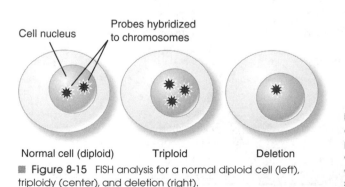

■ **Figure 8-15** FISH analysis for a normal diploid cell (left), triploidy (center), and deletion (right).

■ **Figure 8-16** FISH analysis using distinct probes to detect a translocation. A normal nucleus has two signals from each probe (top). A translocation involving the two chromosomes combines the two probe colors (middle). Dual fusion probes confirm the presence of the translocation by also giving a signal from the reciprocal breakpoint (bottom).

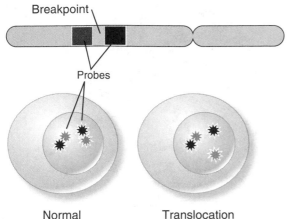

■ **Figure 8-17** Break-apart probes bind to the chromosome flanking the translocation breakpoint region. Normal cells will display the combination signal (bottom left), and a translocation will separate the probe signals (bottom right).

of any chromosome. Combinations of centromeric probes and region-specific probes are often used to confirm deletions or amplifications in specific chromosomes. Addition of a CEN probe to dual color probes comprises a tricolor probe and serves as a control for amplification or loss of one of the chromosomes involved in the translocation. For example, the IGH/MYC CEP 8 Tri-color Dual Fusion Translocation Probe (Abbott Molecular) is a mixture of a 1.5-Mb–labeled probe, complementary to the immunoglobulin heavy chain region (IGH) of chromosome 14, an approximately 750-kb distinctly labeled probe complementary to the *myc* gene on chromosome 8, and a CEN to chromosome 8.

Each chromosome arm has a unique set of repeat sequences located just before the end of the chromosome, called the **telomere** (Fig. 8-18). These sequences have been studied to develop a set of DNA probes specific to the telomeres of all human chromosomes. **Telomeric probes** are useful for the detection of chromosome structural abnormalities, such as cryptic translocations or small deletions that are not easily visualized by standard karyotyping.

Because interphase cells for FISH do not require culturing of the cells and stimulating division to get metaphase spreads, as is required for standard karyotyping, interphase FISH is valuable for analysis of cells that do not divide well in culture, including fixed cells.[27,28] Furthermore, because hundreds of cells are analyzed microscopically using FISH, the sensitivity of detection is higher than that of metaphase procedures, which commonly examine 20 spreads. A limitation of FISH, however, is the inability to identify chromosomal changes other than those at the specific binding region of the probe(s). In contrast, karyotyping, a more generic method, can detect any chromosomal change that causes changes in chromosomal size, number, or banding pattern within the sensitivity limits of the procedure.

Preparation of the sample is critical in interphase FISH analysis, both to permeabilize the cells for optimal probe-target interaction and to maintain cell morphology.[29] Optimal results are obtained if fresh interphase cells are incubated overnight (aging) after deposition on slides. After aging overnight, cells are treated with protease to minimize interference from cytoplasmic proteins and fixed with 1% formaldehyde to stabilize the nuclear morphology. Before DNA denaturation, the cells are dehydrated in graded concentrations of ethanol. Paraffin-embedded tissues are dewaxed in xylene before protease and formaldehyde treatment.

The quality of the probe also needs to be checked and its performance validated before use. Fluorescent probes (DNA with covalently attached fluorescent dyes) are usually purchased from vendors, which may also supply compatible hybridization reagents and controls. Nevertheless, the probe performance should be observed on control tissue before use on patient samples. Under a fluorescent microscope with the appropriate color distinction filters, the signal from the probe should be bright, specific to the target in the cell nuclei, and free of high background noise. Probes differ in their signal characteristics and intensities; the technologist should become familiar with what to expect from a given probe on different types of tissues.

■ **Figure 8-18** The binding sites for telomeric probes are unique sequences just next to the telomeric associated repeats and telomeric repeat sequences at the ends of chromosomes.

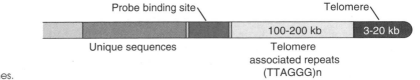

As in Southern and Northern blotting procedures, both probe and target must be denatured prior to hybridization. The amount of time taken to hybridize and use Cot-1 DNA (Invitrogen; placental DNA enriched for repetitive sequences to reduce nonspecific binding) or facilitators such as dextran sulfate (to increase the effective probe concentration) depends on the sequence complexity of the probe (see Chapter 6, "Analysis and Characterization of Nucleic Acids and Proteins"). A 10-nanogram to 1-microgram probe may be used in a hybridization volume of 3 to 10 μL. The hybridization of the probe on the target cells is performed at 37° to 42°C in a humidified chamber. The slides are cover-slipped and sealed to optimize the hybridization conditions.

Following hybridization and rinsing off of unbound probe, the sample is observed microscopically. The probe signals should be visible from entire intact nuclei. Adequate numbers of cells must be visible, but crowded cells where the nuclei and signals overlap do not yield accurate results. Furthermore, different tissue types have different image qualities and characteristics that must also be taken into account when assessing the FISH image. Another complication to FISH analysis is **photobleaching** (fading) or loss of probe signal emission (10^5 photons/second) due to photochemical destruction of the fluorophore molecules. For this reason, FISH slides should not be subjected to prolonged light exposure.

Metaphase FISH

Metaphase analysis has been enhanced by the development of fluorescent probes that bind to metaphase chromosomal regions or to whole chromosomes. Probes that cover the entire chromosome, or **whole chromosome paints**, are valuable for detecting small or complex rearrangements that are not apparent by regular chromosome banding (Fig. 8-19). By mixing combinations of five fluors and using special imaging software, **spectral karyotyping** can distinguish all 23 chromosomes by chromosome-specific colors.[30] This type of analysis is used to detect abnormalities that affect multiple chromosomes, as is sometimes found in cancer cells or immortalized cell lines.[31–33] Telomeric and centromeric probes are also applied to metaphase chromosomes (Fig. 8-20) to detect aneuploidy and structural abnormalities.

Preparation of chromosomes for metaphase FISH procedures begins with the culture of cells for 72 hours.

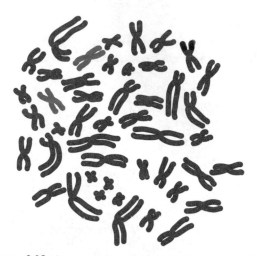

■ **Figure 8-19** Chromosome painting showing a derivative chromosome formed by movement of a fragment of chromosome 12 (black) to an unidentified chromosome.

About 45 minutes before harvesting, colcemid is added to the cultures to arrest dividing cells in metaphase. The cells are then suspended in a hypotonic medium (0.075 M KCl) and fixed with methanol/acetic acid (3:1). The fixed-cell suspension is applied to an inclined slide and allowed to dry. A second treatment with 70% acetic acid may improve the chromosome spreading and decrease background noise. Condensed chromosome spreads, especially those from cultured metaphases, may be affected by temperature and humidity. Under a phase contrast microscope, the chromosomes should appear well separated with sharp borders. Cytoplasm should not be visible. Once the

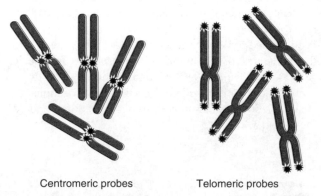

Centromeric probes   Telomeric probes

■ **Figure 8-20** Centromeric (left) and telomeric (right) probes on metaphase chromosomes.

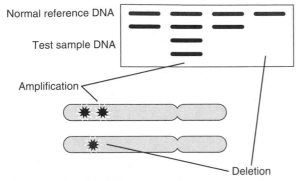

Normal reference DNA

Test sample DNA

Amplification

Deletion

■ **Figure 8-21** In CGH, the test sample is compared with a normal reference sample on a metaphase spread. Normally, test and reference signals are equal. A higher test signal denotes an amplification, and a higher reference signal denotes a deletion.

slide is dried, hybridization proceeds as discussed above for interphase FISH.

Intrachromosomal amplifications or deletions can be detected by **comparative genome hybridization (CGH)**.[34,35] In this method, DNA from test and reference samples is labeled and used as a probe on a normal metaphase chromosome spread (Fig. 8-21). One advantage of CGH is its capability to identify the location of deletions or amplifications throughout the genome.[36] The resolution (precise identification of the amplified or deleted region), however, is not as high as can be achieved with **array CGH** (see Chapter 6).

For CGH, the test DNA is isolated and labeled along with a reference DNA. Two colorimetrically distinct cyanine dyes, commonly Cy3 and Cy5, are used as fluorescent labels for the test and reference DNA. Cy3, which fluoresces at a wavelength of 550 nm, is often represented as "green," and Cy5, which fluoresces in the far-red region of the spectrum (650 to 667 nm), is represented as "red." Derivatives of these dyes, such as Cy3.5, which fluoresces in the red-orange region, are also available. Because these dyes fluoresce brightly and are water-soluble, they have been used extensively for CGH using imaging equipment.

Labeling (attachment of Cy3 or Cy5 dye to the test and reference DNA) is achieved by nick translation or primer extension in which nucleotides covalently attached to the dye molecules are incorporated into the DNA sequences. The dye-nucleotides commonly used for this type of labeling are 5-amino-propargyl-2'-deoxycytidine 5'-triphosphate coupled to the Cy3 or Cy5 fluorescent dye (Cy3-AP3-dCTP, Cy5-AP3-dCTP) or 5-amino-propargyl-2'-deoxyuridine 5'-triphosphate coupled to the Cy3 or Cy5 fluorescent dye (Cy3-AP3-dUTP, Cy5-AP3-dUTP). Separate aliquots of test and reference DNA are labeled with different Cy3 and Cy5 dyes, respectively, before application to a normal metaphase spread. Test DNA is partially digested with DNase to produce fragments that will bind efficiently to the denatured DNA in a metaphase chromosome spread. Figure 8-22 shows an example of results from a CGH analysis.

Despite its utility and versatility in detecting chromosomal abnormalities, CGH does require a dvanced technical expertise. Array CGH is less comprehensive, but more specific, for detection of particular abnormalities.

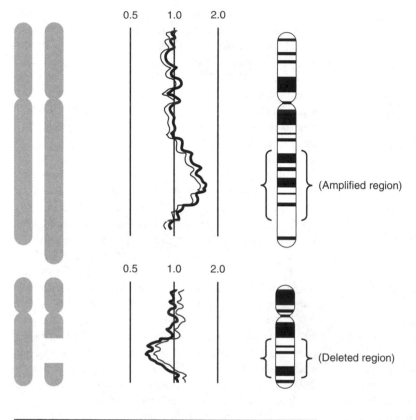

(Amplified region)

(Deleted region)

■ **Figure 8-22** CGH analysis of four chromosomes of cells from a cancer cell line. Amplified or deleted areas are observed where the test and reference signals are not equal. The vertical lines in the center of the diagram represent the ratio of test/reference signals on the chromosomal spread showing excess test or excess reference signal (right idiograms).

• STUDY QUESTIONS •

1. What chromosomal location is indicated by 15q21.1?

2. During interphase FISH analysis for the t(9;22) translocation, one nucleus was observed with two normal signals (one red for chromosome 22 and one green for chromosome 9) and one composite red/green signal. Five hundred other nuclei were normal. What is one explanation for this observation?

3. Is 47; XYY a normal karyotype?

4. Write the numerical and structural chromosomal abnormalities represented by the following genotypes:

   47, XY, +18

   46, XY, del(16)p(14)

   iso(Xq)

   46,XX del(22)q(11.2)

   45, X

5. A chromosome with a centromere located such that one arm of the chromosome is longer than the other arm, is called:
   a. metacentric.
   b. paracentric.
   c. telocentric.
   d. sub-metacentric.

6. A small portion from the end of chromosome 2 has been found on the end of chromosome 15, replacing the end of chromosome 15, which has moved to the end of chromosome 2. This mutation is called a:
   a. reciprocal translocation.
   b. inversion.
   c. deletion.
   d. robertsonian translocation.

7. Phytohemagglutinin is added to a cell culture when preparing cells for karyotyping. The purpose of the phytohemagglutinin treatment is to:
   a. arrest the cell in metaphase.
   b. spread out the chromosomes.

c. fix the chromosomes on the slide.

d. stimulate mitosis in the cells.

8. A centromeric probe is used to visualize chromosome 21. Three fluorescent signals are observed in the cell nuclei when stained with this probe. These results would be interpreted as consistent with:

a. a normal karyotype.

b. Down syndrome.

c. Klinefelter syndrome.

d. technical error.

9. Cells were harvested from a patient's blood, cultured to obtain chromosomes in metaphase, fixed onto a slide, treated with trypsin, and then stained with Giemsa. The resulting banding pattern is called:

a. G banding.

b. Q banding.

c. R banding.

d. C banding.

10. A FISH test with a centromere 13 probe is ordered for a suspected case of Patau syndrome (trisomy 13). How many signals per nucleus will result if the test is positive for Patau syndrome?

11. What would be the results if a centromere 13 probe was used on a case of Edward syndrome (trisomy 18)?

12. Angelman syndrome is caused by a microdeletion in chromosome 15. Which method, karyotyping or metaphase FISH, is better for accurate detection of this abnormality? Why?

13. The results of a CGH analysis of Cy3 (green)-labeled test DNA with Cy5 (red)-labeled reference DNA on a normal chromosome spread revealed a bright red signal along the short arm of chromosome 3. How is this interpreted?

a. 3p deletion

b. 3q deletion

c. 3p amplification

d. 3q amplification

14. A break-apart probe is used to detect a translocation. The results of FISH analysis show two signals in 70% of the nuclei counted and three signals in 30% of the nuclei. Is there a translocation present?

15. What FISH technique is most useful for detection of multiple complex genomic mutations?

References

1. Murray A. How to compact DNA. *Science* 1998; 282:425–427.

2. Black B, Foltz DR, Chakravarthy S, et al. Structural determinants for generating centromeric chromatin. *Nature* 2004;430(6999):578–582.

3. Gassmann R, Vagnarelli P, Hudson D, et al. Mitotic chromosome formation and the condensin paradox. *Experimental Cell Research* 2004;296(1):35–42.

4. Berger S. The histone modification circus. *Science* 2001;292:64–65.

5. Richmond TJ. The structure of DNA in the nucleosome core. *Nature* 2003;423(6936):145–150.

6. Porter I, Khoudoli GA, Swedlow JR. Chromosome condensation: DNA compaction in real time. *Current Biology* 2004,14(14):R554–R556.

7. Hirano T, Mitchison TJ. A heterodimeric coiled-coil protein required for mitotic chromosome condensation in vitro. *Cell* 1994;79(3):449–458.

8. Kinoshita E, van der Linden E, Sanchez H, Wyman C. RAD50, an SMC family member with multiple roles in DNA break repair: How does ATP affect function? *Chromosome Research* 2009;17:277–288.

9. Hudson D, Ohta S, Freisinger T, et al. Molecular and genetic analysis of condensin function in vertebrate cells. *Molecular and Cellular Biology* 2008;19:3070–3079.

10. Waye J, Willard HF. Chromosome-specific alpha satellite DNA: Nucleotide sequence analysis of the 2.0 kilobase pair repeat from the human X chromosome. *Nucleic Acids Research* 1985;13(8): 2731–2743.

11. Caspersson T, Zech L, Johansson C. Differential banding of alkylating fluorochromes in human chromosomes. *Experimental Cell Research* 1970;60:315–319.

12. Lewin B. Gene Expression 2, vol. 2. Cambridge, MA: John Wiley & Sons, 1980.

13. Seabright M. A rapid banding technique for human chromosomes. *Lancet* 1971;2:971–972.

14. Seabright M. The use of proteolytic enzymes for the mapping of structural rearrangements in the chromosomes of man. *Chromosoma* 1972;36: 204–210.

15. Burkholder G, Weaver M. DNA protein interactions and chromosome binding. *Experimental Cell Research* 1977;110:251–262.

16. Dutrillaux B, Lejeune J. Sur une nouvelle technique d'analyse du caryotype human. *Comptes Rendus de l'Academie des Sciences Paris* 1971;272: 2638–2640.

17. Bobrow M, Madan, K. The effects of various banding procedures on human chromosomes studied with acridine orange. *Cytogenetics and Cell Genetics* 1973;12:145–156.

18. Arrighi F, Hsu TC. Localization of heterochromatin in human chromosomes. *Cytogenetics* 1971;10: 81–86.

19. Jagielski M, Zaleska M, Kaluzewski S, et al. Applicability of DAPI for the detection of mycoplasms in cell cultures. *Medycyna dojwiadczalna i mikrobiologia* 1976;28(2):161–173.

20. Schweizer D, Ambros P, Anderle M. Modification of DAPI banding on human chromosomes by prestaining with a DNA-binding oligopeptide antibiotic, distamycin A. *Experimental Cell Research* 1978;111:327–332.

21. Gustashaw K. Chromosome stains. In MJ B, ed. The ACT Cytogenetics Laboratory Manual, 2nd ed. New York: Raven Press, Ltd., 1991.

22. Grimm D. Genetics: Disease backs cancer origin theory. *Science* 2004;306(5695):389.

23. Mayall B, Carrano AV, Moore DH, Rowley JD. Quantification by DNA-based cytophotometry of the 9q+/22q-chromosomal translocation associated with chronic myelogenous leukemia. *Cancer Research* 1977;37:3590-3593.

24. Volpi E, Bridger JM: FISH glossary: an overview of the fluorescence in situ hybridization technique. *Biotechnology* 2008;45:385–399.

25. Juliusson G, Oscier DG, Fitchett M. Prognostic subgroups in B-cell chronic lymphocytic leukemia defined by specific chromosomal abnormalities. *New England Journal of Medicine* 1990;323: 720–724.

26. John S, Erming T, Jeffrey S, et al. High incidence of chromosome 13 deletion in multiple myeloma detected by multiprobe interphase FISH. *Blood* 2000;96(4):1505–1511.

27. Gellrich S, Ventura R, Jones M, et al. Immunofluorescent and FISH analysis of skin biopsies. *American Journal of Dermatopathology* 2004;26(3):242–247.

28. Cook J. Paraffin section interphase fluorescence in situ hybridization in the diagnosis and classification of non-Hodgkin lymphomas. *Diagnostic Molecular Pathology* 2004;13(4):197–206.

29. Van Stedum S, King W. Basic FISH techniques and troubleshooting. *Methods in Molecular Biology* 2002;204:51–63.

30. Macville M, Veldman T, Padilla-Nash H, et al. Spectral karyotyping, a 24-colour FISH technique for the identification of chromosomal rearrangements. *Histochemical Cell Biology* 1997;108 (4–5):299–305.

31. Kakazu N, Abe T. Cytogenetic analysis of chromosome abnormalities in human cancer using SKY. *Experimental Medicine* 1998;16:1638–1641.

32. Liang J, Ning Y, Wang R, et al. Spectral karyotypic study of the HL-60 cell line: Detection of complex rearrangements involving chromosomes 5, 7, and 16 and delineation of critical region of deletion on 5q31.1. *Cancer Genetics and Cytogenetics* 1999;113:105–109.

33. Mehra S, Messner H, Minden M, et al. Molecular cytogenetic characterization of non-Hodgkin lymphoma cell lines. *Genes Chromosomes and Cancer* 2002;33(3):225–234.

34. Lapierre J, Cacheux V, Da Silva F, et al. Comparative genomic hybridization: Technical development and cytogenetic aspects for routine use in clinical laboratories. *Annales de Genetique* 1998;41(1): 56–62.

35. Wienberg J, Stanyon R. Comparative painting of mammalian chromosomes. *Current Opinion in Genetics and Development* 1997;7(6):784–791.

36. Kytola S, Rummukainen J, Nordgren A, et al. Chromosomal alterations in 15 breast cancer cell lines by comparative genomic hybridization and spectral karyotyping. *Genes, Chromosomes and Cancer* 2000;28:308–317.

Gene Mutations

OBJECTIVES

- Compare phenotypic consequences of different types of point mutations.

- Distinguish detection of known mutations from scanning for unknown mutations.

- Discuss methods used to detect point mutations.

- Determine which detection methods are appropriate for screening of new mutations or detection of previously identified mutations.

- Describe gene mutation nomenclature for expressing sequence changes at the DNA, RNA, and protein levels.

Gene mutations include deletions, insertions, inversions, translocations, and other changes that can affect one base pair to hundreds or thousands of base pairs. Large differences in DNA sequence will likely have a significant effect on protein sequence. Alterations of a single or a few base pairs, or **point mutations**, will have a range of effects on protein sequence. Refer to the genetic code in Chapter 3, "Proteins," Figure 3-7, to see how a difference of one or a few base pairs may or may not change the encoded amino acid.

Types of Gene Mutations

Because there is more than one codon for most of the amino acids, DNA sequence changes do not necessarily change amino acid sequence. This is an important concept for interpreting results of mutation analyses. Substitution of one nucleotide with a different nucleotide may be **silent**, that is, not change the amino acid sequence (Table 9.1). **Conservative substitutions** may change the amino acid sequence, but the replacement and the original amino acid have similar biochemical properties (e.g., leucine for valine), and the change will not drastically affect protein function. In contrast, a **nonconservative substitution** results in the replacement of an amino acid with a biochemically different amino acid (e.g., proline for glutamine), which changes the biochemical nature of the protein. A **nonsense substitution** mutation terminates proteins prematurely when a nucleotide substitution produces a

stop codon instead of an amino acid codon. About 11% of disease-related gene lesions are nonsense mutations.[1]

Insertion or deletion of other than a multiple of three nucleotides results in a **frameshift mutation**, throwing the triplet code out of frame. The amino acids in the chain after the frameshift mutation are affected, as the triplet code will include new combinations of three nucleotides. The genetic code is structured such that frameshifts often terminate protein synthesis prematurely because a stop codon appears sooner in the out-of-frame coding sequence than it would in a nonmutated reading frame.

Nonconservative, nonsense, and frameshift mutations will generate different phenotypes, depending on where they occur along the protein sequence. Point mutations in the end of a coding region may have minimal consequences, whereas mutations at the beginning of a coding sequence are more likely to result in drastic alterations or even effective deletion of the protein coding region.

These factors are important when interpreting results of mutation analyses. Merely finding a change in a test DNA sequence does not guarantee an altered phenotype. Furthermore, screening methods designed to detect point mutations over large sequence regions may not detect the specific sequence alterations and, therefore, cannot distinguish among silent, conservative, and nonconservative changes. For inherited or recurring diseases, the specific change in the DNA may be ascertained from a family history or previous analysis.

Detection of Gene Mutations

Some, mostly inherited, disease-associated sequence changes in DNA occur frequently, for example, for the factor V Leiden mutation and the hemochromatosis C282Y, H63D, and S65C mutations. Also, increasing

Table 9.1 **Types of Point Mutations**

DNA Sequence	Amino Acid Sequence	Type of Mutation
ATG CAG GTG ACC TCA GTG	M Q V T S V	None
ATG CAG GT<u>T</u> ACC TCA GTG	M Q V T S V	Silent
ATG CA<u>A</u> GTG ACC TCA GTG	M Q L T S V	Conservative
ATG C<u>C</u>G GTG ACC TCA GTG	M <u>P</u> V T S V	Nonconservative
ATG CAG GTG ACC T<u>G</u>A GTG	M Q V T ter	Nonsense
ATG CAG GTG A<u>A</u>C CTC AGT G	M Q V <u>N</u> <u>L</u> <u>S</u>	Frameshift

---

Advanced Concepts

The nature of the genetic code is such that frameshift mutations lead to a termination codon within a small number of codons. This characteristic might have evolved to protect cells from making long nonsense proteins. It is a useful parameter to identify open reading frames in DNA.

numbers of specific single nucleotide polymorphisms (SNPs, see Chapter 10, "DNA Sequencing") are being mapped close to disease genes. These changes, although outside of the disease gene, are detected as specific sequence changes frequently inherited along with the disease phenotype.

Some diseases are associated with many possible mutations in a single gene. For instance, there are more than 600 disease-associated mutations in the cystic fibrosis transmembrane regulator (*CFTR*) gene, and more than 2000 cancer susceptibility mutations have been reported in the *BRCA1* and *BRCA2* genes. Furthermore, unknown numbers of gene mutations are yet to be discovered. Detection of mutations in large genes requires screening across thousands of base pairs to detect a single altered nucleotide. To date, other than sequencing, there is no genomewide scanning procedure that can identify yet unreported mutations.[2] However, in some cases, biochemical-based methods are used to detect or quantify the altered protein product, as described below.

Biochemical Methods

Biochemical methods are used to directly analyze the change in protein structure or function rather than to search for potential point mutations such as with gene mutation analyses. This type of testing is also useful for metabolic defects where several genes are involved in the disease phenotype and the actual protein or amino acid alterations can be detected using biochemical methods. Commonly used biochemical methods include immunoassays that detect the presence of hormones, drugs, antibodies, cancer biomarkers, and other metabolites in blood, urine, or other biological fluids. In addition, automated methods based on high-performance liquid or gas chromatography (GC) and mass spectrometry (MS) are also frequently used; these are described below.

Immunoassays

Immunoassays are flexible, potentially high-throughput methods for detecting a variety of analytes. These methods involve the use of specific antibodies or other ligands to detect the presence of the target molecules (Fig. 9-1). For this type of assay, plate wells, strips, or capillaries coated with capture antibody are exposed to test fluid (serum, plasma, or urine) that is diluted in the appropriate assay buffer. If the analyte is present in the test fluid, it will bind

to the immobilized antibody. After rinsing away unbound material, detection antibodies covalently linked to **alkaline phosphatase** or horseradish peroxidase are introduced. The unbound antibody conjugates are washed away and a substrate is added that will generate chemiluminescence, fluorescence, or color signals. Variations of this assay include immobilization of the antigen to detect target antibodies in the test fluid. The antibodies are then detected using anti-human antibody conjugates. This test is useful in detection of antibodies against infectious agents.

EIA methods are liquid handling techniques that have been effectively automated. Today, there are over 40 EIA analyzers on the market that have varying capabilities. Turbidimetry (latex agglutination), chemiluminescence, and magnetic particle methods are supported on these instruments. Most work with the 96-well plate format and there are preoptimized reagent sets designed for a wide variety of analytes.

High-Performance Liquid Chromatography (HPLC)

HPLC is the basis for separation/analysis instruments such as amino acid analyzers. Migration rates of molecules differ with varying combinations of HPLC component and

---

Historical Highlights

Enzyme immunoassays (EIA) and enzyme-linked immunosorbent assays (ELISA) are modifications of an earlier technique called radioimmunoassay (RIA) that was first reported as a method to detect insulin in plasma.[3] A significant concern for RIA and its later variations was the radioactive hazards from iodine 131 (^{131}I), even when it was replaced with less toxic ^{125}I. In 1970, chemical methods were designed that coupled enzymes (alkaline phosphatase and others) with the antibodies to the analyte. These enzymes would then produce a signal from a color or light-producing substrate. In 1971, Engvall and Perlmann reported the use of ELISA to detect immunoglobulin G in rabbit serum.[4] That same year, van Weemen and Schurs demonstrated the use of EIA to quantify human chorionic gonadotropin concentrations in urine.

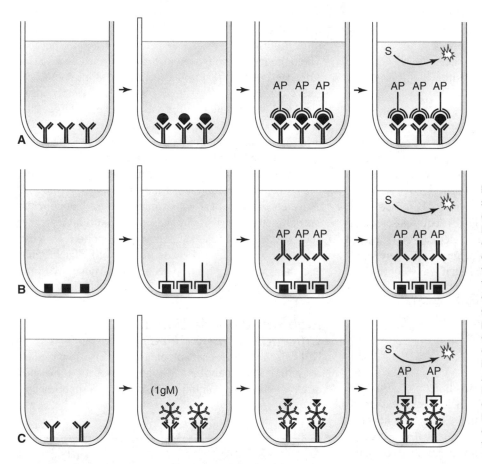

Figure 9-1 Enzyme immunoassay formats for antigen detection (A, C) and antibody detection (B). For direct antigen detection, antibody specific for the target analyte is immobilized in plate wells. If present, antigen binds to the antibody and is detected with a secondary antibody conjugated to enzyme (AP, alkaline phosphatase). For antibody detection, antigen is immobilized and bound to specific antibody, if present, which is detected with AP-conjugated secondary antibody. Antigen may also be detected with immobilized antibodies to IgM or IgG, which will capture antigen for detection with enzyme conjugate.

detectors. HPLC consists of two phases, a column with a mobile phase or a solvent that flows through a stationary phase or solid support. The solvent chemistry is selected so that it interacts more strongly with samples to slow migrations or more weakly to speed their migrations. Organic solvent in the mobile phase may be the same throughout the column (isocratic) or of increasing strength (gradient). In the stationary phase the solvent will also interact with the sample and affect migration speed. Mutated or missing molecules can thus be distinguished from normal migration patterns.

Stationary phases of HPLC differ depending on the application. Size exclusion columns are comprised of porous beads that exclude larger molecules and retain smaller molecules inside of the beads so that the larger molecules are eluted faster than the smaller molecules (Fig. 9-2). Normal and reverse phases separate on the basis of hydrophilicity, with lipophilic molecules eluting

faster, or hydrophobicity, with lipophilic molecules eluting slower. In ion exchange, ions in the sample are retained as counterions to charged groups that are permanently attached to the stationary phase. Changing the chemical properties of the mobile phase will selectively elute the trapped sample ions. Another selective solid phase, affinity, is designed to immobilize specific ions while other ions are washed through. The selected ion is eluted by changing the mobile phase conditions.

When a test sample is dissolved in the mobile phase, it is introduced to HPLC by injection with a syringe through an injection port in the column. Pumps will force the sample through the column, and elutions are monitored by a detector that produces a readout of signal peaks as the sample components elute. There are many types of detectors, depending on the characteristics of the sample, including light scattering, refractive index, uv light absorption, and mass spectrometry. The retention

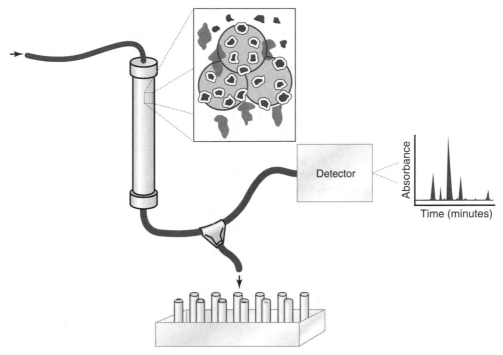

■ **Figure 9-2** Liquid chromatography is separation of molecules in solution through interaction with a solid support in the column. Separated molecules are detected directly or collected fractions are further analyzed by mass spectrometry.

time and size of peaks indicate the type and amount of sample components. HPLC may be used to separate nucleic acids as well as proteins.[5]

Gas Chromatography

In gas chromatography (GC), which is an automated method of analysis, the mobile phase is an inert gas and the stationary phase is a high-boiling-point liquid that is absorbed to an inert solid support in the column (Fig. 9-3). The sample is introduced to the column and vaporized into a gas. The inert gas carries the sample through the column. The strength of the interaction or dissolution of the sample components into the liquid phase will result in varying retention times in the column. The effluent from the column is monitored by a detector, such as a flame ionization detector, that is sensitive to organic molecules. Alternatively, GC may be coupled to a mass spectrometer. GC is used for detection of drugs and poisons and their metabolites in biological samples.[6,7]

Mass Spectrometry

A mass spectrometer converts molecules to ions that can be moved in a magnetic field based on their charge and

mass. In this automated method, an ion source sends high-energy electrons that hit the target sample molecules, separating them into ions, usually cations with the loss of one or two electrons. The ions themselves may further fragment into smaller ions and neutral particles. This collection of particles is accelerated and focused into a beam through a magnetic field. The ions are

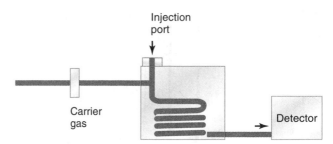

■ **Figure 9-3** Gas chromatography (gas-liquid chromatography) is separation of vaporized sample through a column of inert carrier gas and liquid stationary phase that differentially adsorbs molecules. The sample is injected through the injection port and the separated molecules are recorded by the detector.

deflected by the magnetic field according to their mass and charge. By varying the magnetic field strength, different ions are aimed at a detector. The readout of the instrument is a spectrum with the mass/charge value on the x axis and the abundance of the ion on the y axis (Fig. 9-4). A given compound can therefore be identified by its characteristic spectrum or set of peaks.

A variety of ionization methods have been developed for mass spectrometry (MS). In electrospray ionization (ESI), a test sample is converted into a fine spray of charged droplets that are electrostatically directed to the mass spectrometer inlet through a vacuum where ions are released and drawn through electrostatic lenses to the MS inlet. Another ionization method, matrix-assisted laser desorption/ionization (MALDI),[8] produces ions by firing a laser pulse into a surface coated with material that generates a positive ion (A+) from the peptide (Fig. 9-5). A high positive charge on the plate surface repulses the ion, which flies to the detector. High-molecular-weight molecules are identified using time of flight with MALDI ionization (MALDI-TOF). If the ions are allowed to drift in the flight tube, they will separate according to mass/charge ratio so that the lighter ions travel faster and reach the detector before the heavier ions do (Fig. 9-6). An extension of MALDI, surface-enhanced

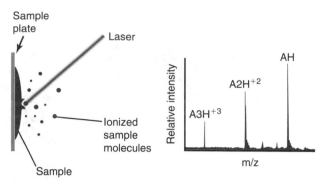

■ **Figure 9-5** In MALDI spectrophotometry, sample is adhered to the matrix on a sample plate, ionized (protonated), and released by laser bombardment. The ionized molecules are separated in an electric field by mass and charge. A sample molecule (A) will have multiple protonated species (AH, A2H, A3H).

laser desorption/ionization (SELDI), combined with time of flight (SELDI-TOF) offers flexibility in the identification and quantification of peptides.[9] With these techniques it is possible to analyze almost any class of molecule. Further information about the basic structure of a compound is gained by three-dimensional quadrupolar electric fields, tandem MS (MS/MS), and hybrid instruments such as MALDI-TOF/TOF. The resolution of these instruments is sufficient to identify amino acid sequences in peptides.

Nucleic Acid Analyses

Biochemical detection and/or characterization of proteins using the biochemical methods just described is one area of molecular analysis. These methods may be part of a clinical chemistry laboratory menu or performed as

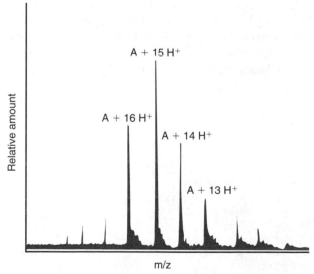

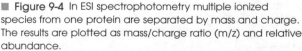

■ **Figure 9-4** In ESI spectrophotometry multiple ionized species from one protein are separated by mass and charge. The results are plotted as mass/charge ratio (m/z) and relative abundance.

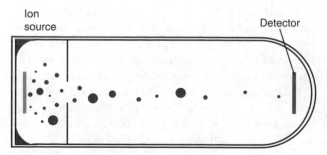

■ **Figure 9-6** In MALDI-TOF spectrophotometry, the ionized molecules are accelerated at a fixed point and allowed to drift through the flight tube to the detector. The time of flight is determined by the mass/charge ratio of the molecules.

molecular diagnostics. Mutation detection by analysis of nucleic acids is considered the classical molecular methodology. Nucleic acid analysis is performed on a variety of specimen types. Inherited mutations are detected from the most convenient and noninvasive specimen material, such as blood or buccal cells. Somatic mutations are often more challenging to find because cells harboring mutations may be only a small fraction of the total specimen that consists of mostly normal cells. Polymerase chain reaction (PCR) amplification, which is part of many procedures, has simplified mutation detection, especially from limiting specimens. PCR or other amplification methods, however, must be performed under conditions that minimize the introduction of mutations in the course of amplification.

Interpretation of the results of mutation analyses may also be challenging. Mutation scanning by methods that do not indicate the primary sequence change do not differentiate between silent, conservative, and nonconservative mutations. The actual effect on phenotype is left to posttest interpretation of supporting clinical data and patient family history. Mutations discovered through this type of scanning may be subjected to sequence analysis to confirm and further characterize the mutated region. (See Chapter 10, "DNA Sequencing.")

Although it is the most definitive method for detecting mutations, DNA sequencing may not be appropriate, especially for high-throughput procedures. A number of techniques have been designed for detection of DNA mutations from single base-pair changes to large chromosomal rearrangements without having to determine the primary DNA sequence. Some of these methods are described below.

Sequence detection methods can be generally classified according to three broad approaches: *hybridization-based* methods, **sequence (polymerization)-based** methods, and enzymatic or **chemical cleavage** methods. Brief descriptions of representative methods are presented in the following sections. The methods selected are currently used or proposed for use in clinical applications. A summary of the methods discussed in this chapter is shown in Table 9.2.

Hybridization-Based Methods

Single-Strand Conformation Polymorphism
Single-strand conformation polymorphism (SSCP)[9–11] is based on the preference of DNA (as well as RNA) to exist in a double-stranded, rather than single-stranded, state. In the absence of a complementary strand, nucleic acids form intrastrand duplexes to attain as much of a double-stranded condition as possible. Each folded strand forms a three-dimensional structure, or **conformer**, the shape of which is determined by the primary sequence of the folded strand. The migration of the single-stranded conformers in polyacrylamide gels under precisely controlled denaturing and temperature conditions distinguishes sequence variants.

For SSCP, dilute concentrations of short, double-stranded PCR products, optimally 100 to 400 base pairs (bp) long, are denatured (e.g., in 10 to 20 mM NaOH, 80% formamide for 5 minutes at 95°C; or 10 to 20 mM NaOH, 0.004 mM EDTA, 10% formamide for 5 minutes at 55°C to 60°C) followed by rapid cooling. Because the diluted single strands cannot easily find their **homologous** partners, they fold by intrastrand hybridization, forming three-dimensional conformers. The shape of the conformer depends on the complementary nucleotides available for hydrogen bonding and folding. A single base difference in the DNA sequence can cause the conformer to fold differently. These conformers are resolved in a polyacrylamide gel or by capillary electrophoresis with strict temperature control.[12] The speed of migration depends on the shape as well as the size of the conformer. Differences in the shape of the conformers (kinks, loops, bubbles, and tails) are caused by sequence differences in the DNA single strand (Fig. 9-7). The band or peak patterns are detected by silver stain, radioactivity, or fluorescence. To avoid renaturation of homologous partners, a low concentration of products after denaturation must be maintained. As a consequence, less sensitive stains such as ethidium bromide are not often used for this assay. Band or peak patterns different from those of normal sequence-control conformers prepared simultaneously with the test conformers indicate the presence of gene mutations.

SSCP is reported to detect 35% to 100% of putative mutations.[13] The assay can be sensitive enough to detect mutations in samples containing as low as 5% potentially mutant cells,[14] although specimens that are at least 30% potentially mutant cells produce more reliable results. This requirement is satisfied in inherited mutations, as at least 50% of cells of a specimen will potentially carry a mutation. However, for somatic mutations, such as the analysis of tumor cells, the potentially mutant cells may be mixed with or surrounded by a vast majority of normal

Table 9.2 **Summary of Mutation Detection Methodologies**

Method[*]	Target[†] (bp)	Accuracy[‡] (%)	Specificity[§] (%)	Sensitivity[‖] (%)	Laboratory Application[¶]	Reference[#]
Sequencing	>1000	100	100	10-20	C, R	Chapter 10
SSCP	50–400	70–100	80–100	5–20	C, R	141, 142
DGGE	200–500	95–100	90–100	1–15	R	143, 144
TTGE	200–1000	95–100	90–100	1–10	R	145, 146
ASO	Defined	100	90–100	5–20	C, R	41, 147
HR-MCA	Defined	95–100	95–100	1–5	C, R	45, 49, 148
MIP	Defined, multiplex	100	95–100		R	56, 155, 156
HA, DHPLC	50–1000	95–100	85–100	5–20	C, R	60, 64, 65, 68, 149–154
Array Technology	Defined, multiplex	95–100	80–100	1–5	C, R	68, 70
SSP	Defined	98–100	95–100	0.0005	C, R	86, 158
ddF	40–600	85–100	70–100	1–15	R	88, 89
Allelic discrimination	Defined	95–100	90–100	0.0001	C,R	48, 80, 81
Dye terminator	Defined	98–100	95–100	5–10	R	93, 95, 159
PTT	500–2500	95–100	85–100	10–20	R	107, 160
PCR-RFLP	Defined	100	100	0.01–1	C, R	111, 157
BESS	200–600				R	116, 161
NIRCA	500–1000	85–90	80–90	5–10	R	117, 162, 163
Invader	Defined, multiplex	100	95–100		C, R	127, 164
CCM	40–30,000	85–100		0.01–1	R	2

[*]See text. Data are from methods done under optimal conditions.
[†]Optimal length of sequence that can be screened accurately; defined methods target a single nucleotide or site; multiplex methods target multiple defined types in the same reaction.
[‡]Concordance with direct sequencing or other assays reported in the references.
[§]True positive detection of mutations without concurrent false-positive.
[‖]Detection of one mutant target in a background of normal targets.
[¶]C: Presently used in clinical applications; R: Research applications.
[#]Also see references in text.

cells or tissue. Therefore, a cell suspension that is at least 30% tumor cells or a microdissection of solid tumor tissue from fixed or frozen sections is recommended.

Because SSCP works more accurately on some genes than others, modifications of the SSCP procedure have been developed, for instance, using RNA instead of DNA (**RNA-SSCP** or **rSSCP**)[15,16] or using **restriction endonuclease fingerprinting (REF-SSCP).**[17] rSSCP or REF-SSCP methods, although more sensitive, are more difficult to interpret and not in general use.

Denaturing Gradient Gel Electrophoresis

Denaturing gradient gel electrophoresis (DGGE) exploits differences in denaturation between a normal and mutated DNA helix caused by as few as one base-pair difference in a sequence. The contribution of the

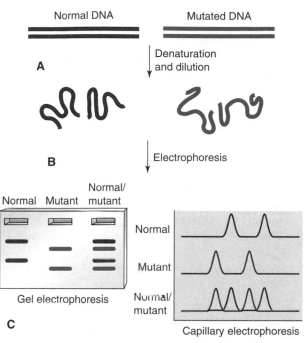

Normal DNA   Mutated DNA

A

Denaturation
and dilution

B

Electrophoresis

Normal   Mutant   Normal/
                  mutant

Gel electrophoresis

C

Normal

Mutant

Normal/
mutant

Capillary electrophoresis

■ **Figure 9-7** Single-strand conformation polymorphism analysis. Double-stranded PCR products (A) of normal or mutant sequences are denatured and form conformers (B) through intrastrand hydrogen bonding. These conformers can be resolved (C) by gel (left) or capillary (right) electrophoresis.

attraction between successive bases on the same DNA strand (stacking) can affect denaturation of double-stranded DNA.[18–20] For DGGE, double-stranded DNA fragments 200 to 700 bp in length are prepared by PCR amplification of test sequences or by restriction digestion. The fragments are separated on polyacrylamide gels containing a gradient of concentrations of urea and formamide. A 100% denaturant solution is 7 M urea and 40% formamide. Gradients range from 15% to 90% denaturant, usually with a 10% to 20% difference between the high denaturant concentration at the bottom of the gel and the low denaturant concentration at the top of the gel for a given analysis. **Gradient gels** can be prepared manually or with special equipment (gradient makers).

As the double-stranded DNA fragment moves through the gel, the denaturing conditions increase, sequences reach their denaturing point, and the complementary

strands begin to denature. Domains of the sequences with different melt characteristics denature at different points in the gradient. The formation of single-stranded areas of the denaturing duplex slows migration of the fragment through the gel matrix from the point of the initial denaturation. Differences in the DNA sequence result in denaturation at different positions in the gel so that the band of a mutated DNA band shifts to a different position in the gel as compared with the normal DNA band. Complete strand separation is prevented by naturally occurring or artificially placed GC-rich sequences (**GC clamps**). These can be conveniently placed at the ends of PCR products by using primers tailed on the 5' end with a 40-bp GC sequence.

Two gradient orientations are used in DGGE. The gradient can increase horizontally across the gel, that is, perpendicularly to the direction of sample migration (perpendicular DGGE), or the gradient can increase vertically, parallel to the direction of sample migration (parallel DGGE; Fig. 9-8). In the perpendicular DGGE, a mixture of samples is loaded across the entire gel in a single well and a sigmoid curve of migration is observed, corresponding to the denaturing characteristics of the sequences. This type of gradient is used to establish the more defined gradient conditions used in parallel DGGE. For parallel DGGE, a smaller gradient is used; samples are loaded in single lanes and analyzed by lane comparison.

Because relatively high concentrations of DNA are used for this assay, detection with ethidium bromide is sufficient to visualize the results of the electrophoresis. Specific regions within large sequence areas may be visualized by blotting the bands in the DGGE gel to a nitrocellulose membrane and probing for the specific

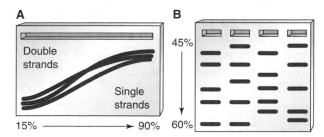

A   B

Double
strands   45%

Single
strands

15% ——————→ 90%   60%

■ **Figure 9-8** Schematic of perpendicular (A) DGGE and parallel (B) DGGE.

sequence (Southern blot). As with SSCP, DGGE gels are analyzed for banding patterns in the test specimens that differ from banding patterns of the control sequences.

DGGE has been used to detect tumor suppressor gene mutations,[21] clonality,[22] and population polymorphisms.[23] In *genomic DGGE*,[24] in which restriction fragments of genomic DNA rather than PCR products are separated on a gradient gel and then blotted and probed as a Southern blot, any area of the genome can be probed for mutations.

Allele-Specific Oligomer Hybridization

Allele-specific hybridization, or **allele-specific oligomer hybridization (ASO)**, utilizes the differences in melting temperatures of short sequences of about 20 bases with one or two mismatches and those with no mismatches. Synthetic single-stranded probes with the normal or mutant target DNA sequence are used for this assay. At

---

Advanced Concepts

DGGE requires a significant amount of preparatory work to optimize conditions for detection of a particular gene mutation. Originally performed on restriction fragments, PCR products are now used for DGGE. Primers are chosen so that the region to be screened for mutations has one or two discrete melting domains (excluding the GC clamp) because more than two domains may give a complex pattern that is difficult to interpret. The GC clamp should be positioned adjacent to the highest melting domain. Design of the primers and the melt characteristics of the resulting product require inspection of the sequence to be screened for mutations. The optimal gradient and gel running conditions must also be established. Initially, sample sequences are separated on a wide gradient (20% to 80% formamide) to find the area where the sequence migrations are most distinct. This area will define a narrower gradient (e.g., 30% to 55% gradient) for use in the actual test. The gel running conditions must be strictly controlled for reproducible results. If either run time or temperature, for instance, is not optimal, resolution of differing sequences may be lost.

Advanced Concepts

Two methods that are similar in design to DGGE are constant gradient gel electrophoresis (CDGE)[25,26] and temporal temperature gradient gel electrophoresis (TTGE).[27,28]

CDGE requires the initial determination of optimal denaturant concentrations for a particular target mutation. This is ascertained by perpendicular DGGE or by using computer programs designed to predict the melting characteristics of a given nucleotide sequence for a range of temperature and denaturing conditions. The sample is then run at the one optimal combination of denaturant concentration and temperature. As parameters must be set in this manner, CDGE is used for detecting known mutations rather than for screening for unknown mutations. CDGE has been extended to capillary electrophoresis (constant denaturant capillary electrophoresis), which increases the speed and resolution of the separation.[29] CDGE has been used to detect mutations in cancer genes.[30] Compared with SSCP, DGGE has less sensitivity for detecting mutations in genes that are rich in GC content.[31]

TTGE is similar to CDGE in that specific concentrations of formamide and urea are used to denature DNA duplexes. In TTGE, unlike CDGE, differences in denaturation are resolved by slowly raising the temperature of the gel during migration, for example, 63°C to 68°C at 1.7°C/hour. This provides a wider range of denaturing conditions such that fragments requiring different denaturant compositions by CDGE can be resolved on a single gel by TTGE. This technique has been used in cancer,[32,33] genetic,[34,35] and industrial[36,37] applications.

---

specific annealing temperatures and conditions (stringency), a probe will not bind to a near complementary target sequence with one or two mismatched bases, whereas a probe with a perfect complementary sequence will bind. ASO is a **dot blot** method, similar to the Southern blot method that uses an immobilized target and a labeled probe in a solution. The dot blot method has been used to test for known, frequently occurring

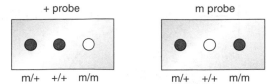

■ **Figure 9-9** Allele-specific oligomer hybridization. Three samples are spotted on two membranes. One membrane is probed with a labeled oligomer of the normal sequence (+ probe, left) and the other with a labeled oligomer containing the mutation (m probe, right). A normal sample (+/+) hybridizes with the normal oligomer only. A homozygous mutant sample (m/m) hybridizes with the mutant oligomer only. A heterozygous mutant sample (m/+) hybridizes with both oligomers.

mutations, for example, in the *BRCA1* and *BRCA2* gene mutations frequently observed in inherited breast cancer[38] and the p16 gene mutations in familial melanoma.[39]

The ASO procedure begins with amplification of the gene region of interest by PCR. After the PCR product is spotted onto nitrocellulose or nylon membranes, the membranes are soaked in a high salt NaOH denaturation solution. The DNA on the membranes is neutralized with dilute acid and permanently affixed to the membrane by baking or ultraviolet cross-linking. Labeled probes matching the normal and mutated sequences are then hybridized to the membranes in separate reactions under specific stringency conditions (Fig. 9-9). Some protocols recommend addition of an unlabeled probe directed at the nontarget sequence to the labeled targeted probe in order to increase binding specificity.[40] Hybridization can

take 2 to 12 hours. Following hybridization, the free probe is rinsed from the membrane, and the probe signal is detected over the spots containing sequences matching that of the probe (Fig. 9-10). This method has been used in clinical testing for detection of specific mutations and polymorphisms and for typing of organisms. ASO is also used in the clinical laboratory for tissue typing (sequence-specific oligonucleotide probe hybridization; see Chapter 15, "DNA-Based Tissue Typing").

ASO analysis also may be carried out as a **reverse dot blot** in a 96-well plate format similar to capture probe methods developed for infectious disease testing, for example, *Chlamydia trachomatis* (Amplicor CT/NG; Roche) and *Mycobacterium tuberculosis* (Amplicor MTB; Roche). For mutation analysis, mutant or normal probes are immobilized on the membrane. The sequence to be tested is amplified by PCR with one regular and one biotinylated primer. The denatured biotinylated products are then exposed to the immobilized probes under conditions set so that only the exact complementary sequences hybridize. Unbound products are washed away, and those that remain bound are detected with a conjugated horseradish peroxidase-antibiotin Fab fragment and exposure to a chromogenic or chemiluminescent substrate. Generation of a color reaction indicates the binding of the test DNA to the normal or mutant probe. This method has been proposed for detection of frequently occurring mutations such as factor V Leiden.[41] HLA typing of multiple alleles on a single specimen using the Luminex Tag-It® technology is based on ASO hybridization (see Chapter 15, "DNA-Based Tissue Typing").

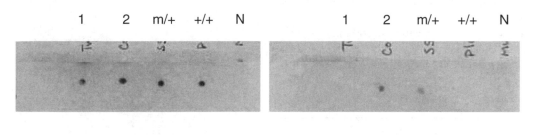

■ **Figure 9-10** Autoradiography results of an allele-specific oligomer hybridization using chemiluminescent detection. One normal (1) sample and one heterozygous mutant (2) sample are shown with a heterozygous mutant control (m/+), a normal control (+/+), and a negative control (N).

Melt Curve Analysis

Like DGGE and related methods, **melt curve analysis (MCA)** exploits the sequence- and stacking-directed denaturation characteristics of DNA duplexes.[42] The method is a postamplification step of real-time PCR.[43,44] PCR amplicons generated in the presence of a DNA-specific fluorescent dye, such as ethidium bromide, SYBR Green, or LC Green, are heated at a rate of about 0.3°C/sec. The dyes, specific for double-stranded DNA, initially yield a high signal because the DNA is mostly double-stranded at the low temperature. As the temperature rises, the DNA duplexes begin to separate into single strands, losing dye accordingly. The fluorescent signal gives a pattern as shown in Fig. 9-11. Sequence differences result in different melting characteristics and T_ms (where there are equal amounts of double- and single-stranded DNA) for each sequence. The T_m is illustrated as a peak, plotting the derivative (speed of decrease) of fluorescence versus temperature. Results are interpreted by the temperature peak placement with respect to the temperature on the x axis. Specimens with identical sequences should yield overlaying peaks at the expected T_m, whereas specimens containing different sequences will yield two or more peaks at different temperatures (Fig. 9-12).

MCA of PCR products using nonspecific dyes is a simple and cost-effective way to screen for sequence differences. These dyes are not sequence-specific, however, and do not distinguish between the target amplicon and extraneous products in the PCR reaction, such as primer dimers or misprimed amplicons. Although the target sample should be identifiable by its T_m, such unintended products can complicate the melt curve and confuse interpretation.

Specificity is increased by using high-resolution melt curve analysis (HR-MCA),[45–47] which uses fluorescent resonance energy transfer (FRET) probes that hybridize

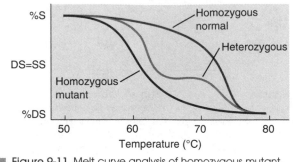

■ Figure 9-11 Melt curve analysis of homozygous mutant, heterozygous, and normal PCR products.

next to one another across the sequence position being analyzed. See Chapter 7, "Nucleic Acid Amplification" for more information on FRET probes. The probes fluoresce only when bound to the target sequence because FRET fluorescence relies on the transfer of energy from a donor fluorescent molecule (fluor) on one probe to an acceptor fluor on the other probe. As the temperature increases, the probes dissociate at a specific T_m. When the probes dissociate from the target, the donor is no longer close to the acceptor and the fluorescence drops. If the target sequence has a mismatch between the target and the probe, hydrogen bonding is perturbed between the two strands of the double helix. The mismatch decreases the dissociation temperature, compared with matched or complementary sequences. A T_m lower than that of the probe and its perfect complement, therefore, indicates the presence of a mutation, or sequence difference, between the probe reference sequence and the test sequence.

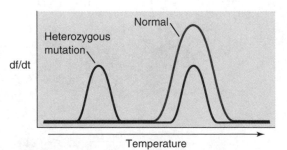

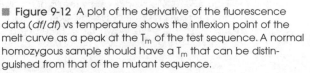

■ Figure 9-12 A plot of the derivative of the fluorescence data (*df/df*) vs temperature shows the inflexion point of the melt curve as a peak at the T_m of the test sequence. A normal homozygous sample should have a T_m that can be distinguished from that of the mutant sequence.

FRET is most frequently performed with two probes; however, single-probe systems have been developed. The single probe is designed to fluoresce much more brightly when hybridized to the target. The fluorescence is lost on dissociation (Fig. 9-13). Another modification that is reported to improve the sensitivity of MCA is the covalent attachment of a minor groove binder (MGB) group to the probe. The MGB, dihydrocyclopyrroloindole tripeptide, folds into the minor groove of the duplex formed by hybridization of the terminal 5 to 6 bp of the probe with the template. This raises the melting temperature of the probe, especially one with high A/T content. The T_m of a 12- to 18-bp MGB conjugated probe has hybridization properties equivalent to that of a 25- to 27-bp non-MGB probe.[48]

Special instrumentation is required for MCA and HR-MCA. Thermal cyclers with fluorescent detection, such as the Roche LightCycler and the ABI 7000 series, have melt curve options that can be added to the thermal cycling program. Although the Roche LightTyper and the Idaho Technologies HR-1 perform MCA only, they can process more samples per unit time than the Roche Light Cycler and Idaho Technologies thermal cycler systems.[49] Melt curve methodology has been proposed for a variety of clinical laboratory applications, such as detection of DNA polymorphisms[50–52] and typing of microorganisms.[53,54] Naturally occurring sequence variation must be considered in performing MCA, as it can complicate interpretation of the test.[55]

Inversion Probe Assay

The molecular inversion probe system is a method for detection of single nucleotide polymorphisms (SNPs) in DNA.[56] The molecular inversion probe is a linear probe containing two target-specific regions, one at each end; primer binding sites; and a 20-nucleotide-long unique sequence tag (Fig. 9-14). The probe hybridizes to the target sequence, the two ends flanking the potential SNP being tested. In four separate reactions, A, C, T, or G is added along with DNA polymerase and DNA ligase to

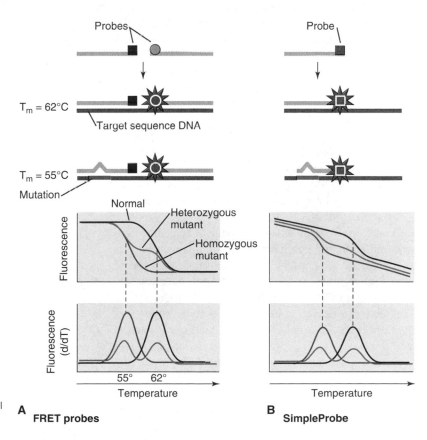

■ **Figure 9-13** Melt curve analysis with FRET probes (left) and SimpleProbe (right). A mismatch between the target and probe will lower the T_m of the duplex.

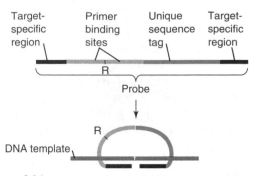

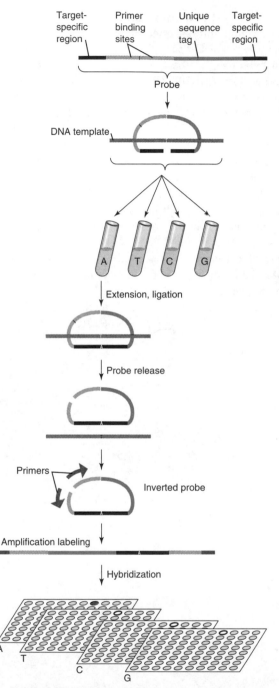

■ **Figure 9-14** The molecular inversion probe is designed to recognize specific genomic targets on the template. A restriction site R is for release of the probe after template-dependent circularization. A unique sequence tag identifies that target by its location of hybridization on a microarray.

the probe-target hybridization reaction (Fig. 9-15). A one-base extension and ligation of the probe occurs only in the tube containing the nucleotide complementary to the SNP site on the template.

Once the probe is ligated and circularized, it is released from the target and relinearized with a single-stranded exonuclease. Fluorescently labeled primers complementary to the cut site will amplify the probe to produce a product that is "inverted" with respect to the regions complementary to the target. Amplicons will be present only in the tube(s) containing the nucleotide matching the template. The contents of each tube are hybridized to one of four identical microarrays, probing for the unique sequence tag that identifies the genomic location of the polymorphism. Fluorescence will emit from the ligated and amplified probe bound to one of the arrays, that is, the one corresponding to the nucleotide added to the probe.

The inversion probe assay is capable of screening multiple mutations or polymorphisms simultaneously as a multiplex inversion probe assay.[57] Because each probe has a unique sequence tag to identify it in the array step and common PCR primer sites, thousands of probes can be added to a single set of four reactions with genomic DNA (500 ng) in four wells of a 96-well plate. Each of the probes will be successfully ligated in one of the four nucleotide-extension reactions. As the PCR primer sites are the same for all probes, one set of primers can amplify all ligated probes. The amplicons are then hybridized to microarrays by the unique sequence tags, which identify their genomic locations.

■ **Figure 9-15** Molecular inversion probe procedure (only one of four reactions shown). Closure of the hybridized circular probe occurs only in the presence of the nucleotide complementary to the template. The circular probe from each tube is released, cut, amplified, and labeled for hybridization to one of four arrays. Each probe hybridizes to one of the four arrays, depending on the original template sequence.

Although the original multiplex inversion probe assay method used four separate identical microarrays, one for the amplified products of each extension reaction, with four-color dye technology, hybridization of all four reactions is performed on the same microarray. The location of the array position identifies the location of the mutation. The color identifies the nucleotide at that location. This assay is one of the high-throughput methods used in the Human Haplotype Mapping Project (see Chapter 11, "DNA Polymorphisms and Human Identification").

Heteroduplex Analysis

Solution hybridization and electrophoresis of test nucleic acid fragments mixed with reference nucleic acid fragments can reveal mutations. To form **heteroduplexes**, nonidentical double-stranded DNA duplexes are heated to a temperature that results in complete denaturation of the double-stranded DNA (e.g., 95°C) and then slowly cooled (e.g., –1°C/4 to 20 sec). Heteroduplexes are formed when single strands that are not completely complementary hybridize to one another. (Heteroduplexes are also formed when test PCR products amplified from genetically heterozygous specimens are denatured and renatured.) The heteroduplexes migrate differently than do **homoduplexes** through polyacrylamide or agarose gels (Fig. 9-16). The presence of bands different from a homozygous reference control is indicative of mutations. Gel-based heteroduplex methods have been designed for HIV typing[58] and hematological testing.[59]

Conformation-sensitive gel electrophoresis is a **heteroduplex analysis** method in which the heteroduplexes are resolved on a 1,4-bis (acroyl) piperazine gel with ethylene glycol and formamide as mildly denaturing solvents to optimize conformational differences.[60,61] This method was intended for screening large genes for mutations and polymorphisms. The use of fluorescent detection increases sensitivity and throughput of the assay.

Heteroduplexes are also resolved by denaturing high-performance liquid chromatography (DHPLC). This version of heteroduplex analysis is performed on PCR products, ideally 150 to 450 bp in length. The amino acid analog **betaine** is sometimes added to the heteroduplex mixture to minimize the differences in stability of AT and GC base pairs, increasing the sensitivity of detection.[62] HPLC separation is then performed on a 25% to 65% gradient of acetonitrile in triethylammonium acetate at the melting temperature of the PCR product. The

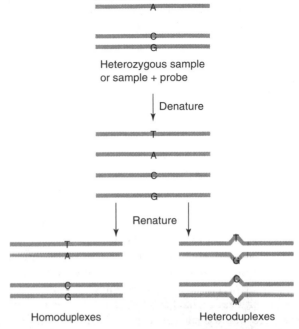

■ Figure 9-16 Heteroduplex analysis is performed by mixing sample amplicons with a reference amplicon, denaturing, and slowly renaturing. If the sample contains mutant sequences, a fraction of the renatured products will be heteroduplexes. These structures can be resolved from homoduplexes by electrophoresis.

heteroduplexes elute ahead of the homoduplexes as the denaturing conditions intensify. The migrating homoduplexes and heteroduplexes are detected by absorbance at 260 nm or by fluorescence. HPLC methods are reported to be more sensitive than gel methods, with greater capacity for screening large numbers of samples.[63–65] Although gel-based heteroduplex analyses are routinely used in the clinical laboratory, HPLC analysis of heteroduplexes is still being evaluated as a mutation screening method in the clinical laboratory.[66,67]

Array Technology

Single base-pair resolution by hybridization differences is achievable with **high-density oligonucleotide arrays** (see Chapter 6, "Analysis and Characterization of Nucleic Acids and Proteins"). These methods are similar to comparative genome hybridization but focus on a single gene with higher resolution, as in ASO procedures. Mutation analysis of the p53 tumor suppressor gene by array analysis has sensitivity and specificity similar to that of direct sequencing.[68] The advantage of array methods is the large number of inquiries (potential sequence mutations or SNPs) that can be tested simultaneously.

Arrays are also designed to test multiple genes for sequence mutations. To do this type of analysis, the test DNA is fragmented by treatment with DNase before binding to the complementary probes on the array. If the sample fragments are too large (not treated with DNase), a single base-pair mismatch has minimal effect on hybridization, so the fragment binds to multiple probes and the specificity of detection is lost. An example of one type of hybridization format, **standard tiling**, is shown in Figure 9-17.[68] In this format, the base substitution in the immobilized probe is always in the twelfth position from its 3' end. Commonly occurring mutations are targeted in another type of format, **redundant tiling**, in which the same mutation is placed at different positions in the probe (at the 5' end, in the middle, or at the 3' end). After hybridization of the fluorescently labeled sample DNA, the fluorescent signal is read on a scanner with appropriate software and the mutations are identified as indicated by which probes are bound. Although not performed routinely in clinical laboratories, a number of applied methods have been developed using high-density oligonucleotide and microelectronic arrays.[69–72]

Bead array technology utilizes sets of color-coded polystyrene beads in suspension as the solid matrix. In an extension of the FlowMetrix system,[73] 100 sets of beads are dyed with distinct fluorochrome mixes. Each set is coated with oligonucleotide probes corresponding to a genetic locus or gene region. In this technology 10^5 or more probes are attached to each 3- to 6-micron-diameter bead. When labeled test samples are hybridized to the beads through complementary probe sequences, the combination of bead color and test label reveals the presence or absence of a mutation or polymorphism. The advantage of this arrangement is that multiple loci can be tested simultaneously from small samples. Up to 100 analytes are tested in a single well of a microtiter plate. This method requires a flow cytometry instrument, Luminex, that excites and reads the emitted fluorescence as the beads flow past a detector. This technology has been applied to antibody detection and infectious diseases and is used in tissue typing and in other clinical applications.[74–76]

Sequencing (Polymerization)-Based Methods

Sequence-Specific (Primer) PCR

Sequence-specific (primer) PCR (SSP-PCR) is commonly used to detect point mutations and other single-nucleotide polymorphisms. There are numerous modifications to the method, which involve careful design of primers such that the primer 3' end falls on the nucleotide to be analyzed. Unlike the 5' end, the 3' end of a primer must match the template perfectly to be extended by *Taq* polymerase (Fig. 9-18). By designing primers to end on a mutation, the presence or absence of product is interpreted as the presence or absence of the mutation.

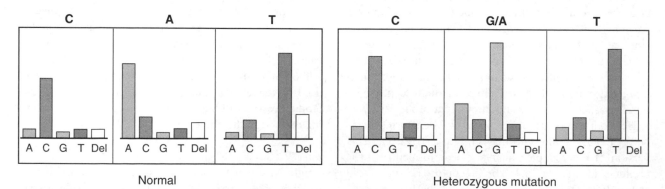

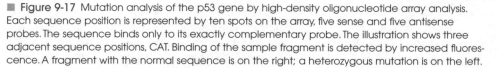

■ Figure 9-17 Mutation analysis of the p53 gene by high-density oligonucleotide array analysis. Each sequence position is represented by ten spots on the array, five sense and five antisense probes. The sequence binds only to its exactly complementary probe. The illustration shows three adjacent sequence positions, CAT. Binding of the sample fragment is detected by increased fluorescence. A fragment with the normal sequence is on the right; a heterozygous mutation is on the left.

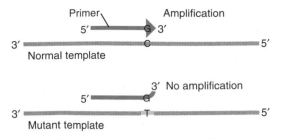

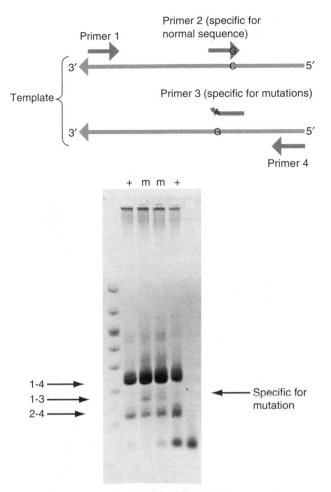

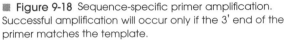

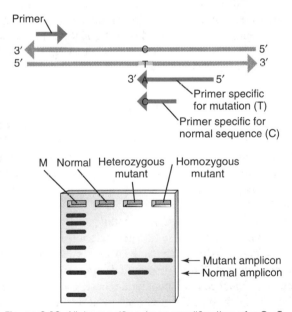

Figure 9-18 Sequence-specific primer amplification. Successful amplification will occur only if the 3' end of the primer matches the template.

In a modification of SSP-PCR, normal and mutant sequences are distinguished from one another by making either the normal or the mutant primer longer, resulting in differently sized products, depending on the sequence of the template (Fig. 9-19). Alternatively, primers can be multiplexed[38] (Fig. 9-20). Multiplexed SSP-PCR was originally called amplification refractory

Figure 9-19 Allele-specific primer amplification of a C→T mutation. A longer primer is designed with the mutated nucleotide (A) at the 3' end. This primer is longer and gives a larger amplicon than the primer binding to the normal sequence (top). The resulting products can be distinguished by their size on an agarose gel (bottom). First lane: molecular weight marker; second lane: a normal sample; third lane: a heterozygous mutant sample; fourth lane: a homozygous mutant.

Figure 9-20 Multiplex allele-specific PCR. The mutation (C→A) is detected by an allele-specific primer (3) that ends at the mutation. Primers 3 and 4 would then produce a mid-sized fragment (1-3). If there is no mutation, a normal primer (2) binds and produces a smaller fragment (2-4). Primers 1 and 4 always amplify the entire region (1-4).

mutation system PCR or tetra primer PCR.[77,78] Sequence-specific PCR is routinely used for high-resolution HLA typing (Chapter 15, "DNA-Based Tissue Typing") and for detection of commonly occurring mutations.

A high-throughput application of bead array technology (Illumina bead array)[79] uses sequence-specific PCR (Fig. 9-21). In this assay, primers tailed at the 5' end with locus-specific sequences and allele-specific sequences (A or G in Fig. 9-21) are used to amplify the test DNA.

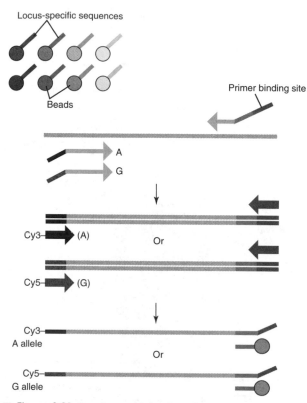

■ **Figure 9-21** Bead array technology. Beads colored with distinct fluorescent dyes (upper left) are covalently attached to the probe sequences, each color of bead attached to a probe representing a specific locus. In a sequence-specific PCR, test DNA is amplified with tailed primers. The tailed PCR products are amplified in a second reaction to generate labeled amplicons that will bind to specific beads, according to the gene locus. The combination of bead label and the hybridized amplicon label reveals whether there is a mutant or normal allele at that locus.

Each resulting PCR product will have an allele-specific sequence at one end and a locus-specific sequence at the other end. The PCR products are subsequently amplified in a second round using Cy3 or Cy5 (fluorescently) labeled 5' primers, complementary to the sequences introduced by the tailed primers in the first round. These amplicons are then hybridized to the locus-specific sequences covalently attached to the bead array. The bead color (locus) combined with Cy3 or Cy5 fluorescence (allele) types the allele at each locus. This system is one of the technologies used in the Human Haplotype Mapping Project.

Allelic Discrimination with Fluorogenic Probes

Thermal cyclers with fluorescent detection support **allelic discrimination** with fluorogenic probes. This method, an extension of the 5' nuclease real-time PCR assay, uses two probes labeled with different fluors (Fig. 9-22). Each probe matches either the normal or mutant sequence. The probe matching the test sequence is digested by the enzyme, releasing the reporter dye. The presence of the corresponding fluorescent signals indicates whether the test sequence is normal or mutant, that is, whether the probe matched and hybridized to the test sequence. In the example shown in Figure 9-22, the probe complementary to the normal sequence is labeled with FAM dye; the probe complementary to the mutant sequence is labeled with VIC dye. If the test sequence is normal, FAM fluorescence will be high, and VIC fluorescence will be low. If the test sequence is mutant, VIC will be high and FAM will be low. If the sequence is heterozygous, both VIC and FAM will be high. Negative controls show no VIC or no FAM. This assay has the advantage of interrogating multiple samples simultaneously and has been proposed as a practical high-throughput laboratory method.[80,81] It has been used in research applications in genetics and infectious disease.[82–86]

Dideoxy DNA Fingerprinting

Dideoxy DNA fingerprinting (ddF) is a modified chain termination sequencing procedure (see Chapter 10, "DNA Sequencing," for a description of **dideoxy chain termination** sequencing). Dideoxynucleotides lack the 3' hydroxyl group necessary for formation of the phosphodiester bond and elongation of the DNA chain (see Chapter 1, "DNA"). For this analysis, a single dideoxynucleotide is used to generate a series of terminated fragments that are resolved in one lane of a polyacrylamide gel. The ddF method resolves normal and mutant sequences by nucleotide base differences that result in the absence of a normal band or presence of an additional band (informative dideoxy component).

Dideoxynucleotide triphosphates (ddNTP) terminate DNA synthesis (see Chapter 10, "DNA Sequencing"). For example, dideoxy guanosine triphosphate added to a DNA synthesis reaction terminates copying of the template at each C residue on the template. If the template sequence has a mutation that replaces another nucleotide

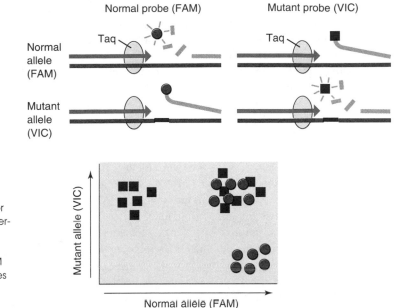

Figure 9-22 Allelic discrimination. Probes, complementary to either the normal sequence (left) or the mutant sequence (right), are labeled with different fluors, for example, FAM and VIC, respectively. The *Taq* exonuclease functions only if the probe is matched to the sequence being tested. High FAM indicates normal sequence, and high VIC indicates mutant sequence. If both fluors are detected, the test sample is heterozygous.

with C (or substitutes a C residue for another nucleotide), an additional fragment terminated by ddG will be present on the gel (Fig. 9-23). Furthermore, fragments terminated at C residues beyond the mutation migrate with altered mobility due to the base change. Whereas the additional fragment is absolute, the altered mobility is subject to gel conditions and temperature, just as with SSCP. Each of the four dideoxynucleotides will be used in this assay, depending on the nature of the sequence changes under study. This assay was introduced as an improvement in sensitivity over SSCP and other screening methods.[87]

The basic ddF procedure screens only one strand of the template duplex. By adding two primers instead of one, simultaneous termination reactions on both strands are generated in **bidirectional** dideoxy fingerprinting.[88] Although the band patterns produced by this method are more complex, mutations that might be missed on one strand will be detected in the complementary strand. Both ddF and bi-ddF can be performed using capillary electrophoresis as well as gel electrophoresis.[89,90]

Dye Terminator Incorporation
Multiplex assays have been designed using limited incorporation of fluorescently labeled dideoxynucleotide

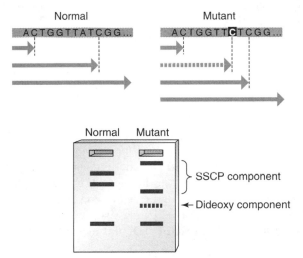

Figure 9-23 Dideoxy fingerprinting detection of an A>C mutation. ddG added to the synthesis reaction terminates copies of the template at each opportunity to add G (opposite C in the template). An additional termination product will be generated from the mutant template (dotted line). This fragment will be detected as an extra band on the gel (dideoxy component). The subsequent larger terminated fragments will have a 1-bp difference from the normal ones, which may affect migration (SSCP component).

triphosphates. In one method, fluorescent polarization-template–directed dye terminator incorporation (FP-TDI),[91] primers are designed to hybridize on the test sequence up to the nucleotide being tested (Fig. 9-24). Two fluorescence-labeled terminator dideoxynucleotides corresponding to the alleles to be typed serve as primers for a single-base extension reaction. For example, one nucleotide is labeled with the fluorescent dye, 6-carboxy-X-rhodamine (ROX,) or 9-(2-carboxyphenyl)-3,6-diamino-3H-xanthylium chloride (R110), and the other is labeled with the dye 5- or 6-carboxy-tetramethyl rho-damine (TAMRA), as in the figure, ROX-ddCTP and TAMRA-ddUTP. The remaining two terminators, ddATP and ddGTP, are also present, although in unlabeled form, to prevent misincorporations. No deoxy nucleotides (dNTPs) are present. If a labeled ddNTP is incorporated onto the primer, the polarized signal of that dye increases as it becomes part of the larger oligonucleotide.[92] The samples are read twice on a fluorometer, with filters corresponding to each of the dyes used. Instrument software calculates the polarization from the raw data and produces a numerical report. Although this procedure is compatible with mutation detection, its present use is in single-nucleotide polymorphism analysis.[93]

Another extension/termination assay is *Homogeneous MassExtend* or *MassArray.*[94,95] In this method, mass spectrometry is used to detect extension products terminated by specific dye-labeled dideoxynucleotides. An example is shown in Figure 9-25. All four deoxynucleotides and one dideoxynucleotide (e.g., ddT) are added to the extension reaction. Depending on the allele in the test sequence, A or C in the example, the primer will either incorporate ddTTP and terminate at the A in the template or continue to the next A in the template sequence, producing a larger extension product. The products are then analyzed by mass spectrometry to distinguish their sizes. Like FP-TDI, this method can detect

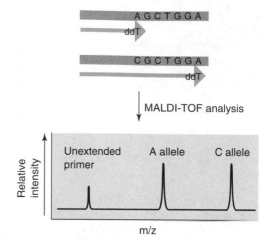

■ **Figure 9-25** Sequenom MassExtend uses matrix-assisted desorption/ionization–time-of-flight mass spectrometry to detect extension products of different sizes (mass).

large numbers of mutations or polymorphisms simultaneously. The system does, however, require expensive instrumentation. Because of their high-throughput detection capabilities, both FP-TDI and MassExtend were used in the Human Haplotype Mapping Project. Mutation detection by mass spectrometry may become more practical in the clinical laboratory as new methods are developed.[96–101]

Protein Truncation Test

Nonsense or frameshift mutations cause premature **truncation** of proteins. The **protein truncation test** (also called **in vitro synthesized protein** or **in vitro transcription/translation**) is designed to detect truncated proteins as an indication of the presence of DNA mutations.[102] This procedure uses a PCR product containing the area of the gene likely to have a truncating DNA mutation. The PCR product is transcribed and translated in vitro using commercially available coupled transcription/translation systems. When the peptide products of the reaction are resolved by polyacrylamide gel electrophoresis, bands below the normal control bands, representing truncated translation products, are indicative of the presence of DNA mutations (Fig. 9-26). This procedure has been used to detect mutations associated with breast cancer,[103,104] cystic fibrosis,[105] familial adenosis polyposis,[106] retinoblastoma,[107] and many other diseases. Due to its technical complexity and

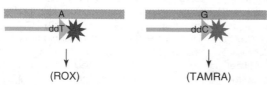

■ **Figure 9-24** FP-TDI detection of an A or G allele of a gene sequence. The color of the polarized fluorescence detected indicates which dideoxynucleotide is incorporated and, therefore, the nucleotide on the test template.

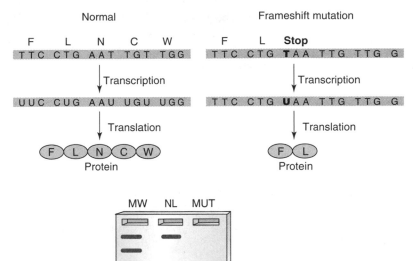

Figure 9-26 A frameshift mutation (top right) results in a truncated protein synthesized in vitro from a PCR product. The truncated peptide is resolved by polyacrylamide gel electrophoresis (bottom). Results from analysis of a homozygous mutant sample (MUT) and a normal sample (NL) are shown.

sample quality demands, however, PTT has had limited use as a clinical test.

Enzymatic and Chemical Cleavage Methods

Restriction Fragment Length Polymorphisms

If a mutation changes the structure of a restriction enzyme target site or changes the size of a fragment generated by a restriction enzyme, restriction fragment length polymorphism (RFLP) analysis can be used to detect the sequence alteration. Analysis of RFLPs in genomic DNA by Southern blot is described in Chapter 6, "Analysis and Characterization of Nucleic Acids and Proteins." To perform PCR-RFLP, the region surrounding the mutation is amplified, and the mutation is detected by cutting the amplicon with the appropriate restriction enzyme (Fig. 9-27). Mutations may inactivate a naturally occurring restriction site or generate a new restriction site so that digestion of the PCR product results in cutting of the mutant amplicon but not the normal control amplicon or vice versa. Although straightforward, PCR-RFLP requires careful design, as rare polymorphisms have been reported to confound RFLP results.[108] Several PCR-RFLP methods are widely used for detection of

commonly occurring mutations, such as factor V Leiden[109] and HFE mutations. PCR-RFLP has also been used for HLA typing (see Chapter 15, "DNA-Based Tissue Typing").

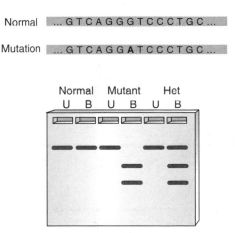

Figure 9-27 PCR-RFLP. The normal sequence (top line) is converted to a *Bam*H1 restriction site (GGATCC) by a G>A mutation. The presence of the mutation is detected by testing the PCR product with *Bam*H1. The bottom panel shows the predicted gel patterns for the homozygous normal, homozygous mutant, and heterozygous samples uncut (U) or cut with *Bam*H1 (B).

PCR-RFLP can be multiplexed to detect more than one gene mutation simultaneously. This has been practical for detection of separate gene mutations that affect the same phenotype, for example, factor V Leiden and prothrombin.[110] Alternatively, a combination of SSP-PCR and PCR-RFLP is also applied to simultaneous detection of mutations in more than one locus. An example is shown in Figure 9-28, in which a primer designed to produce a restriction site in the amplicon is used for each gene in a multiplex PCR. In the example, the primers are designed to generate a *Hind*III site in the amplicons. The PCR reaction and the *Hind*III digestion are performed in the same tube, and the products are separated on one lane of the gel.[111–113] This procedure is used in clinical analysis of factor V Leiden and prothrombin mutations.

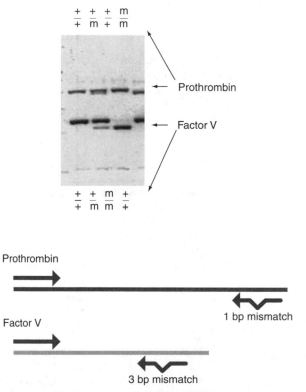

Figure 9-28 Multiplex PCR with mutagenic primers to detect mutations in factor V and prothrombin. The primer sequences are designed to generate a *Hind*III site in the PCR product if the mutations are present. The prothrombin and factor V PCR products are different sizes that can be resolved on the gel in a single lane.

Heteroduplex Analysis with Single-Strand Specific Nucleases

The detection sensitivity of heteroduplex analysis can be increased by using single-strand-specific nucleases (e.g., S1 nuclease) that cleave heteroduplexes at the mispaired bases.[114] PCR amplifications and heteroduplex formation were described in the earlier section on heteroduplex analysis. After cooling, the heteroduplexes are digested with a single-strand-specific nuclease. Digested heteroduplexes (but not homoduplexes) yield smaller fragments that are resolved on an agarose gel (Fig. 9-29). In addition to detecting mutations, the fragment sizes are used to estimate the placement of the mutation within the amplified sequence.

Base Excision Sequence Scanning

Base excision sequence scanning (BESS) is PCR amplification in the presence of small amounts of deoxyuridine triphosphate (dUTP) added to the reaction mix, followed by treatment with excision enzymes that cleave the fragment at the dU sites.[115] For example, the sequence to be scanned is amplified in a standard PCR reaction containing a mixture of 0.2 mM dNTPs and 0.015 mM dUTP. One of the primers in the PCR reaction has a fluorescent or radioactive label. With given ratios of dNTP/dUTP and an amplicon of given size, an average of 1 dU is incorporated into each amplicon. After the PCR reaction, the

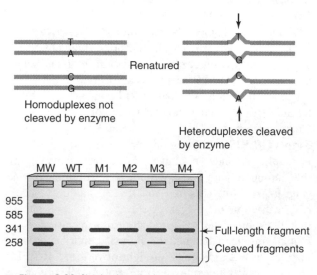

Figure 9-29 Single-stranded endonucleases cleave mispaired regions of heteroduplexes (top). The cleaved fragments are resolved by agarose gel electrophoresis.

amplicons are digested with uracil-*N*-glycosylase and *Escherichia coli* endonuclease IV to remove the uracils and cut the sugar-phosphate backbone of the DNA. Mutations affecting AT base pairs in the test sequence will be revealed by the incorporation of dU and subsequent fragmentation of the amplicon at the site of dU incorporation. The fragments can then be resolved by gel or capillary electrophoresis (Fig. 9-30). Premixed reagents for this assay are available (BESS T-Scan, Epicentre Technologies).

An extension of this method, the BESS G-Tracker, is designed to interrogate G residues in the test sequence.[116] The amplicons, dissolved in a G modification reagent, are subjected to a photoreaction with visible light. A proprietary enzyme mix will then fragment the amplicons at the positions of the modified G residues. Interpretation of the electrophoresis fragment patterns is the same as described above for the T-Scan. BESS is reported to have less optimization requirements than SSCP and ddF. Even so, the complex optimization and interpretation required for BESS preclude its wide use as a clinical test method.

Nonisotopic RNase Cleavage Assay

Nonisotopic RNase cleavage assay (NIRCA) is a heteroduplex analysis using duplex RNA.[117] The sequences to be scanned are amplified using primers tailed with promoter sequences of 20 to 25 bp. T7 or SP6 phage RNA polymerase promoters are most often used for this purpose. Following amplification, the PCR products with the promoter sequences are used as templates for in vitro synthesis of RNA with the T7 or SP6 RNA polymerase enzymes. This reaction yields a large amount of double-stranded RNA (Fig. 9-31). The transcripts are denatured at 95°C and then renatured by cooling to room temperature. If a mutation is present, heteroduplexes form between normal and mutant transcripts. These mismatches in the RNA are targets for cleavage by RNase enzymes. A mixture of single-strand-specific *E. coli* RNase I and *Aspergillus* RNase T1 cleaves different types of mismatches. The remaining double-stranded RNA fragments can then be separated by agarose gel electrophoresis. As in DNA heteroduplex analysis, the size of the RNA fragments indicates the placement of the mutation. NIRCA has been applied to screening of several clinical targets, including factor IX,[117] p53,[118] Jak2 kinase,[119] and BRCA1.[120,121]

Invader Assay

Invader, a method developed by Third Wave Technologies, is based on the characteristic enzymatic activity of the proprietary enzyme Cleavase.[122–124] Premixed reagents including Cleavase are added to a standard 96-well plate along with the test specimens (sample DNA or PCR products) and controls. Cleavase recognizes the structure formed by hybridization of the normal or mutant probes to the test sequences. During an isothermal

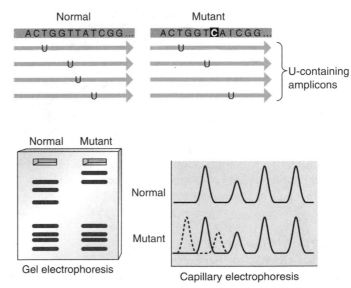

■ **Figure 9-30** Base excision sequence scanning. Uracil-containing amplicons yield different digestion fragments, depending on the sequence of the template. Gel (left) or capillary (right) electrophoresis patterns are depicted.

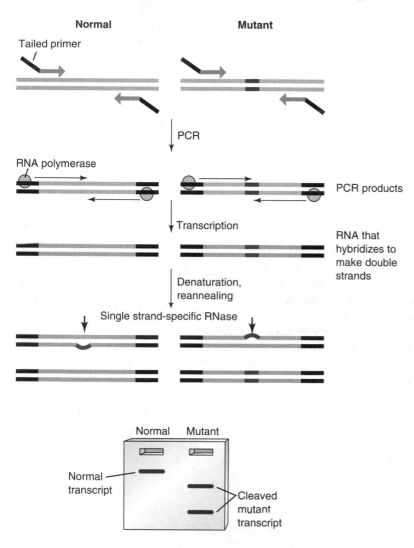

Normal   **Mutant**

Tailed primer

PCR

RNA polymerase

PCR products

Transcription

RNA that hybridizes to make double strands

Denaturation, reannealing

Single strand-specific RNase

Normal   Mutant

Normal transcript

Cleaved mutant transcript

■ **Figure 9-31** NIRCA analysis. Normal (left) and mutant (right) transcription templates covering the area to be screened are produced by PCR with tailed primers carrying promoter sequences. RNA polymerase then transcribes the PCR products. The transcripts are denatured and reannealed, forming heteroduplexes between normal and mutant transcripts. RNase cleavage products can be resolved on native agarose gels.

incubation, if the probe and test sequence are complementary, two enzymatic cleavage reactions occur, ultimately resulting in a fluorescent signal (Fig. 9-32). The signal can be read by a standard fluorometer. The advantages of this method are the short hands-on time and optional PCR amplification. This method has been applied to several areas of clinical molecular diagnostics including genetics,[124] hemostasis,[125–127] and infectious disease.[128,129]

Chemical Cleavage

Chemical cleavage of mismatches (CCM) exploits the differential susceptibility of specific base mismatches to chemical modification.[130] Mismatched cytosines and thymines are modified by hydroxylamine and osmium tetroxide, respectively. For CCM, a labeled normal probe is hybridized to the test sequence; the resulting duplex is treated chemically to modify the bases. Subsequent exposure to a strong reducing agent, piperidine, separates the sugar-phosphate backbone of the DNA at the site of the modified bases. The fragments are resolved by polyacrylamide gel electrophoresis. CCM detects only AA, CC, GG, TT, AC, AG, CT, and GT mismatches. The ability to detect mutations is extended by using both the sense and antisense strands of the probe. CCM, although highly sensitive, is not attractive for routine analysis due to the

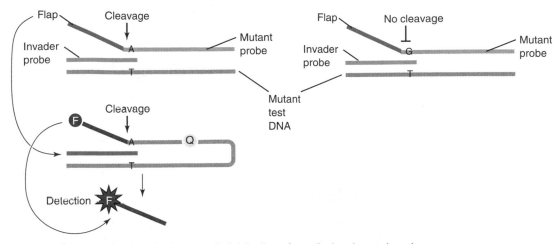

■ **Figure 9-32** Invader single-color assay. Hybridization of supplied probe and anchor sequences to the input template (upper left) forms a structure that is the substrate for the cleavage enzyme. The enzyme removes the flap sequences, which form another hybridization structure with the labeled probe. The second cleavage releases the fluorescent dye from the vicinity of the quencher on the probe, a fluorescent signal. If the template does not match the probe in the first hybridization (upper right), no cleavage occurs.

hazardous chemicals required and laborious procedure. Still, it is used in some research applications,[131,132] and there have been efforts to automate the process.[133]

The DNA endonucleases, T4E7 and T7E1 from bacteriophages T4 and T7, also cleave mismatches in DNA.[134] The plant endonuclease CEL 1, with properties similar to the single-stranded nuclease S1, has also been described.[2] Although this method has a higher background noise than chemical cleavage, it has greater potential for automation and routine use. Commercial kits for this procedure are available (Amersham-Pharmacia). Another commercial enzyme, Surveyor® (Transgenomics), is a member of the CEL nuclease family. It cuts both strands of DNA at a mismatch site without regard to the bases involved in the mismatch. This system has been proposed as a screening method for single-base alterations.[135]

Other Methods

The challenges of clinical laboratory requirements for robust, accurate, and sensitive assays have driven the discovery of new techniques and modification of existing techniques.[86,136–138] As a consequence, many methods have been devised, especially for high-throughput screening. SSCP was probably the most commonly used mutation screening method in clinical laboratories, but it became apparent from the use of SSCP that a single procedure may not be ideal for all genes. Hence the development of DGGE, TTGE, DHPLC, and other methods. Combinations of methods have also been proposed to increase sensitivity and detection, such as RFLP and SSCP. As the field of molecular diagnostics grows, the development of high-throughput methods has become a main focus. Array-based methods (Chapter 6, "Analysis and Characterization of Nucleic Acids and Proteins") and massive parallel sequencing methods (Chapter 10, "DNA Sequencing") potentially provide the specific multiplex detection and sensitivity required for clinical applications; however, instrument and reagent costs are still relatively high for these technologies. Overall, the method selected will depend on available instrumentation, the genetic target, and the nature of the mutation.

A summary of the methods described in this chapter is outlined in Table 9.2. Performance of each method varies, depending on the specimen, template sequence, and type of mutation to be detected. For instance, T-BESS or some chemical cleavage methods that detect only mutations involving specific nucleotides can have 100% accuracy and specificity for these mutations but 0% for mutations affecting other nucleotides. Procedures that are developed by targeting a specific mutation will perform for that target but may not work as well for other targets. For instance, hybridization methods generally detect mutations in GC-rich sequence environments more accurately than in AT-rich sequences. Methods designed to detect defined targets have the best accuracy and specificity; however, they detect only the targeted mutation. Screening methods are required for discovery of new mutations, but these mutations have to be confirmed by other methods or direct sequencing (Chapter 10, "DNA Sequencing").

Gene Mutation Nomenclature

Accurate testing and reporting of gene mutations require a descriptive and consistent system of expressing mutations and polymorphisms. Recommendations have been reported and generally accepted.[139,140] This section features general descriptive terms for basic alterations and structures.

For DNA and cDNA, the first nucleotide of the first amino acid in the sequence, usually A of ATG for methionine, is designated as position +1. The preceding nucleotide is position +1. There is no nucleotide position 0. Nucleotide changes are expressed as the position or nucleotide interval, the type of nucleotide change, the changed nucleotide, the symbol >, and finally the new nucleotide. For example, consider a nucleotide reference sequence: ATGCGTCACTTA. A substitution of a T for a C at position 7 in the DNA sequence (mutant sequence ATGCGTTACTTA) is expressed as 7C>T. A deletion of nucleotides 6 and 7, ATGCG ACTTA, is expressed as 6_7del or 6_7delTC. An insertion of a TA between nucleotides 5 and 6, ATGCGTATCACTTA, is denoted 5_6insTA.

Duplications are a special type of insertion. For example, a duplication of nucleotides 4 and 5, ATGCGCGTCACTTA, is expressed as 4_5dupCG. An insertion with a concomitant deletion, **indel**, has three alternate descriptive terms. For example, if TC at positions 6 and 7 of ATGCGTCACTTA is deleted from the reference sequence and GACA is inserted, the altered sequence, ATGCGGACAACTTA, is denoted 6_7delTCinsGACA, 6_7delinsGACA, or 6_7>GACA. Inversion of nucleotides is designated by the nucleotides affected, inv, and the number of nucleotides inverted. For example, inversion of GCGTCAC starting at position 3 to position 9 in the reference sequence (ATCACTGCGTTA) is 3_9inv7.

Gene mutations in recessive diseases, where both alleles are affected, are indicated by the designation of each mutation separated by +. Thus, a 2357C>T mutation in one allele of a gene and a 2378delA mutation in the other allele on the homologous chromosome is written [2357C>T] + [2378CdelA]. This is distinct from two mutations in the same allele, which is written as [2357C>T; 2378CdelA].

Mutations in introns of genomic DNA are indicated by the position of the mutation in the genomic sequence of the DNA or the position from the end of the coding sequence + the position in the intron. Thus, a G>T mutation 5 nucleotides into intron 2 that starts after the 91st nucleotide of exon 2 is designated as 91+5G>T or c.91+5G>T for coding sequence. If this same base change was at the 356th nucleotide in the genomic sequence, an alternative designation would be 356G>T or g.356G>C for genomic sequence.

At the protein level, numbering begins with the initial amino acid, methionine, in the protein sequence designated +1. The single-letter code has been used to convey protein sequence, but because of potential confusion with the single-letter designations, three-letter denotations are also acceptable (see Chapter 3, "Proteins," Table 3.1). Stop codons are designated by X in either case. Amino acid changes are described by the amino acid changed, the position, and the new amino acid. Consider the protein sequence methionine-arginine-histidine-leucine, or MRHL. If the second amino acid, arginine (R), was substituted by tyrosine (Y), the mutation of the new amino acid sequence, MYHL, would be R2Y. A nonsense mutation in codon 3, mutant sequence MRX, would be written H3X. Deletion of the arginine and histidine, ML, would be R2_H3del or R2_H3del2. Insertions are denoted by the amino acid interval, ins, and the inserted amino acids. For instance, insertion of amino acids glycine (G), alanine (A), and threonine (T), making the altered amino acid sequence MRGATHL, is indicated by R2_H3insGAT or, alternatively, R2_H3ins3. A short notation for frameshift mutations is the amino acid, its position, and fs. A frameshift mutation affecting the histidine residue changing the amino acid sequence to MRCPLRGWX is simply H3fs. The length of the shifted open reading frame is indicated by adding X and the position of the termination codon. H3CfsX7 is a frameshift in codon 3 that changes a histidine to a cysteine and new reading frame ending in a stop at the seventh codon.

To distinguish between mutation nomenclature referring to genomic DNA, coding (complementary or copy) DNA, mitochondrial DNA, RNA, or protein sequences, a prefix of g., c., m., r., and p. are recommended, respectively. Furthermore, RNA sequences are written in lowercase letters. For example, c.89T>C in the coding DNA would be r.89u>c in RNA.

Complex changes and multiple concurrent mutations are reported as they occur. Some mutations, even with sequence information, cannot be positively determined and must be inferred, for example, additions or deletions of repeat units in repeated sequences. For these changes, it is assumed that the 3'-most repeat is the one affected, and the alteration is noted for that position. Updates and further clarifications of mutation nomenclature are continually being addressed. Current information and descriptors for more complex changes are available at http://www.genomic.unimelb.edu.au/mdi/mutnomen/.

Gene Names

Gene nomenclature is different from gene names or sequence designation. The HUGO gene nomenclature committee has set rules for reporting or publishing gene names.[165] Gene names should be capitalized and set in italics with no hyphens. Protein names are not italicized or completely capitalized. For example, the *KRAS* gene codes for the K-Ras protein and the *TP53* gene codes for the protein, p53. Thus a report will contain the official gene name and the appropriately named change in the DNA sequence, if present. (See Chapter 16, "Quality Assurance and Quality Control in the Molecular Laboratory.")

• STUDY QUESTIONS •

1. What characteristic of the genetic code facilitates identification of open reading frames in DNA sequences?

2. Compare and contrast EIA with western blots for detection of protein targets.

3. On a size exclusion column, large molecules will elute_____ (before/after) small molecules.

4. MALDI methods separate ions by
   a. molecular volume.
   b. mass.
   c. charge.
   d. mass and charge.

5. What is a heteroduplex?

6. Exon 4 of the HFE gene from a patient suspected to have hereditary hemachromatosis was amplified by PCR. The G to A mutation, frequently found in hemachromatosis, creates an *Rsa*1 site in exon 4. When the PCR products are digested with *Rsa*1, what results (how many bands) would you expect to see if the patient has the mutation if no other *Rsa*1 sites are naturally present in the PCR product?

7. Which of the following methods would be practical to use to screen a large gene for mutations?
   a. SSP-PCR
   b. SSCP
   c. PCR-RFLP
   d. DGGE
   e. FP-TDI

8. What is the effect on the protein when a codon sequence is changed from TCT to TCC?

9. A reference sequence, ATGCCCTCTGGC, is mutated in malignant cells. The following mutations in this sequence have been described:

   ATGCGCTCTGGC

   ATGCCCTC - -GC

   ATAGCCTCTGGC

   ATGTCTCCCGGC

   Express these mutations using the accepted gene nomenclature (A = nucleotide position 1).

10. A reference peptide, MPSGCWR, is subject to inherited alterations. The following peptide sequences have been reported:

    MPS<u>T</u>GCWR

    MPSG<u>X</u>

    MPSGCW<u>LVT</u>GX

    MPSG<u>R</u>

    MPSGCW<u>GCW</u>R

    Express these mutations using the accepted nomenclature (M = amino acid position 1).

References

1. Mort M, Ivanov D, Cooper DN, et al. A meta-analysis of nonsense mutations causing human genetic disease. *Human Mutation* 2008;29:1037–1047.

2. Yeung A, Hattangadi D, Blakesley L, et al. Enzymatic mutation detection technologies. *BioTechniques* 2005; 38(5):749–758.

3. Yalow R, Berson SA. Immunoassay of endogenous plasma insulin in man. *Clinical Investigation* 1960;39:1157–1175.

4. Engvall E, Perlmann P. Enzyme-linked immunosorbent assay (ELISA). Quantitative assay of immunoglobulin G. *Immunochemistry* 1971;8:871–874.

5. Xiang Z, Tang AG, Ren YP, et al. Simultaneous determination of serum tryptophan metabolites in patients with systemic lupus erythematosus by high performance liquid chromatography with fluorescence detection. *Clinical Chemistry and Laboratory Medicine* 2010;48:513–517.

6. Kasumov T, Huang H, Chung YM, et al. Quantification of ceramide species in biological samples by liquid chromatography-electrospray tandem mass spectrometry. *Analytical Biochemistry* 2010;401:154–161.

7. Skrzypczak M, Heinritz W, Schulz AM, et al. Evaluation of IP-RP-HPLC for length determination of the trinucleotide repeat fragments in Huntington's disease. *Journal of Chromatographic Science* 2010;48:55–58.

8. Chace D. Mass spectrometry in newborn and metabolic screening: Historical perspective and future directions. *Journal of Mass Spectrometry* 2009;44: 163–170.

9. Orita M, Iwahana H, Kanazawa H, et al. Detection of polymorphisms of human DNA by gel electrophoresis as single-strand conformation polymorphisms. *Proceedings of the National Academy of Sciences* 1989;86:2766–2770.

10. Orita M, Suzuki Y, Sekiya T, et al. Rapid and sensitive detection of point mutations and DNA polymorphisms using the polymerase chain reaction. *Genomics* 1989;5:874–879.

11. Hayashi K. A simple and sensitive method for detection of mutations in the genomic DNA. *PCR Methods and Applications* 1991;1:34–38.

12. Atha D, Wenz H-M, Morehead H, et al. Detection of p53 point mutations by single strand conformation polymorphism: Analysis by capillary electrophoresis. *Electrophoresis* 1998;19:172–179.

13. Ellison J, Dean M, Goldman D. Efficacy of fluorescence-based PCR-SSCP for detection of point mutations. *BioTechniques* 1993;15:684–691.

14. Soong R, Iacopetta BJ. A rapid nonisotopic method for the screening and sequencing of p53 gene mutations in formalin-fixed, paraffin-embedded tumors. *Modern Pathology* 1997;10:252–258.

15. Sarkar G, Sommer SS. Screening for mutations by RNA single-strand conformation polymorphism (rSSCP): Comparison with DNA-SSCP. *Nucleic Acids Research* 1992;20(4):871–878.

16. Bisceglia L, Grifa A, Zelante L, et al. Development of RNA-SSCP protocols for the identification and screening of CFTR mutations: Identification of two new mutations. *Human Mutation* 1994;4(2): 136–140.

17. Liu Q, Sommer SS. Restriction endonuclease fingerprinting (REF): A sensitive method for screening mutations in long contiguous segments of DNA. *BioTechniques* 1995;18(3):470–477.

18. Fodde RLM. Mutation detection by denaturing gradient gel electrophoresis (DGGE). *Human Mutation* 1994;3(2):83–94.

19. Fisher S, Lerman LS. Length-independent separation of DNA restriction fragments in two-dimensional gel electrophoresis. *Cell* 1979;16:191–200.

20. Fischer S, Lerman LS. DNA fragments differing by single base-pair substitutions are separated in denaturing gradient gels: Correspondence with melting theory. *Proceedings of the National Academy of Sciences* 1983;80(6):1579–1583.

21. Hayes V, Bleeker W, Verind E, et al. Comprehensive TP53-denaturing gradient gel electrophoresis

mutation detection assay also applicable to archival paraffin embedded tissue. *Diagnostic Molecular Pathology* 1999;8(1):2–10.

22. Brady S, Magro CM, Diaz-Cano SJ, et al. Analysis of clonality of atypical cutaneous lymphoid infiltrates associated with drug therapy by PCR/DGGE. *Human Pathology* 1999;30(2):130–136.

23. Miller K, Ming TJ, Schulze AD, et al. Denaturing gradient gel electrophoresis (DGGE): A rapid and sensitive technique to screen nucleotide sequence variation in populations. *BioTechniques* 1999;27: 1016–1030.

24. Burmeister M, diSibio G, Cox DR, et al. Identification of polymorphisms by genomic denaturing gradient gel electrophoresis: Application to the proximal region of human chromosome 21. *Nucleic Acids Research* 1991;19(7):1475–1481.

25. Borresen A, Hovig E, Smith-Sorensen B, et al. Constant denaturant gel electrophoresis as a rapid screening technique for p53 mutations. *Proceedings of the National Academy of Sciences* 1991;88:8405–8409.

26. Smith-Sorensen B, Hovig E, Andersson B, et al. Screening for mutations in human HPRT cDNA using the polymerase chain reaction (PCR) in combination with constant denaturant gel electrophoresis (CDGE). *Mutation Research* 1992;269(1):41–53.

27. Yoshino K, Nishigaki K, Husimi Y. Temperature sweep gel electrophoresis: A simple method to detect point mutations. *Nucleic Acids Research* 1991;19:3153.

28. Wiese U, Wulfert M, Prusiner S, et al. Scanning for mutations in the human prion protein open reading frame by temporal temperature gradient gel electrophoresis. *Electrophoresis* 1995;16: 1851–1860.

29. Khrapko K, Hanekamp JS, Thilly WG, et al. Constant denaturant capillary electrophoresis (CDCE): A high resolution approach to mutational analysis. *Nucleic Acids Research* 1994;22:364–369.

30. Borresen A-L, Hovig E, Smith-Sorensen B, et al. Mutation analysis in human cancers using PCR and constant denaturant gel electrophoresis (CDGE). *Advances in Molecular Genetics* 1991;4:63–71.

31. Sheffield V, Beck JS, Kwitek AE, et al. The sensitivity of single-strand conformation polymorphism analysis for the detection of single base substitutions. *Genomics* 1993;16(2):325.

32. Taniere P, Martel-Planche G, Maurici D, et al. Molecular and clinical differences between adenocarcinomas of the esophagus and of the gastric cardia. *American Journal of Pathology* 2001; 158(1):33–40.

33. Lindforss U, Zetterquist H, Papadogiannakis N, et al. Persistence of *K-ras* mutations in plasma after colorectal tumor resection. *Anticancer Research* 2005;25:657–661.

34. Balogh KPA, Patocs A, Majnik J, et al. Genetic screening methods for the detection of mutations responsible for multiple endocrine neoplasia type 1. *Molecular Genetics and Metabolism* 2004;83(1–2): 74–81.

35. Bor M, Balogh K, Pusztai A, et al. Genetic screening of exon 12 of the hydroxymethylbilane synthase enzyme of patients with acute intermittent porphyria. *Journal of Physiology* 2000;526:111P.

36. Hernan-Gomez SEJ, Espinosa JC, Ubeda JF. Characterization of wine yeasts by temperature gradient gel electrophoresis (TGGE). *FEMS Microbiology Letters* 2000;193(1):45–50.

37. Tominaga T. Rapid identification of pickle yeasts by fluorescent PCR and microtemperature-gradient gel electrophoresis. *FEMS Microbiol Letters* 2004; 238(1):43–48.

38. Struewing J, Hartge P, Wacholder S, et al. The risk of cancer associated with the 185delAG and 5382insC mutations of *BRCA1* and the 6174delT mutation of *BRCA2* among Ashkenazi Jews. *New England Journal of Medicine* 1997;336(20):1401–1408.

39. Hussussian C, Struewing JP, Goldstein AM, et al. Germline p16 mutations in familial melanoma. *Nature Genetics* 1994;8:15–21.

40. Roa B, Boyd AA, Volcik K, et al. Ashkenazi Jewish population frequencies for common mutations in *BRCA1* and *BRCA2*. *Nature Genetics* 1996;14: 185–187.

41. Ørum H, Jakobsen MH, Koch T, et al. Detection of the factor V Leiden mutation by direct allele-specific hybridization of PCR amplicons to photoimmobilized locked nucleic acids. *Clinical Chemistry* 1999;45:1898–1905.

42. Wittwer C, Gudrun HR, Gundry CN, et al. High-resolution genotyping by amplicon melting analysis using LC Green. *Clinical Chemistry* 2003;49(6): 853–860.

43. Ririe K, Rasmussen RP, Wittwer CT. Product differentiation by analysis of DNA melting curves during the polymerase chain reaction. *Analytical Biochemistry* 1997;245:154–160.

44. Lay M, Wittwer CT. Real-time fluorescence genotyping of factor V Leiden during rapid cycle PCR. *Clinical Chemistry* 1997;43:2262–2267.

45. Reed G, Wittwer CT. Sensitivity and specificity of single-nucleotide polymorphism scanning by high-resolution melting analysis. *Clinical Chemistry* 2004;50(10):1748–1754.

46. Lyon E. Mutation detection using fluorescent hybridization probes and melting curve analysis. *Expert Reviews in Molecular Diagnostics* 2001;1(1): 92–101.

47. Pals G. Detection of a single base substitution in single cells by melting peak analysis using dual color hybridization probes. In Dietmaier W, Wittwer C, Sivasubramanian N, eds. Rapid Cycle Real-Time PCR Methods and Applications. Springer-Verlag, Berlin, 2002, pp. 77–84.

48. Kutyavin I, Afonina IA, Mills A, et al. 3+-minor groove binder-DNA probes increase sequence specificity at PCR extension temperatures. *Nucleic Acids Research* 2000;28(2):655–661.

49. Bennett C, Campbell MN, Cook CJ, et al. The LightTyper: High-throughput genotyping using fluorescent melting curve analysis. *BioTechniques* 2003;34(6):1288–1292.

50. de Kok J, Wiegerinck ET, Giesendorf BA, et al. Rapid genotyping of single nucleotide polymorphisms using novel minor groove binding DNA oligonucleotides (MGB probes). *Human Mutation* 2002;19(5):554–559.

51. Van Hoeyveld EHF, Massonet C, Moens L, et al. Detection of single nucleotide polymorphisms in the mannose-binding lectin gene using minor groove binder-DNA. *Journal of Immunological Methods* 2004;287:227–230

52. Belousov Y, Welch RA, Sanders S, et al. Single nucleotide polymorphism genotyping by two-colour melting curve analysis using the MGB Eclipse Probe System in challenging sequence environment. *Human Genomics* 2004;1(3):209–217.

53. Fujigaki H, Takemura M, Takahashi K, et al. Genotyping of hepatitis C virus by melting curve analysis with SYBR Green I. *Annals of Clinical Biochemistry* 2004;41(2):130–132.

54. Zhou M, Veenstra TD. Mass spectrometry: m/z 1983–2008. *BioTechniques* 2008;44:667–669.

55. Vorderwülbecke S, Cleverley S, Weinberger SR, Wiesner A. Protein quantification by the SELDI-TOF-MS–based ProteinChip® System. *Nature Methods* 2005;2:393–395.

56. Hardenbol P, Baner J, Jain M, et al. Multiplexed genotyping with sequence-tagged molecular inversion probes. *Nature Biotechnology* 2003;21(6): 673–678.

57. Hardenbol P, Yu F, Belmont J, et al. Highly multiplexed molecular inversion probe genotyping: Over 10,000 targeted SNPs genotyped in a single tube assay. *Genome Research* 2005;15(2):269–275.

58. Belda F, Barlow KL, Clewley JP. Subtyping HIV-1 by improved resolution of heteroduplexes on agarose gels. *Journal of Acquired Immune Deficiency Syndromes & Human Retrovirology* 1997;16(3):218–219.

59. Gonzalez M, Gonzalez D, Lopez-Perez R, et al. Heteroduplex analysis of VDJ amplified segments from rearranged IgH genes for clonality assessments in B-cell non-Hodgkin's lymphoma: A comparison between different strategies. *Haematologica* 1999;84(9):779–784.

60. Ganguly A, Rock MJ, Prockop DJ. Conformation-sensitive gel electrophoresis for rapid detection of single-base differences in double-stranded PCR products and DNA fragments: Evidence for solvent-induced bends in DNA heteroduplexes. *Proceedings of the National Academy of Sciences* 1993;90: 10325–10329.

61. Ganguly A. An update on conformation sensitive gel electrophoresis. *Human Mutation* 2002;19(4): 334–342.

62. Rees W, Yager TD, Korte J, et al. Betaine can eliminate the base pair composition dependence of DNA melting. *Biochemistry* 1993;32(1):137–144.

63. O'Donovan M, Oefner PJ, Robers SC, et al. Blind analysis of denaturing high-performance liquid chromatography as a tool for mutation detection. *Genomics* 1998;15(1):44–49.

64. Keller G, Hartmann A, Mueller J, et al. Denaturing high-pressure liquid chromatography (DHPLC) for the analysis of somatic p53 mutations. *Laboratory Investigation* 2001;81(12):1735–1737.

65. Narayanswami G, Taylor PD. Improved efficiency of mutation detection by denaturing high-performance

liquid chromatography using modified primers and hybridization procedure. *Genetic Testing* 2001;5(1):9–16.

66. Schollen E, Dequeker E, McQuaid S, et al. Diagnostic DHPLC quality assurance (DDQA): A collaborative approach to the generation of validated and standardized methods for DHPLC-based mutation screening in clinical genetics laboratories. *Human Mutation* 2005;25(6):583–592.

67. Stone B, Burrows J, Schepetiuk S, et al: Rapid detection and simultaneous subtype differentiation of influenza: A viruses by real time PCR. *Journal of Virological Methods* 2004;117:103–112.

68. Wen W, Bernstein L, Lescallett J, et al. Comparison of TP53 mutations identified by oligonucleotide microarray and conventional DNA sequence analysis. *Cancer Research* 2000;60(10):2716–2722.

69. Moutereau S, Narwa R, Matheron C, et al. An improved electronic microarray-based diagnostic assay for identification of MEFV mutations. *Human Mutation* 2004;23(6):621–628.

70. Lopez-Crapez E, Livache T, Marchand J, et al. *K-ras* mutation detection by hybridization to a polypyrrole DNA chip. *Clinical Chemistry* 2001;47:186–194.

71. Fedrigo O, Naylor G. A gene-specific DNA sequencing chip for exploring molecular evolutionary change. *Nucleic Acids Research* 2004;32(3):1208–1213.

72. Anderson T, Werno AM, Beynon KM, et al. Failure to genotype Herpes Simplex Virus by real-time PCR assay and melting curve analysis due to sequence variation within probe binding sites. *Journal of Clinical Microbiology* 2003;41:2135–2137.

73. Fulton R, McDade RL, Smith PL, et al. Advanced multiplexed analysis with the FlowMetrix system. *Clinical Chemistry* 1997;43(9):1749–1756.

74. Martins T. Development of internal controls for the Luminex instrument as part of a multiplex seven-analyte viral respiratory antibody profile. *Clinical and Diagnostic Laboratory Immunology* 2002;9(1):41–45.

75. Bortolin S, Black M, Modi H, et al. Analytical validation of the tag-it high-throughput microsphere-based universal array genotyping platform: Application to the multiplex detection of a panel of thrombophilia-associated single-nucleotide polymorphisms. *Clinical Chemistry* 2004;50(11):2028–2036.

76. Biagini R, Sammons DL, Smith JP, et al. Comparison of a multiplexed fluorescent covalent microsphere immunoassay and an enzyme-linked immunosorbent assay for measurement of human immunoglobulin G antibodies to anthrax toxins. *Clinical and Diagnostic Laboratory Immunology* 2004;11(11):50–55.

77. Ye S, Humphries S, Green F. Allele-specific amplification by tetra-primer PCR. *Nucleic Acids Research* 1992;20(5):1152.

78. Ye S, Dhillon S, Ke X, et al. An efficient procedure for genotyping single nucleotide polymorphisms. *Nucleic Acids Research* 2001;29(17):e88 1–8.

79. Oliphant A, Barker DL, Stuelpnagel JR, et al. Bead array technology: Enabling an accurate, cost-effective approach to high-throughput genotyping. *BioTechniques* 2002;32:s56–s61.

80. Louis M, Dekairelle AF, Gala JL. Rapid combined genotyping of factor V, prothrombin and methylenetetrahydrofolate reductase single nucleotide polymorphisms using minor groove binding DNA oligonucleotides (MGB probes) and real-time polymerase chain reaction. *Clinical Chemistry and Laboratory Medicine* 2004;42:1364–1369.

81. Behrens M, Lange R. A highly reproducible and economically competitive SNP analysis of several well characterized human mutations. *Clinical Laboratory* 2004;50(5–6):305–316.

82. Osgood-McWeeneya D, Galluzzi JR, Ordovas JM. Allelic discrimination for single nucleotide polymorphisms in the human scavenger receptor class B type 1 gene locus using fluorescent probes. *Clinical Chemistry* 2000;46:118–119.

83. Gopalraj R, Zhu H, Kelly JF, et al. Genetic association of low density lipoprotein receptor and Alzheimer's disease. *Neurobiology and Aging* 2005;26(1):1–7.

84. Hughes D, Ginolhac SM, Coupier I, et al. Common *BRCA2* variants and modification of breast and ovarian cancer risk in *BRCA1* mutation carriers. *Cancer Epidemiology Biomarkers and Prevention* 2005;14(1):265–267.

85. Campsall P, Au NH, Prendiville JS, et al. Detection and genotyping of varicella-zoster virus by TaqMan allelic discrimination real-time PCR. *Journal of Clinical Microbiology* 2004;42(4):1409–1413.

86. Easterday W, Van Ert MN, Zanecki S, et al. Specific detection of *Bacillus anthracis* using TaqMan

mismatch amplification mutation assay. *BioTechniques* 2005;38(5):731–735.

87. Lancaster J, Berchuck A, Futreal PA, et al. Dideoxy fingerprinting assay for *BRCA1* mutation analysis. *Molecular Carcinogenesis* 1997;19(3):176–179.

88. Liu Q, Feng J, Sommer SS. Bidirectional dideoxy fingerpringing (Bi-ddF): A rapid method for quantitative detection of mutations in genomic regions of 300–600 bp. *Human Molecular Genetics* 1993;5(1):107–114.

89. Larsen L, Johnson M, Brown C, et al. Automated mutation screening using dideoxy fingerprinting and capillary array electrophoresis. *Human Mutation* 2001;18(5):451–457.

90. Larsen L, Christiansen M, Vuust J, et al. High throughput mutation screening by automated capillary electrophoresis. *Combinatorial Chemistry and High Throughput Screening* 2000;3:393–409.

91. Hsu T, Chen X, Duan S, et al. Universal SNP genotyping assay with fluorescence polarization detection. *BioTechniques* 2001;31(3):560–570.

92. Chen X, Levine L, Kwok P-Y. Fluorescence polarization in homogeneous nucleic acid analysis. *Genome Research* 1999;9(5):492–498.

93. Xiao M, Latif SM, Kwok P-Y. Kinetic FP-TDI assay for SNP allele frequency determination. *BioTechniques* 2003;34(1):190–197.

94. Leushner J, Chiu NH. Automated mass spectrometry: A revolutionary technology for clinical diagnostics. *Molecular Diagnostics* 2000;5(4):341–348.

95. Jurinke C, Oeth P, van den Boom D. MALDI-TOF mass spectrometry: A versatile tool for high-performance DNA analysis. *Molecular Biotechnology* 2004;26(2):147–164.

96. Hung K, Sun X, Ding H, et al. A matrix-assisted laser desorption/ionization time-of-flight–based method for screening the 1691G: A mutation in the factor V gene. *Blood Coagulation and Fibrinolysis* 2002;13(2):117–122.

97. Stanssens P, Zabeau M, Meersseman G, et al. High-throughput MALDI-TOF discovery of genomic sequence polymorphisms. *Genome Research* 2004;14(1):126–133.

98. Tost J, Gut IG. Genotyping single nucleotide polymorphisms by MALDI mass spectrometry in clinical applications. *Clinical Biochemistry* 2005;38(4): 335–350.

99. Buyse I, McCarthy SE, Lurix P, et al. Use of MALDI-TOF mass spectrometry in a 51-mutation test for cystic fibrosis: Evidence that 3199del6 is a disease-causing mutation. *Genetics in Medicine* 2005;6(5):426–430.

100. Li Q, Li LY, Huang SW, et al. Rapid genotyping of known mutations and polymorphisms in beta-globin gene based on the DHPLC profile patterns of homoduplexes and heteroduplexes. *Clinical Biochemistry* 2008;41:681–687.

101. Jackson E, Sievert AJ, Gai X, et al. Genomic analysis using high-density single nucleotide polymorphism-based oligonucleotide arrays and multiplex ligation-dependent probe amplification provides a comprehensive analysis of INI1/SMARCB1 in malignant rhabdoid tumors. *Clinical Cancer Research* 2009;15:1923–1930.

102. Roest P, Roberts RG, Sugino S, et al. Protein truncation test (PTT) for rapid detection of translation-terminating mutations. *Human Molecular Genetics* 1993;2:1719–1721.

103. Zikan M, Pohlreich P, Stribrna J. Mutational analysis of the *BRCA1* gene in 30 Czech ovarian cancer patients. *Journal of Genetics* 2005;84(1):63–67.

104. Hogervorst F, Cornelis R, Bout M, et al. Rapid detection of *BRCA1* mutations by the protein truncation test. *Nature Genetics* 1995;10:208–212.

105. Romey M, Tuffery S, Desgeorges M, et al. Transcript analysis of CFTR frameshift mutations in lymphocytes using the reverse transcription-polymerase chain reaction technique and the protein truncation test. *Human Genetics* 1996;98(3):328–332.

106. van der Luijt R, Khan PM, Vasen H, et al. Rapid detection of translation-terminating mutations at the adenomatous polyposis coli (APC) gene by direct protein truncation test. *Genomics* 1994; 20(1):1–4.

107. Tsai T, Fulton L, Smith BJ, et al. Rapid identification of germline mutations in retinoblastoma by protein truncation testing. *Archives of Ophthalmology* 2004;122:239–248.

108. Gold B, Hanson M, Dean M. Two rare confounding polymorphisms proximal to the factor V Leiden mutation. *Molecular Diagnostics* 2001;6(2): 137–140.

109. DiSiena M, Intres R, Carter DJ. Factor V Leiden and pulmonary embolism in a young woman

taking an oral contraceptive. *American Journal of Forensic Medical Pathology* 1998;19(4): 362–367.

110. Baris I, Koksal V, Etlik O. Multiplex PCR-RFLP assay for detection of factor V Leiden and pro-thrombin G20210A. *Genetic Testing* 2004;8(4):381.

111. Lucotte G, Champenois T. Duplex PCR-RFLP for simultaneous detection of factor V Leiden and pro thrombin G20210A. *Molecular and Cellular Probes* 2003;17(5):267–269.

112. Huber S, McMaster KJ, Voelkerding KV. Analyti-cal evaluation of primer engineered multiplex polymerase chain reaction–restriction fragment length polymorphism for detection of factor V Leiden and prothrombin G20210A. *Journal of Molecular Diagnostics* 2000;2:153–157.

113. Welbourn J, Maiti S, Paley J. Factor V Leiden detection by polymerase chain reaction–restriction fragment length polymorphism with mutagenic primers in a multiplex reaction with Pro G20210A: A novel technique. *Hematology* 2003;8(2):73–75.

114. Howard J, Ward J, Watson JN, et al. Heteroduplex cleavage analysis using S1 nuclease. *BioTechniques* 1999;27(1):18–19.

115. Hawkins G, Hoffman LM. Base excision sequence scanning. *Nature Biotechnology* 1997;15(8):803–804.

116. Hawkins G, Hoffman LM. Rapid DNA mutation identification and fingerprinting using base excision sequence scanning. *Electrophoresis* 1999; 20(6):1171–1176.

117. Goldrick M, Kimball GR, Liu Q, et al. NIRCA: A rapid robust method for screening for unknown point mutations. *BioTechniques* 1996;21(1): 106–112.

118. Macera M, Godec CJ, Sharma N, et al. Loss of heterozygosity of the TP53 tumor suppressor gene and detection of point mutations by the non-isotopic RNAse cleavage assay in prostate cancer. *Cancer Genetics and Cytogenetics* 1999;108(1): 42–47.

119. Levine A, Figueiredo JC, Lee W, et al. Genetic variability in the MTHFR gene and colorectal can-cer risk using the colorectal cancer family registry. *Cancer Epidemiology Biomarkers and Prevention* 2010;19:89–100.

120. Shen D, Wu Y, Subbarao M, et al. Mutation analy-sis of *BRCA1* gene in African-American patients

with breast cancer. *Journal of the National Medical Association* 2000;92(1):29–35.

121. Shen D, Wu Y, Chillar R, et al. Missense alter-ations of *BRCA1* gene detected in diverse cancer patients. *Anticancer Research* 2000;20: 1129–1132.

122. Lyamichev V, Mast AL, Hall JG, et al. Polymorphism identification and quantitative detection of genomic DNA by invasive cleavage of oligonucleotide probes. *Nature Biotechnology* 1999;17(3):292–296.

123. Hall J, Eis PS, Law SM, et al. Sensitive detection of DNA polymorphisms by the serial invasive signal amplification reaction. *Proceedings of the National Academy of Sciences* 2000;97:8272–8277.

124. Kwiatkowski RW, de Arruda M, Neri B. Clinical, genetic, and pharmacogenetic applications of the Invader assay. *Molecular Diagnostics* 1999;4(4): 353–364.

125. Hessner M, Budish MA, Friedman KD. Genotyp-ing of factor V G1691A (Leiden) without the use of PCR by invasive cleavage of oligonucleotide probes. *Clinical Chemistry* 2000;46(8):1051–1056.

126. Patnaik M, Dlott JS, Fontaine RN, et al. Detection of genomic polymorphisms associated with venous thrombosis using the invader biplex assay. *Journal of Molecular Diagnostics* 2004;6(2):137–144.

127. Ryan D, Nuccie B, Arvan D. Non-PCR-dependent detection of the factor V Leiden mutation from genomic DNA using a homogeneous invader microtiter plate assay. *Molecular Diagnostics* 1999;4(2):135–144.

128. Hjertner B, Meehan B, McKillen J, et al. Adapta-tion of an invader assay for the detection of African swine fever virus DNA. *Journal of Virological Methods* 2005;124(1–2):1–10.

129. Honisch C, Mosko M, Arnold C, et al. Replacing reverse line-blot hybridization spoligotyping of the mycobacterium tuberculosis complex. *Journal of Clinical Microbiology* 2010;48(5):1520–1526.

130. Cotton R, Rodrigues NR, Campbell RD. Reactiv-ity of cytosine and thymine in single base-pair mismatches with hydroxylamine and osmium tetroxide and its application to the study of muta-tions. *Proceedings of the National Academy of Sciences* 1988;85(12):4397–4401.

131. Fuhrmann M, Oertel W, Berthold P, et al. Removal of mismatched bases from synthetic genes by

enzymatic mismatch cleavage. *Nucleic Acids Research* 2005;33(6):e58.

132. Freson K, Peerlinck K, Aguirre T, et al. Fluorescent chemical cleavage of mismatches for efficient screening of the factor VIII gene. *Human Mutation* 1999;11(6):470–479.

133. Rowley G, Saad S, Gianelli F, et al. Ultrarapid mutation detection by multiplex, solid-phase chemical cleavage. *Genomics* 1995;30:574–582.

134. Inganäs M, Byding S, Eckersten A, et al. Enzymatic mutation detection in the P53 gene. *Clinical Chemistry* 2000;46:1562–1573.

135. Qiu P, Shandilya H, D'Alessio JM, et al. Mutation detection using Surveyor nuclease. *BioTechniques* 2004;36(4):702–707.

136. Tessitore A, Di Rocco ZC, Cannita K, et al. High sensitivity of detection of TP53 somatic mutations by fluorescence-assisted mismatch analysis. *Genes Chromosomes Cancer* 2002; 35(1):86–91.

137. Benoit N, Goldenberg D, Deng SX, et al. Colorimetric approach to high-throughput mutation analysis. *BioTechniques* 2005;38(4):635–639.

138. Espasa M, Gonzalez-Martin J, Alcaide F, Aragon LM, et al. Direct detection in clinical samples of multiple gene mutations causing resistance of *Mycobacterium* tuberculosis to isoniazid and rifampicin using fluorogenic probes. *Journal of Antimicrobial Chemotherapy* 2005;55:860–865.

139. Antonarakis S, Nomenclature Working Group. Recommendations for a nomenclature system for human gene mutations. *Human Mutation* 1998;11:1–3.

140. den Dunnen J, Antonarakis SE. Mutation nomenclature extensions and suggestions to describe complex mutations. *Human Mutation* 2000;15:7–12.

141. Barros F, Lareu MV, Salas A, et al. Rapid and enhanced detection of mitochondrial DNA variation using single-strand conformation analysis of superposed restriction enzyme fragments from polymerase chain reaction-amplified products. *Electrophoresis* 1997;18(1):52–54.

142. Hayashi K, Yandell DW. How sensitive is PCR-SSCP? *Human Mutation* 1993;2(5):338–346.

143. Fodde R, Losekoot M. Mutation detection by denaturing gradient gel electrophoresis (DGGE). *Human Mutation* 1994;3(2):83–94.

144. Hanekamp J, Thilly WG, Chaudhry MA. Screening for human mitochondrial DNA polymorphisms with denaturing gradient gel electrophoresis. *Human Genetics* 1996;98:243–245.

145. Chen T-J, Boles RG, Wong L-JC. Detection of mitochondrial DNA mutations by temporal temperature gradient gel electrophoresis. *Clinical Chemistry* 1999;45:1162–1167.

146. Wang Y, Helland A, Holm R, et al. TP53 mutations in early-stage ovarian carcinoma: Relation to long-term survival. *British Journal of Cancer* 2004;90:678–685.

147. Wallace R, Shaffer J, Murphy RF, et al. Hybridization of synthetic oligodeoxyribonucleotides to phi chi 174 DNA: The effect of single base-pair mismatch. *Nucleic Acids Research* 1979;6(11):3543.

148. Stamer U, Bayerer B, Wolf S, et al. Rapid and reliable method for cytochrome P450 2D6 genotyping. *Clinical Chemistry* 2002;48(9):1412–1417.

149. Yamanoshita O, Kubota T, Hou J, et al. DHPLC is superior to SSCP in screening p53 mutations in esophageal cancer tissues. *International Journal of Cancer* 2005;114(1):74–79.

150. Premstaller A, Oefner PJ. Denaturing HPLC of nucleic acids. *PharmaGenomics* 2003;20: 21–37.

151. Metaxa-Mariatou V, Papadopoulos S, Papadopoulou E, et al. Molecular analysis of GISTs: Evaluation of sequencing and dHPLC. *DNA and Cell Biology* 2004;23(11):777–782.

152. Hecker K, Taylor PD, Gjerde DT. Mutation detection by denaturing DNA chromatography using fluorescently labeled polymerase chain reaction products. *Analytical Biochemistry* 1999;272: 156–164.

153. Bahrami A, Dickman MJ, Matin MM, et al. Use of fluorescent DNA-intercalating dyes in the analysis of DNA via ion-pair reversed phase denaturing high-performance liquid chromatography. *Analytical Biochemistry* 2002;309:248–252.

154. Heller M, Forster AH, Tu E. Active microeletronic chip devices which utilize controlled electrophoretic fields for multiplex DNA hybridization and other genomic applications. *Electrophoresis* 2000;21(1):157–164.

155. Johnson DC, Corthals S, Ramos C, et al. Genetic associations with thalidomide mediated venous thrombotic events in myeloma identified using targeted genotyping. *Blood* 2008; 112(13): 4924–4934.

156. Schiffman JD, Wang Y, McPherson LA, et al. Molecular inversion probes reveal patterns of 9p21 deletion and copy number aberrations in childhood leukemia. *Cancer Genetics and Cytogenetics* 2009;193(1):9–18.

157. Gohring K, Feuchtinger T, Mikeler E, et al. Dynamics of the emergence of a human cytomegalovirus UL97 mutant strain conferring ganciclovir resistance in a pediatric stem-cell transplant recipient. *Journal of Molecular Diagnostics* 2009;11(4)364–368.

158. Juszczynski P, Woszczek G, Borowiec M, et al. Comparison study for genotyping of a single-nucleotide polymorphism in the tumor necrosis factor promoter gene. *Diagnostic Molecular Pathology* 2002;11(4):228–233.

159. Ellis M. "Spot-on" SNP genotyping. *Genome Research* 2000;10(7):895–897.

160. Geisler J, Hatterman-Zogg MA, Rathe JA, et al. Ovarian cancer *BRCA1* mutation detection: Protein truncation test (PTT) outperforms single-strand conformation polymorphism analysis (SSCP). *Human Mutation* 2001;18(4):337–344.

161. Brieger A, Trojan J, Raedle J, et al. Identification of germline mutations in hereditary nonpolyposis colorectal cancer using base excision sequence scanning analysis. *Clinical Chemistry* 1999;45:1564–1567.

162. Matsuno N, Nanri T, Kawakita T, et al. A novel FLT3 activation loop mutation N841K in acute myeloblastic leukemia. *Leukemia* 2005;19:480–481.

163. Waldron-Lyncha F, Adamsa C, Shanahanb F, et al. Genetic analysis of the 3′ untranslated region of the tumour necrosis factor shows a highly conserved region in rheumatoid arthritis–affected and –unaffected subjects. *Journal of Medical Genetics* 1999;36:214–216.

164. Hessner M, Friedman KD, Voelkerding K, et al. Multisite study for genotyping of the factor II (prothrombin) G20210A mutation by the Invader assay. *Clinical Chemistry* 2001;47:2048–2050.

165. http://www.gene.ucl.ac.uk/nomenclature/.

DNA Sequencing

OBJECTIVES

- Compare and contrast the chemical (Maxam/Gilbert) and the chain termination (Sanger) sequencing methods.

- List the components and the molecular reactions that occur in chain termination sequencing.

- Discuss the advantages of dye primer and dye terminator sequencing.

- Derive a text DNA sequence from raw sequencing data.

- Describe examples of alternative sequencing methods, such as bisulfite sequencing and pyrosequencing.

- Define bioinformatics, and describe electronic systems for the communication and application of sequence information.

- Recount the events of the Human Genome Project.

DNA sequence information (the order of nucleotides in the DNA molecule) is used in the medical laboratory for a variety of purposes, including detecting mutations, typing microorganisms, identifying human haplotypes, and designating polymorphisms. Ultimately, targeted therapies will be directed at abnormal DNA sequences detected by these techniques.[1]

Direct Sequencing

The importance of knowing the order, or sequence, of nucleotides on the DNA chain was appreciated in the earliest days of molecular analysis. Elegant genetic experiments with microorganisms indirectly detected molecular changes at the nucleotide level.

Indirect methods of investigating nucleotide sequence differences are still in use today. Molecular techniques, from Southern blot to the mutation detection methods described in Chapter 9, "Gene Mutations," are aimed at identifying nucleotide changes. Without knowing the nucleotide sequence of the targeted areas, results from many of these methods would be difficult to interpret; in fact, some methods would not be useful at all. Direct determination of the nucleotide sequence, or DNA sequencing, is the most definitive molecular method to identify genetic lesions.

Manual Sequencing

Direct determination of the order, or sequence, of nucleotides in a DNA polymer is the most specific and direct method for identifying genetic lesions (mutations) or polymorphisms, especially when looking for changes affecting only one or two nucleotides. Two types of sequencing methods were concurrently developed in the 1970s: **Maxam-Gilbert sequencing**[2] and **Sanger sequencing**.[3]

Chemical (Maxam-Gilbert) Sequencing
The Maxam-Gilbert chemical sequencing method was developed by Allan M. Maxam and Walter Gilbert. Maxam-Gilbert sequencing requires a double- or single-stranded version of the DNA region to be sequenced, with one end radioactively labeled.

For sequencing, the labeled fragment, or **template**, is aliquotted into four tubes. Each aliquot is treated with a different chemical with or without high salt (Fig. 10-1). Upon addition of a strong reducing agent, such as 10%

piperidine, the single-stranded DNA will break at specific nucleotides (Table 10.1).

After the reactions, the piperidine is evaporated, and the contents of each tube are dried and resuspended in formamide for gel loading. The fragments are then separated by size on a denaturing polyacrylamide gel (Chapter 5, "Resolution and Detection of Nucleic Acids"). The denaturing conditions (formamide, urea, and heat) prevent the single strands of DNA from hydrogen bonding with one another or folding up so that they

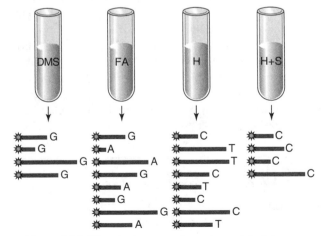

■ Figure 10-1 Chemical sequencing proceeds in four separate reactions in which the labeled DNA fragment is selectively broken at specific nucleotides. (DMS-dimethylsulphate; FA-formic acid; H-hydrazine; H + S = hydrazine + salt)

Table 10.1   **Specific Base Reactions in Maxam-Gilbert Sequencing**

Chain breaks at:	Base Modifier	Reaction	Time (min at 25°C)
G	Dimethylsulphate	Methylates G	4
G + A	Formic acid	Protonates purines	5
T + C	Hydrazine	Splits pyrimidine rings	8
C	Hydrazine + salt	Splits only C rings	8

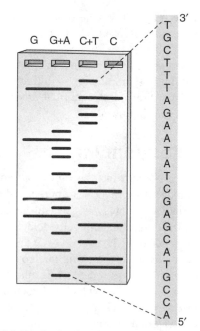

■ **Figure 10-2** Products of a Maxam-Gilbert sequencing reaction. The gel is read from the bottom to the top. The size of the fragments gives the order of the nucleotides. The nucleotides are inferred from the lane in which each band appears. A or T is indicated by bands that appear in the G + A lane or C + T lane, respectively, but not in the G lane or the C lane. G is present in the G + A lane and the G lane. C is present in the C + T lane and the C lane.

migrate through the gel strictly according to their size. The migration speed is important because single-base resolution is required to interpret the sequence properly.

After electrophoresis, the gel apparatus is disassembled; the gel is removed to a sheet of filter paper; and it is dried on a gel dryer. The dried gel is exposed to light-sensitive film. Alternatively, wet gels can be exposed directly. An example of Maxam-Gilbert sequencing results is shown in Figure 10-2. The sequence is inferred from the bands on the film. The smallest (fastest-migrating) band represents the base closest to the labeled end of the fragment. The lane in which that band appears identifies the nucleotide. Bands in the purine (G + A) or pyrimidine (C + T) lane are called based on whether they are also present in the G- or C-only lanes. Note how the sequence is read from the bottom (5' end of the DNA molecule) to the top (3' end of the molecule) of the gel.

Although Maxam-Gilbert sequencing is a relatively efficient way to determine short runs of sequence data, the method is not practical for high-throughput sequencing of long fragments. In addition, the hazardous chemicals hydrazine and piperidine require more elaborate precautions for use and storage. This method was therefore

replaced by the dideoxy chain termination sequencing method for most sequencing applications.

Dideoxy Chain Termination (Sanger) Sequencing

Dideoxy chain termination (Sanger) sequencing is a modification of the DNA replication process. A short, synthetic, single-stranded DNA fragment (primer) complementary to sequences just 5' to the region of DNA to be sequenced is used for priming dideoxy sequencing reactions (Fig. 10-3). For detection of the products of the sequencing reaction, the primer may be attached covalently at the 5' end to a ^{32}P-labeled nucleotide or a fluorescent dye-labeled nucleotide. An alternative detection strategy is to incorporate ^{32}P- or ^{35}S-labeled deoxynucleotides in the nucleotide sequencing reaction mix. The alternative detection strategy is called **internal labeling**.

Just as in the in vivo DNA replication reaction, an in vitro DNA synthesis reaction would result in polymerization

---

Advanced Concepts

Polyacrylamide gels from 6% to 20% are used for sequencing. Bromophenol blue and xylene cyanol loading dyes are used to monitor the migration of the fragments. Run times range from 1 to 2 hours for short fragments (up to 50 bp) to 7 to 8 hours for longer fragments (more than 150 bp).

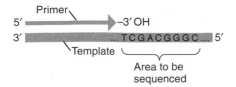

■ **Figure 10-3** Manual dideoxy sequencing requires a single-stranded version of the fragment to be sequenced (template). Sequencing is primed with a short synthetic piece of DNA complementary to bases just before the region to be sequenced (primer). The sequence of the template will be determined by extension of the primer in the presence of dideoxynucleotides.

of deoxynucleotides to make full-length copies of the DNA template (DNA replication is discussed in Chapter 1, "DNA"). For sequencing, modified **dideoxynucleotide (ddNTP)** derivatives are added to the reaction mixture. Dideoxynucleotides lack the hydroxyl

Historical Highlights

The original dideoxy chain termination sequencing methods used in the late 1970s into the early 1980s required a single-stranded template. Templates up to a few thousand bases long could be produced using **M13** bacteriophage, a bacterial virus with a single-stranded DNA genome. This virus replicates by infecting *Escherichia coli*, in which the viral single-stranded circular genome is converted to a double-stranded plasmid called the replication factor (RF). The plasmid codes for viral gene products that use the bacterial transcription and translation machinery to make new single-stranded genomes and viral proteins. To use M13 for template preparation, the RF was isolated from infected bacteria, cut with restriction enzymes, and the fragment to be sequenced was ligated into the RF (Fig. 10-4). When the recombined RF was reintroduced into the host bacteria, M13 continued its life cycle producing new phages, some of which carried the inserted fragment. When the phages were spread on a lawn of host bacteria, plaques (clear spaces) of lysed bacteria formed by phage replication contained pure populations of recombinant phage. The single-stranded DNA was then isolated from the phage by picking plugs of agar from the plaques and boiling them.

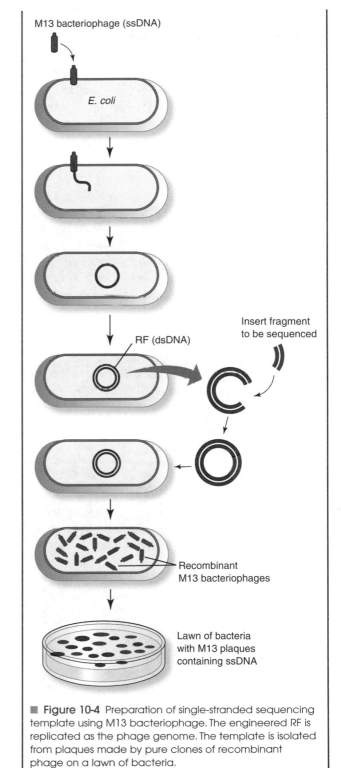

■ **Figure 10-4** Preparation of single-stranded sequencing template using M13 bacteriophage. The engineered RF is replicated as the phage genome. The template is isolated from plaques made by pure clones of recombinant phage on a lawn of bacteria.

Advanced Concepts

Because of extensive use of M13, a primer that hybridizes to M13 sequences could be used to sequence any fragment. This primer, the **M13 universal primer**, is still used in some applications, even though the M13 method of template preparation is no longer practical.

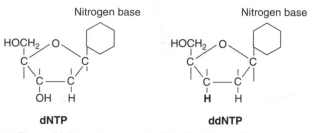

■ **Figure 10-5** A dideoxynucleotide (right) lacks the hydroxyl group on the 3' ribose carbon that is required for formation of a phosphodiester bond with the phosphate group of another nucleotide.

group found on the 3' ribose carbon of the deoxynucleotides (dNTPs; Fig. 10-5). DNA synthesis will stop upon incorporation of a ddNTP into the growing DNA chain (chain termination) because without the hydroxyl group at the 3' sugar carbon, the 5'-3' phosphodiester bond cannot be established to incorporate a subsequent nucleotide. The newly synthesized chain will terminate, therefore, with the ddNTP (Fig. 10-6).

For manual dideoxy sequencing, a 1:1 mixture of template and primer is placed into four separate reaction tubes in sequencing buffer containing the sequencing enzyme and ingredients necessary for the polymerase activity (Fig. 10-7). Mixtures of all four dNTPs and one of the four ddNTPs are then added to each tube, with a different ddNTP in each of the four tubes.

The ratio of ddNTPs/dNTPs is critical for generation of a readable sequence. If the concentration of ddNTPs is too high, polymerization will terminate too frequently early along the template. If the ddNTP concentration is too low, infrequent or no termination will occur. In the beginning days of sequencing, optimal ddNTP/dNTP ratios were determined empirically (by experimenting with various ratios). Modern sequencing reagent mixes have preoptimized nucleotide mixes.

With the addition of DNA polymerase enzyme to the four tubes, the reaction begins. After about 20 minutes, the reactions are terminated by addition of a stop buffer. The stop buffer consists of 20 mM EDTA to chelate

Advanced Concepts

PCR products are often used as sequencing templates. It is important that the amplicons to be used as sequencing templates are free of residual components of the PCR reaction, especially primers and nucleotides. These reactants can interfere with the sequencing reaction and lower the quality of the sequencing ladder. PCR amplicons are cleaned using solid phase (column or bead) matrices, alcohol precipitation, or enzymatic digestion with **alkaline phosphatase**. Alternatively, amplicons can be run on an agarose gel and the bands eluted. The alternative method provides not only a clean template but also confirmation of the product being sequenced. It is especially useful when the PCR reactions are not completely free of misprimed bands or primer dimers (see Chapter 7, "Nucleic Acid Amplification").

Advanced Concepts

Manganese (Mn^{++}) may be added to the sequencing reaction to promote equal incorporation of all dNTPs by the polymerase enzyme.[6,7] Equal incorporation of the dNTPs makes for uniform band intensities on the sequencing gel, which eases interpretation of the sequence. Manganese increases the relative incorporation of ddNTPs as well, which will enhance the reading of the first part of the sequence by increasing intensity of the smaller bands on the gel. Modified nucleotides, deaza-dGTP and deoxyinosine triphosphate (dITP), are also added to sequencing reaction mixes to deter secondary structure in the synthesized fragments. Such additives as Mn^{++}, deaza-dGTP, and dITP are supplied in commercial sequencing buffers.

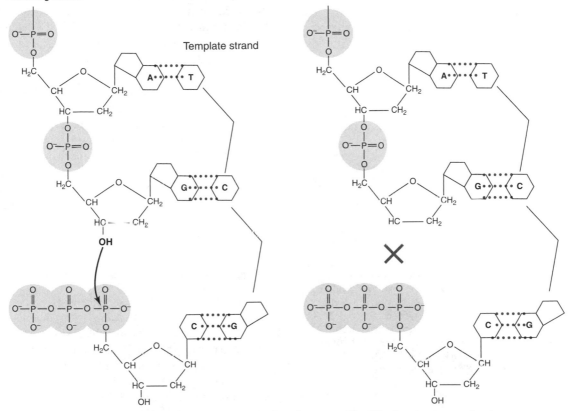

Growing strand

Template strand

■ **Figure 10-6** DNA replication (left) is terminated by the absence of the 3′ hydroxyl group on the dideoxyguanosine nucleotide (ddG, right). The resulting fragment ends in ddG.

cations and stop enzyme activity, formamide to denature the products of the synthesis reaction, and gel loading dyes (bromophenol blue and/or xylene cyanol). It is important that all four reactions are carried out for equal times. Maintaining equal reaction times will provide consistent band intensities in all four lanes of the sequencing gel sequence, which facilitates final reading of the sequence.

The sets of synthesized fragments are then loaded onto a denaturing polyacrylamide gel (see Chapter 5, "Resolution and Detection of Nucleic Acids," for more details about polyacrylamide gel electrophoresis). The products of each of the four sequencing reactions are loaded into adjacent lanes, labeled A, C, G, or T, corresponding to the ddNTP in the four reaction tubes. Once the gel is dried and exposed to x-ray film, the fragment patterns are visualized by the signal on the ^{32}P-labeled primer or nucleotide. All fragments from a given tube will end in

the same ddNTP; for example, all the fragments synthesized in the ddCTP tube end in C.

The four-lane gel electrophoresis pattern of the products of the four sequencing reactions is called a **sequencing ladder** (Fig. 10-8). The ladder is read to deduce the DNA sequence. From the bottom of the gel, the smallest (fastest-migrating) fragment is the one in which synthesis terminated closest to the primer. The identity of the ddNTP at a particular position is determined by the lane in which the band appears. If the smallest band is in the ddATP lane, then the first base is an A. The next larger fragment is the one that was terminated at the next position on the template. The lane that has the next larger band identifies the next nucleotide in the sequence. In the figure, the next largest band is found in the ddGTP lane, so the next base is a G. The sequence is thus read from the bottom (smallest, 5′-most) to the top (largest, 3′-most) fragments

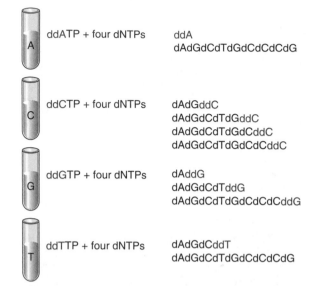

A	ddATP + four dNTPs	ddA dAdGdCdTdGdCdCdCdG
C	ddCTP + four dNTPs	dAdGddC dAdGdCdTdGddC dAdGdCdTdGdCddC dAdGdCdTdGdCdCddC
G	ddGTP + four dNTPs	dAddG dAdGdCdTddG dAdGdCdTdGdCdCdCddG
T	ddTTP + four dNTPs	dAdGdCddT dAdGdCdTdGdCdCdCdG

■ **Figure 10-7** Components required for DNA synthesis (template, primer, enzyme, buffers, dNTPs) are mixed with a different ddNTP in each of four tubes (left). With the proper ratio of ddNTPs/dNTPs, the newly synthesized strands of DNA will terminate at each opportunity to incorporate a ddNTP. The resulting synthesis products are a series of fragments ending in either A (ddATP), C (ddCTP), G (ddGTP) or T (ddTTP). This collection of fragments is the sequencing ladder.

across or within lanes to determine the identity and order of nucleotides in the sequence.

Depending on the reagents and gel used, the number of bases per sequence read averages 300 to 400. Advances in enzyme and gel technology have increased this capability to over 500 bases per read. Sequencing reads are lengthened by loading the same ladders in intervals of 2 to 6 hours so that the larger bands are resolved with longer (e.g., 8-hour) migrations, whereas smaller bands will be resolved simultaneously in a 1- to 2-hour migration that was loaded 6 to 7 hours later.

Sequencing technology has been improved significantly from the first manual sequencing procedures. Recombinant polymerase enzymes[4,5] with in vitro removal of the exonuclease activity are faster and more processive (i.e., they stay with the template longer, producing longer sequencing ladders). In addition, these engineered enzymes more efficiently incorporate ddNTPs and nucleotide analogs such as dITP (deoxyinosine triphosphate) or 7-deaza-dGTP, which are used to deter secondary structure (internal folding and hybridization) in the

template and sequencing products. Furthermore, most sequencing methods in current use are performed with double-stranded templates, eliminating the requirement for preparation of single-stranded versions of the DNA to be sequenced.

Using heat-stable enzymes, the sequencing reaction can be performed in a thermal cycler (**cycle sequencing**). With cycle sequencing, timed manual starting and stopping of the sequencing reactions are not necessary. The labor savings in this regard increase the number of reactions that can be performed simultaneously; for example, a single operator can run 96 sequencing reactions (i.e., sequence 24 fragments) in a 96-well plate. Finally, improvements in fluorescent dye technology have led to the automation of the sequencing process and, more importantly, sequence determination.

Automated Fluorescent Sequencing

The chemistry for automated sequencing is the same as described for manual sequencing, using double-stranded templates and cycle sequencing. Because cycle sequencing (unlike manual sequencing) does not require sequential addition of reagents to start and stop the reaction, cycle sequencing is more easily adaptable to high-throughput applications and automation.[8] Universal systems combine automation of DNA isolation of the template and setup of the sequencing reactions.

Electrophoresis and reading of the sequencing ladder is also automated. A requirement for automated reading of the DNA sequence ladder is the use of fluorescent

---

Advanced Concepts

Fluorescent dyes used for automated sequencing include fluorescein, rhodamine, and Bodipy (4,4-difluoro-4-bora-3a,4a-diaza-*s*-indacene) dye derivatives that are recognized by commercial detection systems.[9,10] Automated sequence readers excite the dyes with a laser and detect the emitted fluorescence at predetermined wavelengths. More advanced methods have been proposed to enhance the distinction between the dyes for more accurate determination of the sequence.[11]

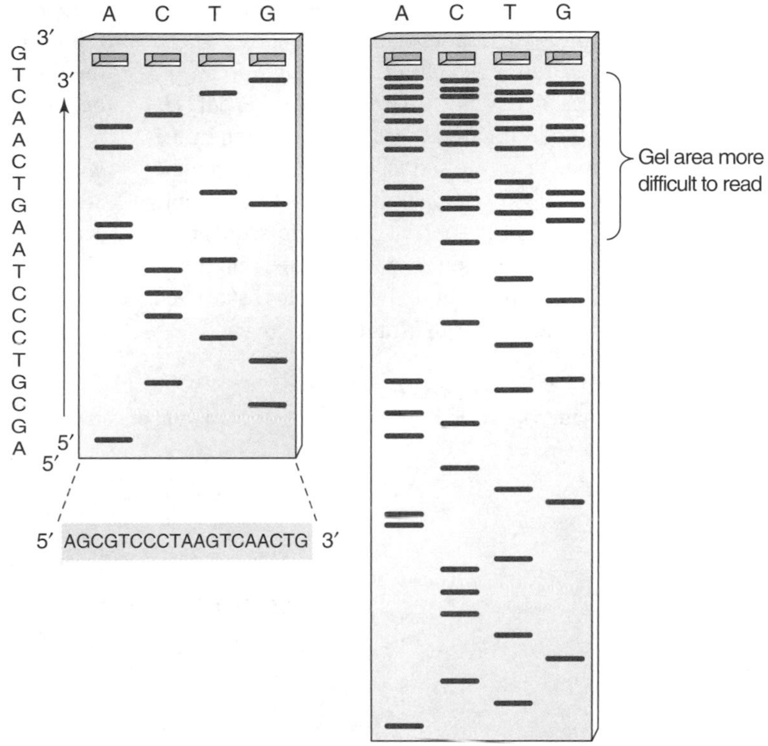

Figure 10-8 A sequencing ladder is read from the bottom of the gel to the top. The smallest (fastest-migrating) fragment represents the first nucleotide attached to the primer by the polymerase. Since that fragment is in lane A, from the reaction that contained ddATP (left), the sequence read begins with A. The next largest fragment is in lane T. The sequence, then, reads AT. The next largest fragment is in lane C, making the sequence ATC, and so forth up the gel. Larger bands on a sequencing gel can sometimes be compressed, limiting the length of sequence that can be read on a single gel run (right).

dyes instead of radioactive nucleotides to label the primers or sequencing fragments.

Fluorescent dyes used for sequencing have distinct "colors," or peak wavelengths of fluorescence emission, that can be distinguished by automated sequencers. The advantage of having four distinct colors is that all four of the reaction mixes can be read in the same lane of a gel or on a capillary. Fluorescent dye color rather than lane placement will assign the fragments as ending in A, T, G, or C in the sequencing ladder (Fig. 10-9).

Approaches to Automated Sequencing

There are two approaches to automated fluorescent sequencing: **dye primer** and **dye terminator** sequencing (Fig. 10-10). The goal of both approaches is the same: to label the fragments synthesized during the sequencing reaction according to their terminal ddNTP. Thus, fragments ending in ddATP, read as A in the sequence, will be labeled with a "green" dye; fragments ending in ddCTP, read as C in the sequence, will be labeled with a "blue" dye; fragments ending in ddGTP, read as G in the sequence, will be labeled with a "black" or "yellow" dye;

and fragments ending in ddTTP, read as T in the sequence, will be labeled with a "red" dye. This facilitates reading of the sequence by the automated sequence.

In dye primer sequencing, the four different fluorescent dyes are attached to four separate aliquots of the primer. The dye molecules are attached covalently to the

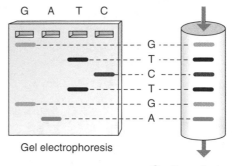

Figure 10-9 Instead of four gel lanes (left) fluorescent fragments can be run in a single gel lane or in a capillary (right). Note that the sequence of nucleotides, AGTCTG, read by lane in the slab gel is read by color in the capillary.

5' end of the primer during chemical synthesis, resulting in four versions of the same primer with different dye labels. The primer labeled with each "color" is added to four separate reaction tubes, one each with ddATP, ddCTP, ddGTP, or ddTTP, as shown in Figure 10-10. After addition of the remaining components of the sequencing reaction (see the section above on manual sequencing) and of a heat-stable polymerase, the reaction is subjected to cycle sequencing in a thermal cycler. The products of the sequencing reaction are then labeled at the 5' end, the dye color associated with the ddNTP at the end of the fragment.

Dye terminator sequencing is performed with one of the four fluorescent dyes covalently attached to each of the ddNTPs instead of to the primer. The primer is unlabeled. A major advantage of this approach is that all four sequencing reactions are performed in the same tube (or well of a plate) instead of in four separate tubes. After addition of the rest of the reaction components and cycle sequencing, the product fragments are labeled at the 3' end. As with dye primer sequencing, the "color" of the dye corresponds to the ddNTP that terminated the strand.

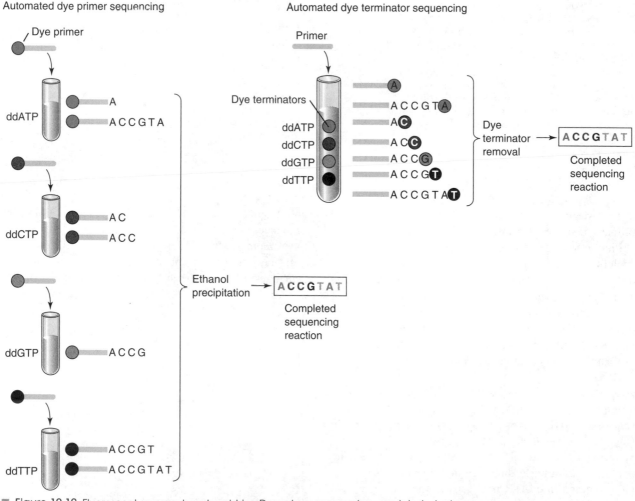

■ **Figure 10-10** Fluorescent sequencing chemistries. Dye primer sequencing uses labeled primers (A). The products of all four reactions are resolved together in one lane of a gel or in a capillary. Using dye terminators (B), only one reaction tube is necessary, since the fragments can be distinguished directly by the dideoxynucleotides on their 3' ends.

Preparation of the Sequencing Ladder

After a sequencing reaction using fluorescent dye terminators, excess dye terminators must be removed from the sequencing ladder. Sequencing ladders are cleaned with columns or beads or by ethanol precipitation. Most spin columns or bead systems bind the sequencing fragments to allow removal of residual sequencing components by rinsing with buffers. Another approach is to bind the dye terminators onto specially formulated magnetic beads and recover the DNA ladder from the supernatant as the beads are held by a magnet applied to the outside of the tube or plate.

The fragments of the sequencing ladder should be completely denatured before running on a gel or capillary. Denaturing conditions (50°C to 60°C, formamide, urea denaturing gel) are maintained so that the fragments are resolved strictly according to size. Secondary structure affects migration speed and lowers the quality of the sequence. Before loading in a gel or capillary instrument, sequence ladders are cleaned, as described above, to remove residual dye terminators, precipitated, and resuspended in formamide. The ladders are heated to 95°C to 98°C for 2 to 5 minutes and placed on ice just before loading.

Electrophoresis

The four sets of sequencing products in each reaction are loaded onto a single gel lane or capillary. The fluorescent dye colors, rather than lane assignment, distinguish which nucleotide is at the end of each fragment. Running all four reactions together not only increases throughput but also eliminates lane-to-lane migration variations that

Advanced Concepts

DNA sequences with high GC content are sometimes difficult to read due to intrastrand hybridization in the template DNA. Reagent preparations that include 7-deaza-dGTP (2'-deoxy-7-deazaguanosine triphosphate) or deoxyinosine triphosphate instead of standard dGTP improve the resolution of bands in regions that exhibit GC band compressions, or bunching of bands close together so that they are not resolved, followed by several bands running farther apart.

affect accurate reading of the sequence. The migrating fragments pass a laser beam and a detector in the automated sequencer. The laser beam excites the dye attached to each fragment, causing the dye to emit fluorescence that is captured by the detector. The detector converts the fluorescence to an electrical signal that is recognized by computer software as a flash or peak of color.

Fluorescent detection equipment yields results as an **electropherogram**, rather than a gel pattern. Just as the gel sequence is read from the smallest (fastest-migrating) fragments to the largest, the automated sequencer reads, or "calls," the bases from the smallest (fastest-migrating) fragments that first pass the detector to the largest based on the dye emission wavelength; that is, the instrument calls the base by the "color" of the fluorescence of the fragment as it passes the detector. The readout from the instrument is a series of peaks of the four fluorescent dyes as the bands of the sequencing ladder migrate by the detector. The software assigns one of four colors—red, black, blue, or green—associated with each of the fluorescent dyes and a text letter to the peaks for ease of interpretation.

As with manual sequencing, the ratio of ddNTPs/dNTPs is key to the length of the sequence read (how much of the template sequence can be determined). Too many ddNTPs will result in a short sequence read. Too low a concentration of ddNTPs will result in loss of sequence data close to the primer but give a longer read, because the sequencing enzyme will polymerize further down the template before it incorporates a ddNTP into the growing chain. The quality of the sequence (height and separation of the peaks) improves away from the primer and begins to decline at the end. At least 400 to 500 bases can be easily read with most sequencing chemistries.

Sequence Interpretation

Interpretation of sequencing data from a dye primer or dye terminator reaction depends on the quality of the electropherogram, which, in turn, depends on the quality of the template, the efficiency of the sequencing reaction, and the cleanliness of the sequencing ladder. Failure to clean the sequencing ladder properly results in bright flashes of fluorescence (**dye blobs**) that obliterate parts of the sequence read (Fig. 10-11). Poor starting material results in a poor-quality sequence that cannot be read accurately (Fig. 10-12). Clear, clean sequencing ladders

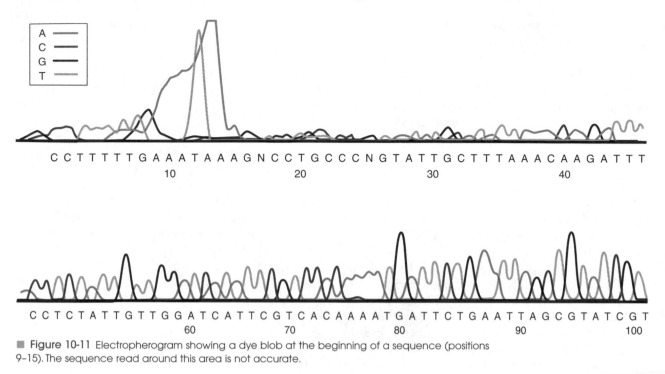

■ **Figure 10-11** Electropherogram showing a dye blob at the beginning of a sequence (positions 9–15). The sequence read around this area is not accurate.

are read accurately by the automated reader, and a text sequence is generated. Sequencing software indicates the certainty of each base call in the sequence. Software programs can compare two sequences or test sequences with reference sequences to identify mutations or polymorphisms. Less than optimal sequences are not accurately readable by automated detectors but may be readable by an experienced operator.

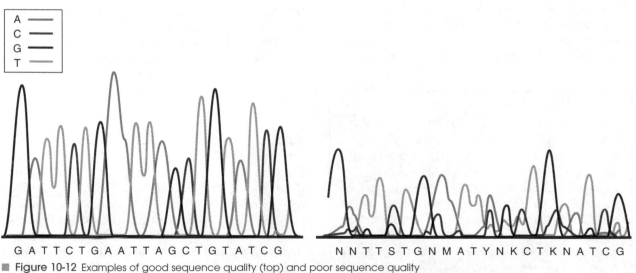

■ **Figure 10-12** Examples of good sequence quality (top) and poor sequence quality (bottom). Note the clean baseline on the good sequence; that is, only one color peak is present at each nucleotide position. Automatic sequence reading software will not accurately call a poor sequence. Compare the text sequences below the two scans.

It is important to sequence both complementary strands of DNA to confirm sequence data. This is critical for confirmation of mutations or polymorphisms in a sequence (Fig. 10-13). Alterations affecting a single base pair may be subtle on an electropherogram, especially if the alteration is in the heterozygous form, or mixed with normal reference sequence. Ideally, a heterozygous mutation appears as two peaks of equal height but different colors directly on top of one another, that is, at the same position in the electropherogram. The overlapping peaks should be about half the height of the rest of the sequence. Heterozygous deletions or insertions (e.g., the *BRCA* frameshift mutations) affect all positions of the sequence downstream of the mutation (Fig. 10-14) and, thus, are more easily detected. Somatic mutations in clinical specimens are sometimes difficult to detect as they may be diluted by normal sequences that mask the somatic change.

Several software programs have been written to interpret and apply sequence data from automatic sequencers. Software that collects the raw data from the instrument is supplied with automated sequencing instruments. Software that interprets, compares, or otherwise manipulates sequence data is sometimes supplied with a purchased instrument or available on the Internet.[12] A representative sample of these applications is shown in Table 10.2.

Pyrosequencing

Chain termination sequencing is the most widely used method to determine DNA sequence. Other methods have been developed that yield the same information but not with the throughput capacity of the chain termination method. **Pyrosequencing** is an example of a method designed to determine a DNA sequence without having to make a sequencing ladder.[13,14] This procedure relies on the generation of light (luminescence) when nucleotides are added to a growing strand of DNA (Fig. 10-15). With this system, there are no gels, fluorescent dyes, or ddNTPs.

The pyrosequencing reaction mix consists of a single-stranded DNA template, sequencing primer, sulfurylase and luciferase, plus the two substrates adenosine 5' phosphosulfate (APS) and luciferin. One of the four dNTPs is added in a predetermined order to the reaction. If the nucleotide is complementary to the base in the template strand next to the 3' end of the primer, DNA polymerase extends the primer. Pyrophosphate (PPi) is released with the formation of the phosphodiester bond between the dNTP and the primer. The PPi is converted to ATP by sulfurylase that is used to generate a luminescent signal by luciferase-catalyzed conversion of luciferin to oxyluciferin.

The process is repeated with each of the four nucleotides again added sequentially to the reaction. The generation of a signal indicates which nucleotide is the next correct base in the sequence. Results from a pyrosequencing reaction, a **pyrogram**, consist of single peaks of luminescence associated with the addition of the complementary nucleotide (Fig. 10-15). If a sequence contains a repeated nucleotide, for instance, GTTAC, the results would be dG peak, dT peak (double the height of the dG peak), dA peak, dC peak.

Pyrosequencing is most useful for short- to moderate-sequence analysis. It is therefore used mostly for mutation

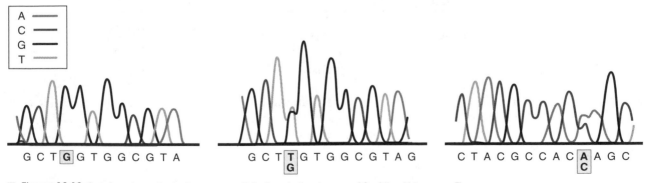

■ Figure 10-13 Sequencing of a heterozygous G to T mutation in exon 12 of the *Kras* gene. The normal codon sequence is GGT (right). The heterozygous mutation (GT, center) is confirmed in the reverse sequence (CA, right).

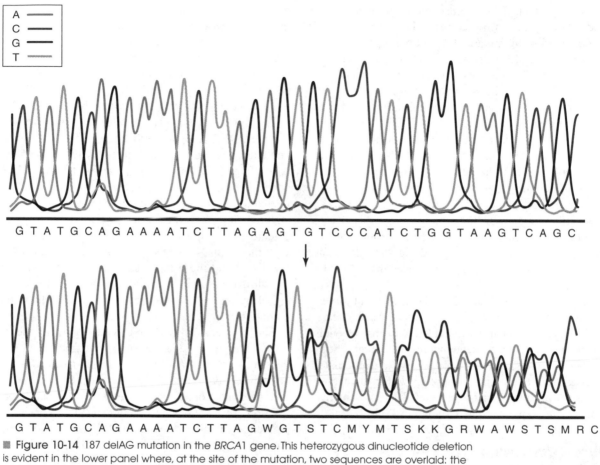

GTATGCAGAAAATCTTAGAGTGTCCCATCTGGTAAGTCAGC

GTATGCAGAAAATCTTAGWGTSTCMYMTSKKGRWAWSTSMRC

■ **Figure 10-14** 187 delAG mutation in the *BRCA*1 gene. This heterozygous dinucleotide deletion is evident in the lower panel where, at the site of the mutation, two sequences are overlaid: the normal sequence and the normal sequence minus two bases.

Table 10.2 **Software Programs Commonly Used to Analyze and Apply Sequence Data**

Software	Name	Application
BLAST	Basic Local Alignment Search Tool	Compares an input sequence with all sequences in a selected database
GRAIL	Gene Recognition and Assembly Internet Link	Finds gene-coding regions in DNA sequences
FASTA	FAST-All derived from FAST-P (protein) and FAST-N (nucleotide) search algorithms	Rapidly aligns pairs of sequences by sequence patterns rather than individual nucleotides
Phred	Phred	Reads bases from original trace data and recalls the bases, assigning quality values to each base
Polyphred	Polyphred	Identifies single-nucleotide polymorphisms (SNPs) among the traces and assigns a rank indicating how well the trace at a site matches the expected pattern for an SNP

Table 10.2 **Software Programs Commonly Used to Analyze and Apply Sequence Data—cont'd**

Software	Name	Application
Phrap	Phragment Assembly Program	Uses user-supplied and internally computed data quality information to improve accuracy of assembly in the presence of repeats
TIGR Assembler	The Institute for Genomic Research	Developed by TIGR as an assembly tool to build a consensus sequence from smaller-sequence fragments
Factura	Factura	Identifies sequence features such as flanking vector sequences, restriction sites, and ambiguities
SeqScape	SeqScape	Provides mutation and SNP detection and analysis, pathogen subtyping, allele identification, and sequence confirmation
Assign	Assign	Identifies alleles for haplotyping
Matchmaker	Matchmaker	Identifies alleles for haplotyping

Step 1

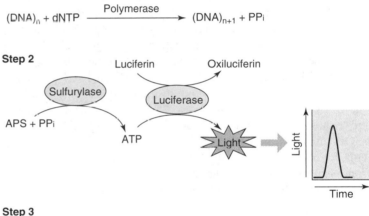

$$(DNA)_n + dNTP \xrightarrow{\text{Polymerase}} (DNA)_{n+1} + PPi$$

Step 2

Step 3

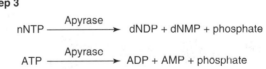

$$nNTP \xrightarrow{\text{Apyrase}} dNDP + dNMP + phosphate$$

$$ATP \xrightarrow{\text{Apyrase}} ADP + AMP + phosphate$$

■ **Figure 10-15** Pyrosequencing is analysis of pyrophosphate (PPi) released when a nucleotide base (dNTP) is incorporated into DNA (top left). The released PPi is a cofactor for ATP generation from adenosine 5' phosphosulfate (APS). Luciferase plus ATP converts luciferin to oxyluciferin with the production of light, which is detected by a luminometer. The system is regenerated with apyrase that degrades residual free dNTP and dATP (Step 3). As nucleotides are added to the system one at a time, the sequence is determined by which of the four nucleotides generates a light signal.

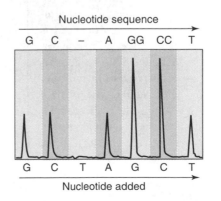

or single nucleotide polymorphism (SNP) detection and typing rather than for generating new sequences. It has been used for applications in infectious disease typing[15,16] and HLA typing.[17]

Bisulfite DNA Sequencing

Bisulfite DNA sequencing, or methylation-specific sequencing, is a modification of chain termination sequencing designed to detect methylated nucleotides.[18,19] Methylation of cytosine residues to 5-methyl cytosines in DNA is an important part of regulation of gene expression and chromatin structure (see Chapter 2, "RNA"). Methylated DNA is also involved in cell differentiation and is implicated in a number of diseases, including several types of cancer.

For bisulfite sequencing, 2 to 4 µg of genomic DNA is cut with restriction enzymes to facilitate denaturation. The enzymes should not cut within the region to be sequenced. The restriction digestion products are resolved on an agarose gel, and the fragments of the size of interest are purified from the gel. DNA from fixed tissue may be used directly without restriction digestion. The DNA is denatured with heat (97°C for 5 minutes) and exposed to bisulfite solution (sodium bisulfite, NaOH, and hydroquinone) for 16 to 20 hours. Buffer systems, for example, the Qiagen EpiTect, that protect DNA from bisulfite damage may be used to increase the yield of converted DNA. During the incubation with bisulfite, the cytosines in the reaction are deaminated, converting them to uracils, whereas the 5-methyl cytosines are unchanged.

After the reaction, the treated template is cleaned, precipitated, and resuspended for use as a template for PCR amplification. The primers used for amplification may have to be altered to accommodate C to U changes in the primer binding sites caused by the bisulfite treatment. The PCR amplicons are then sequenced in standard sequencing methods. Methylation is detected by comparing the treated sequence with an untreated sequence and noting where in the treated sequence CG base pairs are not changed to TA; that is, the sequence will be altered relative to the reference sequence at the unmethylated C residues. An example of pyrosequencing of bisulfite converted DNA is shown in Figure 10-16, where the height of the cytosine peaks relative to the thymine (uracil) peaks indicates the percent methylation.

Nonsequencing detection methods have also been devised to detect DNA methylation, such as using methylation-sensitive restriction enzymes or enzymes with recognition sites generated or destroyed by the C to U changes. Other methods use PCR primers that will bind only to the converted or nonconverted sequences so that the presence or absence of PCR product indicates the methylation status. These methods, however, are not always applicable to detection of methylation in unexplored sequences. As the role of methylation and epigenetics in human disease is increasingly recognized, bisulfite sequencing has become a popular method in the research laboratory. Clinical tests have been devised using this strategy as well.[20,21]

RNA Sequencing

The sequences of RNA transcripts are, for the most part, complementary to their DNA templates. Post-transcriptional processing of RNA, however, changes the RNA sequence relative to its encoding DNA. Alternative splicing and RNA editing may further modify the RNA sequence. Early methods to sequence RNA made use of ribonucleases to cut end-labeled RNA at specific nucleotides.[22] Today, a frequently used approach is to determine RNA transcript sequence from complementary DNA. This method, however, is prone to error, mostly from the cDNA synthesis step.[23–25]

Advanced Concepts

Pyrosequencing requires a single-stranded sequencing template. Methods using streptavidin-conjugated beads have been devised to easily prepare the template. First the region of DNA to be sequenced is PCR-amplified with one of the PCR primers covalently attached to a biotin molecule. The double-stranded amplicons are then immobilized onto the beads and denatured with NaOH. After several washings to remove the nonbiotinylated complementary strand (and all other reaction components), the sequencing primer is added and annealed to the pure single-stranded DNA template.

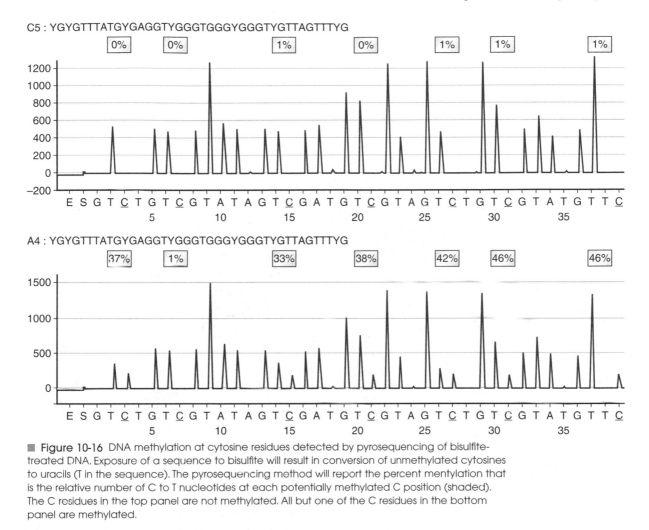

Figure 10-16 DNA methylation at cytosine residues detected by pyrosequencing of bisulfite-treated DNA. Exposure of a sequence to bisulfite will result in conversion of unmethylated cytosines to uracils (T in the sequence). The pyrosequencing method will report the percent methylation that is the relative number of C to T nucleotides at each potentially methylated C position (shaded). The C residues in the top panel are not methylated. All but one of the C residues in the bottom panel are methylated.

A method to directly sequence RNA has been proposed based on single-molecule sequencing technology and virtual terminator nucleotides.[26,27] In this method, mRNA is captured by immobilized polydT DNA (Fig. 10-17). For those RNA species without polyA tails, an initial treatment with polyA polymerase is performed to add a 3' A-tail. The 3' ends of the captured RNA are chemically blocked to prevent extension in the sequencing step. The four reversibly dye-labeled nucleotides, VT-T, -A, -C, and -G, are added. An image is taken, and the extension inhibitors are cleaved and alternating C, T, A, or G nucleotides are added with imaging, cleavage, and rinsing between each nucleotide addition. After repeating this process many times (e.g., 120 cycles) the collected

images are aligned and used to build the sequence from each poly(dT) anchor.

Next Generation Sequencing

Data obtained from sequence analysis is best interpreted in context with population norms and variations; however, few large sequence analyses are repeated for multiple individuals. Although array studies have been applied to this type of analysis, even the most dense oligo array does not provide whole genome sequence data with single base-pair resolution. Next generation sequencing is designed to sequence large numbers of templates simultaneously, yielding not just one, but hundreds of

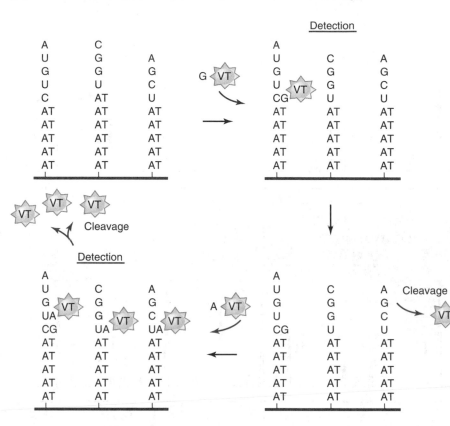

■ **Figure 10-17** Sequencing of RNA captured by natural or appended polyA tails is determined by the position of each RNA on the solid matrix. Reversibly labeled virtual terminator (VT) nucleotides are added in turn to the growing sequence and detected. After detection, the label is cleaved and the next nucleotide is added, detected, and so forth.

thousands of sequences in a run that takes a few hours. The goal of next generation sequencing is to achieve the sequence of the human genome for a minimal cost ($1,000), making genomic studies a routine component of both research and clinical analysis.

Next generation sequencing includes technologies such as the 454 FLX pyrosequencer (Roche), the Illumina Cluster bead array system (Luminex), the HeliScope single-molecule sequencing system (Helicos Bioscience), and SOLiD sequencing by ligation (Applied Biosystems).[28] Next generation sequencing requires novel methods of template preparation, such as emulsion PCR and bridge PCR (see Chapter 7, "Nucleic Acid Amplification") or single-molecule capabilities (Fig. 10-18). Powerful computer data assembly systems are required to organize the massive amounts of sequence information that is generated. These technologies can be used not only to sequence multiple whole genomes but also to investigate populations of small genomes such as microbial diversity.[29] Ongoing challenges with massive sequencing include the integration of technologies and the compromising of accuracy for throughput.[30,31]

Bioinformatics

Information technology has had to encompass the vast amount of data arising from the growing numbers of sequence discovery methods, especially direct sequencing and array technology. This deluge of information requires careful storage, organization, and indexing of large amounts of data. **Bioinformatics** is the merger of biology with information technology. Part of the practice in this field is biological analysis **in silico**, that is, by computer rather than in the laboratory. Bioinformatics dedicated specifically to handling sequence information is a form of **computational biology**. A list of some of the terms used in bioinformatics is shown in Table 10.3. The handling of the mountains of data being generated requires continual renewal of stored data, and a number of database programs are available for this purpose.[32]

Standard expression of sequence data is important for the clear communication and organized storage of sequence data. In some cases, such as in heterozygous mutations, there may be more than one base or mixed bases at the same position in the sequence. Polymorphic

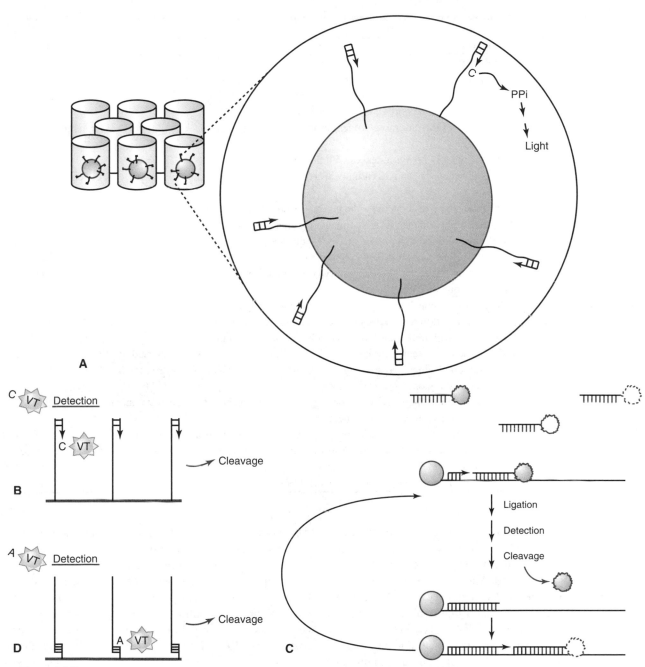

■ **Figure 10-18** Four approaches to next generation sequencing are shown. 454 sequencing (A) is a pyrosequencing method performed on templates attached to beads through emulsion PCR. Templates for Illumina sequencing (B) are produced by bridge PCR. The sequencing is performed using virtual terminators (VT), detection, and cleavage. SOLiD sequencing (C) also uses templates immobilized on bead matrices, with a smaller bead (1 um) than 454 sequencing. Labeled 8-base oligonucleotides are sequentially hybridized to the template. If an oligonucleotide sequence is complementary to the template, the oligonucleotide is ligated, the label detected, and then cleaved. HeliScope sequencing (D) differs from the other approaches in that the sample DNA is not amplified before sequencing. It is performed similar to RNA sequencing as explained in Figure 10-17.

Table 10.3 **Bioinformatics Terminology**

Term	Definition
Identity	The extent to which two sequences are the same
Alignment	Lining up two or more sequences to search for the maximal regions of identity in order to assess the extent of biological relatedness or homology
Local alignment	Alignment of some portion of two sequences
Multiple sequence alignment	Alignment of three or more sequences arranged with gaps so that common residues are aligned together
Optimal alignment	The alignment of two sequences with the best degree of identity
Conservation	Specific sequence changes (usually protein sequence) that maintain the properties of the original sequence
Similarity	The relatedness of sequences, the percent identity or conservation
Algorithm	A fixed set of commands in a computer program
Domain	A discreet portion of a protein or DNA sequence
Motif	A highly conserved short region in protein domains
Gap	A space introduced in alignment to compensate for insertions or deletions in one of the sequences being compared
Homology	Similarity attributed to descent from a common ancestor
Orthology	Homology in different species due to a common ancestral gene
Paralogy	Homology within the same species resulting from gene duplication
Query	The sequence presented for comparison with all other sequences in a selected database
Annotation	Description of functional structures, such as introns or exons in DNA or secondary structure or functional regions to protein sequences
Interface	The point of meeting between a computer and an external entity, such as an operator, a peripheral device, or a communications medium
GenBank	The genetic sequence database sponsored by the National Institutes of Health
PubMed	Search service sponsored by the National Library of Medicine that provides access to literature citations in Medline and related databases
SwissProt	Protein database sponsored by the Medical Research Council (United Kingdom)

or heterozygous sequences are written as **consensus sequences**, or a family of sequences, with proportional representation of the polymorphic bases. The International Union of Pure and Applied Chemistry and the International Union of Biochemistry and Molecular Biology (IUB) have assigned a universal nomenclature for mixed, degenerate, or wobble bases (Table 10.4). The base designations in the IUB code are used to communicate consensus sequences and for computer input of polymorphic sequence data.

The Human Genome Project

From the first description of its double helical structure in 1953 to the creation of the first recombinant molecule in

the laboratory in 1972, DNA and the chemical nature of the arrangement of its nucleotides attracted great interest. Gradually, this information began to accumulate, first regarding simple microorganisms and then partially in lower and higher eukaryotes. The deciphering of the human genome is a hallmark of molecular biology. It is a benchmark in the ongoing discovery of the molecular basis for disease and the groundwork of molecular diagnostics. In the process of solving the human DNA sequence, genomes of a variety of clinically significant organisms have also been deciphered, advancing typing and predicting infectious disease treatment outcomes.

The first complete genome sequence of a clinically important organism was that of Epstein-Barr virus, published in 1984.[33] The 170,000–base-pair sequence was

Table 10.4 **IUB Universal Nomenclature for Mixed Bases**

Symbol	Bases	Mnemonic
A	Adenine	Adenine
C	Cytosine	Cytosine
G	Guanine	Guanine
T	Thymine	Thymine
U	Uracil	Uracil
R	A, G	puRine
Y	C, T	pYrimidine
M	A, C	aMino
K	G, T	Keto
S	C, G	Strong (3 H bonds)
W	A, T	Weak (2 H bonds)
H	A, C, T	Not G
B	C, G, T	Not A
V	A, C, G	Not T
D	A, G, T	Not C
N	A, C, G, T	aNy
X, ?	Unknown	A or C or G or T
O, -	Deletion	

determined using the M13 template preparation/chain termination manual sequencing method. In 1985 and 1986, the possibility of mapping or sequencing the human genome was discussed at meetings at the University of California, Santa Cruz; Cold Spring Harbor, New York; and the Department of Energy in Santa Fe, New Mexico. The idea was controversial because of the risk that the $2 to $5 billion cost of the project might not justify the information gained, most of which would be sequences of "junk," or non-gene-coding DNA. Furthermore, there was no available technology up to the massive task. The sequencing automation and the computer power necessary to assemble the 3 billion bases of the human genome into an organized sequence of 23 chromosomes was not yet developed.

Nevertheless, several researchers, including Walter Gilbert (of Maxam-Gilbert sequencing), Robert Sinsheimer, Leroy Hood, David Baltimore, David Botstein, Renato Dulbecco, and Charles DeLici, saw that the project was feasible because technology was rapidly advancing toward full automation of the process. In 1982, Akiyoshi Wada had proposed automated sequencing machinery and had gotten support from Hitachi Instruments. In

1987, Smith and Hood announced the first automated DNA sequencing machine.[34] Advances in the chemistry of the sequencing procedure, described in the first sections of this chapter, were accompanied by advances in the biology of DNA mapping, with methods such as pulsed field gel electrophoresis,[35,36] restriction fragment length polymorphism analysis,[37] and transcript identification.[38] Methods were developed to clone large (500 kbp) DNA fragments in artificial chromosomes, providing long contiguous sequencing templates.[39] Finally, application of capillary electrophoresis to DNA resolution[40–42] made the sequencing procedure even more rapid and cost-efficient.

With these developments in technology, the Human Genome Project was endorsed by the National Research Council. The National Institutes of Health (NIH) established the Office of Human Genome Research with James Watson as its head. Over the next 5 years, meetings on policy, ethics, and cost of the project resulted in a plan to complete 20 Mb of sequence of model organisms by 2005 (Table 10.5). To organize and compare the growing amount of sequence data, the **Basic Local Alignment Search Tool** and Gene Recognition and Assembly Internet Link algorithms were introduced in 1990.[43,44]

For the human sequence, the decision was made to use a composite template from multiple individuals rather than a single genome from one donor. Human DNA was donated by 100 anonymous volunteers; only 10 of these genomes were sequenced. Not even the volunteers knew

Table 10.5 **Model Organisms Sequenced During the Human Genome Project**

Organism	Genome Size (Mb)	Estimated Number of Genes
Epstein-Barr virus	0.17	80
Mycoplasma genitalium	0.58	470
Haemophilus influenzae	1.8	1740
Escherichia coli K-12	4.6	4377
E. coli O157	5.4	5416
Saccharomyces cerevisiae	12.5	5770
Drosophila melanogaster	180	13,000
Caenorhabditis elegans	97	19,000
Arabidopsis thaliana	100	25,000

if their DNA was used for the project. To ensure accurate and high-quality sequencing, all regions were sequenced 5 to 10 times.

A second project started with the same goal. In 1992, Craig Venter left the NIH to start The Institute for Genomic Research (TIGR). Venter's group completed the first sequence of a free-living organism (*Haemophilus influenzae*)[45] and the sequence of the smallest free-living organism (*Mycoplasma genitalium*).[46] Venter established a new company named Celera and proposed to complete the human genome sequence in 3 years for $300 million, faster and cheaper than the NIH project. Meanwhile, Watson had resigned as head of the NIH project and was replaced by Francis Collins. In response, the Wellcome Trust doubled its support of the NIH project. The NIH moved its completion date from 2005 to 2003, with a working draft to be completed by 2001. Thus began a competitive effort on two fronts to sequence the human genome.

The two projects approached the sequencing differently (Fig. 10-19). The NIH method (**hierarchal shotgun sequencing**) was to start with sequences of known regions in the genome and "walk" further away into the chromosomes, always aware of where the newly generated sequences belonged in the human genome map. Venter and the researchers working with Celera—Gene Meyers, Jane Rogers, Robert Millman, John Sulston, and Todd Taylor—had a different idea. Their approach (*whole genome shotgun sequencing*) was to start with 10 equivalents of the human genome cut into small fragments and randomly sequence the lot. Then, powerful computers would find overlapping sequences and use those to assemble the billions of bases of sequence into their proper chromosomal locations.

Initially, the Celera approach was met with skepticism. The human genome contains large amounts of repeated sequences (see Chapter 11, "DNA Polymorphisms and Human Identification"), some of which are very difficult to sequence and even more difficult to map properly. A random sequencing method would repeatedly cover areas of the genome that are more easily sequenced and miss more difficult regions. Moreover, assembly of the whole sequence from scratch with no chromosomal landmarks would take a prohibitive amount of computer power. Nonetheless, Celera began to make headway (some

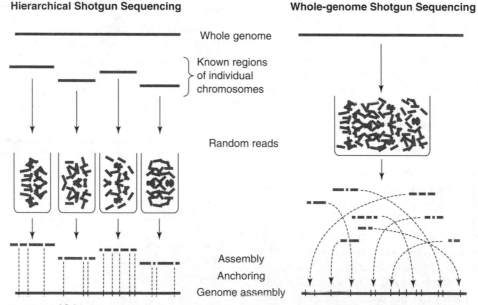

■ **Figure 10-19** Comparison of two approaches for sequencing of the human genome. The hierarchal shotgun approach taken by the NIH (left) was to sequence from known regions so that new sequences could easily be located in the genome. The Celera whole-genome shotgun approach (right) was to sequence random fragments from the entire genome and then to assemble the complete sequence with computers.

alleged with the help of the publicly published sequences from the NIH), and eventually the NIH project modified its approach to include both methods.

Over the next months, some efforts were made toward combining the two projects, but these efforts broke down over disagreements over database policy and release of completed sequences. The result of the competition was that the rough draft of the sequence was completed by both projects earlier than either group had proposed, in June 2000. A joint announcement was made, and both groups published their versions of the genome, the NIH version in the journal *Nature*[47] and the Celera version in the journal *Science*.[48]

The sequence completed in 2000 was a rough draft of the genome; that is, there were still areas of missing sequence and sequences yet to be placed. Only chromosomes 21 and 22, the smallest of the chromosomes, had been fully completed. In the ensuing years, the finished sequences of each chromosome have been released (Table 10.6).

Remaining errors, gaps, and complex gene rearrangements will take years to resolve.[49] Detailed analysis of an individual genome will require sequencing of both homologs of each chromosome.[50] Even with the rough draft, interesting characteristics of the human genome were revealed. The size of the entire genome is 2.91 Gbp (2.91 billion base pairs). The genome was initially calculated as 54% AT, 38% GC, with 8% of the bases still to be determined. Chromosome 2 is the most GC-rich chromosome (66%), and chromosome X has the fewest GC base pairs (25%). A most surprising discovery was that the number of genes, estimated to be from 20,000 to 30,000, was much lower than expected. The average size of a human gene is 27 kbp. Chromosome 19 is the most gene-rich per unit length (23 genes/Mbp). Chromosomes 13 and Y have the fewest genes per base pair (5 genes/Mbp). Only about 2% of the sequences code for genes. Thirty to 40% of the genome consists of repeat sequences. There is one single base difference between two random individuals found approximately every 1000 bases along the human DNA sequence. More detailed information, databases, references, and updated information are available at http://www.ncbi.nlm.nih.gov/.

The promise of the Human Genome Project for molecular diagnostics can be appreciated with the example of the discovery of the gene involved in cystic fibrosis. Seven years of work were required for discovery of this gene.

Table 10.6 **Completed Chromosomes**

Chromosome	Completion Date
21	December 1999
22	May 2000
20	December 2001
14	January 2003
Y	June 2003
7	July 2003
6	October 2003
13	March 2004
19	March 2004
10	May 2004
9	May 2004
5	September 2004
16	December 2004
18	January 2005
X	March 2005
2	April 2005
4	April 2005
8	January 2006
11	March 2006
15	March 2006
12	March 2006
17	April 2006
3	April 2006
1	May 2006

With proper mapping information, a gene for any disease can now be found by computer, already sequenced, in a matter of minutes. Of course, all genetic diseases are not due to malfunction of a single gene. In fact, most diseases and normal states are driven by a combination of genes as well as by environmental influences. Without the rich information afforded by the sequence of the human genome, identification of these multicomponent diseases would be almost impossible. Ten years after the announcement of the completion of the Human Genome Project, almost 200 human genomes have been sequenced. Although the information gathered from the sequencing effort has not yielded the benefits to human health expected at the start of the project, it has increased the appreciation of the vast complexity of genes and their regulation.[51]

Another project has been launched to further define the relationship between gene sequence and disease. This is the Human Haplotype Mapping, or HapMap, Project.

The goal of this project is to find blocks of sequences that are inherited together, marking particular traits and possibly disease-associated genetic lesions. (A description of this project is presented in Chapter 11.) The HapMap Project has revealed more than 100 disease-associated regions of the genome, covering commonly occurring conditions such as coronary artery disease and diabetes.

Data from the HapMap Project will be extended by the 1000 Genomes Project. In this project, the genomes of over 1000 unidentified individuals will be sequenced using next generation sequencing technologies in laboratories in the United States, United Kingdom, China, and Germany. The resulting sequence data will be an extensive catalog of human sequence variation. In addition to SNPs identified by the HapMap Project, the 1000 Genomes Project will provide a resource of structural variants and their haplotypes.

The technology developed as part of the Human Genome Project has made sequencing a routine method in the clinical laboratory. Small, cost-effective sequencers are available for rapid sequencing. In the clinical laboratory, sequencing is actually resequencing, or repeated analysis of the same sequence region, to detect mutations or to type microorganisms, making the task even more routine. The technology continues to develop, reducing the cost and labor of sequencing larger and larger areas, so that several regions can be sequenced to detect multicomponent diseases or to predict predisposition to disease. Accurate and comprehensive sequence analysis is one of the most promising areas of molecular diagnostics.

• STUDY QUESTIONS •

1. Read 5' to 3' the first 15 bases of the sequence in the gel on the right in Figure 10-8 (p. 229).

2. After an automated dye primer sequencing run, the electropherogram displays consecutive peaks of the following colors:

   red, red, black, green, green, blue, black, red, green, black, blue, blue, blue

   If the computer software displays the fluors from ddATP as green, ddCTP as blue, ddGTP as black, and ddTTP as red, what is the sequence of the region given?

3. A dideoxy sequencing electropherogram displays bright (high, wide) peaks of fluorescence, obliterating some of the sequencing peaks. What is the most likely cause of this observation? How might it be corrected?

4. In a manual sequencing reaction, the sequencing ladder on the polyacrylamide gel is very bright and readable at the bottom of the gel, but the larger (slower-migrating) fragments higher up are very faint. What is the most likely cause of this observation? How might it be corrected?

5. In an analysis of the p53 gene for mutations, the following sequences were produced. For each sequence, write the expected sequence of the opposite strand that would confirm the presence of the mutations detected.

   5'TATCTGTTCACTTGTGCCCT3' (Normal)

   5'TATCTGTTCATTTGTGCCCT3' (Homozygous substitution)

   5'TATCTGT(T/G)CACTTGTGCCCT3' (Heterozygous substitution)

   5'TATCTGTT(C/A)(A/C)(C/T)T(T/G)(G/T)(T/G) (G/C)CC(C/T)(T/...3' (Heterozygous deletion)

6. A sequence, TTGCTGCGCTAAA, may be methylated at one or more of the cytosine residues. After bisulfite sequencing, the following results are obtained:

   Bisulfite treated: TTGCTGTGCTAAA

   Untreated: TTGCTGCGCTAAA

   Write the sequence showing the methylated cytosines as C^{Me}.

7. In a pyrosequencing readout, the graph shows peaks of luminescence corresponding to the addition of the following nucleotides:

   dT peak, dC peak (double height), dT peak, dA peak

   What is the sequence?

8. Why is it necessary to add adenosine residues in vitro to ribosomal RNA before capture for sequencing?

9. Which of the following is not next generation sequencing?
   a. 454 sequencing
   b. tiled microarray
   c. SOLID system
   d. Illumina Genome Analyzer

10. Which of the following projects would require mass array sequencing?
    a. Mapping a mutation in the hemochromatosis gene
    b. Sequencing a viral genome
    c. Characterization of a diverse microbial population
    d. Typing a single bacterial colony

References

1. Amos J, Grody W. Development and integration of molecular genetic tests into clinical practice: The US experience. *Expert Review of Molecular Diagnostics* 2004;4(4):465–477.

2. Maxam A, Gilbert W. Sequencing end-labeled DNA with base-specific chemical cleavage. *Methods in Enzymology* 1980;65:499–560.

3. Sanger F, Nicklen S, Coulson AR. DNA sequencing with chain terminating inhibitors. *Proceedings of the National Academy of Sciences* 1977;74:5463–5467.

4. Tabor S, Richardson CC. Selective inactivation of the exonuclease activity of bacteriophage T7 DNA polymerase by in vitro mutagenesis. *Journal of Biological Chemistry* 1989;264(11):6447–6458.

5. Elie C, Salhi S, Rossignol JM, et al. A DNA polymerase from a thermoacidophilic archaebacterium: Evolutionary and technological interests. *Biochimica Biophysica Acta* 1988;951(2–3):261–267.

6. Tabor S, Richardson CC. Effect of manganese ions on the incorporation of dideoxynucleotides by bacteriophage T7 DNA polymerase and *E. coli* DNA polymerase I. *Proceedings of the National Academy of Sciences* 1989;86:4076–4080.

7. Tabor S, Richardson CC. Sequence analysis with a modified bacteriophage T7 DNA polymerase: Effect of pyrophorolysis and metal ions. *Journal of Biological Chemistry* 1990;265:8322–8328.

8. Hilbert H, Schafer A, Collasius M, et al. High-throughput robotic system for sequencing of microbial genomes. *Electrophoresis* 1998;19(4):500–503.

9. Smith L, Sanders JZ, Kaiser RJ, et al. Fluorescence detection in automated DNA sequence analysis. *Nature* 1986;32(6071):674–679.

10. Metzker ML, Lu J, Gibbs RA. Electrophoretically uniform fluorescent dyes for automated DNA sequencing. *Science* 1996;271:1420–1422.

11. Lewis E, Haaland WC, Nguyen F, et al. Color-blind fluorescence detection for four-color DNA sequencing. *Proceedings of the National Academy of Sciences* 2005;102(15):5346–5351.

12. Carr I, Robinson JI, Dimitriou R, et al. Inferring relative proportions of DNA variants from sequencing electropherograms. *Bioinformatics* 2009;25:3244–3250.

13. Ronaghi M, Uhlen M, Nyren P. A sequencing method based on real-time pyrophosphate. *Science* 1998;281(5375):363–365.

14. Nyren M, Pettersson B, Uhlen M. Solid phase DNA minisequencing by an enzymatic luminometric inorganic pyrophosphate detection assay. *Analytical Biochemistry* 1993;208:171–175.

15. Unemo M, Olcen P, Jonasson J, et al. Molecular typing of *Neisseria gonorrhoeae* isolates by pyrosequencing of highly polymorphic segments of the porB gene. *Journal of Clinical Microbiology* 2004;42:2926–2934.

16. Cebula T, Brown EW, Jackson SA, et al. Molecular applications for identifying microbial pathogens in the post-9/11 era. *Expert Review of Molecular Diagnostics* 2005;5(3):431–445.

17. Ramon D, Braden M, Adams S, et al. Pyrosequencing: A one-step method for high resolution HLA typing. *Journal of Translational Medicine* 2003;1:9.

18. Fraga M, Esteller M. DNA methylation: A profile of methods and applications. *BioTechniques* 2002;33(3):632–649.

19. Shiraishi M, Hayatsu H. High-speed conversion of cytosine to uracil in bisulfite genomic sequencing analysis of DNA methylation. *DNA Research* 2004;11(6):409–415.

20. Weller M, Stupp R, Reifenberger G, et al. MGMT promoter methylation in malignant gliomas: Ready for personalized medicine? *Nature Review Neurology* 2010;6:39–51.

21. Mikeska T, Bock C, El-Maarri O, et al. Optimization of quantitative MGMT promoter methylation analysis using pyrosequencing and combined

bisulfite restriction analysis. *Journal of Molecular Diagnostics* 2007;9:368–381.

22. Perbal B. A Practical Guide to Molecular Cloning, 2nd ed. New York: John Wiley & Sons, 1988, pp. 641–653.

23. Gubler U. Second-strand cDNA synthesis: Classical method. *Methods in Enzymology* 1987;152:325–329.

24. Cocquet J, Chong A, Zhang G, et al. Reverse transcriptase template switching and false alternative transcripts. *Genomics* 2006;88:127–131.

25. Roberts J, Preston BD, Johnston LA, et al. Fidelity of two retroviral reverse transcriptases during DNA-dependent DNA synthesis in vitro. *Molecular and Cellular Biology* 1989;9:469–476.

26. Braslavsky I, Hebert B, Kartalov E, et al. Sequence information can be obtained from single DNA molecules. *Proceedings of the National Academy of Sciences* 2003;100:3960–3964.

27. Ozsolak F, Platt AR, Jones DR, et al. Direct RNA sequencing. *Nature* 2009;461:814–818.

28. Rothberg J, Leamon JH. The development and impact of 454 sequencing. *Nature Biotechnology* 2008;26:1117–1124.

29. Mardis E. The impact of next-generation sequencing technology on genetics. *Trends in Genetics* 2008;24(3):133–141.

30. Pop M, Salzberg SL. Bioinformatics challenges of new sequencing technology. *Trends in Genetics* 2008;24:142–149.

31. Fuller C, Middendorf LR, Benner SA, Church GM, Harris T, Huang X, Jovanovich SB, Nelson JR, Schloss JA, Schwartz DC, Vezenov DV. The challenges of sequencing by synthesis. *Nature Biotechnology* 2009;27:1013–1023.

32. Wheeler D, Barrett T, Benson DA, et al. Database resources of the National Center for Biotechnology Information. *Nucleic Acids Research* (database issue) 2005;33(D39–D45).

33. Baer R, Bankier AT, Biggin MD, et al. DNA sequence and expression of the B95-8 Epstein-Barr virus genome. *Nature* 1984;310(5974):207–211.

34. Hood LE, Hunkapiller MW, Smith LM. Automated DNA sequencing and analysis of the human genome. *Genomics* 1987;1:201–212.

35. Schwartz D, Cantor CR. Separation of yeast chromosome-sized DNAs by pulsed field gradient gel electrophoresis. *Cell* 1984;37(1):67–75.

36. Van der Ploeg L, Schwartz DC, Cantor CR, et al. Antigenic variation in *Trypanosoma brucei* analyzed by electrophoretic separation of chromosome-sized DNA molecules. *Cell* 1984;37(1):77–84.

37. Donis-Keller H, Green P, Helms C, et al. A genetic linkage map of the human genome. *Cell* 1987;51(2): 319–337.

38. Green E, Mohr RM, Idol JR, et al. Systematic generation of sequence-tagged sites for physical mapping of human chromosomes: Application to the mapping of human chromosome 7 using yeast artificial chromosomes. *Genomics* 1991;11(3): 548–564.

39. Riethman H, Moyzis RK, Meyne J, et al. Cloning human telomeric DNA fragments into *Saccharomyces cerevisiae* using a yeast-artificial-chromosome vector. *Proceedings of the National Academy of Sciences* 1989;86(16):6240–6244.

40. Luckey J, Drossman H, Kostichka AJ, et al. High-speed DNA sequencing by capillary electrophoresis. *Nucleic Acids Research* 1990;18(15): 4417–4421.

41. Karger A. Separation of DNA sequencing fragments using an automated capillary electrophoresis instrument. *Electrophoresis* 1996;17(1):144–151.

42. Chen D, Swerdlow HP, Harke HR, et al. Low-cost, high-sensitivity laser-induced fluorescence detection for DNA sequencing by capillary gel electrophoresis. *Journal of Chromatography* 1991;559(1–2):237–246.

43. Altschul S, Gish W, Miller W, et al. Basic local alignment search tool. *Journal of Molecular Biology* 1990;215(3):403–410.

44. Xu Y, Mural RJ, Uberbacher EC. Constructing gene models from accurately predicted exons: An application of dynamic programming. *Computer Applications in the Biosciences* 1994;10(6):613–623.

45. Fleischmann R, Adams MD, White O, et al. Whole-genome random sequencing and assembly of *Haemophilus influenzae*. *Science* 1995;269: 496–512.

46. Fraser C, Gocayne JD, White O, et al. The minimal gene complement of *Mycoplasma genitalium*. *Science* 1995;270(5235):397–403.

47. Lander E, Linton LM, et al. Initial sequencing and analysis of the human genome. *Nature* 2001; 409(6822):860–921.

48. Venter J, Adams MD, et al. The sequence of the human genome. *Science* 2001;291(5507): 1304–1351.

49. Dolgin E. The genome finishers. *Nature* 2009;462: 843–845.

50. Levy S, Sutton G, Ng PC, et al. The diploid genome sequence of an individual human. *PLoS Biology* 2007;5:2113–2145.

51. Hayden E. Life is complicated. *Nature* 2010;464: 664–667.

Techniques in the Clinical Laboratory

Chapter **11**

DNA Polymorphisms and Human Identification

OBJECTIVES

- Compare and contrast different types of polymorphisms.
- Define restriction fragment length polymorphisms and discuss how they are used in genetic mapping, parentage testing, and human identification.
- Describe short tandem repeat structure and nomenclature.
- Describe gender identification using the amelogenin locus.
- Explain matching probabilities and the contribution of allele frequencies to the certainty of matching.
- Describe the use of Y-STR in forensic and lineage studies.
- Give examples of the use of STR for bone marrow engraftment monitoring.
- Show how STR may be used for quality assurance of histological sections.

OBJECTIVES—cont'd

- Define single nucleotide polymorphisms and their potential use in disease gene mapping.
- Discuss mitochondrial DNA typing.

As discussed in Chapter 8, "Chromosomal Structure and Chromosomal Mutations," polymorphisms are DNA sequences that differ from the sequences of a majority of a population but are still shared by a certain percentage. These sequences range from a single base pair to thousands of base pairs.

Types of Polymorphisms

The probability of polymorphic DNA in humans is great due to the relatively large size of the human genome, 98% of which does not code for genes. At the nucleotide-sequence level, it is estimated that genome sequences differ by 1 nucleotide every 1000 to 1500 bases. These single nucleotide differences, or **single nucleotide polymorphisms** (**SNPs**), may occur in gene-coding regions or in intergenic sequences (see Chapter 3, "Proteins and the Genetic Code," for the nature of the genetic code and Chapter 8, "Chromosomal Structure and Chromosomal Mutations," for a discussion of silent and conservative mutations in coding regions).

Polymorphisms are more frequent in some areas of the genome than in others. The human leukocyte antigen (HLA) locus is a familiar example of a highly polymorphic region of human DNA. The variable nucleotide sequences in this locus code for peptides that establish self-identity of the immune system. The extent of similarity or compatibility between immune systems of transplant recipients and potential donors can thus be determined by comparing DNA sequences (see Chapter 15, "DNA-Based Tissue Typing"). HLA typing may also be used for exclusion in human identification tests.

Some human sequence polymorphisms affect many base pairs. Large blocks of repeated sequences may be inverted, deleted, or duplicated from one individual to another. **Long interspersed nucleotide sequences (LINES)** are highly repeated sequences, 6 to 8 kbp in length, that contain RNA polymerase promoters and open reading frames related to the reverse transcriptase of retroviruses. There are more than 500,000 of these LINE-1 (L1) elements, making up more than 15% of the human genome. There are even more **short interspersed nucleotide sequences (SINES)** scattered over the genome. SINES, 0.3 kbp in size, are present in over 1,000,000 copies per genome. SINES include **Alu elements**, named for harboring recognition sites for the *Alu*I restriction enzyme. LINES and SINES are also known as mobile elements or transposable elements. They are copied and spread by recombination and reverse transcription and may be responsible for formation of **pseudogenes** (intronless, nonfunctional copies of active genes) throughout the human genome. Shorter blocks of repeated sequences also undergo expansion or shrinkage through generations. Examples of the latter are **short tandem repeats (STRs)** and **variable number tandem repeats (VNTRs).**

Single nucleotide polymorphisms, larger sequence variants, and tandem repeats can be detected by observing changes in the restriction map of a DNA region. Analysis of restriction fragments by Southern blot reveals **restriction fragment length polymorphisms (RFLPs).** Particular types of polymorphisms, specifically SNPs, VNTRs, STRs, and RFLPs, are routinely used in the laboratory (Table 11.1).

Table 11.1 **Types of Useful Polymorphisms and Laboratory Methods**

Polymorphism	Structure	Detection Method
RFLP	One or more nucleotide changes that affect the size of restriction enzyme products	Southern blot
VNTR	Repeats of 10–50 base sequences in tandem	Southern blot, PCR
STR	Repeats of 1–10 base sequences in tandem	PCR
SNP	Alterations of a single nucleotide	Sequencing, other

RFLP Typing

The first polymorphic RFLP was described in 1980. RFLPs were the original DNA targets used for gene mapping, human identification, and parentage testing. RFLPs are observed as differences in the sizes and number of fragments generated by restriction enzyme digestion of DNA (Fig. 11-1) Fragment sizes may vary as a result of changes in the nucleotide sequence in or between the recognition sites of a restriction enzyme. Nucleotide changes may also destroy, change, or create restriction enzyme sites, altering the number of fragments.

The first step in using RFLPs is to construct a restriction enzyme map of the DNA region under investigation. (Construction of restriction maps is described in Chapter 6,

"Analysis and Characterization of Nucleic Acids and Proteins.") Once the restriction map is known, the number and sizes of the restriction fragments of a test DNA region cut with restriction enzymes are compared with the number and sizes of fragments expected based on the restriction map. Polymorphisms are detected by observing fragment numbers and sizes different from those expected from the reference restriction map. An example of a polymorphism in a restriction site is shown in Figure 11-2. In a theoretical linear piece of DNA, loss of the recognition site for the enzyme (*Bgl*II in the figure) results in alteration of the size and number of bands detected after gel electrophoresis.

Initially, RFLP typing in humans required the use of the Southern blot technique (see Chapter 5, "Resolution

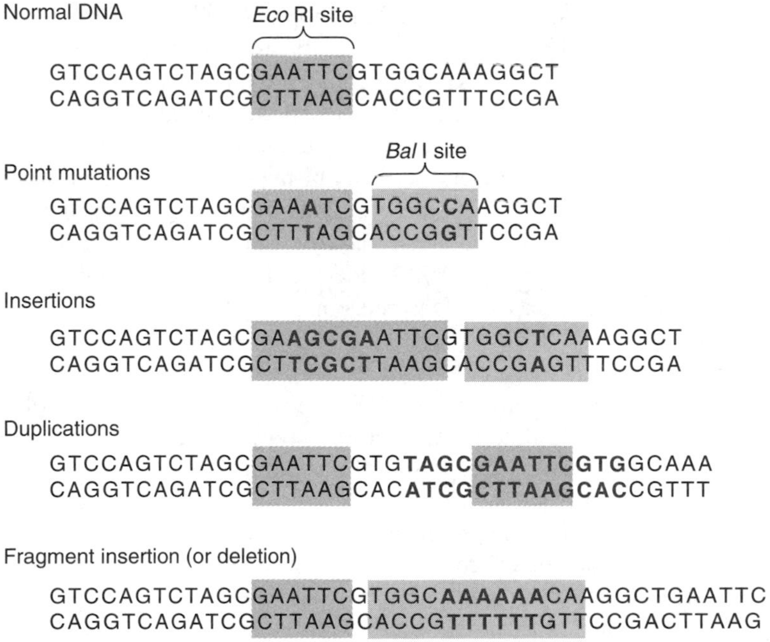

Figure 11-1 Types of DNA sequence alterations that change restriction fragment lengths. The normal sequence (top) has an *Eco* R1 site (GAATTC). Single base changes (point mutations, second line) can destroy the *Eco*R1 site or create a new restriction site, as can insertions, duplications, or deletions of any number of bases (third through fifth lines). Insertions, duplications, and deletions between two restriction sites change fragment size without affecting the restriction sites themselves.

Normal DNA   *Eco* RI site

```
GTCCAGTCTAGCGAATTCGTGGCAAAGGCT
CAGGTCAGATCGCTTAAGCACCGTTTCCGA
```

Point mutations   *Bal* I site

```
GTCCAGTCTAGCGAAATCGTGGCCAAGGCT
CAGGTCAGATCGCTTTAGCACCGGTTCCGA
```

Insertions

```
GTCCAGTCTAGCGAAGCGAATTCGTGGCTCAAAGGCT
CAGGTCAGATCGCTTCGCTTAAGCACCGAGTTTCCGA
```

Duplications

```
GTCCAGTCTAGCGAATTCGTGTAGCGAATTCGTGGCAAA
CAGGTCAGATCGCTTAAGCACATCGCTTAAGCACCGTTT
```

Fragment insertion (or deletion)

```
GTCCAGTCTAGCGAATTCGTGGCAAAAAACAAGGCTGAATTC
CAGGTCAGATCGCTTAAGCACCGTTTTTTGTTCCGACTTAAG
```

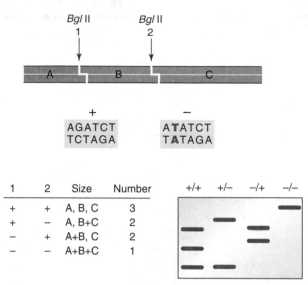

Figure 11-2 A linear piece of DNA with two polymorphic *Bgl* II restriction enzyme sites, designated as 1 and 2, will yield different fragment sizes, depending on the presence of neither, either, or both of the restriction sites. For instance a G→T mutation will change the sequence of the normal site (+) to one not recognized by the enzyme (−). The presence or absence of the polymorphic sites is evident from the number and size of the fragments after cutting the DNA with *Bgl* II (bottom right).

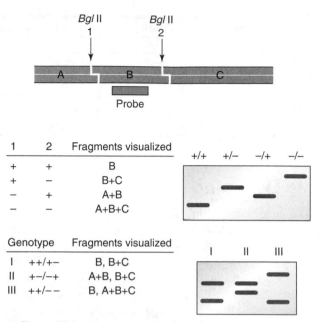

Figure 11-3 Using a Southern blot to probe for RFLP. With the same region shown in Figure 11-2, only the fragments with complementary sequences to a probe to the B region (top) can be visualized. The bottom panel shows a diploid genotype where homologous chromosomes carry different RFLP alleles.

and Detection of Nucleic Acids"). DNA was cut with restriction enzymes, resolved by gel electrophoresis, and blotted to a membrane. Probes to specific regions of DNA containing potential RFLPs were then hybridized to the DNA on the membrane to determine the size of the resulting bands. Figure 11-3 shows the pattern of bands resulting from a Southern blot analysis of the RFLP in the linear fragment from Figure 11-2. Note that not all of the restriction fragments are detected by the probe, yet the three polymorphisms can still be identified.

DNA is inherited as one chromosome complement from each parent. Each chromosome carries its polymorphisms so that the offspring inherits a combination of the parental polymorphisms. When visualized as fragments that hybridize to a probe of a polymorphic region, the band patterns represent the combination of RFLPs inherited from each parent. Due to recombination and random assortment, each person has a unique set of RFLPs, half inherited maternally and half paternally. Every genotype will yield a descriptive band pattern, as shown in Figure 11-3.

Over many generations, mutations, intra- and inter-chromosomal recombination, gene conversion, and other genetic events have increased the diversity of DNA sequences. One consequence of this genetic diversity is that a single **locus**, that is, a gene or region of DNA, will have several versions, or **alleles**. Human beings are diploid with two copies of every locus. In other words, each person has two alleles of each locus. If these alleles are the same, the locus is **homozygous**; if the two alleles are different, the locus is **heterozygous**.

Depending on the extent of diversity or polymorphism of a locus, any two people can share the same alleles or have different alleles. More closely related individuals are likely to share more alleles than unrelated persons. In the examples shown in Figure 11-3, (+ +), (+ −), (− +), and (− −) describe the presence (+) or absence (−) of *Bgl*II sites making up four alleles of the locus detectable by Southern blot. In the illustration, genotypes I and II both have the (+ −) allele on one chromosome, but genotype I has (+ +), and genotype II has (− +) on the other chromosome. This appears in the Southern blot results as one band of equal size between the two genotypes and one band that is a different size. Two individuals can share both alleles at a single locus, but the chances of two individuals, except for identical twins, sharing the same alleles decrease 10-fold with each additional locus tested.[1]

More than 2000 RFLP loci have been described in human DNA. The uniqueness of the collection of polymorphisms in each individual is the basis for human identification at the DNA level. Detection of RFLP by Southern blot made positive paternity testing and human identification possible for the first time. RFLP protocols for human identification in most North American laboratories used the restriction enzyme *Hae*III for fragmentation of genomic DNA. Many European laboratories used the *Hin*fI enzyme. These enzymes cut DNA frequently enough to reveal polymorphisms in multiple locations throughout the genome. To regulate results from independent laboratories, the Standard Reference Material (SRM) DNA Profiling Standard for RFLP analysis was released in 1992. The SRM supplies cell pellets, genomic DNA, gel standards, precut DNA, electrophoresis materials, molecular-weight markers, and certified values for final analysis. These materials, currently provided by the National Institute of Standards and Technology (NIST), were designed to maintain reproducibility of the RFLP process across laboratories.

Genetic Mapping with RFLPs

Polymorphisms are inherited in a Mendelian fashion, and the locations of many polymorphisms in the genome are known. Therefore, polymorphisms can be used as landmarks, or markers, in the genome to determine the location of other genes. In addition to showing clear family history or direct identification of a genetic factor, one can confirm that a disease has a genetic component by demonstrating a close genetic association or linkage to a known marker. Formal statistical methods are used to determine the probability that an unknown gene is located close to a known marker in the genome. The more frequently a particular polymorphism is present in persons with a disease phenotype, the more likely the affected gene is located close to the polymorphism. This is the basis for linkage mapping and one of the ways genetic components of disease are identified.

Historical Highlights

Mary Claire King used RFLP to map one of the genes mutated in inherited breast cancer.[2,3] Following extended families with high incidence of breast and ovarian cancer, she found particular RFLP always present in affected family members. Because the location in the genome of the RFLP was known (17q21), the *BRCA1* gene was thereby mapped to this position on the long arm of chromosome 17.

RFLP and Parentage Testing

In diploid organisms, chromosomal content is inherited half from each parent. This includes the DNA polymorphisms located throughout the genome. Taking advantage of the unique combination of RFLP in each individual, one can infer a parent's contribution of alleles to a son or daughter from the combination of alleles in the child and those of the other parent. The fragment sizes of an individual are a combination of those from each parent, as illustrated in Figure 11-4. In a paternity test, the alleles or fragment sizes of the offspring and the mother are

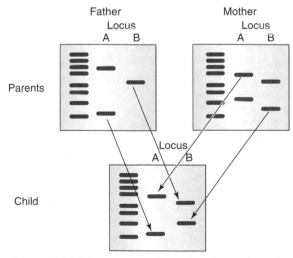

■ **Figure 11-4** RFLP inheritance. Two different genetic regions, or loci, are shown, locus A and locus B. There are several versions or alleles of each locus. Note that the father is heterozygous at locus A and homozygous at locus B. The alleles in the child will be a combination of one allele from each parent.

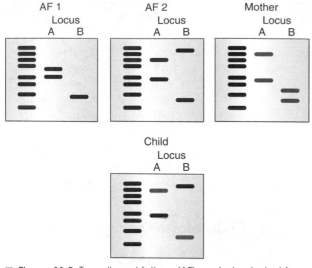

Figure 11-5 Two alleged fathers (AF) are being tested for paternity of the child whose partial RFLP profile is shown in the bottom gel. The mother's alleles are shown in green. One AF (AF1) is excluded from paternity, as he cannot supply the child's paternal allele at locus B.

Human Identification Using RFLP

The first genetic tool used for human identification was the ABO blood group antigens. Although this type of analysis could be performed in a few minutes, the discrimination power was low. With only four possible groups, this method was only good for **exclusion** (elimination) of a person as a source of biological material and was informative only in 15% to 20% of cases. Analysis of the polymorphic HLA loci could add a higher level of discrimination, with exclusion in 90% of cases. Testing both ABO and HLA could exclude a person in 97% of cases but still did not provide positive identification.

The initial use of DNA as an identification tool relied on RFLP detectable by Southern blot. As shown in Figure 11-1, RFLP can arise from a number of genetic events, including point mutations in the restriction site, mutations that create a new restriction site, and insertion or deletion of repeated sequences (tandem repeats). The insertion or deletion of nucleotides occurs frequently in repeated sequences in DNA.

Tandem repeats of sequences of all sizes are present in genomic DNA (Fig. 11-6). Repeats of eight or more nucleotides are called variable number tandem repeats (VNTRs), or **minisatellites**. These repeats are large enough so that loss or gain of one repeat can be resolved by gel electrophoresis of a restriction enzyme digest. The frequent cutters, *Hae*III (recognition site GGCC) or *Hinf*I (recognition site GANTC), generate fragments that are small enough to resolve those that contain different numbers of repeats and thereby give an informative pattern by Southern blot.

The first human DNA profiling system was introduced by the United Kingdom Forensic Science Service in 1985 using Alec Jeffreys' Southern blot **multiple locus probe (MLP)-RFLP** system.[4] This method utilized three to five probes to analyze three to five loci on the same blot.

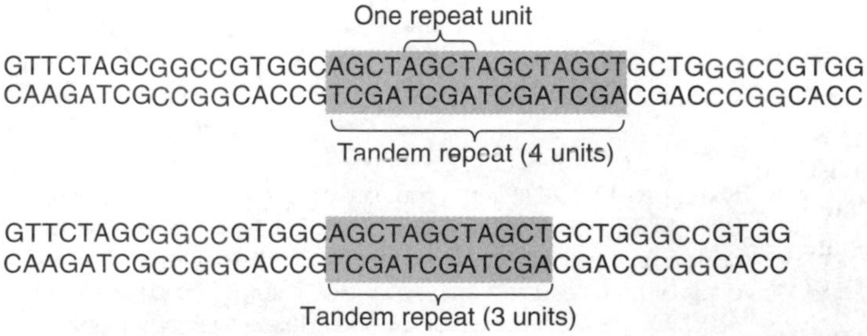

analyzed. The remaining fragments (the ones that do not match the mother) have to come from the father. Alleged fathers are identified based on the ability to provide the remaining alleles **(inclusion)**. Aside from possible mutations, a difference in just one allele may exclude paternity.

A simplified RFLP paternity test is shown in Figure 11-5. Of the two alleged fathers shown, only one could supply the fragments not supplied by the mother. In this example, only two loci are shown. A parentage test requires analysis of at least eight loci. The more loci tested, the higher the probability of positive identification of the father.

```
                        One repeat unit
GTTCTAGCGGCCGTGGCAGCTAGCTAGCTAGCTGCTGGGCCGTGG
CAAGATCGCCGGCACCGTCGATCGATCGATCGACGACCCGGCACC
                        Tandem repeat (4 units)


GTTCTAGCGGCCGTGGCAGCTAGCTAGCTGCTGGGCCGTGG
CAAGATCGCCGGCACCGTCGATCGATCGACGACCCGGCACC
                        Tandem repeat (3 units)
```

Figure 11-6 A tandem repeat is a direct repeat 1 to >100 nucleotides in length. The one shown has a 4-bp repeat unit (AGCT). A gain or loss of repeat units forms a different allele. Different alleles are detected as variations in fragment size on digestion with *Hae* III (GGCC recognition sites).

Results of probing multiple loci at once produced patterns that were highly variable between individuals but that required some expertise to optimize and interpret. In 1990, **single locus probe (SLP)** systems were established in Europe and North America.[5,6] Analysis of one locus at a time yielded simpler patterns, which were much easier to interpret, especially in cases where specimens might contain DNA from more than one individual (Fig 11-7).

The RFLP Southern blot technique required 100 ng to 1 μg of relatively high quality DNA, 1 to 20 kbp in size. Furthermore, large, fragile 0.7% gels were required to achieve adequate band resolution, and the ^{32}P-based probe system could take 5 to 7 days to yield clear results. After visually inspecting the band patterns, profiles were subjected to computer analysis to accurately size the restriction fragments and apply the results to an established matching criterion. RFLP is an example of a **continuous allele system** in which the sizes of the fragments define alleles. Therefore, precise band sizing was critical to the accuracy of the results. A match implied inclusion, which was refined by determination of the genotype frequency of each allele in the general or local population. This process established likelihood of the same genotype occurring by chance. The probability of two people having the same set of RFLP, or **profile**, becomes lower and lower as more loci are analyzed.

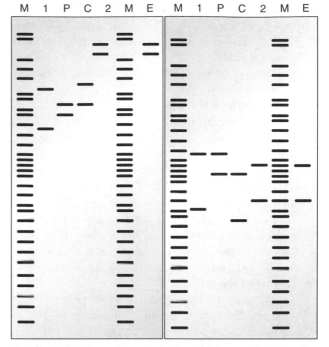

■ **Figure 11-7** Example of RFLP crime evidence using two single-locus probes. M are molecular weight markers, 1 and 2 are suspects, C is the child victim, and P is the parent of the child victim. E is evidence from the crime scene. For both loci probed, suspect 2 "matches" the evidence found at the crime scene. Positive identification of suspect 2 requires further determination of the frequencies of these specific alleles in the population and the probability of matching them by chance.

Historical Highlights

Professor Sir Alec John Jeffreys, a British geneticist, first developed techniques for **genetic profiling**, or **DNA fingerprinting**, using RFLP to identify humans. The technique has been used in forensics and law enforcement to resolve paternity and immigration disputes and can be applied to nonhuman species, for example, in wildlife population genetics. The initial application of this DNA technique was in a regional screen of human DNA to identify the rapist and killer of two girls in Leicestershire, England, in 1983 and 1986. Colin Pitchfork was identified and convicted of murder after samples taken from him matched semen samples taken from the two dead girls.

STR Typing by PCR

The first commercial and validated PCR-based typing test specifically for forensic use was the HLA DQ alpha system, now called DQA1, developed by Cetus Corporation in 1986.[7] This system could distinguish 28 DQA1 types. With the addition of another commercial system, the Polymarker (PM) system, the analyst could type five additional genetic markers. The PM system is a set of primers complementary to sequences flanking **short tandem repeats (STRs)**, or **microsatellites**. STRs are similar to VNTRs (minisatellites) but have repeat units of 1 to 7 base pairs. (The upper limit of repeat unit size for STR varies from 7 to 10 bp, depending on different texts and reports.) Because of the increased power of discrimination and ease of use of STR, the HLA DQA forensic DNA amplification and typing kit was discontinued in 2002.

The tandem repeat shown in Figure 11-6 is an STR with a 4-bp repeat unit, AGCT. Occasionally, STRs contain repeat units with altered sequences, or **microvariants**, repeat units missing one or more bases of the repeat. These differences have arisen through mutation or other genetic events.

In contrast to VNTRs, the smaller STRs are efficiently amplified by PCR, easing specimen demands significantly. Long, intact DNA fragments are not required to detect the STR products; therefore, degraded or otherwise less-than-optimal specimens are potentially informative. The amount of specimen required for STR analysis by PCR is reduced from 1 μg to 10 ng, a key factor for forensic analysis.[9] Furthermore, PCR procedures shorten the analysis time from several weeks to 24 to 48 hours. Careful design of primers and amplifications facilitated multiplexing and automation of the process.[10]

STR alleles are identified by PCR product size. Primers are designed to produce amplicons of 100 to 400 bp in which the STRs are embedded (Fig. 11-8). The sizes of the PCR products are influenced by the number of embedded repeats. If one of each primer pair is labeled with a fluorescent marker, the PCR product can be analyzed in fluorescent detection systems. Silver-stained gels may also be used; however, capillary electrophoresis with fluorescent dyes is the preferable method, especially for high-throughput requirements.

Advanced Concepts

At least three to seven RFLP probes were originally required to determine genetic identity. Available probes included G3, MS1, MS8, MS31, and MS43, which were subclones of Jeffreys' multilocus probes 33.6 and 33.15 and pYNH24m, MS205, and MS621.[8] Single-locus probes MS1, MS31, MS43, G3, and YNH24 were used by Cellmark in the O.J. Simpson trial in 1996.

A further development of **STR analysis** was the design of **MINI-STR**.[11] These STR are amplified with PCR primers located closer to the tandem repeat than in the standard STR. Compared with standard STR products, the small amplicons are more efficiently produced from such challenging starting material as fixed tissue[12] and degraded specimens.[13]

To perform genotyping, test DNA is mixed with the primer pairs, buffer, and polymerase to amplify the test loci. A control DNA standard is also amplified. Following amplification, each sample PCR product is combined with **allelic ladders** (sets of fragments representing all possible alleles of a repeat locus) and **internal size standards** (molecular-weight markers) in formamide for

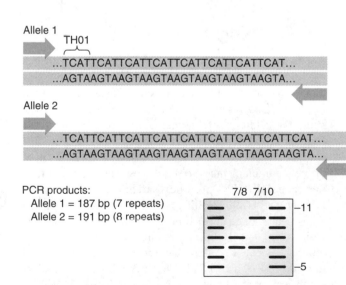

Allele 1

TH01

...TCATTCATTCATTCATTCATTCATTCATTCAT...
...AGTAAGTAAGTAAGTAAGTAAGTAAGTAAGTA...

Allele 2

...TCATTCATTCATTCATTCATTCATTCATTCATTCAT...
...AGTAAGTAAGTAAGTAAGTAAGTAAGTAAGTAAGTA...

PCR products:
   Allele 1 = 187 bp (7 repeats)
   Allele 2 = 191 bp (8 repeats)

7/8 7/10

—11

—5

■ **Figure 11-8** Short tandem repeat TH01 (repeat unit TCAT) linked to the human tyrosine hydroxylase gene on chromosome 11p15.5. Primers are designed to amplify short regions containing the tandem repeats. Allelic ladders consisting of all alleles in the human population (flanking lanes in the gel shown at bottom right) are used to determine the number of repeats in the locus by the size of the amplicon. The two alleles shown contain 7 and 8 repeats. If these alleles were found in a single individual, that person would be heterozygous for TH01 with a genotype of 7/8. Compare the 7/8 genotype pattern with the 7/10 genotype gel pattern.

Advanced Concepts

Theoretically, the minimal sample requirement for polymerase chain reaction analysis is a single cell. A single cell has approximately 6 pg of DNA. This number is derived from the molecular weight of A/T and G/C base pairs (617 and 618 g/mol, respectively). There are about 3 billion base pairs in one copy of the human genome; therefore, for one genome copy:

$$3 \times 10^9 \text{ bp} \times 618 \text{ g/mol/bp} = 1.85 \times 10^{12} \text{ g/mol}$$

$$1.85 \times 10^{12} \text{ g/mol} \times 1 \text{ mol}/6.023 \times 10^{23}$$
$$\text{molecules} = 3.07 \times 10^{-12} \text{ g} = 3 \text{ pg}$$

A diploid cell has two genome copies, or 6 pg of DNA. One ng (1000 pg) of DNA should, therefore, contain 333 copies (1000 pg/3pg/genome copy) of each locus.

electrophoresis. After electrophoresis, detection and analysis software will size and identify the alleles. In contrast to RFLPs and VNTRs, STRs are **discrete allele systems** in which a finite number of alleles are defined by the number of repeat units in the tandem repeat (see Fig. 11-8). Several available commercial systems consist of labeled primers for 1 to more than 16 loci. The allelic ladders in these reagent kits allow accurate identification of the sample alleles (Fig. 11-9).

Advances in fluorescence technology have increased the ease and sensitivity of STR allele identification (Fig. 11-10). Although capillary electrophoresis is faster and more automated than gel electrophoresis, a single run through a capillary of single dye-labeled products can resolve only loci whose allele ranges do not overlap. The number of loci that can be resolved on a single run was increased by the use of multicolor dye labels. Primer sets labeled with dyes that can be distinguished by their emission wavelength generate products that are resolved according to fluorescent color as well as size (Fig. 11-11).

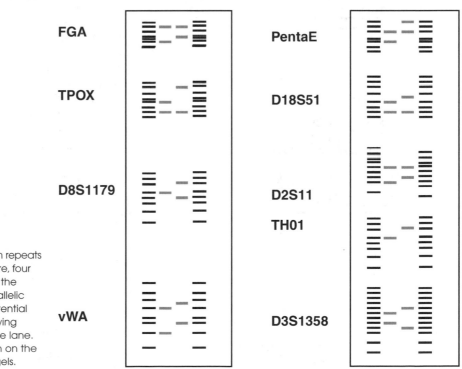

■ Figure 11-9 Multiple short tandem repeats can be resolved on a single gel. Here, four and five different loci are shown on the left and right gels, respectively. The allelic ladders show that the ranges of potential amplicon sizes do not overlap, allowing resolution of multiple loci in the same lane. Two individual genotypes are shown on the second and third lanes of the two gels.

Advanced Concepts

Commercial primer sets are designed with "stuffer" sequences to modify the size of the PCR products so that the range of alleles for four to five loci can be resolved by electrophoresis. The product size for a given allele will, therefore, not always be the same with primers from different commercial sources.

Test DNA amplicons, allelic ladders, and size standards for multiple loci are thus run simultaneously through each capillary. Genotyping software, such as GeneMapper (Applied Biosystems), STaR Call, and FMBIO Analysis Software (Hitachi Software Engineering), provide automated resolution of fluorescent dye colors and genotyping by comparison with the size standards and the allelic ladder.

STR by gel electrophoresis

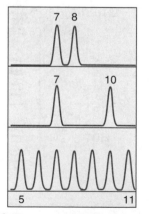

STR by capillary electrophoresis

■ **Figure 11-10** STR analysis by capillary gel electrophoresis. Instead of bands on a gel (top), peaks of fluorescence on an electropherogram reveal the PCR product sizes (bottom). Alleles (7, 8, or 10) are determined by comparison with allelic ladders run through the capillary simultaneously with the sample amplicons.

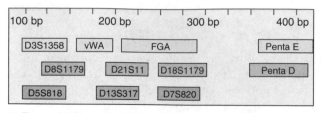

■ **Figure 11-11** An illustration of the ranges of allele peak locations for selected STRs. By labeling primers with different fluorescent dye colors (FAM, JOE, and NED), STRs with overlapping size ranges can be resolved by color. The molecular-weight markers (bottom) are labeled with the fluorescent dye ROX.

As in RFLP testing, an STR "match" is made by comparing profiles followed by probability calculations. The AmpliType HLA DQa Forensic DNA Amplification and Typing Kit (Promega) has been used in conjunction with the PM system to generate highly discriminatory allele frequencies. For example, the chance of a set of alleles occurring in two unrelated individuals at random is 1 in 10^6 to 7×10^8 Caucasians or 1 in 3×10^6 to 3×10^8 African Americans.

STR Nomenclature

The International Society for Forensic Genetics recommended nomenclature for STR loci in 1997.[14] STRs within genes are designated according to the gene name; for example, TH01 is in intron 1 of the human tyrosine hydroxylase gene on chromosome 11, and TPOX is in intron 10 of the human thyroid peroxidase gene on chromosome 2. These STRs do not have any phenotypic effect with respect to these genes. Non-gene-associated STRs are designated by the D#S# system. D stands for DNA; the following number designates the chromosome where the STR is located (1-22, X or Y). S refers to a unique segment, followed by a number registered in the International Genome Database (GDB). See Table 11.2 for some examples.

STRs are present all over the genome. Some of the STR loci commonly used for laboratory investigation are shown in Table 11.2. A comprehensive collection of STR information is available at http://cstl.nist.gov/biotech/strbase.

Gender Identification

The **amelogenin locus** is a very useful marker often analyzed along with STR. The amelogenin gene, which

Table 11.2 **STR Locus Information*[71]**

STR	Locus	Chromosome Sequence	Repeat	Alleles[†]
CD4	Locus between CD4 and triosephosphate isomerase	12p	AAAAG[‡]	4, 6, 7, 8, 8+, 9, 10, 11, 12, 13, 14, 15
CSF1PO	c-fms protooncogene for CSF-1 receptor	5q	TAGA	6, 7, 8, 9, 10, 11, 12, 13, 14, 15
D3S1358		3p	TCTA[§]	8, 9, 10, 11, 12, 13, 14, 15, 15+, 15.2, 16, 16+, 16.2, 17, 17+, 17.1, 18, 18.3, 19, 20
D5S818		5q	AGAT	7, 8, 9, 10, 11, 12, 13, 14
D7S829		7q	GATA	7, 8, 9, 10, 11, 12, 13, 14, 15
D8S1179	Sequence tagged site	8q	TCTA	7, 8, 9, 10, 11, 12, 13, 14, 15, 16, 17, 18, 19
D13S317		13q	TATC	7, 8, 9, 10, 11, 12, 13, 14, 15
D16S539		16q	GATA	5, 8, 9, 10, 11, 12, 13, 14, 15
D18S51	Sequenced tagged site	18q	GAAA	7, 8, 9, 10, 11, 12, 13, 14, 15, 16, 17, 18, 19, 20, 21, 22, 23, 24, 25, 26, 27
D21S11[‖]		21q	TCTG	24, 25, 26, 27, 28, 29, 30, 31, 32, 33, 34, 35, 36, 37, 38 F13A01
F13A01	Coagulation factor IX	6p	GAAA	3.2, 4, 5, 6, 7, 8, 9, 10, 11, 12, 13, 14, 15, 16
F13B	Factor XIII b	1q	TTTA	6, 7, 8, 9, 10, 11, 12
FESFPS	c-fes/fps protooncogene	15q	ATTT	7, 8, 9, 10, 11, 12, 13, 14
HPRTB	Hypoxanthine phosphoribosyl-transferase	Xq	TCTA	6, 7, 8, 9, 10, 11, 12, 13, 14, 15, 16, 17
LPL	Lipoprotein lipase	8p	TTTA	7, 8, 9, 10, 11, 12, 13, 14
TH01	Tyrosine hydroxylase	11p	TCAT	5, 6, 7, 8, 9, 9.3, 10, 11
TPOX	Thyroid peroxidase	2p	TGAA	6, 7, 8, 9, 10, 11, 12, 13
vWA	Von Willebrand factor	12p	TCTA	11, 12, 13, 14, 15, 16, 17, 18, 19, 20, 21
PentaD		21q	AAAGA	2.2, 3.2, 5, 7, 8, 9, 10, 11, 12, 13, 14, 15, 16, 17
PentaE		15q	AAAGA	5, 6, 7, 8, 9, 10, 11, 12, 13, 14, 15, 16, 17, 18, 19, 20, 20.3, 21, 22, 23, 24

*http://www.cstl.nist.gov/div831/strbase/index.htm.

[†]Some alleles have units with 1, 2, or 3 missing bases.

[‡]In an alternate 8-repeat allele, one repeat sequence is AAAGG.

[§]In alternate 15-, 16-, or 17-repeat alleles, one repeat sequence is TCTG.

[‖]D21S11 has multiple alternate alleles.

is not an STR, is located on the X and Y chromosomes. Its function is required for embryonic development and tooth maturation. The polymorphism is located in the second intron of the amelogenin gene. The Y allele of the gene is six base pairs larger in this region than in the X allele. Amplification and electrophoretic resolution reveals two bands or peaks for males (XY) and one band or peak for females (XX, Fig. 11-12). Some commercially available sets will contain primers to amplify the amelogenin polymorphism in addition to the STR primer sets.

Analysis of Test Results

Analysis of polymorphisms at multiple loci results in very high levels of discrimination (Table 11.3). Discovery of the same set of alleles from different sources or shared alleles between allegedly related individuals is

Advanced Concepts

The GDB is overseen by the Human Genome Nomenclature Committee, a part of the Human Genome Organization (HUGO) located at University College, London. HUGO was established in 1989 as an international association of scientists involved in human genetics. The goal of HUGO is to promote and sustain international collaboration in the field of human genetics. The GDB was originally used to organize mapping data during the earliest days of the Human Genome Project (see Chapter 10, "DNA Sequencing"). With the release of the human genome sequences and the development of polymerase chain reaction (PCR), the number of laboratories doing genetic testing has grown significantly. The GDB is still widely used as a source of information about PCR primers, PCR products, polymorphisms, and genetic testing. Information from GDB is available at http://www.ncbi.nlm.nih.gov/sites/genome.

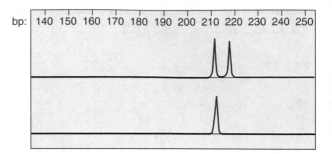

■ **Figure 11-12** Males are heterozygous for the amelogenin locus (XY, top), and females are homozygous for this locus (XX, bottom). Amplification of amelogenin will produce a male-specific 218-bp product (Y allele) in addition to the 212-bp product found on the X chromosome (X allele).

Advanced Concepts

In 1997 the Federal Bureau of Investigation adopted 13 "core" loci as the Combined DNA Indexing System (**CODIS**). The loci are TPOX on chromosome 2, D3S1358 on chromosome 3, FGA on chromosome 4, D5S818 and CSF1PO on chromosome 5, D7S820 on chromosome 7, D8S1179 on chromosome 8, TH01 on chromosome 11, vWA on chromosome 12, D13S317 on chromosome 13, D16S539 on chromosome 16, D18S51 on chromosome 18, D21S11 on chromosome 2, and the amelogenin locus on the X and Y chromosomes. The National Institute of Standards and Technology supplies Standard Reference Material that certifies values for 22 STR loci, including CODIS and markers used by European forensic laboratories. Profiler Plus (Life Technologies/Applied Biosystems) and PowerPlex (Promega) primer mixes include the CODIS loci.

strong evidence of identity, paternity, or relatedness. Results from such studies, however, must be expressed in terms of the background probability of chance matches.

DNA testing results in peak or band patterns that must be converted to genotype (allele identification) for comparison of results between laboratories. As described above, an STR **locus genotype** is defined by the number of repeats in the alleles. For instance, if the locus genotype in Figure 11-8 represented homologous chromosomes from an individual, the locus would be heterozygous, with 7 repeats on one chromosome and 8 repeats on the other. This locus would thus be designated 7/8 or 7,8. A homozygous locus (where both homologous chromosomes carry the same allele) is designated by the single number of repeats of that allele; for instance, 7/7 or 7,7. Some reports use a single number, such as 6 or 7, to designate a homozygous locus. Microvariant alleles containing partial repeat units are indicated by the number of

Table 11.3 **Matching Probability of STR Genotypes in Different Subpopulations**

	African American	White American	Hispanic American
8 loci	1/274,000,000	1/114,000,000	1/145,000,000
†9 loci	$1/5.18 \times 10^9$	$1/1.03 \times 10^9$	$1/1.84 \times 10^9$
*10 loci	$1/6.76 \times 10^{10}$	$1/9.61 \times 10^{10}$	
†12 loci	$1/4.61 \times 10^{12}$		
†14 loci	$1/6.11 \times 10^{17}$	$1/9.96 \times 10^{17}$	$1/1.31 \times 10^{17}$
†16 loci	$1/7.64 \times 10^{17}$	$1/9.96 \times 10^{17}$	$1/1.31 \times 10^{17}$

*AmpliSTR Identifiler Kit (Applied Biosystems)
†PowerPlex Systems (Promega)

complete repeats followed by a decimal point and then the number of bases in the partial repeat. For example, the 9.3 allele of the TH01 locus has 9 full 4-base-pair repeat units and 1 repeat unit with 3 base pairs. Microvariants are detected as bands or peaks very close to the full-length allele (Fig. 11-13).

The genotype, or profile, of a specimen is the collection of alleles in all the locus genotypes tested. To determine the extent of certainty that one profile matches another, the occurrence of the detected genotype in the general or a defined population must be assessed.

A matching genotype is not necessarily an absolute determination of the identity of an individual. **Genetic**

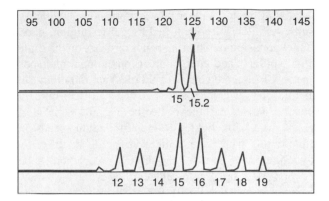

■ Figure 11-13 A microvariant allele (15.2, top) migrates between the full-length alleles (15 and 16 on the allelic ladder, bottom).

concordance is a term used to express the situation where all locus genotypes (alleles) from two sources are the same. Concordance is interpreted as inclusion of a single individual as the donor of both genotypes. Two samples are considered different if at least one locus genotype differs (**exclusion**). An exception is paternity testing, in which mutational events may generate a new allele in the offspring, and this difference may not rule out paternity.

Advanced Concepts

Alec Jeffreys' DNA profiling was the basis for the National DNA Database (NDNAD) launched in Britain in 1995. Under British law, the DNA profile of anyone convicted of a serious crime is stored on a database. This database includes 5.2% of the UK population (compared with 0.5% of the population in the U.S. database). Over 3.4 million DNA profiles are held in the database, accounting for a majority of the known active offender population. Nearly 60% of crime scene profiles submitted to the NDNAD were matched to a subject profile between 2008 and 2009. Created by the DNA Identification Act of 1994, the National DNA Index System (NDIS) is the federal level of the Combined DNA Indexing System (CODIS) used in the United States. There are three levels of CODIS: the Local DNA Index System (LDIS), State DNA Index System (SDIS), and NDIS. At the local level, CODIS software maintained by the Federal Bureau of Investigation (FBI) is used in sizing alleles as the assay is performed. This information may be applied locally and/or submitted to the SDIS. At the state level, interlaboratory searching occurs. The state data may be sent to the NDIS. The SDIS and NDIS must adhere to the quality assurance standards recommended by the FBI. The original entries to these databases were RFLP profiles; all future entries will be STR profiles. As of February 2010, the NDIS contained over 7,940,321 offender profiles and 306,028 forensic profiles.

Advanced Concepts

Artifact air bubbles, crystals, and dye blobs, as well as sample contaminants, temperature variations, and voltage spikes, can interfere with consistent band migration during electrophoresis. In addition, amplification artifacts occur during PCR. Some polymerases add an additional nontemplate adenine residue to the 3' end of the PCR product. If this 3' nucleotide addition does not include all the amplified products, a mixed set of amplicons will result in extra bands or peaks located very close together.

Stutter is another anomaly of PCR amplification, in which the polymerase may miss a repeat during the replication process, resulting in two or more different species in the amplified product. These also appear as extra bands or peaks. Generally, the larger the repeat unit length, the less stutter is observed. These or other aberrant band patterns confuse the analysis software and can result in the miscalling of alleles.

Matching requires clear and unambiguous laboratory results. As alleles are identified by gel resolution, good intragel precision (comparing bands or peaks on the same gel or capillary) and intergel precision (comparing bands or peaks of separate gels or capillaries) are important. In general, intergel precision is less stringent than intragel precision. This is not unexpected because the same samples may run with slightly different migration speeds on different gels. Since some microvariant alleles differ by only a single base pair (see Fig. 11-13), precision must be less than ±0.5 bp. Larger alleles, however, may show larger variation. The TH01 9.3 allele described above is an example. This allele must be distinguished from the 10 allele, which is a single base pair larger than the 9.3 allele.

To establish the identity of peaks from capillary electrophoresis (or peaks from densitometry tracings of gel data), the peak is assigned a position relative to some landmark within the gel lane or capillary, such as the loading well or the start of migration. Upon replicate resolutions of a band or peak, electrophoretic variations from capillary to capillary, lane to lane, or gel to gel may occur. Normalization of migration is achieved by relation of the migration of the test peaks to the simultaneous migration of size standards. Size standards can be internal (in the same gel lane or capillary) or external (in a separate gel lane). Even with normalization, however, tiny variations in position, height, and area of peaks or gel bands may persist. If the same fragments are run repeatedly, a distribution of observed sizes can be established. An acceptable range of sizes in this distribution is a **bin**. A bin can be thought of as an uncertainty window surrounding the mean position of multiple runs of each peak or band. All bands or peaks, therefore, that fall within this window are considered identical. Collection of all peaks or bands within a characteristic distribution of positions and areas is called **binning**.[15,16] Bins for each allele can be established manually in the laboratory. Alternatively, commercially available software has been designed to automatically bin and identify alleles.

All peaks within a bin are interpreted as representative of the same allele of a locus. Each band or peak in a genotype is binned and identified according to its migration characteristics. The group of bands or peaks makes up the characteristic pattern or profile of the specimen.

Advanced Concepts

Binning may be performed in different ways using replicate peak heights and positions. To calculate the probability that two peaks are representative of the same allele, the proportion of alleles that fall within the uncertainty window (bin) must be determined. This proportion is represented exactly in fixed bins and approximated in floating bins. The fixed bin approach is an approximation of the more conservative floating bin approach.[15,17] An alternative assessment of allele certainty is the use of **locus-specific brackets.** In this approach, artificial "alleles" are designed to run at the high and low limit of the expected allele size. Identical alleles are expected to fall within this defined bracket.[16]

Matching of Profiles

The number of loci tested must be taken into consideration in genotyping analysis. The more loci analyzed, the higher the probability that the locus genotype positively identifies an individual (**match probability**; see Table 11.3). Degraded, compromised, or mixed samples will affect the match probability, as all loci may not yield clear, informative results. Criteria for interpretation of results and determination of a true allele are established by each laboratory. These criteria should be based on validation studies and results reported from other laboratories. Periodic external proficiency testing is performed to confirm the accuracy of test performance.

Results from the analysis of polymorphisms are used to determine the probability of identity or inheritance of genetic markers or to **match** a particular marker or marker pattern. To establish the identity of an individual by an allele of a locus, the chance that the same allele could arise in the population randomly must be taken into account.

The frequency of a set of alleles or a genotype in a population is the product of the frequency of each allele separately (the **product rule**). The product rule can be applied because of **linkage equilibrium**. Linkage equilibrium assumes that the observed frequencies of haplotypes in a population is concordant with haplotype frequencies predicted by multiplying together the frequency of

Advanced Concepts

The certainty of a matching pattern increases with decreased frequency of alleles in the general population. Under defined conditions, the relative frequency of two alleles in a population remains constant. This is **Hardy-Weinberg equilibrium**, or the Hardy-Weinberg Law.[18] The population frequency of two alleles, p and q, can be expressed mathematically as

$$p^2 + 2pq + q^2 = 1.0$$

This equilibrium assumes a large population with random mating and no immigration, emigration, mutation, or natural selection. Under these circumstances, if enough individuals are assessed, a close approximation of the true allele frequency in the population can be determined

individual genetic markers in each haplotype and that loci are not associated with one another (genetically linked) in the genome. The overall frequency (OF) of a locus genotype consisting of *n* loci can be calculated as:

$$OF = F_1 \times F_2 \times F_3 \times \ldots F_n$$

where $F_{1 \ldots n}$ represents the frequency of each individual allele in the population.

Individual allele frequencies are determined by data collected from testing many individuals in general and defined populations. For example, at locus penta D on chromosome 21, the 5 allele has been previously determined to occur in 1 of 10 people in a theoretical population.

Advanced Concepts

In contrast to linkage equilibrium, **linkage disequilibrium (LD)** is discordance of the observed frequencies of haplotypes in a population and the predicted haplotype frequencies. LD indicates that markers are physically close to one another on the chromosomal DNA so that minimal recombination occurs between them, meaning they are linked. LD is used for mapping genetic loci.

At locus D7S829 on chromosome 7, the 8 allele has been previously observed in 1 of 50 people in the same population. The overall frequency of the profile containing the loci penta D 5 allele and D7S829 8 allele would be $1/10 \times 1/50 = 1/500$. That is, that genotype or profile would be expected to occur in 1 out of every 500 randomly chosen members of that population. As should be apparent, the more loci tested, the greater the certainty that the profile is unique to a single individual in that population; that is, the overall frequency of the profile is very low. The overall frequencies in Table 11.3 illustrate this point.

Allele frequencies differ between **subpopulations** or ethnic groups. Different allele frequencies in subpopulations are determined through study of each ethnic group.[19] As can be seen from the data in Table 11.3, there are differences in the polymorphic nature of alleles in different subpopulations.

When profile identification requires comparing the genotype of an unknown specimen with a known reference sample—for example, the genotype of evidence from a crime and the genotype of an individual from a database—the determination that the two genotypes match (are from the same person) is expressed in terms of a **likelihood ratio**. The likelihood ratio is the comparison of the probability that the two genotypes came from the same person with the probability that the two genotypes came from different persons, taking into account allele frequencies and linkage equilibrium in the population. A high likelihood ratio greater than 1 is an indication that the probability is more likely, whereas a likelihood ratio of less than 1 indicates that the probability is less likely. If a likelihood ratio is [1/(1/1000)] = 1000, the tested genotypes are 1000 times more likely to have come from the same person than from two randomly chosen members of the population. Or, in a random sampling of 100,000 members of a population, 100 people (100,000/1000) with the same genotype might be found.

A simplified illustration can be made from the penta D and D7S829 example above. Suppose the penta D 5 (1/10 allele frequency) and D7S829 8 (1/50 allele frequency) profiles were discovered in a specimen from an independent source. The likelihood that the penta D 5/D7S829 8 profile came from the tested individual is 1, having been directly determined. The likelihood that the same profile could come from someone else in the population is 1/500. The likelihood ratio is 1/(1/500), or 500. The specimen material is 500 times more likely to have come from the tested individual than from some other person in the population.

When comparing genotypes with those in a database looking for a match, it is important to consider whether the database is representative of a population or subpopulation, as allele frequencies will be different in differently defined groups. It is also important to consider whether the population is homogeneous (a random mixture) with respect to the alleles tested. Familial searches and forensic applications involving mass disasters or other complex mixtures of DNA involve analysis of partial or uncertain DNA genotypes. More advanced analyses are required for defining the likelihood in these cases.[20]

Allelic Frequencies in Paternity Testing

A paternity test is designed to choose between two hypotheses: The test subject is not the father of the tested child (H_0), or the test subject is the father of the tested child (H_1). Paternity is first assessed by observation of shared alleles between the alleged father and the child (Fig. 11-14). Identity of shared alleles is a process of matching, as described above for identity testing.

A **paternity index**, or likelihood ratio of paternity, is calculated for each locus in which the alleged father and the child share an allele. The paternity index is an expression of how many times more likely the child's allele is inherited from the alleged father than by random occurrence of the allele in the general population. An allele that occurs frequently in the population has a low paternity index; a rare allele has a high paternity index. Table 11.4 shows the paternity index for each of four loci.

Advanced Concepts

Peter Gill developed a forensic DNA identification method for minimal samples called low copy number analysis.[21] In contrast to standard DNA analysis that requires approximately 200 pg DNA, low copy number analysis is reportedly performed on less than 100 pg DNA (about 16 diploid cells). The method involves increasing the number of PCR cycles for amplification and fastidiously cleaned work areas. Although used in over 21,000 serious criminal cases since the 1990s, the validity of this technique has been questioned in recent appeal cases.[22] Assaying limited amounts of starting material may result in peak drop-outs (failed amplification of an allele) or drop-ins (mispriming of an allele). Furthermore, the heightened detection limit required for low amounts of target DNA raises the risk of contamination.[22]

The FESFPS 13 allele is rarer than the D 16S539 9 allele. In this example, the child is 5.719 times more likely to have inherited the 9 allele of locus D16S539 from the alleged father than from another random man in the population. Similarly, the child is 15.41 times more likely to have inherited the 13 allele of FESFPS from the alleged father than by random occurrence. When each tested locus is on a different chromosome (not linked), the inheritance or occurrence of each allele can be considered

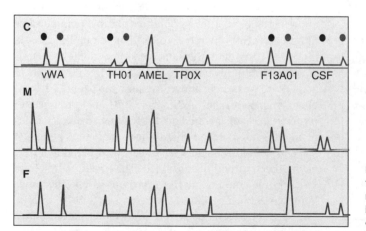

■ **Figure 11-14** Electropherogram showing results from five STR loci and the amelogenin locus for a child (C), mother (M), and father (F). Note how the child has inherited one of each allele from the mother (black dots) and one from the father (green dots).

Advanced Concepts

Thomas Bayes proposed a theory to predict the chance of a future event based on the observation of the frequency of that event in the past. Bayes's theorem was found among his papers in an article entitled "An Essay Towards Solving a Problem in the Doctrine of Chances" by the Reverend Thomas Bayes published by The Royal Society in 1763 (*Philosophical Transactions of the Royal Society*, volume 53, pp. 370–418, 1763). The article had been published posthumously. In it, Bayes developed his theorem about conditional probability:

$$P(A|B) = P(A) \times P(B|A)/P(B)$$

That is, the probability that A will occur, given that B has occurred (posterior odds), is equal to the probability that B has occurred given that A has occurred (**prior odds**) times the quotient of the separate probabilities of A and B (likelihood ratio). Bayes's theorem is used in paternity testing and genetic association studies.[23]

an independent event. The paternity index for each locus, therefore, can be multiplied together to calculate the **combined paternity index (CPI)**, which summarizes and evaluates the genotype information. The CPI for the data shown in Table 11.4 is

$$CPI = 5.719 \times 8.932 \times 15.41 \times 10.22 = 8044.931$$

This data indicates that the child is 8045 times more likely to have inherited the four observed alleles from the alleged father than from another man in the population.

If a paternal allele does not match between the alleged father and the child, H_1 for that allele is 0. One might

assume, therefore, that the nonmatching allele paternity index of 0 would make the CPI 0. This is not the case. Nonmatching alleles between the alleged father and the child found at one locus (exclusion) is traditionally not regarded as a demonstration of nonpaternity because of the possibility of mutation. Although mutations were quite rare in the traditional RFLP systems, analysis of 12 or more STR loci may occasionally reveal one or two mutations resulting in nonmatching alleles even if the man is the father. To account for mutations, the paternity index for nonmatching alleles is calculated as

paternity index for a mutant allele = μ

where μ is the observed mutation rate (mutations/meiosis) of the locus. The American Association of Blood Banks has collected data on mutation rates in STR loci (Table 11.5). Using these data, in the case of a non-matching allele, H_1 is not 0 but μ.

In a paternity report, the combined paternity index is accompanied by the **probability of paternity**, a number calculated from the paternity index (genetic evidence)

Table 11.4 **Example Data From a Paternity Test Showing Inclusion**

Alleged	Child	Father Allele	Shared Allele	Paternity Index
D16S539	8, 9	9, 10	9	5.719
D5S818	10, 12	7, 12	12	8.932
FESFPS	9, 13	13, 14	13	15.41
F13A01	4, 5	5, 7	5	10.22

Table 11.5 **Observed Mutation Rates in Paternity Tests Using STR Loci**

STR Locus	Mutation Rate (%)
D1S1338	0.09
D3S1358	0.13
D5S818	0.12
D7S820	0.10
D8S1179	0.13
D13S317	0.15
D16S539	0.11
D18S51	0.25
D19S433	0.11
D21S11	0.21
CSF1PO	0.16
FGA	0.30
TH01	0.01
TPOX	0.01
VWA	0.16
F13A01	0.05
FESFPS	0.05
F13B	0.03
LPL	0.05
Penta D	0.13
Penta E	0.16

and prior odds (nongenetic evidence). For the prior odds, the laboratory as a neutral party assumes a $^{50}/_{50}$ chance that the test subject is the father. The probability of paternity is, therefore,

$$\frac{CP \times prior\ odds}{(CPI \times prior\ odds) + (1 - prior\ odds)}$$

$$= \frac{CP \times 0.50}{(CPI \times 0.50) + (1 - 0.50)}$$

In the example illustrated previously, the CPI is 8,044.931. The probability of paternity is

$$\frac{8044.931 \times 0.50}{(8044.931 \times 0.50) + 0.50} = 0.999987$$

The genetic evidence (CPI) has changed the probability of paternity (prior odds) of 50% to 99.9987%.

There is some disagreement about the assumption of 50% prior odds. Using different prior odds assumptions changes the final probability of paternity (Table 11.6). As can be observed from the table, however, at a CPI over 100 the differences become less significant.

Sibling Tests

Polymorphisms are also used to generate a probability of siblings or other blood relationships (familial searches).[26] A sibling test is a more complicated statistical analysis than a paternity test.[27,28] A full sibling test is

Table 11.6 Odds of Paternity Using Different Prior Odds Assumptions

| CPI | Prior Odds | | | | |
	10%	25%	50%	75%	90%
5	0.36	0.63	0.83	0.94	0.98
9	0.50	0.75	0.90	0.96	0.98
19	0.68	0.86	0.95	0.98	0.994
99	0.92	0.97	0.99	0.997	0.999
999	0.99	0.997	0.999	0.9997	0.9999

a determination of the likelihood that two people tested share a common mother and father. A half-sibling test is a determination of the likelihood that two people tested share one common parent (mother or father). The likelihood ratio generated by a sibling test is sometimes called a **kinship index**, **sibling index**, or **combined sibling index**.

A test to determine the possibility of an aunt or uncle relationship, also known as **avuncular testing**, measures the probabilities that two alleged relatives are related as either an aunt or an uncle of a niece or nephew. The probability of relatedness is based on the number of shared alleles between the tested individuals. As with paternity and identity testing, allele frequency in the population will affect the significance of the final results. The probabilities can be increased greatly if other known relatives, such as a parent of the niece or nephew, are available for testing. Determination of first- and second-degree relationships is important for genetic studies because linkage mapping of disease genes in populations can be affected by undetected familial relationships.[29]

Y-STR

Unlike conventional STRs (**autosomal STRs**), where each locus is defined by two alleles, one from each parent, **Y-STRs** are represented only once per genome and only in males (Fig. 11-15). A set of Y-STR alleles comprises a **haplotype**, or series of linked alleles always inherited together. This is because the Y chromosome cannot exchange information (recombine) with the X chromosome or another Y chromosome. Thus, marker alleles on the Y chromosome are inherited from generation to generation in a single block. This means that the frequency of entire Y-STR profiles (haplotypes) in a given population can be determined by

---

Advanced Concepts

Based on studies showing that the majority of STR mutations are gains or losses of a single repeat,[24] Charles H. Brenner proposed that the paternity index for a mutant allele must take into account the nature of the mutation, that is, loss or gain of one or more repeats.[25] The loss of one repeat is much more likely in a single mutation event than the loss of two or more repeats. According to Brenner's formula:

Paternity index for a mutant allele = $\mu/(4\ P[Q])$ (for a single repeat difference)

Paternity index for a mutant allele = $\mu/(40\ P[Q])$ (for a two-repeat difference) and so forth.

P(Q) is the frequency or probability of occurrence of the normal allele, Q, in the population.

empirical studies. For example, if a combination of alleles (haplotype) was observed only two times in a test of 200 unrelated males, that haplotype is expected to occur with a frequency of approximately 1 in 100 males tested in the future. The discrimination power of Y-haplotype testing will depend on the number of subjects tested and will always be less definitive than that of autosomal STR.

Despite being a less powerful system for identification, STR polymorphisms on the Y chromosome have unique characteristics that have been exploited for forensic, lineage, and population studies as well as kinship testing.[30] Except for rare mutation events, every male member of a family (brothers, uncles, cousins, and grandfathers) will

have the same Y-chromosome haplotype. Thus Y-chromosome inheritance can be applied to lineage, population, and human migration studies. The **Y-STR/paternal lineage test** can determine whether two or more males have a common paternal ancestor. In addition to family history studies, the results of a paternal lineage test serve as supportive evidence for adoptees and their biological relatives or for individuals filing inheritance and Social Security benefit claims. As Y chromosomes are inherited intact, spontaneous mutations in the DNA sequence of the Y chromosome are used to follow human migration patterns and historical lineages. Y-chromosome genotyping has been used in studies designed to locate the geographical origin of all human beings.[31]

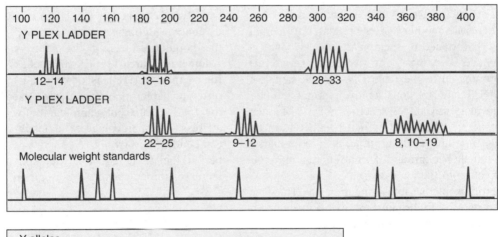

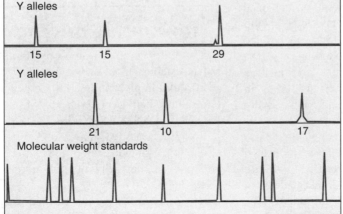

■ **Figure 11-15** Electropherogram showing allelic ladders for six STR loci in the Y-Plex 6 system (top panel) and a single haplotype (bottom panel). Molecular-weight standards are shown at the bottom of each.

As all male relatives in a family will share the same allele combination or profile, the statistical significance of a Y-STR DNA match cannot be assessed by multiplying likelihood ratios as was described above for autosomal STR. Instead of allele frequency used in autosomal STR match calculations, haplotype frequencies are used. Estimation of haplotype frequencies, however, is limited by the number of known Y haplotypes. This smaller data set accounts for the reduced inclusion probabilities and a discrimination rate that is significantly lower than that for autosomal STR polymorphisms. Traditional STR loci are, therefore, preferred for identity or relationship analyses, and the Y-STRs are used to aid in special situations; for instance, in confirming sibship between males who share commonly occurring alleles, that is, have a low likelihood ratio based on traditional STRs.

Y-STRs have been utilized in forensic tests where evidence consists of a mixture of male and female DNA, such as semen, saliva, other body secretions, or fingernail scrapings. For instance in specimens from evidence of rape, the female DNA may be in vast excess (more than 100-fold) compared to the male DNA in the sample.[32] Autosomal STR are not consistently informative under these circumstances. Using Y-specific primers, however, Y-STR can be specifically amplified by PCR from the male-female mixture, resulting in an analyzable marker that has no female background. This affords a more accurate identification of the male donor.

The Y chromosome has a low mutation rate. The overall mutation rate for Y chromosome loci is estimated at 1.72 to 4.27 mutations per thousand alleles.[24,33] Assuming that Y-chromosome mutations generally occur once every 500 generations/locus,[34] for 25 loci, 1 locus should have a mutation every 20 generations (500 generations/ 25 markers = 20 generations). Lineage testing over several generations is made possible by this low mutation rate. It is also useful for missing persons' cases in which reference samples can be obtained from paternally related males.

A list of informative Y-STRs is shown in Table 11.7. Several Y-STRs are located in regions that are duplicated on the Y chromosome. DSY389I and DSY389II are examples of a duplicated locus. A quadruplicated locus, DSY464, has also been reported.[35] Like autosomal STRs,

Y-STRs have microvariant alleles containing incomplete repeats and alleles containing repeat sequence differences. Reagent systems consisting of multiplexed primers for identification of Y-STRs are available commercially: for example, the Powerplex Y System, which contains 12 Y loci (Promega); the AmpliSTR Y-filer, which contains 17 Y loci (Life Technologies/Applied Biosystems); and the Y-Plex 6, which contains 6 Y loci (ReliaGene).

Matching with Y-STRs

Matching probabilities from Y-STR data are determined differently than for the autosomal STR. **Haplotype diversity (HD)** is calculated from the frequency of occurrence of a given haplotype in a tested population. The probability of two random males sharing the same haplotype is estimated at 1-HD; that is, if the haplotype diversity is high, the probability of two random males in the population having the same haplotype is low. Another measure of profile uniqueness, the **discriminatory capacity (DC)**, is determined by the number of different haplotypes seen in the tested population and the total number of samples in the population. DC expresses the percentage of males in a population who can be identified by a given haplotype. Just as the number of loci included in an autosomal STR genotype increases the power of discrimination, DC is increased

---

Advanced Concepts

The European Y chromosome typing community has established a set of Y-STR loci termed the **minimal haplotype** (see http://www.yhrd.org). The minimal haplotype consists of Y-STR markers DYS19, DYS389I, DYS389II, DYS390I, DYS391, DYS392, DYS393, and DYS385.[36] An "extended haplotype" includes all of the loci from the minimal haplotype plus the highly polymorphic dinucleotide repeat YCAII.

Table 11.7 **Y-STR Locus Information**[*72–74]

Y-STR	Repeat Sequence[†]	Alleles
DYS19	$[TAGA]_3 TAGG[TAGA]_n$	10, 11, 12, 13, 14, 15, 16, 17, 18, 19
DYS385	$[GAAA]_n$	7, 8, 9, 10, 11, 12, 13, 14, 15, 16, 16.3, 17, 17.2 17.3, 18, 19, 20, 21, 22, 23, 24, 28
DYS388	$[CAA]_n$	10, 11, 12, 13, 14, 15, 16, 17, 18
DYS389 I[‡]	$[TCTG]_q [TCTA]_r$	9, 10, 11, 12, 13, 14, 15, 16, 17
DYS389 II[‡]	$[TCTG]_n[TCTA]_p[TCTG]_q$ $[TCTA]_r$	26, 27, 28, 28', 29, 29', 29", 29''', 30, 30' 30", 30''', 31, 31', 31", 32, 32', 33, 34
DYS390	$[TCTG]_n[TCTA]_m[TCTG]_p$ $[TCTA]$	17,18, 19, 20, 21, 22, 23, 24, 25, 26, 27, 28
DYS391	$[TCTA]_n$	6, 7, 8, 9, 10, 11, 12, 13, 14
DYS392	$[TAT]_n$	6, 7, 8, 10, 11, 12, 13, 14, 15, 16, 17
DYS393	$[AGAT]_n$	9, 10, 11, 12, 13, 14
DYS426	$[CAA]_n$	6.2, 9, 10, 11, 12, 13, 14
DYS434	$[CTAT]_n$	8, 9, 10, 11
DYS437	$[TCTA]_n[TCTG]_2[TCTA]_4$	13, 14, 15, 16, 17
DYS438		
DYS439	$[TTTTC]_n$	6, 7, 8, 9, 10, 11, 12, 13, 14
DYS439	$[GATA]_n$	9, 10, 11, 12, 13, 14
(Y-GATA-A4)	$[GATA]_n$	9, 10, 11, 12, 13, 14
DYS441	$[CCTT]_n$	8, 10.1, 11, 11.1, 12, 13, 13.1, 14, 14.3, 15, 16, 17, 18, 19, 20
DYS442	$[TATC]_n$	8, 9, 10, 11, 12, 12.1, 13, 14, 15
DYS444	$[TAGA]_n$	9, 10, 11, 12, 13, 14, 15, 16
DYS445	$[TTTA]_n$	6, 7, 8, 9, 10, 10.1, 11, 12, 13, 14
DYS446	$[AGAGA]_n$	8, 9, 10, 11, 12, 13, 14, 15, 15.1, 16, 17, 18, 19, 19.1, 20, 21, 22, 23
DYS447	$[TTATA]_n$	15, 16, 17, 18, 19, 19.1, 20, 21, 22, 22.2, 22.4, 23, 24, 25, 26, 26.2, 27, 28, 29, 30, 31, 32, 33, 34, 35, 36
DYS448	$[AGAGAT]_n$	17, 19, 19.2, 20, 20.2, 20.4, 21, 21.2, 21.4, 22, 22.2, 23, 23.4, 24, 24.5, 25, 26, 27
DYS449	$[GAAA]_n$	23, 23.4, 24, 24.5, 25, 26, 27, 27.2, 28, 28.2, 29, 29.2, 30, 30.2, 31, 32, 32.2, 33, 33.2, 34, 35, 36, 37, 37.3, 38
DYS452	$[TATAC]_n$	24, 24, 25, 26, 27, 28, 29, 30, 31, 32, 33, 34, 35
DYS454	$[TTAT]_n$	6, 7, 8, 9, 10, 11, 12, 13
DYS455	$[TTAT]_n$	7, 8, 9, 10, 11, 12, 13
DYS456	$[AGAT]_n$	11, 12, 13, 14, 15, 16, 17, 18, 19, 20
DYS458	$[CTTT]_n$	12, 12.2, 13, 14, 15, 15.2, 16, 16.1, 16.2, 17, 17.2, 18, 18.2, 19, 19.2, 20, 20.2, 21
DYS460 (Y-GATA-A7.1)	$[ATAG]_n$	7, 8, 9, 10, 10.1, 11, 12, 13

[*]http://www.cstl.nist.gov/div831/strbase/index.htm.
[†]Some alleles contain repeats with 1, 2, or 3 bases missing.
[‡]DYS389 I and II is a duplicated locus.

by increasing the number of loci defining a haplotype. For instance, the loci tested in the Y-Plex 6 system can distinguish 82% of African American males. Using 22 loci raises the DC to almost 99% (Table 11.8).

As there is no recombination between loci on the Y chromosome, the product rule cannot be applied. The results of a Y typing might be reported accompanied by the number of observations or frequency of the analyzed haplotype in a database of adequate size. Suppose a haplotype containing the 17 allele of DYS390 occurs in only 23% of men in a database of 12,400. However, if that same haplotype contains the 21 allele of DYS446, only 6% of the men will have haplotypes containing both the DYS390 17 and DYS446 21 alleles. If the 11 allele of DYS455 and the 15 allele of DYS458 are also present, only 1 out of 12,400 men in the population has a haplotype containing all four alleles. The uniqueness of this haplotype is strong evidence that a match is not the result of a random coincidence, which gives extra support to the hypothesis that an independent source with this haplotype comes from an individual or a paternal relative. Even with a 99.9% DC, however, the matching probability is orders of magnitude lower than that for autosomal STR.

Y-chromosome haplotypes can be used to exclude paternity. Taking into account the mutation rate of each allele, any alleles that differ between the male child and the alleged father are strong evidence for nonpaternity. Conversely, if a Y haplotype is shared between a child and alleged father, a paternity index is calculated in a manner similar to that of the autosomal STR analysis. For example, suppose 6 Y-STR alleles are tested and match between the alleged father and child. If the haplotype has not been observed before in the population, the occurrence of that haplotype in the population database is 0/1200, and the haplotype frequency will be 1/1200, or 0.0008333. The paternity index (PI) is the probability that a man with that haplotype could produce one sperm carrying the haplotype, divided by the probability that a random man could produce one sperm carrying the haplotype. The PI is then 1/0.0008333 = 1200. With a prior probability of 0.5, the probability of paternity is $(1200 \times 0.5)/[(1200 \times 0.5) + 0.5]$, or 99.9%. This result, however, does not exclude patrilineal relatives of the alleged father.

Y-STRs as marker loci for Y-chromosome, or **surname**, tests are used to determine ancestry. For example, a group of males of a strictly male descent line (having the same last name or surname) is expected to be related to a common male ancestor. Therefore, they should all share the same Y-chromosome alleles (except for mutations, which should be minimal, given 1 mutation per 20 generations, as explained above). The Y-chromosome haplotype does not provide information about degree of relatedness, just inclusion or exclusion from the family. An analysis to find a most recent common ancestor (MRCA) is possible, however, using a combination of researched family histories, Y-STR test results, and statistical formulas for mutation frequencies.

Bone Marrow Engraftment Testing Using DNA Polymorphisms

Bone marrow transplantation is a method used to treat malignant and nonmalignant blood disorders as well as some solid tumors. One transplant approach is **autologous** (from self), in which cells from the patient's own bone marrow are removed and stored. The patient then receives high doses of chemotherapy and/or radiotherapy. The portion of marrow previously removed from the patient may also be purged of cancer cells before being returned to the patient. Alternatively, **allogeneic**

Table 11.8 **Discriminatory Capacity of Y-STR Genotypes in Different Subpopulations**[75]

	African American (%)	White American (%)	Hispanic American (%)
*6 loci	82.3	68.9	78.3
†9 loci	84.6	74.8	85.1
‡11 loci	91.3	83.8	90.3
§17 loci	99.1	98.8	98.3
‖20 loci	98.5	97.2	98.6
#22 loci	98.9	99.6	99.3

*Y-Plex 6 (DYS19, DYS390, DYS391, DYS393, DYS389II, and DYS385)
†European minimal haplotype
‡Minimal haplotype + SWGDAM
§AmpliSTR Y-filer as reported by Applied Biosystems
‖Y-STR 20 plex (Minimal haplotype plus DYS388, DYS426, DYS437, DYS439, DYS460, H4, DYS438 DYS447, and DYS448)
#Y-STR 22 plex

transplants (between two individuals) are used. The donor supplies healthy cells to the recipient patient (Fig. 11-16). Donor cells are supplied as bone marrow, peripheral blood stem cells (also called **hematopoietic stem cells**), or umbilical cord blood. To assure successful establishment of the transplanted donor cells, the immune compatibility of the donor and recipient is tested prior to the transplant by HLA typing (see Chapter 15, "DNA-Based Tissue Typing").

In myeloablative transplant strategies, high doses of therapy completely remove the recipient bone marrow, particularly the stem cells that give rise to all the other cells in the marrow (conditioning). The allogeneic or autologous stem cells are then expected to re-establish a new bone marrow in the recipient (**engraftment**). The toxicity of this procedure is reduced by using

Autologous bone marrow transplant

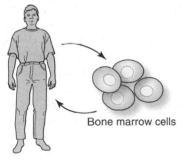

Bone marrow cells

Allogeneic bone marrow transplant

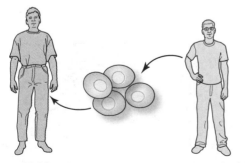

■ **Figure 11-16** In autologous bone marrow transplant (top), bone marrow cells are taken from the patient, purged, and returned to the patient after conditioning treatment. In allogeneic transplant (bottom), bone marrow cells are taken from another genetically compatible individual (donor) and given to the patient.

nonmyeloablative transplant procedures or minitransplants. In this approach, pretransplant therapy will not completely remove the recipient bone marrow. The donor bone marrow is expected to eradicate the remaining recipient cells through recognition of residual recipient cells as foreign to the new bone marrow. This process also imparts a graft-versus-leukemia or **graft-versus-tumor (GVT) effect**, which is a process closely related to **graft-versus-host disease (GVHD)**. The T-cell fraction of the donor marrow is particularly important for engraftment and for GVT effect. Efforts to avoid GVHD by removing the T-cell fraction before infusion of donor cells has resulted in increased incidence of graft failure and relapse.

The first phase of allogeneic transplantation is donor matching, in which potential donors are tested for immunological compatibility. This is performed by examining the human leukocyte antigen (HLA) locus (see Chapter 15, "DNA-Based Tissue Typing") to determine which donor would be most tolerated by the recipient immune system. Donors may be known or related to the patient or anonymous unrelated contributors (**matched unrelated donor [MUD]**).

Stem cells may also be acquired from donated umbilical cord blood. After conditioning and infusion with the donor cells, the patient enters the engraftment phase, in which the donor cells reconstitute the recipient's bone marrow. Once a successful engraftment of donor cells is established, the recipient is a genetic **chimera**; that is, the recipient has body and blood cells of separate genetic origins.

The engraftment of donor cells in the recipient must be monitored, especially in the first 90 days after the transplant. This requires distinguishing between donor cells and recipient cells. Historically, red blood cell phenotyping, immunoglobulin allotyping, HLA typing, karyotyping, and fluorescence in situ hybridization have been used for this purpose. Each of these methods has drawbacks. Some require months before engraftment can be detected. Others are labor-intensive or restricted to sex-mismatched donor-recipient pairs.

DNA typing has become the method of choice for engraftment monitoring.[37,38] Because all individuals, except identical twins, have unique DNA polymorphisms, donor cells are monitored by following donor polymorphisms in the recipient blood and bone marrow. Although RFLP can effectively distinguish donor and recipient cells, the detection of RFLP requires use of the

Advanced Concepts

Chimerism is different from mosaicism. A chimera is an individual carrying two populations of cells that arose from different zygotes. In a **mosaic**, cells arising from the same zygote have undergone a genetic event, resulting in two clones of phenotypically different cells in the same individual.

Southern blot method, which is too labor-intensive and has limited sensitivity for this application. In comparison, small VNTRs and STRs are easily detected by PCR amplification of VNTRs and STRs (see Fig. 11-9), which is preferable because of the increased rapidity and the 0.5% to 1% sensitivity achievable with PCR. Sensitivity can be raised to 0.01% using Y-STR, but this approach is limited to those transplants from sex-mismatched donor-recipient pairs, preferably from a female donor to a male recipient.[39,40]

In the laboratory, there are two parts to engraftment/chimerism DNA testing. Before the transplant, several polymorphic loci in the donor and recipient cells must be screened to find at least one **informative locus**, that is, one locus in which donor alleles differ from the recipient alleles. **Noninformative loci** are those in which the donor and the recipient have the same alleles. In donor-informative loci, donor and recipient share one allele for which the donor is heterozygous and the donor has a unique allele. Conversely, in recipient-informative loci, the unique allele is in the recipient (Fig. 11-17). The

second part of the testing process is the engraftment analysis, which is performed at specified intervals after the transplant. In the engraftment analysis, the recipient blood and bone marrow are tested to determine the presence of donor cells using the informative and/or recipient-informative loci.

Pretransplant analysis and engraftment were measured in early molecular studies by amplification of small VNTRs and resolution of amplified fragments on polyacrylamide gels with silver-stain detection.[41] Before the transplant, the screen for informative loci was based on band patterns of the PCR products, as illustrated in Figure 11-17. After the transplant, analysis of the gel band pattern from the blood or bone marrow of the recipient revealed one of three different states: **full chimerism**, in which only the donor alleles were detected in the recipient; **mixed chimerism**, in which a mixture of donor and recipient alleles was present, or **graft failure**, in which only recipient alleles were detectable (Fig. 11-18).

Currently, the prefered method is PCR amplification of STRs, resolution by capillary electrophoresis, and fluorescent detection. This procedure provides ease of use, accurate quantitation of the percentage of donor/recipient cells, and high sensitivity with minimal sample requirements.

Donor and recipient DNA for allele screening prior to transplant can be isolated from blood or buccal cells. One ng of DNA is reportedly sufficient for the screening of multiple loci; however, 10 ng is a more practical lower

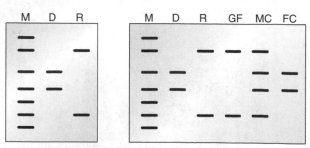

Figure 11-18 Band patterns after PAGE analysis of VNTR. First, before the transplant, several VNTR must be screened to find informative loci that differ in pattern between the donor and recipient. One such marker is shown at left (M = molecular-weight marker, D = donor, R = recipient). After the transplant, the band patterns can be used to distinguish between graft failure (GF), mixed chimerism (MC), or full chimerism (FC).

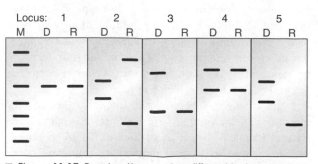

Figure 11-17 Band patterns of five different loci comparing donor (D) and recipient (R) genotypes. The second and fifth loci are informative. The first and fourth loci are noninformative. The third locus is donor-informative.

Advanced Concepts

A more defined condition can be uncovered by cell type separation. Some cell fractions such as granulocytes engraft before others. For example, isolated granulocytes may show full chimerism while the T-cell fraction still shows mixed chimerism. This is a case of **split chimerism**.

limit. Multiple loci can be screened simultaneously using multiplex PCR. Although not validated for engraftment testing, several systems designed for human identification are used for this purpose. Primer sets that specifically amplify Y-STR may also be useful for sex-mismatched donor-recipient pairs. Figure 11-19 shows the five tetramethylrhodamine (TMR)-labeled loci from the PowerPlex® system used for identity testing. A total of nine loci are amplified simultaneously by this set of multiplexed primers. Although multiplex primer systems are optimized for consistent results, all loci may not amplify with equal efficiency in a multiplex reaction. For example, the amelogenin locus in Figure 11-19 did not amplify as well as the other four loci in the multiplex. This is apparent from the lower peak heights in the amelogenin products compared with the products of the other primers.

Although the instrumentation used for this method is the same as that used for sequence analysis (see Chapter 10, "Nucleic Acid Sequencing"), investigating peak sizes and peak areas is distinguished from sequence analysis as **fragment analysis** and sometimes requires adjustment of the instrument or capillary polymer. Automatic detection will generate an electropherogram, as shown in Figure 11-20. Informative and noninformative loci will appear as nonmatching or matching donor and recipient peaks, respectively, and many combinations of donor-recipient peaks are possible. Optimal loci for analysis should be clean peaks without **stutter**, especially stutter peaks that comigrate with informative peaks, nonspecific amplified peaks (misprimes), or other technical artifacts.[42]

Ideally, the chosen locus should have at least one recipient informative allele. This is to assure direct detection of minimal amounts of residual recipient cells. If the recipient is male and the donor is female, the amelogenin locus supplies a recipient-informative locus. Good

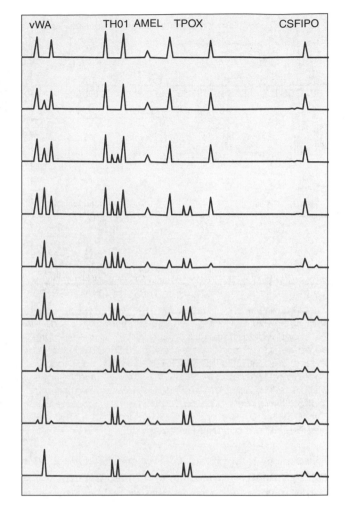

Figure 11-19 Multiplex PCR of DNA mixtures from two unrelated individuals (top and bottom trace) showing peak patterns for vWA, TH01, Amelogenin, TPOX, and CSF1PO loci. The center traces are stepwise mixtures of the two genotypes.

separation (ideally, but not necessarily, by two repeat units) of the recipient and donor alleles is desirable for ease of discrimination in the post-transplant testing. The choices of informative alleles are more limited in related donor-recipient pairs, as they are likely to share alleles. Unrelated donor-recipient pairs, on the other hand, will yield more options.

After the transplant, the recipient is tested on a schedule determined by the clinician or according to consensus recommendations.[43] With nonmyeloablative or reduced-intensity pretransplant protocols, testing is recommended at 1, 3, 6, and 12 months. Because early patterns of

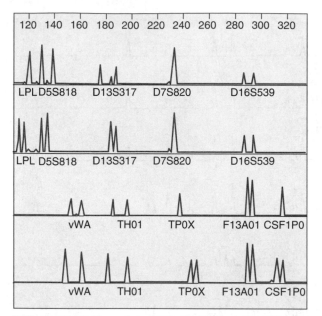

120 140 160 180 200 220 240 260 280 300 320

LPL D5S818   D13S317   D7S820   D16S539

LPL D5S818   D13S317   D7S820   D16S539

vWA   TH01   TPOX   F13A01 CSF1PO

vWA   TH01   TPOX   F13A01 CSF1PO

■ **Figure 11-20** Screening of 16 loci for informative STR alleles. Recipient peak patterns (first, third, and fifth traces) are compared with donor patterns (second, fourth, and sixth traces). The loci are: D3S1358, THO1, D21S11, D18S51, Penta E (top two traces), Amelogenin, vWA, D8S1179, TPOX, FGA (middle traces), D5S818, D13S317, D7S870, D16S539, CSF1PO, and Penta D (bottom two traces). D3S1358, D21S11, Penta E, Amelogenin, FGA, D13S317, D7S820, and D16S539 are informative. THO1 and Penta D are donor-informative.

engraftment may predict GVHD or graft failure after non**myeloblative** treatments, even more frequent blood testing may be necessary, such as at 1, 2, and 3 months after transplant. Bone marrow specimens can most conveniently be taken at the time of bone marrow biopsy following the transplant, with blood specimens taken in intervening periods. Usually, 3 to 5 mL of bone marrow or 5 mL of blood is more than sufficient for analysis; however, specimens collected soon after the transplant may be hypocellular, so larger volumes (5 to 7 mL bone marrow, 10 to 20 mL blood) may be required.

Quantification of percent recipient and donor cells post-transplant is performed using the informative locus or loci selected during the pretransplant informative analysis. The raw data for these calculations are the areas under the peaks generated by the PCR products after amplification. The emission from the fluorescent dyes attached to the primers and thus to the ends of the PCR products is collected as each product migrates

past the detector. The fluorescent signal is converted into fluorescence units by the computer software. The software displays the PCR products as peaks of fluorescence units (y-axis) vs. migration speed (x-axis). The amount of fluorescence in each product or peak is represented as the area under the peak. This number is provided by the software and is used to calculate the percent recipient and donor cells (Fig. 11-21).

There are several formulae for percent calculations, depending on the configuration of the donor and recipient peaks. For homozygous or heterozygous donor and recipient peaks with no shared alleles, the percent recipient cells is equal to $R/(R + D)$, where R is the area under the recipient-specific peak(s) and D is the area under the donor-specific peak(s). Shared alleles, where one allele is the same for donor and recipient (Fig. 11-20), can be dropped from the calculation, and the percent recipient cells is calculated as

$$\frac{R_{(unshared)}}{(R_{(unshared)} + D_{(unshared)})}$$

Chimerism/engraftment results are reported as percent recipient cells and/or percent donor cells in the bone

Advanced Concepts

Positive or negative selection techniques may be used to test specific cell lineages. For example, analysis of the T-cell fraction separately is used to monitor graft-versus-tumor potential. T cells may comprise 10% of peripheral blood leukocytes and 3% of bone marrow cells following allogeneic transplantation. Analysis of unfractionated blood and especially bone marrow where all other lineages are 100% could miss split chimerism in the T-cell fraction. T-lineage-specific chimerism will therefore increase the sensitivity of the engraftment analysis, particularly after nonmyeloablative and immunoablative pretransplant treatments.

T cells are conveniently separated from whole blood using magnetized polymer particles (beads), such as MicroBeads (MicroBeads AS), DynaBeads (Dynal), or EasySep (StemCell Technologies), attached to pan-T antibodies (anti-CD3). To isolate T cells using beads, white blood cells isolated by density gradient centrifugation are mixed with the beads in saline or phosphate-buffered saline and incubated to allow the antibodies on the beads to bind to the CD3 antigens on the T-cell surface. With the beads, T cells are immobilized by a magnet that is applied to the outside of the tube and the supernatant containing non-T cells is decanted. After another saline wash, the T cells are collected and lysed for DNA isolation. It is not necessary to detach the T cells from the beads.

Automated cell sorter systems such as the autoMACS separator (Miltenyi Biotec) may also be used for this purpose. With a positive selection program, the instrument is capable of isolating up to 2×10^8 pure T cells per separation. Unwanted cells can be removed with the depletion programs.

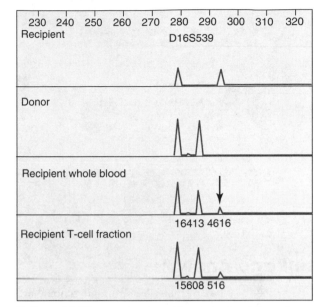

■ Figure 11-21 Postengraftment analysis of an informative locus D16S539. The area (fluorescence units) under the peaks is calculated automatically. The recipient and donor patterns are shown in the first and second trace, respectively. Results from the whole blood and T-cell fraction are shown in the third and fourth traces. For D16S539 the formula, $R_{(unshared)}/(R_{(unshared)} + D_{(unshared)})$ yields $4616/(4616 + 16{,}413) \times 100 = 22\%$ recipient cells in the unfractionated blood (arrow) and $516/(516 + 15{,}608) \times 100 = 3.3\%$ recipient cells in the T-cell fraction.

Time trends may be more important than single-point results following transplantation.

Because cell lineages engraft with different kinetics, testing of blood and bone marrow may yield different levels of chimerism. Bone marrow will contain more myeloid cells, and blood will contain more lymphoid cells. The first determination to be made from engraftment testing is whether donor engraftment has occurred and secondly whether there is mixed chimerism. In mixed chimerism, cell separation techniques may be used to determine which lineages are mixed and which are fully donor. Nonmyeloablative conditioning of the transplant recipients requires monitoring of both myeloid and lymphoid cell engraftment. This information may be determined by positive or negative lineage separation of whole blood (see the Advanced Concepts box that discusses cell lineage) or by testing blood and bone marrow.

marrow, blood, or cell fraction. These results do not reflect the absolute cell number, which could change independently of the donor/recipient ratio. Inability to detect donor or recipient cells does not mean that that cell population is completely absent, as capillary electrophoresis and fluorescent detection methods offer a sensitivity of 0.1% to 1% for autosomal STR markers.

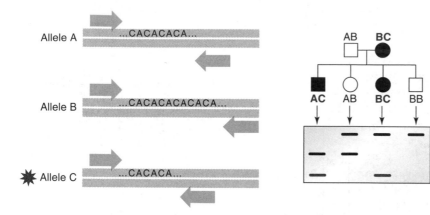

Figure 11-22 Linkage analysis with STRs. Three alleles, A, B, and C, of an STR locus are shown (left). At right is a family pedigree showing assortment of the alleles along with gel analysis of PCR amplification products. Allele C is present in all affected family members. This supports the linkage of this STR with the gene responsible for the disease affecting the family. Analysis for the presence of allele C of this STR may also provide a simple indicator to predict inheritance of the affected gene.

Linkage Analysis

Because the locations of many STRs in the genome are known, these structures can be used to map genes, especially those genes associated with disease. Three basic approaches are used to map genes: family histories, population studies, and sibling analyses.

Family history and analysis of generations of a single family for the presence of a particular STR allele in affected individuals is one way to show association. Family members are tested for several STRs, and the alleles of affected and unaffected members of the family are compared. Assuming normal Mendelian inheritance, if a particular allele of a particular locus is always present in affected family members, that locus must be closely linked to the gene responsible for the phenotype in those individuals (linkage disequilibrium; Fig. 11-22). If the linkage is close enough to the gene (no recombination between the STR and the disease gene), the STR may serve as a convenient target for disease testing. Instead of

testing for mutations in the disease gene, the marker allele is determined. It is easier, for example, to look for a linked STR allele than to screen a large gene for point mutations. The presence of the "indicator" STR allele serves as a genetic marker for the disease (Fig. 11-23).

Another approach to linkage analysis is to look for gene associations in large numbers of unrelated individuals in population studies. Just as with family history studies, close linkage to specific STR alleles supports the genetic proximity of the disease gene with the STR. In this case, however, large numbers of unrelated people are tested for linkage rather than a limited number of related individuals in a family. The results are expressed in probability terms that an individual with the linked STR allele is likely to have the disease gene.

Sibling studies are another type of **linkage analysis**. Monozygotic (identical) and dizygotic (fraternal) twins serve as controls for genetic and environmental studies. Monozygotic twins will always have the same genetic alleles, including disease genes. There should be 100%

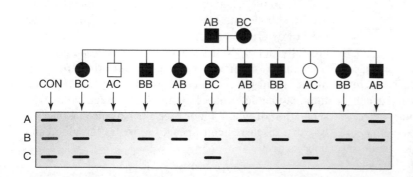

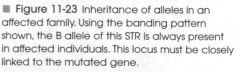

Figure 11-23 Inheritance of alleles in an affected family. Using the banding pattern shown, the B allele of this STR is always present in affected individuals. This locus must be closely linked to the mutated gene.

recurrence risk (likelihood) that if one twin has a genetic disease, the other twin has it, and both should have the same linked STR alleles. Fraternal twins have the same likelihood of sharing a gene allele as any sibling pair. Investigation of adoptive families may also distinguish genetic from environmental or somatic effects.

Quality Assurance for Surgical Sections Using STR

Personnel in the molecular diagnostics laboratory can assist in assuring that surgical tissue sections are properly identified and not contaminated. During processing of tissue specimens, microscopic fragments of tissue may persist in paraffin baths (floaters).[44] These fragments can adhere to subsequent tissue sections, resulting in anomalous appearance of the tissue under the microscope. If a tissue sample is questioned, STR identification can be used to confirm the origin of tissue.[45,46]

For this procedure, the suspect tissue must be carefully removed from the slide by microdissection. Reference DNA isolated from the patient and DNA isolated from the tissue in question are subjected to multiplex PCR. The results are compared for matching alleles. If the tissue in question originated from the patient, all alleles should match. Assuming good-quality data, one nonmatching locus excludes the tissue in question as coming from the reference patient.

An example of such a case is shown in Figure 11-24. A uterine polyp was removed from a patient for microscopic examination. An area of malignant tissue was present on the slide. The pathologists were suspicious about the malignancy as there was no other malignant tissue observed in other sections. The tissue fragment was microdissected from the thin section and tested at nine STR loci. The allelic profile was compared to reference DNA from the patient. The profiles were identical, confirming that the tissue fragment was from the patient.

Single Nucleotide Polymorphisms

Data from the Human Genome Project revealed that the human nucleotide sequence differs every 1000 to 1500 bases from one individual to another.[47] The majority of these sequence differences are variations of single nucleotides, or SNPs. The traditional definition of polymorphism requires

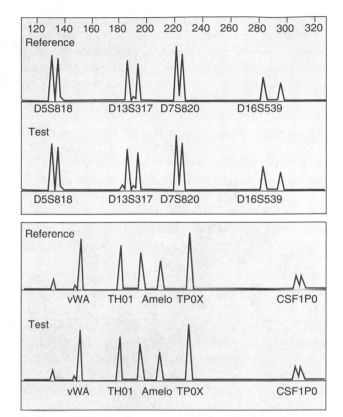

■ Figure 11-24 Quality assurance testing of a tissue fragment. The STR profile of the fragment in question (test) was compared with that of reference DNA from the patient. The alleles matched at all loci, supporting genotypic identity of the test material with the patient.

that the genetic variation be present at a frequency of at least 1% of the population. The International SNP Map Working Group observed that two haploid genomes differ at 1 nucleotide per 1331 bp.[48] This rate, along with the theory of neutral changes expected in the human population, predicts 11 million sites in a genome of 3 billion bp that vary in at least 1% of the world's population. In other words, each individual has 11 million SNPs.

Due to the density of SNPs across the human genome, these polymorphisms were of great interest for genetic mapping, disease prediction, and human identification. The problem was that detection of single base-pair changes was not as easy as detection of STRs, VNTRs, or even RFLPs.

With improving technology, mapping studies are achieving denser coverage of the genome.[49] The most definitive way to detect SNPs has been by direct sequencing. A number of additional methods were subsequently designed to detect single nucleotide polymorphisms (see Chapter 9, "Gene Mutations"). Computer analysis is also required to confirm that the population frequency of the SNPs meets the requirements of a polymorphism. So far, approximately 5 million SNPs have been identified in the human genome. Almost all (99%) of these have no biological effect. Over 60,000, however, are within genes, and some are associated with disease. A familiar example is the single nucleotide polymorphism responsible for the formation of hemoglobin S in sickle cell anemia. SNPs have been classified according to location, relation to coding sequences, and whether they cause a conservative or nonconservative sequence alteration (Table 11.9).

In 1999, the SNP Consortium (TSC) was established as a public resource of SNP data. The original goal of TSC was to discover 300,000 SNPs in 2 years, but the final results exceeded 1.4 million SNPs released into the public domain by the end of 2001. Since SNPs, with their denser coverage of the genome, are especially attractive markers for genetic variation and disease association studies,[50,51] the next phase in SNP analysis is the study of SNPs and SNP frequencies in populations.

The Human Haplotype Mapping (HapMap) Project

Despite the presence of numerous polymorphisms, any two people are 99.5% identical at the DNA sequence level. Understanding the 0.5% difference is important, in part because these differences may be the basis of differences in disease susceptibility and other variations among "normal" human traits. The key to finding the

genetic sources of these variations depends on identification of closely linked markers or landmarks throughout the genome. Genes, RFLPs, VNTRs, STRs, and other genetic structures have been mapped previously; however, long stretches of DNA sequence are yet to be covered with high density. Closely linked markers allow accurate mapping of regions associated with phenotypic characteristics.

Blocks of closely linked SNPs on the same chromosome tend to be inherited together; that is, recombination rarely takes place within these sequences (linkage disequilibrium). The groups of SNPs comprise haplotypes. In the human genome, SNP haplotypes tend to be approximately 20,000 to 60,000 bp of DNA sequence containing up to 60 SNPs (Fig. 11-25). Furthermore, as all of the SNPs in the haplotype are inherited together, the entire haplotype can be identified by only a subset of the SNPs in the haplotype. This means that up to 60,000 bp of sequence can be identified through detection of four or five informative SNPs, or **tag SNPs**.[52]

SNP haplotypes offer great potential for mapping of disease genes. A mutation responsible for a genetic disease originally occurs in a particular haplotype, the **ancestral haplotype**. Over several generations, the disease allele and the SNPs closest to it (the haplotype) tend to be inherited as a group. This haplotype, therefore, should always be present in patients with the disease. The genetic location and the identification of any disease gene can thus be ascertained, by association with a SNP haplotype. There is, therefore, much interest in developing a haplotype map of the entire human genome.

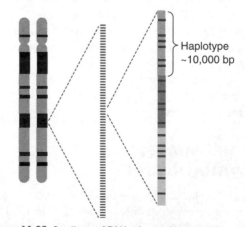

■ **Figure 11-25** Sections of DNA along chromosomes can be inherited as a unit or block of sequence in which no recombination occurs. All the SNPs on that block comprise a haplotype.

Table 11.9 **Types of SNP**

SNP	Region	Alteration
Type I	Coding	Nonconservative
Type II	Coding	Conservative
Type III	Coding	Silent
Type IV	Noncoding 5' UTR*	
Type V	Noncoding 3' UTR	
Type VI	Noncoding, other	

*Untranslated region

To this end, the Human Haplotype Mapping project was initiated in October 2002, with a target completion date of September 2005.[53,54] The goal of the project is to map the common patterns of SNPs in the form of a haplotype map, or HapMap. An initial draft of the HapMap was completed before the deadline date, and a second phase was started to generate an even more detailed map. The new phase increased the density of SNP identification fivefold from 1 SNP per 3000 bases to 1 SNP per 1000 bases, or a total of 3.1 million SNPs, approximately 25% of the estimated 11 million SNPs in the human genome.[55] Finding a haplotype frequently in people with a disease, especially genetically complex diseases such as asthma, heart disease, type II diabetes, or cancer, identifies a genomic region that may contain genes contributing to the condition. The improved detail of the second-phase project (phase II HapMap) is not only advancing efforts to locate specific genes involved in complex genetic disorders but also providing insights into ancestry, recombination, and linkage disequilibrium studies.

To create the HapMap, DNA was taken from 270 blood samples from volunteer donors in Chinese, Japanese, African, and European populations, and SNPs were detected in DNA from each individual and compared. SNP detection is performed by high-throughput detection systems such as Beadarray, Invader, Multiplex Inversion Probe, Fluorescent Polarization-Template Directed Dye Terminator Incorporation, and Homogenous Mass EXTEND (MassArray, Sequenom). (See Chapter 9, "Gene Mutations," for detailed descriptions of these assay methods.) Ultimately, diseases will be identified by a pattern of haplotypes in an individual. This information will lead to therapeutic strategies or predictions of response to treatment. In addition, genetic determinants of normal traits such as longevity or disease resistance may also be uncovered. Laboratory testing for these haplotypes will be relatively simple to perform and interpret compared with the more complex methods that are often required to screen for gene mutations.

Mitochondrial DNA Polymorphisms

Mitochondria contain a circular genome of 16,569 base pairs. The two strands of the circular mitochondrial DNA (mtDNA) chromosome have an asymmetric distribution of Gs and Cs generating a G-rich heavy (H) and a C-rich light (L) strand. Each strand is transcribed from a control region starting at one predominant promoter, P_L on the L strand and P_H on the H strand, located in sequences of the mitochondrial circle called the displacement (D)-loop (Fig. 11-26). The D-loop forms a triple-stranded region with a short piece of H-strand DNA, the 7S DNA, synthesized from the H strand. Bidirectional transcription starts from P_L on the L-strand and P_{H1} and P_{H2} on the H-strand. RNA synthesis proceeds around the circle in both directions. A bidirectional attenuator sequence limits L-strand synthesis and, in doing so, maintains a high ratio of rRNA to mRNA transcripts from the H-strand (see Fig. 11-26). Mature mitochondrial RNAs, 1 to 17, are generated by cleavage of the polycistronic (multiple-gene) transcript at the location of the tRNA genes.

Genes encoded on the mtDNA include 22 tRNA genes, 2 ribosomal RNA genes, and 12 genes coding for components of the oxidation-phosphorylation system. Mutations in these genes are responsible for neuropathies and myopathies[56] (see Chapter 13, "Molecular Detection of Inherited Diseases"). In addition to coding sequences, the mitochondrial genome has two noncoding regions that vary in DNA sequence and are called **hypervariable region I** and **hypervariable region II**, or **HVI** and **HVII** (see Fig. 11-26). The reference mtDNA hypervariable region is the sequence published initially by Anderson, called the **Cambridge reference sequence**, the **Oxford sequence**, or the **Anderson reference**.[57] Polymorphisms are denoted as variations from the reference sequence. Nucleotide sequencing of the mtDNA control region has been validated for the genetic characterization of forensic

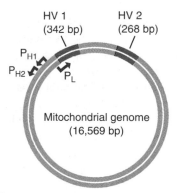

■ **Figure 11-26** The mitochondrial genome is circular. The hypervariable (HV) areas in the control region are shown. Mitochondrial genes are transcribed bidirectionally starting at promoters (P_L, P_{H1}, and P_{H2}).

specimens[58] and disease states[59,60] and for genealogy studies.[61,62]

In contrast to nuclear DNA, including the Y chromosome, mtDNA follows maternal clonal inheritance patterns. With few exceptions,[43,63] mtDNA types (sequences) are inherited maternally. These characteristics make possible collection of reference material for forensic analysis, even in cases in which generations are skipped. For forensic purposes, the quality of an mtDNA match between two mtDNA sources is determined by counting the number of times the mtDNA profile occurs in data collections of unrelated individuals, so the estimate of uniqueness of a particular mtDNA type depends on the size of the reference database.[58] As more mitochondrial DNA sequences are entered into the database, the more powerful the identification by mitochondrial DNA will become.[64]

Mitochondrial nucleotide sequence data are divided into two components, forensic and public. The forensic component consists of anonymous population profiles and is used to assess the extent of certainty of mtDNA identifications in forensic casework. All forensic profiles include, at a minimum, a sequence region in HVI (nucleotide positions 16024 to 16383) and a sequence region in HVII (nucleotide positions 53 to 372). These data are searched through the CODIS program in open case files and missing persons cases. Approximately 610 bp, including the hypervariable regions of mtDNA, are routinely sequenced for forensic analysis. Deviations from the Cambridge reference sequence are recorded as the number of the position and a base designation. For example, a transition from A to G at position 263 would be recorded as 263 G.

The public data consist of mtDNA sequence data from the scientific literature and the GenBank and European Molecular Biology Laboratory databases. The public data have not been subjected to the same quality standards as the forensic data. The public database provides information on worldwide population groups not contained within the forensic data and can be used for investigative purposes.

As all maternal relatives share mitochondrial sequences, the mtDNA of sisters and brothers or mothers and daughters will exactly match in the hypervariable region in the absence of mutations. Therefore, the use of mtDNA polymorphisms is for exclusion. There is

---

Advanced Concepts

A systematic naming scheme identifies mitochondrial profiles in both public and private data sets. A standard 14-character nucleotide sequence identifier is assigned to each profile. The first three characters indicate the country of origin. The second three characters describe the group or ethnic affiliation to which a particular profile belongs. The final six characters are sequential acquisition numbers. For example, profile USA.ASN.000217 designates the 217th nucleotide sequence from an individual of Asian American ethnicity. The population/ethnicity codes for indigenous peoples are numeric and arbitrarily assigned. For example, USA.008.000217 refers to an individual from the Apache tribe sampled from the United States.

---

an average of 8.5 nucleotide differences between mtDNA sequences of unrelated individuals in the hypervariable region. The Scientific Working Group for DNA Methods (SWGDAM) has accumulated a database of more than 4100 mtDNA sequences. The size of this database dictates the level of certainty of exclusion using mtDNA.

SWGDAM has recommended guidelines for the use of mtDNA for identification purposes.[65] The process begins with visual inspection of the specimen. Bone or teeth specimens are examined and ascertained to be of human origin. In the case of hair samples, the hairs are examined microscopically and compared with hairs from a known source. Sequencing is performed only if the specimen meets the criteria of origin and visual matching to the reference source. Before DNA isolation, the specimens are cleaned with detergent or, for bone or teeth, by sanding to remove any possible source of extraneous DNA adhering to the specimen. The cleaned specimen is then ground in an extraction solution. Hair shafts yield mtDNA as do the fleshy pulp of teeth or bone. The dentin layer of old tooth samples will also yield mtDNA. DNA is isolated by organic extraction (see Chapter 4, "Nucleic Acid Extraction Methods") and amplified by PCR (see Chapter 7,

"Nucleic Acid Amplification"). The PCR products are then purified and subjected to dideoxy sequencing (see Chapter 10, "DNA Sequencing"). A positive control of a known mitochondrial sequence is included with every run along with a reagent blank for PCR contamination and a negative control for contamination during the sequencing reaction. If the negative or reagent blank controls yield sequences similar to the specimen sequence, the results are rejected. Both strands of the specimen PCR product must be sequenced.

Raw mitochondrial sequence data are imported into a software program for analysis. With the sequence software, the heavy-strand sequences should be reverse-complemented so that the bases are aligned in the light-strand orientation for strand comparison and base designation.

Occasionally, more than one mtDNA population is present in the same individual. This is called **heteroplasmy**. In point heteroplasmy, two DNA bases are observed at the same nucleotide position. Length heteroplasmy is typically a variation in the number of bases in tracts of like bases (homopolymeric tracts, e.g., CCCCC). A length variant alone cannot be used to support an interpretation of exclusion.[66]

In general, if two or more nucleotide differences occur between a reference and a test sample, the test sample can be excluded as originating from the reference or a maternally related person. One nucleotide difference between the samples is interpreted as an inconclusive result. If the test and reference samples show sequence concordance, then the test specimen cannot be excluded as coming from the same individual or maternal relative as the source of the reference sequence. The conclusion that an individual can or cannot be eliminated as a possible source of mtDNA is reached under conditions defined by each individual laboratory. In addition, evaluation of cases in which heteroplasmy may have occurred is laboratory-defined.

The mtDNA profile of a test sample can also be searched in a population database. Population databases, such as the mtDNA population database and CODIS, are used to assess the weight of forensic evidence, based on the number of different mitochondrial sequences previously identified. The SWGDAM database contains mtDNA sequence information from more than 4100 unrelated individuals. The quality of sequence information

used and submitted for this purpose is extremely important.[67,68] Based on the number of known mtDNA sequences, the probability of sequence concordance in two unrelated individuals is estimated at 0.003. The probability that two unrelated individuals will differ by a single base is 0.014.

Mitochondrial DNA analysis is also used for lineage studies and to track population migrations. As with the Y chromosome, there is no recombination between mitochondria, and polymorphisms arise mostly through mutation. The location and divergence of specific sequences in the HV regions of mitochondria are an historical record of the relatedness of populations.

Because mitochondria are naturally amplified (hundreds per cell and tens of circular genomes per mitochondria) and because of the nuclease- and damage-resistant circular nature of the mitochondrial DNA, mtDNA typing has been a useful complement to other types of DNA identification. Challenging specimens of insufficient quantity or quality for nuclear DNA analysis may still yield useful information from mtDNA. To this end, mtDNA analysis has been helpful for the identification of missing persons in mass disasters or for typing ancient specimens.[69] MtDNA typing can also be applied to quality assurance issues, as described for STR typing of pathology specimens.[70]

CASE STUDY 11 • 1

A 32-year-old woman was treated for mantle cell lymphoma with a nonmyeloablative bone marrow transplant. Before the transplant and after a donor was selected, STR analysis was performed on the donor and the recipient to find informative alleles. One hundred days after the transplant, engraftment was evaluated using the selected STR alleles. The results from one marker, D5S818, are shown in the top panel. One year later, the patient was reevaluated. The results from the same marker are shown in the bottom panel.

(case study continues on page 282)

CASE STUDY 11 • 1—cont'd

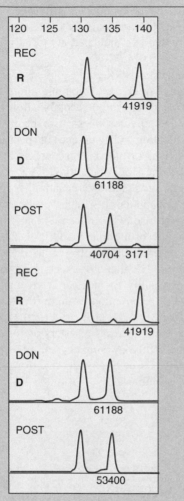

■ Results from engraftment analysis at 100 days (top) and 1 year (bottom) showing marker D5S818. R. recipient; D, donor.

QUESTION: *Was the woman successfully engrafted with donor cells? Explain your answer.*

CASE STUDY 11 • 2

A 26-year-old young man reported to his doctor with joint pain and fatigue. Complete blood count and differential counts were indicative of chronic myelogenous leukemia. The diagnosis was confirmed by karyotyping, showing 9/20 metaphases with the

CASE STUDY 11 • 2—cont'd

t(9;22) translocation. Quantitative PCR was performed to establish a baseline for monitoring tumor load during and following treatment. Treatment with Gleevec and a bone marrow transplant were recommended. The man had a twin brother, who volunteered to donate bone marrow. The two brothers were not sure if they were fraternal or identical twins. Donor and recipient buccal cells were sent to the molecular pathology laboratory for STR informative analysis. The results are shown below.

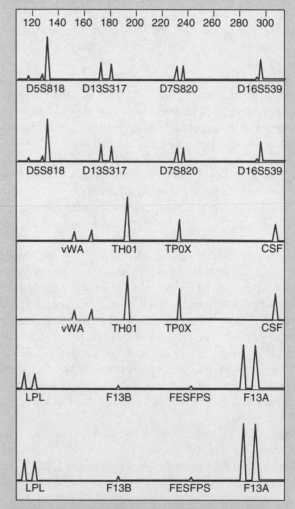

■ STR analysis of two brothers, one who serves as bone marrow donor (D) to the other (R). Twelve loci are shown.

QUESTION: *Were the brothers fraternal or identical twins? Explain your answer.*

CASE STUDY 11 • 3

The pathology department received a fixed paraffin-embedded tissue section with a diagnosis of benign uterine fibroids. Slides were prepared for microscopic study. Only benign fibroid cells were observed on all slides, except one. A small malignant process was observed located between the fibroid and normal areas on one slide. As similar tissue was not observed on any other section, it was possible that the process was a contamination from the embedding process. To determine the origin of the malignant cells, DNA was extracted from the malignant area and compared with DNA extracted from normal tissue from the patient. The results are shown below.

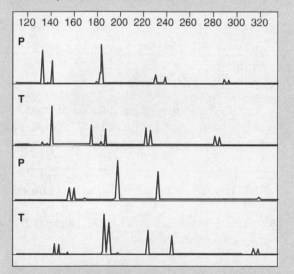

■ STR analysis of suspicious tissue discovered on a paraffin section. Eight loci were tested. P, patient; T, tissue section.

QUESTION: *Were the malignant cells seen in one section derived from the patient, or were they a contaminant of the embedding process? Explain your answer.*

• STUDY QUESTIONS •

1. Consider the following STR analysis.

Locus	Child	Mother	AF1	AF2
D3S1358	15/15	15	15	15/16
vWA	17/18	17	17/18	18
FGA	23/24	22/23	20	24
TH01	6/10	6/7	6/7	9/10
TPOX	11/11	9/11	9/11	10/11
CSF1PO	12/12	11/12	11/13	11/12
D5S818	10/12	10	11/12	12
D13S317	9/10	10/11	10/11	9/11

   a. Circle the child's alleles that are inherited from the father.
   b. Which alleged father (AF) is the biological parent?

2. The following evidence was collected for a criminal investigation.

Locus	Victim	Evidence	Suspect
TPOX	11/12	12, 11/12	11
CSF1PO	10	10, 9	9/10
D13S317	8/10	10, 8/10	9/12
D5S818	9/11	10/11, 9/11	11
TH01	6/10	6/10, 8/10	5/11
FGA	20	20, 20/22	20
vWA	15/17	18, 15/17	15/18
D3S1358	14	15/17, 14	11/12

The suspect is heterozygous at the amelogenin locus.
   a. Is the suspect male or female?
   b. In the evidence column, circle the alleles belonging to the victim.
   c. Should the suspect be held or released?

3. A child and an alleged father (AF) share alleles with the following paternity index.

Locus	Child	AF	Paternity Index for Shared Allele
D5S818	9,10	9	0.853
D8S1179	11	11,12	2.718
D16S539	13,14	10,14	1.782

   a. What is the combined paternity index from these three loci?
   b. With 50% prior odds, what is the probability of paternity from these three loci?

4. Consider the following theoretical allele frequencies for the loci indicated.

Locus	Alleles	Allele Frequency
CSF1PO	14	0.332
D13S317	9,10	0.210, 0.595
TPOX	8,11	0.489, 0.237

   a. What is the overall allele frequency for this genotype, using the product rule?
   b. What is the probability that this DNA found at two sources came from the same person?

5. STR at several loci were screened by capillary electrophoresis and fluorescent detection for informative peaks prior to a bone marrow transplant. The following results were observed.

Locus	Donor Alleles	Recipient Alleles
LPL	7,10	7,9
F13B	8,14	8
FESFPS	10	7
F13A01	5,11	5,11

   Which loci are informative?

6. An engraftment analysis was performed by capillary gel electrophoresis and fluorescence detection. The fluorescence as measured by the instrument under the FESFPS donor peak was 28,118 units, and that under the FESFPS recipient peak was 72,691. What is the percent donor in this specimen?

7. The T-cell fraction from the blood sample in Question 6 was separated and measured for donor cells. Analysis of the FESFPS locus in the T-cell fraction yielded 15,362 fluorescence units under the donor peak and 97,885 under the recipient peak. What does this result predict with regard to T-cell-mediated events such as graft-versus-host disease or graft-versus-tumor?

8. If a child had a Y haplotype including DYS393 allele 12, DYS439 allele 11, DYS445 allele 8, and DYS447 allele 22, what are the predicted Y alleles for these loci of the natural father?

9. Which of these would be used for a surname test: Y-STR, MINI-STR, mitochondrial typing, or autosomal STR?

10. An ancient bone fragment was found and said to belong to an ancestor of a famous family. Living members of the family donated DNA for confirmation of the relationship. What type of analysis would likely be used for this test? Why?

11. What is a biological exception to positive identification by autosomal STR?

12. A partial STR profile was produced from a highly degraded sample. Alleles matched to a reference sample at five loci. Is this sufficient for a legal identification?

13. What is a SNP haplotype? What are tag SNPs?

14. Which of the following is an example of linkage disequilibrium?
   a. Seventeen members of a population of 1000 people have a rare disease and all 17 people have the same haplotype at a particular genetic location on chromosome 3.
   b. Five hundred people from a population of 1000 people have the same SNP on chromosome 3.

15. Why are SNPs superior to STR and RFLP for mapping and association studies?

References

1. Herrin GJ. Probability of matching RFLP patterns from unrelated individuals. *American Journal of Human Genetics* 1993;52:491–497.
2. Hall J, Lee MK, Newman B, et al. Linkage of early-onset familial breast cancer to chromosome 17q21. *Science* 1990;250:1684–1689.
3. King M-C. Localization of the early-onset breast cancer gene. *Hospital Practice* 1991;26:89–94.
4. Gill P, Jeffreys AJ, Werrett DJ. Forensic applications of DNA "fingerprints." *Nature* 1985;318:577–579.
5. Budowle B, Bacchtel FS. Modifications to improve the effectiveness of restriction fragment length polymorphism typing. *Applied and Theoretical Electrophoresis* 1990;1:181–187.

6. Evett I, Gill P. A discussion of the robustness of methods for assessing the evidential value of DNA single locus profiles in crime investigations. *Electrophoresis* 1991;12:226–230.

7. Walsh P, Fildes N, Louie AS, et al. Report of the blind trial of the Cetus Amplitype HLA DQ alpha forensic deoxyribonucleic acid (DNA) amplification and typing kit. *Journal of Forensic Science* 1991; 36:1551–1556.

8. Gomez J, Carracedo A. The 1998–1999 collaborative exercises and proficiency testing program on DNA typing of the Spanish and Portuguese working group of the international society for forensic genetics (GEP-ISFG). *Forensic Science International* 2000;114:21–30.

9. Chakraborty R, Stivers DN, Su B, et al. The utility of short tandem repeat loci beyond human identification: Implications for development of new DNA typing systems. *Electrophoresis* 1999;20:1682–96.

10. Butler J. Forensic DNA Typing: Biology and Technology Behind STR Markers. London: Academic Press, 2001.

11. Gill P, Fereday L, Morling N, et al. The evolution of DNA databases—Recommendations for new European STR loci. *Forensic Science International* 2006;156:242–244.

12. Turrina S, Atzei R, Filippini G, et al. STR typing of archival Bouin's fluid-fixed paraffin-embedded tissue using new sensitive redesigned primers for three STR loci (CSF1P0, D8S1179 and D13S317). *Journal of Forensic and Legal Medicine* 2008;15:27–31.

13. Marjanovic D, Durmic-Pasic A, Kovacevic L, et al. Identification of skeletal remains of Communist Armed Forces victims during and after World War II: Combined Y-chromosome (STR) and MiniSTR approach. *Croation Medical Journal* 2009;50: 296–304.

14. Olaisen B, Bär W, Brinkmann B, et al. DNA recommendations 1997 of the International Society for Forensic Genetics. *Vox Sanguinis* 1998;74:61–63.

15. Leclair B, Frageau CJ, Bowen KL, et al. Precision and accuracy in fluorescent short tandem repeat DNA typing: Assessment of benefits imparted by the use of allelic ladders with the AmpF/STR Profiler Plus kit. *Electrophoresis* 2004;25:790–796.

16. Butler J, Appleby JE, Duewer DL. Locus-specific brackets for reliable typing of Y-chromosome short tandem repeat markers. *Electrophoresis* 2005; 26:2583–2590.

17. Monson K, Budowle B. A comparison of the fixed bin method with the floating bin and direct count methods: Effect of VNTR profile frequency estimation and reference population. *Journal of Forensic Science* 1993;38:1037–1050.

18. Norton H, Neel JV. Hardy-Weinberg equilibrium and primitive populations. *American Journal of Human Genetics* 1965;17:91–92.

19. Hartmann J, Houlihan BT, Keister RS, et al. The effect of ethnic and racial population substructuring on the estimation of multi-locus fixed-bin VNTR RFLP genotype probabilities. *Journal of Forensic Science* 1997;42(2):232–240.

20. Perlin M, Kadane JB, Cotton RW. Match likelihood ratio for uncertain genotypes. *Law, Probability and Risk* 2009;8:289–302.

21. Gill P, Whitaker J, Flaxman C, et al. An investigation of the rigor of interpretation rules for STRs derived from less than 100 pg of DNA. *Forensic Science International* 2000;112:17–40.

22. Gilbert N. DNA's identity crisis. *Nature* 2010;464: 347–348.

23. Whittemore A. Genetic association studies: Time for a new paradigm? *Cancer Epidemiology Biomarkers and Prevention* 2005;14:1359.

24. Brinkmann B, Klintschar M, Neuhuber F, et al. Mutation rate in human microsatellites: Influence of the structure and length of the tandem repeat. *American Journal of Human Genetics* 1998;62:1408–1415.

25. Brenner C. Forensic mathematics, http://dna-view. com/index.html, 2005.

26. Wenk RE, Traver M, Chiafari FA. Determination of sibship in any two persons. *Transfusion* 1996; 36:259–262.

27. Douglas J, Boehnke M, Lange K. A multipoint method for detecting genotyping errors and mutations in sibling-pair linkage data. *American Journal of Human Genetics* 2000;66:1287–1297.

28. Boehnke M, Cox NJ. Accurate inference of relationships in sib-pair linkage studies. *American Journal of Human Genetics* 1997;61:423–429.

29. Epstein M, Duren WL, Boehnke M. Improved inference of relationship for pairs of individuals. *American Journal of Human Genetics* 2000;67(5): 1219–1231.

30. Jobling M, Pandya A, Tyler-Smith C. The Y chromosome in forensic analysis and paternity testing. *International Journal of Legal Medicine* 1997;110:118–124.

31. Sinha S, Budowle B, Chakraborty R, et al. Utility of the Y-STR typing systems Y-PLEXTM 6 and Y-PLEXTM 5 in forensic casework and 11 Y-STR haplotype database for three major population groups in the United States. *Journal of Forensic Science* 2004;49:1–10.

32. Gill P, Brenner C, Brinkmann B, et al. DNA commission of the international society of forensic genetics: Recommendations on forensic analysis using Y-chromosome STRs. *International Journal of Legal Medicine* 2001;114:305–309.

33. Sajantila A, Lukka M, Syvanen AC. Experimentally observed germline mutations at human micro- and mini-satellite loci. *European Journal of Human Genetics* 1999;7:263–266.

34. Heyer E, Puymirat J, Dieltjes P, et al. Estimating Y chromosome specific microsatellite mutation frequencies using deep rooting pedigrees. *Human Molecular Genetics* 1997;6:799–803.

35. Redd A, Agellon AB, Kearney VA, et al. Gene flow from the Indian subcontinent to Australia: Evidence from the Y chromosome. *Forensic Science International* 2002;130:97–111.

36. Roewer L, Krawczak M, Willuweit S, et al. Online reference database of European Y-chromosomal short tandem repeat (STR) haplotypes. *Forensic Science International* 2001; 118:106–113.

37. Van Deerlin V, Leonard DGB. Bone marrow engraftment analysis after allogeneic bone marrow transplantation. *Acute Leukemias* 2000;20:197–225.

38. Thiede C, Florek M, Bornhauser M, et al. Rapid quantification of mixed chimerism using multiplex amplification of short tandem repeat markers and fluorescence detection. *Bone Marrow Transplant* 1999;23:1055–1060.

39. Thiede C. Diagnostic chimerism analysis after allogeneic stem cell transplantation: New methods and markers. *American Journal of Pharmacogenomics* 2004;4:177–187.

40. Leclair B, Frageau CJ, Aye MT, et al. DNA typing for bone marrow engraftment follow-up after allogeneic transplant: A comparative study of current technologies. *Bone Marrow Transplant* 1995;16:43–55.

41. Smith A, Martin PJ. Analysis of amplified variable number tandem repeat loci for evaluation of engraftment after hematopoietic stem cell transplantation. *Reviews in Immunogenetics* 1999; 1:255–264.

42. Thiede C, Bornhauser M, Ehninger G. Evaluation of STR informativity for chimerism testing: Comparative analysis of 27 STR systems in 203 matched related donor recipient pairs. *Leukemia* 2004;18:248–254.

43. Antin J, Childes R, Filipovich AH, et al. Establishment of complete and mixed donor chimerism after allogeneic lymphohematopoietic transplantation: Recommendations from a workshop at the 2001 tandem meetings. *Biology of Blood and Marrow Transplantation* 2001;7: 473–485.

44. Platt E, Sommer P, McDonald L, et al. Tissue floaters and contaminants in the histology laboratory. *Archives of Pathology & Laboratory Medicine* 2009;133:973–978.

45. Hunt J, Swalsky P, Sasatomi E, et al. A microdissection and molecular genotyping assay to confirm the identity of tissue floaters in paraffin-embedded tissue blocks. *Archives of Pathology & Laboratory Medicine* 2003;127:213–217.

46. Junge A, Dettmeyer R, Madea B. Identification of biological samples in a case of contamination of a cytological slide preparation. *Journal of Forensic Science* 2008;53:739–741.

47. Kruglyak L, Nickerson DA. Variation is the spice of life. *Nature Genetics* 2001;27:234–236.

48. Sachidanandam R, Weissman D, Schmidt SC, et al. International SNP Map Working Group: A map of human genome sequence variation containing 1.42 million single nucleotide polymorphisms. *Nature* 2001;409:928–433.

49. Matise T, Sachidanandam R, Clark AG, et al. A 3.9-centimorgan-resolution human single-nucleotide polymorphism linkage map and screening set. *American Journal of Human Genetics* 2003;73: 271–284.

50. Shriver M, Mei R, Parra EJ, et al. Large-scale SNP analysis reveals clustered and continuous patterns of human genetic variation. *Human Genomics* 2005;2:81–89.

51. Tamiya G, Shinya M, Imanishi T, et al. Whole genome association study of rheumatoid arthritis using 27,039 microsatellites. *Human Molecular Genetics* 2005;14(16):2305–2321.

52. Patil N, Berno AJ, Hinds DA, et al. Blocks of limited haplotype diversity revealed by high-resolution scanning of human chromosome 21. *Science* 2001;294:1719–1723.

53. The International HapMap Consortium. The International HapMap Project. *Nature* 2003;426:789–796.

54. The International HapMap Consortium. Integrating ethics and science in the International HapMap Project. *Nature Review Genetics* 2004;5:467–475.

55. The International HapMap Consortium. A second generation human haplotype map of over 3.1 million SNPs. *Nature* 2007;449:851–862.

56. Wick J, Zanni GR. Mitochondrial disease: When the powerhouse goes awry. *Consultant Pharmacist* 2010;25:144–153.

57. Anderson S, Bankier AT, Barrell BG, et al. Sequence and organization of the human mitochondrial genome. *Nature* 1981;290:457–465.

58. Budowle B, Wilson MR, DiZinno JA, et al. Mitochondrial DNA regions HVI and HVII population data. *Forensic Science International* 1999;103: 23–35.

59. Tajima A, Hamaguchi K, Terao H, et al. Genetic background of people in the Dominican Republic with or without obese type 2 diabetes revealed by mitochondrial DNA polymorphism. *Journal of Human Genetics* 2004;49:495–499.

60. van der Walt J, Dementieva YA, Martin ER, et al. Analysis of European mitochondrial haplogroups with Alzheimer disease risk. *Neuroscience Letters* 2004;365:28–32.

61. Nasidze I, Ling EY, Quinque D, et al. Mitochondrial DNA and Y-chromosome variation in the Caucasus. *Annals of Human Genetics* 2004;68:205–221.

62. Shriver M, Kittles RA. Genetic ancestry and the search for personalized genetic histories. *Nature Review Genetics* 2004;5:611–618.

63. Schwartz M, Vissing J. Paternal inheritance of mitochondrial DNA. *New England Journal of Medicine* 2002;347:576–580.

64. Lee Y, Kim WY, Ji M, et al. MitoVariome: A variome database of human mitochondrial DNA. *BMC Genomics* 2009;10:S12.

65. Scientific Working Group on DNA Analysis Methods (SWGDAM). Guidelines for mitochondrial DNA (mtDNA) nucleotide sequence interpretation. *Forensic Science Communications* 2003;5(2):1–5.

66. Stewart JEB, Fisher, CL, Aagaard, PJ, et al. Length variation in HV2 of the human mitochondrial DNA control region. *Journal of Forensic Science* 2001;46:862–870.

67. Bandelt H-J, Salas A, Bravi C. Problems in FBI mtDNA database. *Science* 2004;305:1402–1404.

68. Budowle B, Polanskey D. FBI mtDNA database: A cogent perspective. *Science* 2005;307:845–847.

69. Zupanic I, Gornjak PB, Balazic J. Molecular genetic identification of skeletal remains from the Second World War Konfin I mass grave in Slovenia. *International Journal of Legal Medicine*, 2010; 124(4):307–317.

70. Alonso A, Alves C, Suárez-Mier MP, et al. Mitochondrial DNA haplotyping revealed the presence of mixed up benign and neoplastic tissue sections from two individuals on the same prostatic biopsy slide. *Journal of Clinical Pathology* 2005;58.83–86.

71. Bar W, Brinkman B, Budowle B, et al. DNA recommendations: Further report of the DNA Commission of the ISFH regarding the use of short tandem repeat systems. International Society for Forensic Haemogenetics. *International Journal of Legal Medicine* 1997;110:175–176.

72. Sinha S, Budowle B, Arcot SS, et al. Development and validation of a multiplexed Y-chromosome STR genotyping system, Y-PLEX™ 6, for forensic casework. *Journal of Forensic Science* 2003; 48:1–11.

73. Iida R, Sawazaki K, Ikeda H, et al. A novel multiplex PCR system consisting of Y-STRs DYS441, DYS442, DYS443, DYS444, and DYS445. *Journal of Forensic Science* 2003; 48:1088–1090.

74. Hanson E, Ballantyne J. A highly discriminating 21 locus Y-STR "megaplex" system designed to augment the minimal haplotype loci for forensic casework. *Journal of Forensic Science* 2004;49:1–12.

75. Schoskea R, Vallonea PM, Klinea MC, et al. High-throughput Y-STR typing of U.S. populations with 27 regions of the Y chromosome using two multiplex PCR assays. *Forensic Science International* 2004;139:107–121.

Chapter **12**

Detection and Identification of Microorganisms

OBJECTIVES

- Name the organisms that are common targets for molecular-based laboratory tests.

- Identify advantages and disadvantages of using molecular-based methods as compared with traditional culture-based methods in the detection and identification of microorganisms.

- Differentiate between organisms for which commercially available nucleic acid amplification tests exist and those for which "**home-brew**" polymerase chain reaction (PCR) is used.

- List the genes involved in the emergence of antimicrobial resistance that can be detected by nucleic acid amplification methods.

- Compare and contrast the molecular methods that are used to type bacterial strains in epidemiological investigations.

- Explain the value of controls, in particular amplification controls, in ensuring the reliability of PCR results.

OBJECTIVES—cont'd

• Interpret pulse field gel electrophoresis patterns to determine whether two isolates are related to or different from each other.

The majority of recent microbiological applications for the clinical laboratory are based on the molecular characterization of microorganisms and the development and evaluation of molecular-based laboratory tests of clinical specimens isolated in cultures. Another important application of molecular technology in the clinical microbiology laboratory is in the comparison of biochemically similar organisms in outbreak situations, known as molecular epidemiology, to ascertain whether the isolates have a common or independent source. Clinically important microorganisms include a range of life forms from arthropods to prions, and although molecular-based methods have become routine in clinical microbiology, traditional culture and biochemical testing are still important for the detection and identification of most microorganisms.

In contrast to analysis of phenotypic traits of microorganisms (microscopic and colonial morphologies, enzyme or pigment production, as well as carbohydrate fermentation patterns), the analyte for molecular testing is the genome, transcriptome, or proteome of the microorganism. Bacteria, fungi, and parasites have DNA genomes, whereas viruses can have DNA or RNA genomes. Prions, which cause transmissible encephalopathies such as Creutzfeldt-Jakob disease, consist only of protein.

Microorganisms targeted for molecular-based laboratory tests have been those that are difficult and/or time-consuming to isolate, such as *Mycobacterium tuberculosis*

as well as other species of *Mycobacterium*[1-3]; those that are hazardous with which to work in the clinical laboratory, such as *Histoplasma*[4,5] and *Coccidioides*[6,7]; and those for which reliable laboratory tests are lacking, such as hepatitis C virus (HCV) and Human Immunodeficiency Virus (HIV).[8]

Additionally, molecular-based tests have been developed for organisms that are received in clinical laboratories in high volumes, such as *Streptococcus pyogenes* in throat swabs and *Neisseria gonorrhoeae* and *Chlamydia trachomatis* in genital specimens.[9] Furthermore, genes that confer resistance to **antimicrobial agents** are the targets of molecular-based methodologies, such as *mecA*, which contributes to the resistance of *Staphylococcus aureus* to oxacillin[10]; *vanA*, *vanB*, and *vanC*, which give *Enterococcus* resistance to vancomycin[11]; and *katG* and *inhA*, which mediate *M. tuberculosis* resistance to isoniazid.[12,13]

Finally, characterization of DNA and RNA is being used to find and identify new organisms, such as *Tropheryma whipplei*,[14] and also to further characterize or genotype known organisms, such as species of *Mycobacterium*, HCV, and HIV. Nucleic acid sequence information is used to reclassify bacterial organisms based on 16S rRNA sequence homology, for epidemiological purposes, and to predict therapeutic efficacy.

The molecular methods used in the clinical microbiology laboratory are the same as those that were described previously for the identification of human polymorphisms and those that will be discussed in subsequent chapters for the identification of genes involved in cancer and in inherited diseases. The primary molecular methods used in clinical microbiology laboratories are polymerase chain reaction (PCR)—traditional, real-time, and **reverse transcriptase** PCR (see Chapter 7, "Nucleic Acid Amplification")—as well as sequencing (see Chapter 10, "DNA Sequencing"). An additional method that is used in molecular epidemiology is pulsed field gel electrophoresis (PFGE) (see Chapter 5, "Resolution and Detection of Nucleic Acids") as well as other methods that will be discussed in this chapter. All types of microorganisms serve as targets for molecular-based laboratory tests, from bacteria to viruses, fungi, and parasites. The development of molecular-based methods has been successful for some organisms but not yet for all organisms, as will be discussed in this chapter.

Specimen Collection

As with any clinical test, collection and transport of specimens for infectious disease testing will negatively affect analytical results if proper procedure is not followed. Microbiological specimens may require special handling to preserve the viability of the target organism. Special collection systems have been designed for collection of strict anaerobes, viruses, and other fastidious organisms. Although viability is not as critical for molecular testing, the quality of nucleic acids may be compromised if the specimen is improperly handled. DNA and especially RNA will be damaged in lysed or nonviable cells. Due to the sensitivity of molecular testing, it is also important to avoid contamination that could yield false-positive results.

Collection techniques designed to avoid contamination from the surrounding environment of adjacent tissues apply to molecular testing, especially to those tests that use amplification methods. Sampling must include material from the original infection. The time and site of collection must be optimal for the likely presence of the infectious agent. For example, *Salmonella typhi* is initially present in peripheral blood but not in urine or stool until at least 2 weeks after infection. For classical methods that include culturing of the agent, a sufficient number of microorganisms must be obtained for agar or liquid culture growth. For molecular testing, however, minimum numbers (as few as 50 organisms) can be detected successfully. The quantity of target organisms as well as the clinical implications should be taken into account when interpreting the significance of positive results. Molecular detection can reveal infective agents at levels below clinical significance. Conversely, highly specific molecular methods may miss detection of a variant organism.

Equipment and reagents used for specimen collection are also important for molecular testing (Table 12.1). Blood draws should go into the proper anticoagulant, if one is to be used. (See Chapter 16, "Quality Assurance and Quality Control in the Molecular Laboratory," for a list of anticoagulants and their effect on molecular testing.) Although wooden-shafted swabs may be used for throat cultures, dacron or calcium alginate swabs with plastic shafts have been recommended for collection of bacteria, viruses, and mycoplasma from mucosal surfaces.[15] The plastics are less adherent to the microorganisms and will not interfere with PCR reagents, with the exception of calcium alginate swabs with aluminum shafts, which have been reported to affect PCR amplification.[16] The swab extraction tube system (SETS, Roche Diagnostics) is designed for maximum recovery of microorganisms from swabs by centrifugation (Fig. 12-1).

Table 12.1 **Specimen Transport Systems**

Type	Examples
Sterile containers	Sterile cups, screw-capped tubes, stoppered tubes, Petri dishes
Swabs	Calcium alginate swabs, Dacron swabs, cotton swabs, nasopharyngeal-urogenital swabs, Swab Transport System
Specialty systems	*Neisseria gonorrhoeae* transport systems, SETS
Proprietary systems	Molecular testing, *Neisseria gonorrhoeae* transport systems, STAR buffer[42]
Anaerobic transport systems	Starplex Anaerobic Transport system (Fisher), BBL Vacutainer Anaerobic Specimen Collector
Viral transport systems	BD Cellmatics Viral Transport Pack, BBL Viral Culturette

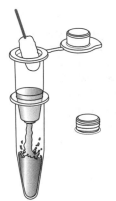

■ **Figure 12-1** The Swab Extraction Tube System (SETS) consists of a punctured inner tube that holds a swab and fits in a cappable outer tube. Under the force of centrifugation, liquid in the swab is forced through the inner tube and into the outer tube, where it can be stored.

Commercial testing kits supply an optimized collection system for a particular test organism. The Clinical and Laboratory Standards Institute has published documents addressing the requirements for transport devices and quality control guidelines. The College of American Pathologists requires documented procedures describing specimen handling, collection, and transport in each laboratory.

Sample Preparation

The isolation of nucleic acids was described in Chapter 4, "Nucleic Acid Extraction Methods." Isolating nucleic acids from microorganisms is similar to isolating nucleic acids from human cells with only a few additional considerations.

First, depending on the microorganism, more rigorous lysis procedures may be required. Mycobacteria and fungi in particular have thick cell walls that are more difficult to lyse than those of other bacteria and parasites. Gram-positive bacteria having a thicker cell wall than gram-negative bacteria and may require more rigorous cell lysis conditions. *Mycoplasma*, on the other hand, lacks a cell wall, and so care must be taken with the sample to avoid spontaneous lysis of the cells and loss of nucleic acids. See Chapter 4 for a description of cell lysis methods.

Advanced Concepts

Biological safety is an important concern for clinical microbiology. Because various collection, transport, and extraction systems inactivate organisms at different times, the technologist should follow the recommendations of the Centers for Disease Control and Prevention (CDC) that call for universal precautions, treating all specimens as if they were infectious throughout the extraction process. Updated guidelines are available from the CDC for the handling of suspected bioterrorism material, for example, the anthrax spores discovered in the United States Postal System in 2001 (http://emergency.cdc.gov/agent/anthrax/environmental-sampling-apr2002.asp). Organisms such as smallpox must be handled only in approved (level 4 containment) laboratories. Molecular testing has eased the requirements for preserving the viability of organisms for laboratory culture. Methods devised to replace the growth of cultures should improve safety levels.

Second, the concentration of organisms within the clinical sample must be considered. Samples should be centrifuged to concentrate the organisms within the fluid from the milliliters of sample that are often received down to microliter volumes that are appropriate for most molecular procedures. Third, inhibitors of enzymes used in molecular analysis may be present in clinical specimens; removal or inactivation of inhibitors might be included in specimen preparation methods. Finally, if RNA is to be analyzed, inactivation or removal of RNases in the sample and in all reagents and materials that come into contact with the sample is important.

Any clinical specimen can be used as a source of microorganism nucleic acid for analysis. Depending on the specimen, however, special preparation procedures may be necessary to allow for optimal nucleic acid isolation, amplification, and analysis. The presence of inhibitors of DNA polymerase has been demonstrated in cerebrospinal fluid; therefore, careful isolation of nucleic acid from other molecules present in the sample will more likely result in an amplifiable sample. Isolation of nucleic acids from blood was discussed in Chapter 4. When processing a whole blood specimen, it is important to remove all of the hemoglobin and other products of metabolized hemoglobin because they have been shown to be inhibitors of DNA polymerase and thus may prevent the amplification of nucleic acid in the sample, resulting in a false-negative PCR result. White blood cells such as lymphocytes can be used as a source of nucleic acid for organisms, primarily viruses that infect these cells. In this case, the cells are isolated from the red blood cells using Ficoll-Hypaque and then lysed. Alternatively, whole blood is processed in automated DNA isolation systems, which effectively remove hemoglobin and other contaminating molecules. Serum and plasma are also used as sources of microorganism nucleic acid.

Sputum is a source of nucleic acid from organisms that cause respiratory tract infections. Acidic polysaccharides present in sputum may inhibit DNA polymerase and thus must be removed. Using a method or an instrument that reliably separates DNA from other cellular molecules is sufficient to remove the inhibitors. Urine, when sent for nucleic acid isolation and amplification, is treated similarly to cerebrospinal fluid; that is, the specimen is centrifuged to concentrate the organisms and then subjected to nucleic acid isolation procedures. Inhibitors of DNA polymerase—nitrate, crystals, hemoglobin, and beta-human chorionic gonadotropin—have been demonstrated in urine as well.[17]

The type of specimen used for molecular testing will also affect extraction and yield of nucleic acid. For example, viral nucleic acid from plasma is easier to isolate than nucleic acid from pathogenic *Enterococcus* in stool specimens. Reagents and devices have been developed to combine collection and extraction of nucleic acid from difficult specimens, for example, stool transport and recovery (STAR, Roche Diagnostics) buffer or the FTA paper systems that inactivate infectious agents and adhere nucleic acids to magnetic beads or paper, respectively.

Quality Control

For any type of medical laboratory procedure, quality control is critical for ensuring the accuracy of patient results. Ensuring the quality of molecular methods themselves is equally important. The sensitivity of molecular methods is high, so even one molecule of target is a potential template. Thus, the integrity of specimens, that is, specimens not contaminated by other organisms or with the products of previous amplification procedures, is critical to avoid inaccurate results. On the other hand, it is equally important to ensure that the lack of a product in an amplification procedure is due to the absence of the target organism and not the presence of inhibitors preventing the amplification of target sequences.

Control substances of known composition are used to monitor the reliability of the method and the input specimen material. The incorporation of **positive controls** shows that an assay system is functioning properly. A **sensitivity control** that is positive at the lower limit of detection demonstrates sensitivity of qualitative assays. Two positive controls, one at the lower limit and the other at the upper limit of detection, are run in quantitative assays to test the dynamic range of the assay. **Reagent blank** or **contamination controls** are critical for monitoring reagents for contamination; the latter contain all of the assay reagents except target sequences and should always be negative. For typing and other studies that might include nontarget organisms, a **negative template control** might also be included. This control will detect the presence of the unwanted target(s), but should not react with the desired target.

With regard to amplification methods that are interpreted by the presence or absence of product, false-negative results can occur due to amplification failure. In order to rule out this type of false-negative result, an **amplification control** aimed at a target that is always present can be incorporated into an amplification assay. The negative template control sample should have a positive amplification control signal, whereas the reagent blank should be negative for amplification. With a positive amplification control, lack of amplification of the target can be more confidently interpreted as a **true negative** result. Amplification controls are usually housekeeping genes or those that are always present in human or microbiological samples. Housekeeping genes that are used as internal controls include prokaryotic genes, such as *groEL*, *rpoB*, *recA*, and *gyrB*,[18] and eukaryotic genes, such as β-actin, glyceraldehyde-3-phosphate, interferon-γ, extrinsic homologous control, human mitochondrial DNA, and peptidylprolyl isomerase A.[15,19]

Internal controls are amplification controls that monitor particular steps of an amplification method. They can be either **homologous extrinsic**, **heterologous extrinsic**, or **heterologous intrinsic** (Fig. 12-2). A homologous

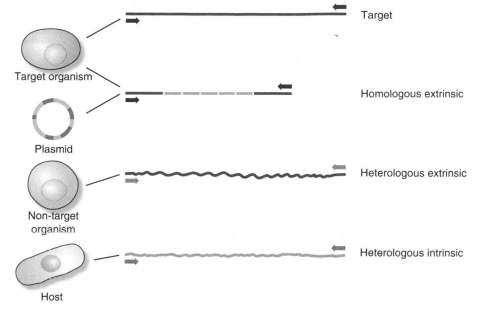

■ **Figure 12-2** Amplification controls and their relationships to the molecular target. Homologous extrinsic controls are a modified version of the target that maintain the target primer binding sites. The homologous intrinsic control may be smaller, larger, or the same size as the target. Heterologous extrinsic controls are obtained from unrelated nontarget organisms and require primers different from those of the target sequences. Heterologous intrinsic controls are similar to heterologous extrinsic controls, except that heterologous intrinsic controls come from host sequences.

extrinsic control is a target-derived control with a non-target-derived sequence insert. This control is added to every sample after nucleic acid extraction and before amplification. The amplification of this control occurs using the same primers as for the target, which is good for ensuring that amplification occurs in the sample but does not control for target nucleic acid degradation during extraction. Heterologous extrinsic controls are non-target-derived controls that are added to every sample before nucleic acid extraction. This control will ensure that the extraction and amplification procedures were acceptable, but a second set of primers must also be added to the reaction for the control to be amplified. Using this control requires that the procedure be optimized so that the amplification of the control does not interfere with the amplification of the target.

Heterologous intrinsic controls are nontarget sequences naturally present in the sample, such as eukaryotic genes in a test for microorganisms. In this case, human gene controls serve to ensure that human nucleic acid is present in the sample in addition to controlling for extraction and amplification. Using this control requires that either two amplification reactions be performed on the sample, one for the control and the other for the target gene, or that the amplification procedure be multiplexed, which may result in interference with the amplification of the target.

In a procedure that detects a microorganism, a positive result states that the organism is present in that sample, whereas a negative result indicates that the organism is not present (at amounts up to the detection limits of the assay). Although most false-positive test results can be eliminated by preventing carryover contamination, another source of false-positive test results that cannot be controlled in the laboratory is the presence of dead or dying microorganisms in the sample of a patient taking antimicrobial agents. In this situation, the nucleic acid–based tests will remain positive longer than culture assays and thus may appear as a false-positive. Repeating the nucleic acid–based assay 3 to 6 weeks after antimicrobial therapy is more likely to yield a true negative result.

False-negative results may be more problematic and arise when the target organism is present but the test result is negative. There are a few reasons for false-negative results on a sample. First, the organism may be present, but the nucleic acid was degraded during collection, transport, and/or extraction. This degradation can be prevented by proper specimen handling, effective transport media, and inhibiting the activity of DNases and RNases that may be present in the sample and in the laboratory. Second, amplification procedures may be inhibited by substances present in the specimen. Hemoglobin, lactoferrin, heparin and other anticoagulants, sodium polyanethol sulfonate (anticoagulant used in blood culture media), and polyamines have been shown to inhibit nucleic acid amplification procedures.[15] Attention to nucleic acid isolation procedures and ensuring optimal purification of nucleic acid from other components of the specimen and extraction reagents will help minimize the presence and influence of inhibitors on the amplification reaction. Experimenting with different commercial nucleic acid extraction systems may result in discovering a system that is optimal for a particular purpose.

Extensive **validation** must be performed on new molecular-based tests that are brought into the laboratory (see Chapter 16, "Quality Assurance and Quality Control in the Molecular Laboratory"). Controls must be tested, and the sensitivity, specificity, and reproducibility of the assay must be determined using reference materials (Madej, 2010 #1200). Proficiency testing of personnel should be performed regularly. The Clinical and Laboratory Standards Institute,[18] Association for Molecular Pathology,[19] and the Food and Drug Administration (FDA) have guidelines for molecular methods in the laboratory.

Selection of Sequence Targets for Detection of Microorganisms

Molecular methods are based on sequence hybridization or recognition using known nucleic acid sequences (primers or probes). These tests are extremely sensitive and specific but are limited by the choice of target sequences for primer or probe hybridization. The primary nucleotide sequence of many clinically important microorganisms is now known. Sequences are available from the National Center for Biological Information (NCBI) or from published literature. The specificity of molecular methods targeting these sequences depends on the primers or probes that must hybridize to the chosen point in the genome of the microorganism.

Choosing a sequence target is critical for the specificity of a molecular test (Fig. 12-3). Many microorganisms share the same sequences in evolutionarily conserved genes. These sequences would not be used for detection of specific strains as they are likely to cross-react over a range of organisms. Sequences unique to the target organism are therefore selected. Some organisms such as HIV have variable sequences within the same species.

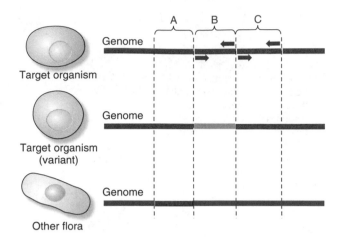

■ Figure 12-3 Selection of target sequences for a nucleic acid test. The genomes of three organisms—the test target, a variant or different type of the test target, and another nontarget organism—are depicted. Sequence region A is not specific to the target organism and is, therefore, not an acceptable area for probe or primer binding to detect the target. Sequences B and C are specific to the target. Sequence B is variable and can be used to detect and type the target, although some variants may escape detection. Sequence C will detect variants of the target organism but cannot be used for determining the type.

Such variations may be informative in, for instance, determining drug resistance or for epidemiological information; however, not all types would be detected by a single sequence. The variable sequences may be included in the probe or primer areas to differentiate between types. These type-specific probes/primers are used in a confirmatory test after an initial test using probes or primers directed to a sequence shared by all types.

In addition to their strain or species specificity, the target sequences must meet technical requirements for hybridization conditions. Primers should have similar annealing temperatures and yield amplicons of appropriate size. Probes must hybridize specifically under the conditions of the procedure. Sequence differences can be distinguished using sequence-specific probes or primers (see Chapter 6, "Analysis and Characterization of Nucleic Acids and Proteins" and Chapter 7, "Nucleic Acid Amplification").

Probe design includes decisions as to the length of the probe, whether the probe is DNA, RNA, or protein; how the probe is labeled; and, for nucleic acid probes, the length of sequences included in the probe. The source of the probe is also important, as probes must be replenished and perform consistently over long-term use.

Probes are manufactured synthetically or biologically by cloning (see Chapter 6). Synthetic oligonucleotides may be preferred for known sequences where high specificity is required. Primer design includes the length and any modifications of the primers and type of signal generation for quantitative PCR. (Refer to Chapters 6 and 7 for further discussion of hybridization and amplification methods.)

Many tests currently used in molecular microbiology are supplied as commercially designed systems, including prevalidated probes and/or primers. Several of these methods are FDA-approved or FDA-cleared (Table 12.2). An updated list of the currently available FDA-approved

tests is available at The American Society for Investigative Pathology at ampweb.org.

Manufacturers of these commercial reagents specify requirements for quality assurance, including controls and assay limitations. Each system must be validated on the type of specimen used for clinical testing, including serum, plasma, cerebrospinal and other body fluids, tissue, cultured cells, and organisms. In addition to the commercial reagent sets, many professionals working in medical laboratories have developed in-house laboratory protocols (home-brew tests) for most of the analyses that they perform. Primers are designed based on sequence information that has been published, the reagents are

Table 12.2 **FDA-Approved/Cleared Test Methods**

Target Organism	Methods[*]
Cytomegalovirus	NASBA, Hybrid capture
Hepatitis C virus (HCV), qualitative	TMA, PCR
HCV, quantitative	bDNA
Human immunodeficiency virus (HIV), quantitative	bDNA, NASBA, RTPCR
HIV resistance testing	Sequencing
Hepatitis B virus/IICV/IIIV screening for blood donations	TMA, PCR, RTPCR
Human papillomavirus	Hybrid capture
Chlamydia trachomatis (CT)	Hybrid capture, TMA, hybridization protection assay, PCR, SDA
Neisseria gonorrhoeae (NG)	Hybrid capture, TMA, hybridization protection assay, PCR, SDA
CT/NG	Hybrid capture, TMA, hybridization protection assay, PCR, SDA
Gardnerella, Trichomonas vaginalis, Candida	Hybridization
Group A Streptococci	Hybridization protection assay
Group B Streptococci	Hybridization protection assay, real-time PCR
Legionella pneumophila	SDA
Methicillin-resistant *Staphylococcus aureus*	Real-time PCR, PNA FISH
Mycobacterium tuberculosis	TMA, PCR
Bacillus anthracis	Real-time PCR
Candida albicans and *Candida* spp.	PNA FISH
Clostridium difficile	PNA FISH
Enterococcus faecalis	PNA FISH
Escherichia coli and *Pseudomonas aeruginosa*	PNA FISH
Escherichia coli, Klebsiella pneumoniae, and *Pseudomonas aeruginosa*	PNA FISH
Francisella tularensis	PNA FISH
Mycobacteria spp., different fungi and bacteria culture confirmation	HPA
Staphylococcus aureus	PNA FISH
Vancomycin resistance	Real-time PCR

[*]See Chapters 7 and 9 for detailed description of these methods.

bought separately, and the procedures are developed and optimized within the individual laboratory.

Molecular Detection of Microorganisms

Molecular-based methods that have been used to detect and identify bacteria include hybridization and nucleic acid sequence–based amplification procedures. (See Chapter 7 for explanations of these methods.) Product detection is accomplished by a variety of methods, including Southern blot hybridization (see Chapter 6), agarose gel electrophoresis (see Chapter 5), PCR (see Chapter 7), sequencing (see Chapter 10, "DNA Sequencing"), enzyme immunoassay, dot blot hybridization (see Chapter 6), and restriction enzyme analysis (see Chapter 6).

Real-time PCR, or quantitative PCR (qPCR), is used frequently for detection of infectious agents, as it provides a sensitive assay with more information than is available from conventional PCR. The quantitative capability of qPCR allows distinction of subclinical levels of infection (qualitatively positive by conventional

PCR) from higher levels with pathological consequences. Furthermore, qPCR programs can be designed to provide closed-tube sequence or typing analysis by adding a melt curve temperature program following the amplification of the target (Fig. 12-4). Like conventional PCR, qPCR is performed on DNA extracted directly from clinical specimens, including viral, bacterial, and fungal pathogens.

Designing a qPCR method requires selecting a target gene unique to the specimen or specimen type for which primers and probes can be designed. The DNA-specific dye, SYBR Green, can be used in place of probes if the amplicon is free of artifact, such as misprimes or primer dimers (see Chapter 7). The probe types most often used include fluorescent energy transfer hybridization probes and hydrolysis (TaqMan) probes.

The requirement for probes in addition to primers increases the complexity of the design process. Instrument software and several websites offer computer programs that automatically design primers and probes on submitted sequences. Commercial primer and probe sets are also available for purchase in kit form. A variety of gene targets have been used for qPCR detection of a

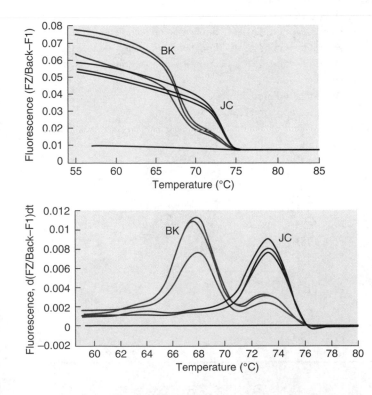

■ **Figure 12-4** Melt curve analysis of BK and JC viruses. BK and JC are differentiated from one another by differences in the T_m* of the probe specific for each viral sequence. Fluorescence from double-stranded DNA decreases with increasing temperature and DNA denaturation to single strands (top panel). Instrument software will present a derivative of the fluorescence (bottom panel) where the T_ms (67°–68°C for BK and 73°–74°C for JC) are observed as peaks.

number of organisms. A list of examples of targets and probes is available in a comprehensive review by Espy et al.[20]

Useful genes for qPCR methods include ribosomal RNA (rRNA), both 16S and 23S, and housekeeping genes such as *groEL*, *rpoB*, *recA*, and *gyrB*.[20] The 16S rRNA is a component of the small subunit of the prokaryotic ribosome, and the 23S rRNA is a component of the large subunit of the prokaryotic ribosome. Analysis of 16S rRNA is performed to determine the evolutionary and genetic relatedness of microorganisms and is driving changes in microorganism nomenclature.[21] The rDNA that encodes the rRNA consists of alternating regions of conserved sequences and sequences that vary greatly from organism to organism. The conserved sequences encode the loops of the rRNA and can be used as a target to detect all or most bacteria. Sequences that have a great amount of heterogeneity encode the stems of the rRNA and can be used to detect a specific genus or species of bacteria.[18] Ribosomal RNA was the original target of many bacterial molecular-based assays, but because of the instability and difficulty in analyzing RNA, current assays amplify and detect rDNA sequences.

Bacteria

Respiratory Tract Pathogens

Bacteria that cause respiratory tract disease account for significant morbidity and mortality levels around the world. Many of these organisms are ubiquitous in the environment and are endemic (native to a certain region or population group) even in higher socioeconomic countries. Bacteria in the respiratory tract are easily transmitted by contact with infected respiratory secretions. Laboratory detection and identification of these organisms by nonmolecular methods often lack sensitivity and/or are time-consuming. Because of their importance in causing human disease and the lack of sensitive, rapid laboratory tests, developing molecular-based assays that can detect and identify bacterial pathogens directly in respiratory specimens has been a priority (see Table 12.3).

Bordetella pertussis

B. pertussis is an upper-respiratory-tract pathogen that is the causative agent of whooping cough. The organism is endemic worldwide and is transmitted via direct contact with infected respiratory secretions. Children ages 1 through 5 are the primary targets of *B. pertussis*. In 1947, vaccination against *B. pertussis* was implemented in the United States, and cases of whooping cough in the target age group decreased significantly. Infections in infants younger than age 1 increased, however, after the vaccination program was started because the infants had not received the full series of three shots. Recently, outbreaks of pertussis have been identified in adolescents and adults in whom the immunity provided by the vaccine waned. A booster vaccine has been developed and is now recommended for adolescents ages 10 to 18. Still, the incidence rate remains highest among infants younger than age 1, with 55.2 cases per 100,000 population. Thus, despite the availability of a vaccine, *B. pertussis* is a significant pathogen, responsible for an estimated 50 million cases of pertussis and 300,000 deaths per year.[22]

One of the problems associated with reducing the incidence of *B. pertussis* related disease has been the lack of reliable culture methods that consistently allow for the isolation of *B. pertussis* from clinical samples. *B. pertussis* is a highly fastidious organism that requires special isolation conditions. Therefore, it very early became a target for the development of molecular-based assays. Once the *B. pertussis* genome was characterized, species-specific target sequences were identified and used to generate primers for PCR assays. Target sequences for *B. pertussis* are located in the IS*481* insertion sequence, the pertussis toxin gene promoter region, the adenylate cyclase gene, and species-specific porin protein structural genes.[23]

Chan and colleagues noted the amount of time required to perform and report results from a PCR assay as compared with the amount of time required for *B. pertussis* to be detected in culture. They reported that results from PCR assays were available in 2.3 days (where the assay was only performed 3 to 5 days/week), whereas positive culture results were not available for 5.1 days (where cultures were performed and read 6 days/week).[24]

While molecular-based assays have clearly and repeatedly been shown to have significantly higher sensitivity rates, there are still some concerns about the performance and interpretation of these assays. The major genetic target for primer binding in PCR assays detecting *B. pertussis* is IS*481*. This insertion sequence is also found in *Bordetella holmesii*, and thus the presence of *B. holmesii* in a clinical specimen can give false-positive results

Table 12.3 **Typical Respiratory Tract Organisms Targeted by Molecular-Based Detection Methods**[23,24]

Organism	Specimen Source	Gene Target	Traditional Diagnostic Methods
Mycoplasma pneumoniae	Bronchoalveolar lavage	16S rRNA	Culture
		16S rDNA	Serology
		Species-specific protein gene	
		P1 adhesion gene	
Chlamydophila pneumoniae	Respiratory	Cloned Pst I fragment	Culture
	Throat	16S rRNA	
	Artherosclerotic lesions	MOMP	
Legionella	Deep respiratory secretions	5S rRNA *mip* gene	Culture
	Serum	16S rRNA	Antigen detection
	Buffy coat		
	Urine		
Bordetella pertussis	Nasopharyngeal	IS 481	Culture
		Adenylate cyclase gene	DFA
		Porin gene	
		Pertussis toxin promoter region	
Streptococcus pneumoniae	Blood	DNA polymerase gene	Culture
	CSF	*plyA* (pneumolysin)	
	Serum	*lytA* (autolysin)	
	Sputum	*pbp2a* (penicillin-binding protein)	
		pbp2b	
		pspA (pneumococcal surface protein)	
Mycobacterium tuberculosis	Sputum	16S rRNA	Culture
	Bronchoalveolar lavage		
	Bronchial washings		
	Gastric aspirates		

when *B. pertussis* is the target.[25] The amplification and detection of another insertion sequence, IS*1001*, can be used to discriminate between *B. pertussis* and *B. holmesii*. IS*1001* is used as a target to detect *Bordetellaparapertussis* in clinical samples primarily, but IS*1001* is also found in *B. holmesii* and not in *B. pertussis*. IS*481* sequences are not seen in *B. parapertussis*. Amplifying both insertion sequence targets greatly increases the specificity of the assay for all three species.[26]

A standardized or FDA-approved, commercially available PCR test for *B. pertussis* is not yet available. Quality assurance programs to assess interlaboratory performance of PCR and real-time PCR assays for *B. pertussis* have been reported in European laboratories.[27,28] In the United States, the College of American Pathologists offers proficiency tests for *Bordetella* as well as other respiratory viruses. Primer and probe ASR for *B. pertussis* and *B. parapertussis* detection by real-time PCR targeting IS*481* and IS*1001,* respectively, are available from Cepheid.

Legionella pneumophila

L. pneumophila is the cause of Legionnaires' disease, a lower-respiratory-tract infection that was first diagnosed in men attending an American Legion convention in Philadelphia in 1976. Since their first identification, *Legionella* species have been found in water, both in the environment as well as in air conditioners and hot water tanks in various types of buildings. *Legionella* species infections range from asymptomatic to fatal and are the third most common cause of community-acquired pneumonias.[22,29]

Laboratory diagnosis of *Legionella* includes culture of bronchoalveolar lavage (BAL) samples on buffered citrate yeast extract media, direct fluorescent antibody (DFA) stain, enzyme immunoassay for urinary antigen, immunochromatographic assay for urinary antigen, and serology, which is only useful retrospectively. PCR assays are available for the direct detection of *Legionella* in respiratory tract specimens that are highly specific (88% to 100% specificity), but they are not more sensitive than the traditional culture assays, with reported sensitivities ranging from 64% to 100%.[30] Thus far, primers for *Legionella* nucleic acid amplification have targeted the macrophage infectivity potentiator (*mip*) gene and 16S and 5S rRNA genes. The 5S rRNA primers and early primers against 16S rRNA sequences have been associated with the reported low sensitivity and specificity mostly because the primers did not amplify all of the clinically relevant species of *Legionella*. Recent reports of PCR detection of *L. pneumophila* and *Legionella* species in BAL using different primers targeting 16S rRNA genes, however, did demonstrate amplification of multiple species of *Legionella*, but the assays are still in the developmental stages.[31,32]

Mycobacterium tuberculosis

M. tuberculosis is an important cause of respiratory tract infections worldwide, with infections causing significant levels of morbidity and mortality. The diagnosis of tuberculosis (TB) may take prolonged periods, during which the patient may spread the organism to other people. The genome of *M. tuberculosis* has been sequenced and has 4,411,529 bp with about 4000 genes that encode proteins and 50 RNA-encoding genes.[23] Of these, more than 250 genes encode enzymes involved in the metabolism of fatty acids, compared with just 50 genes with the same function that are found in *Escherichia coli*. The genomes of different isolates of *M. tuberculosis* do not vary to any great extent, and most variation is due to the movement of insertion elements rather than to point mutations.[33]

For many years, TB was diagnosed by mycobacterial smears and culture. Whereas a fluorochrome stain has increased sensitivity compared with the Kinyoun and Ziehl-Neelsen stains for detecting mycobacteria directly in clinical specimens, the sensitivity of smears in general for mycobacteria is 22% to 80%.[34] At least 10^4 organisms/mL are required in order to see mycobacteria in a smear, and then only 60% of those smears are read as positive.[35] Cultures for *M. tuberculosis* are more sensitive than smears and are able to detect 10^1 to 10^2 organisms/mL of specimen; however, they are still problematic due to the slow in vitro growth of the organism, which may not be isolated for 2 to 3 weeks after specimen collection.[36] Liquid-based culture systems have improved the detection rate of mycobacteria to a few days, depending on the organism load.

Once mycobacteria are detected growing in a culture, they must be speciated. The traditional method for speciation is biochemical testing, which can take a few weeks to perform. Mycolic acid analysis by high-performance liquid chromatography has been used to identify mycobacterial species either in a smear-positive specimen or from the growth in liquid or on solid media,[37] but it is not performed in most laboratories.

In 1990, mycobacterial identification was revolutionized with the development of DNA probe assays by GenProbe, Inc. The AccuProbe family of tests is available for the identification of *M. tuberculosis* complex (*tuberculosis*, *bovis*, and *africanum*), *M. avium-intracellulare*, *M. kansasii*, and *M. gordonae*. These tests detect mycobacterial-specific sequences of 16S rRNA when the rRNA forms a hybrid complex with reagent probe DNA. The hybrid rRNA-DNA complexes are detected in a luminometer that measures chemiluminescence given off by the acridinium ester attached to the DNA probe. The AccuProbe assay can be performed on colonies growing on solid media or from the growth in liquid media. Combining isolation of mycobacteria in a liquid-based medium with identification of species using AccuProbe has decreased the length of time required for detection and identification of *M. tuberculosis* in particular by at least 3 weeks.[38]

Although DNA probes greatly simplify and reduce the time involved in identifying mycobacterial species as compared with traditional biochemical testing, their sensitivity is not great enough to use them for detection of mycobacteria directly in a clinical specimen. Nucleic acid amplification methodologies have led to the development of laboratory tests in which *M. tuberculosis* can be detected directly in a clinical specimen with reliable sensitivity and specificity. Two such tests are available: the Amplified *M. tuberculosis* Direct test (AMTD®; GenProbe) and the AMPLICOR *M. tuberculosis* PCR test (AMPLICOR MTB; Roche).

GenProbe's AMTD test is FDA-approved for the direct detection of *M. tuberculosis* in smear-positive and smear-negative respiratory tract samples. The assay can also be performed on nonrespiratory samples with slight modification, although it is not yet FDA-approved for this use. The test uses transcription-mediated amplification (see Chapter 7) to amplify 16S rRNA present in a concentrated clinical sample. The amplified rRNA is detected using the same DNA probe as that used in the DNA probe assays described above and measures the chemiluminescence of rRNA-DNA hybrids. The sensitivity of the AMTD test when compared with smear and culture of smear-positive respiratory samples was 100% and 83% for specimens that had a negative smear.[39] Amplification and detection can be performed in 3.5 hours in a single tube and have 100% specificity for *M. tuberculosis* complex. When inhibitors are present in the clinical sample as well as when only a few organisms are present in the sample, however, the AMTD test is subject to false-negative results. The incorporation of internal controls and ensuring the amplification of the control in a valid test help to decrease the likelihood of false-negative samples.

The AMPLICOR MTB test is a kit-based PCR assay used for the detection of *M. tuberculosis* complex directly in a clinical specimen.[40] Cells are lysed in the sample, releasing mycobacterial DNA. The DNA is then denatured, and primers complementary to a 584-bp region of 16S rRNA that is common to all mycobacteria hybridize to target sequences. Next, DNA polymerase makes a copy of the target DNA, and dUTP and uracil-N-glycosylase are added to prevent carryover contamination. Finally, product detection is accomplished using a DNA probe specific for *M. tuberculosis* complex and a avidin–horseradish peroxidase conjugate–tetramethyl benzidine substrate system. The AMPLICOR MTB test takes 6.5 to 8 hours to complete and has a sensitivity of 55.3% in smear-negative samples and 94.7% sensitivity in smear-positive samples.[41] The different sensitivities reflect the importance of organism burden in the sample in yielding a positive result, even in a highly sensitive assay.

PCR tests targeting the species-specific sequences, such as IS*6110* and 16S rRNA, allow detection of *M. tuberculosis* from fresh, frozen, or fixed tissue. PCR-positive samples are hybridized with genus-specific and species/complex-specific probes. Real-time PCR assays have also been developed for *M. tuberculosis* detection with primers and probes targeting rRNA internal transcribed spacer elements in *M. tuberculosis*.[41,42]

Chlamydophila (Chlamydia) pneumoniae

C. pneumoniae is an obligate intracellular pathogen that causes 10% of community-acquired pneumonias and has been implicated in atherosclerosis and coronary artery disease. The prevalence of *C. pneumoniae* worldwide is high, with 70% of people having antibodies against *C. pneumoniae* by age 50.[43] *C. pneumoniae* typically causes pharyngitis, bronchitis, and mild pneumonia. Analysis of chlamydial 16S and 23S rRNA sequences has led to the suggestion that the genus *Chlamydia* should be split such that *pneumoniae* is a species of a newly named genus, *Chlamydophila*.[44]

The traditional laboratory method used for the detection of *C. pneumoniae* in respiratory samples is culture of the organism on cell lines in a shell vial culture system. Culture, however, is insensitive and dependent on obtaining and inoculating fresh clinical samples containing infected host cells onto the cell lines. Because reliable laboratory methods for the detection of *C. pneumoniae* are lacking, several groups have developed molecular-based assays targeting detection of *C. pneumoniae* in clinical samples. The RealAccurate™ *M. pneumoniae* + *C. pneumoniae* Duplex PCR kit (PathoFinder) simultaneously detects both pathogens in respiratory samples. Earlier assays lacked the sensitivity and specificity necessary for utilization in routine clinical testing.[45,46]

Mycoplasma pneumoniae

M. pneumoniae is a *Mollicute,* a bacterium that lacks a cell wall and is the smallest in size and genome of the free-living organisms. *M. pneumoniae* is the most common cause of community-acquired pneumonia, causing 20% of these infections. Laboratory diagnosis of *M. pneumoniae* is accomplished primarily by culture of respiratory tract secretions on special media, but serological tests are also available. For culture, specimens must be inoculated into a mycoplasma transport medium; *M. pneumoniae* grows very slowly, taking up to 4 weeks to be detected.

M. pneumoniae has been a target for the development of numerous molecular-based assays.[46] Genes targeted by amplification procedures include the P1 adhesion gene, 16S rRNA, the ATPase operon genes, and the gene (*tuf*) that encodes elongation factor 2. Amplification methodologies range from multiplex, nested, and real-time PCR to NASBA and Qβ-replicase. Primer design and amplification procedures for the nucleic acid of *M. pneumoniae* are well documented[47–50]; however, when amplification assays are compared with isolation of *M. pneumoniae* in culture, the molecular-based methods detect many more positives than do culture methods. Compared with serological test results, the nucleic acid–based tests have a sensitivity ranging from 77% to 94% and a specificity ranging from 97% to 100%, depending on the study.[46] Nucleic acid and culture results correlate better when the samples come from patients who have current lower-respiratory-tract infections than when the samples come from healthy individuals.[45] Respiratory secretions collected from healthy individuals that are positive in the nucleic acid assay yet negative by culture suggest the persistence of inviable organisms after an infection or asymptomatic carriage of low numbers of organisms. Thus, just as with any other laboratory test, the results of nucleic acid amplification procedures should be evaluated with respect to patient symptoms, history, and other laboratory test results.

Despite the problems with the development, implementation, and interpretation of molecular-based assays for *M. pneumoniae*, *L. pneumophila*, *B. pertussis*, and *C. pneumoniae* individually, multiplex nucleic acid amplification tests offer promise of sensitive, specific, and rapid detection leading to improved treatment and reduced hospital stays.[51–53]

Streptococcus pneumoniae

S. pneumoniae is the major cause of community-acquired pneumonia and is also a common cause of bacteremia, sepsis, otitis media, and meningitis.[23] Target age groups for infections causing disease are infants and toddlers younger than age 3 and adults older than age 65. *S. pneumoniae* has been found colonizing in the respiratory tracts of people ages 0 to 65, although the highest rates of carriage are seen in children younger than age 15. The virulence of *S. pneumoniae* in people at the extremes of age is due to the lack of an adequate immune response in these age groups.

Traditional laboratory detection of *S. pneumoniae* is by culture of clinical samples. The organism is fastidious yet grows well on media, such as chocolate agar and trypticase soy agar, with 5% sheep red blood cells. Because the organism can be found colonizing the oropharynx, the significance of its isolation in expectorated sputum that is contaminated with oral secretions is questionable. This fact makes the sensitivity of the culture of sputum for *S. pneumoniae* difficult to assess.

Molecular-based tests targeting *S. pneumoniae* have attempted to detect *S. pneumoniae* in a variety of clinical samples by targeting a variety of genes (see Table 12.3). Unfortunately, the results have been mixed, and amplification methods such as PCR are still not recommended as a method for diagnosing *S. pneumoniae* infections.

In a study comparing the specificity of four different PCR assays for identifying *S. pneumoniae*, primers specific for the autolysin (*lytA*) genes had 100% specificity for *S. pneumoniae*.[54] In another report, PCR assays targeting the pneumococcal pneumolysin gene were sensitive down to 10 colony-forming units per milliliter. The same PCR assay performed on serum was positive in 13% to 30% of healthy children; the serum of healthy adults ages 18 to 50 was negative in all of the subjects tested, suggesting that a positive PCR on an adult would be a **true positive** result, whereas on a child younger than age 16 it might be a false-positive result due to upper-respiratory-tract colonization. Thus, although PCR is specific for *S. pneumoniae*, the clinical significance of a positive PCR assay is questionable because a significant portion of the population (especially children) is colonized with the organism and PCR cannot discern between colonization and infection.[55]

Urogenital Tract Pathogens

Neisseria gonorrhoeae and *Chlamydia trachomatis* were among the first organisms to be targeted for detection in clinical specimens by molecular methods. The molecular methods are so well characterized for these two organisms that they are used almost exclusively in the detection of the nucleic acid of *N. gonorrhoeae* and *C. trachomatis*. Other sexually transmitted bacteria are considered good targets for the development of molecular-based methods because traditional laboratory methods of detection and identification for these organisms either lack sensitivity or are time-consuming. Table 12.4 summarizes the

Table 12.4 Typical Genital Tract Organisms Targeted by Molecular-Based Detection Methods[25,60]

Organism	Specimen Sources	Traditional Diagnostic Methods	Gene Target
Treponema pallidum	Genital ulcers	Serological (indirect and direct)	TpN44.5a
	Blood	Direct antigen detection (dark field, DFA)	TpN19
	Brain tissue		TpN39
	Cerebrospinal fluid		p01A
	Amniotic fluid		TpN47
	Placenta		16S rRNA
	Umbilical cord		*polA*
	Fetal tissue		
	Serum		
Mycoplasma genitalium	Urine	Culture	MgPa (adhesion gene)
	Urethral		rDNA gene
	Vaginal		
	Cervical		
Mycoplasma hominis	Genital tract	Culture	16S rRNA
	Amniotic fluid		
Ureaplasma urealyticum	Genital tract	Culture	16S rRNA
	Amniotic fluid		Urease gene
Haemophilus ducreyi		Gram stain	1.1 kb target
		Culture	*groEL* gene
		Serological	Intergenic spacer between 16S and 23S rDNA
			p27
			16S rDNA gene
Neisseria gonorrhoeae	Urine	Culture	*omp* III gene
	Urethral		*opa* gene
	Cervical		Cytosine DNA methyltrans-ferase gene
	Thin preparation vials		
			cPPB gene
			Site-specific recombinase gene
Chlamydia trachomatis	Urine	Culture	MOMP
	Urethral	EIA	16S RNA
	Cervical	DFA	
	Thin preparation vials		
	Conjunctiva		

molecular-based tests that have been described for the bacteria that cause genital tract infections.

Neisseria gonorrhoeae and Chlamydia trachomatis

N. gonorrhoeae and *C. trachomatis* are the two most common causes of sexually transmitted disease. Disease caused by *N. gonorrhoeae*, called gonorrhea, is associated with dysuria and urethral discharge in men and cervicovaginal discharge in women. *N. gonorrhoeae* can also cause pharyngitis and anorectal infections. *C. trachomatis* causes a nongonococcal urethritis and is asymptomatic in 50% to 66% of men and women. *N. gonorrhoeae* and *C. trachomatis* are often found together in coinfections, so it is prudent to rule out both organisms when considering whether one is present.[56]

Traditional laboratory diagnosis of *N. gonorrhoeae* entails culture of endocervical or urethral swabs onto chocolate agar and selective, enriched media such as modified Thayer Martin. For male urethral swabs, Gram stain alone with the observation of gram-negative diplococci is diagnostic by itself for *N. gonorrhoeae* (sensitivity = 90% to 95%; specificity = 95% to 100%).[57] For female endocervical swabs or other specimen types from males and females, Gram stain alone is not diagnostic (sensitivity = 50% to 70% for endocervical). *N. gonorrhoeae* is fastidious, and the specimen has to be transported in a specialized medium or plated directly onto media at the bedside. Delays in culturing the specimen are associated with false-negative cultures. Plates are examined daily for 72 hours for the presence of colonies resembling *Neisseria*, which are identified by biochemical testing.

Laboratory diagnosis of *C. trachomatis* is more problematic. *C. trachomatis* is an obligate intracellular pathogen; thus, when collecting specimens for isolation of *C. trachomatis*, it is critical that the practitioner scrape the endocervix or urethra to ensure the collection of host columnar epithelial cells that harbor the organisms. *C. trachomatis* is extremely labile, and clinical specimens sent to the laboratory for culture must be placed in a chlamydial transport medium to maintain the viability of the chlamydia. Culture of specimens for *C. trachomatis* is typically performed on McCoy cells in a shell vial system. The specimen is inoculated onto the cell line, the vial is incubated for 48 to 72 hours, and the cells are harvested and stained with a fluoresceinated antibody that has specificity for *C. trachomatis*.

Cultures for *N. gonorrhoeae* and *C. trachomatis* have been considered the gold standard, but when compared with nucleic acid amplification assays, the sensitivity of culture for *N. gonorrhoeae* is 85% to 100% and for *C. trachomatis* it is 80%.[9] Nucleic acid amplification assays have the additional advantages of being rapid, and testing can be batched and automated, resulting in further savings for the laboratory. The first molecular-based assay available for *N. gonorrhoeae* and *C. trachomatis* was AccuProbe from Gen-Probe, Inc. The AccuProbe is a nonamplification-based nucleic acid hybridization method that detects the rRNA of an organism by using an acridinium-labeled single-stranded DNA probe. The sensitivity of the AccuProbe for *N. gonorrhoeae* as compared with culture is 100%, with a specificity of 99.5%. For *C. trachomatis*, the sensitivity of AccuProbe is 67% to 96% (specimen quality is the reason for the variability), and specificity is 96% to 100%.[9] Although the DNA probes have comparable sensitivities and specificities to culture methods, laboratory professionals quickly implemented AccuProbe in their laboratories for the detection of *N. gonorrhoeae* and *C. trachomatis* because the assay is faster than culture and the same swab can be used for the detection of both *N. gonorrhoeae* and *C. trachomatis*.

Numerous nucleic acid amplification assays on the market target *N. gonorrhoeae* and *C. trachomatis*. The commercially available assays include target amplification assays, such as COBAS AMPLICOR CT/NG PCR (Roche), BD ProbeTecET strand displacement amplification (Becton Dickinson), and APTIMA COMBO II transcription mediated amplification (Gen-Probe). One hybrid capture signal amplification assay, called Rapid Capture System II for GC and CT (Digene), is also available. The nucleic acid amplification assays are performed on urethral or cervical swabs, urine, and, in some cases, on ThinPrep transport vials that are used to collect cervical cells for Papanicolaou smears. The sensitivity of all of the amplification methods is excellent and ranges from 93% to 100%, with specificity ranging from 99% to 100%.[9] The ability to use urine as a specimen to screen for the presence of *N. gonorrhoeae* and *C. trachomatis* has many advantages. The acceptability of the ThinPrep vials for *N. gonorrhoeae* and *C. trachomatis* testing means that one specimen can be collected from women for Papanicolaou smear, *N. gonorrhoeae*, *C. trachomatis*, and human papillomavirus.

In general, molecular-based assays are the major method for detection of *N. gonorrhoeae* and *C. trachomatis*. The assays are sensitive, specific, and rapid and have the potential to be fully automated. The only situation in which molecular-based testing is not acceptable for the detection of *N. gonorrhoeae* and *C. trachomatis* is in suspected child abuse cases. For these children, cultures may be performed in conjunction with molecular-based assays. Another consideration is laboratory testing to confirm the cure of an infection. As with any infectious organism and molecular-based test, the nucleic acid is detectable in a clinical sample whether the organism is dead or alive. A sample should not be taken for 3 to 4 weeks after treatment if the practitioner wants to see if the therapy was effective. Collection of samples and testing too soon after treatment will result in positive results after cultures on the same specimen have become negative.

Treponema pallidum

The spirochete *T. pallidum* subspecies *pallidum*, is the causative agent of syphilis, a sexually transmitted disease that results in the formation of a chancre at the site of inoculation (primary syphilis). If left untreated, the organism disseminates through the body, damaging tissues. The patient may progress into the other stages of disease: secondary syphilis (disseminated rash), latent syphilis (asymptomatic period), and tertiary syphilis (central nervous system and cardiovascular manifestations).

Laboratory diagnosis of syphilis is limited to serological testing, in which patients are typically screened (rapid plasma reagin [RPR] and venereal disease research laboratory [VDRL] tests) initially for the presence of antibodies against cardiolipin (a normal component of host membranes) and followed up with testing for the presence of antibodies against *T. pallidum* (TP-PA test; Fujirebio) to confirm infection. *T. pallidum* cannot be grown in vitro. Enzyme immunoassay–based tests are available to detect anti–*T. pallidum* antibodies. The EIA tests prepared using more immunologically relevant antigens have consistently higher sensitivity (97% to 100%) and specificity (98% to 100%) for patients in all stages of syphilis. Laboratories that have adopted the EIA assays use them to screen patients for syphilis and the RPR to monitor effectiveness of treatment and diagnose reinfection.[58]

RPR and VDRL are limited in that, when reactive, they are not specific for syphilis, and the sensitivity of these tests in very early (77% to 100%) and late (73%) syphilis is low.[58] The serological tests that detect *T. pallidum* antibodies are limited by their inability to differentiate between current and past infections; generally, once someone has syphilis, he or she will always have anti-*T. pallidum* antibodies. The RPR test, though, can be used to diagnose reinfections because titers of anticardiolipin antibodies will decrease to nonreactive following successful treatment of the organism and increase again with reinfections.

Several PCR assays have been developed and tested for the direct detection of *T. pallidum* DNA in genital ulcers, blood, brain tissue, cerebrospinal fluid, serum, and other samples, with varying sensitivities (1 to 130 organisms).[59] Amplification of the *T. pallidum* DNA polymerase I gene (*polA*) resulted in a detection limit of about 10 to 25 organisms; when tested on genital ulcers, a sensitivity of 95.8% and a specificity of 95.7% were reported.[60] In another test of PCR for the detection of *T. pallidum* in anogenital or oral ulcers, the authors found that PCR was 94.7% sensitive and 98.6% specific; the positive predictive value was 94.7%, and the negative predictive value was 98.6% in patients who had primary syphilis. The sensitivity and positive predictive value may be lower in secondary syphilis.[61] Qualitative real-time PCR assays for *T. pallidum* that require less than 1 mL of blood or other body fluid are presently in use in medical laboratories. One such assay using Taqman technology reportedly has a sensitivity of 80.39% and a specificity of 98.40% when directly compared with serology.[62]

Haemophilus ducreyi

H. ducreyi is a fastidious gram-negative coccobacillus that is the causative agent of chancroid. *H. ducreyi* is rarely found in the United States; it causes more infections in lower socioeconomic countries, especially in Africa, Asia, and Latin America. Laboratory diagnosis of *H. ducreyi* is difficult because the organism does not grow well in vitro and requires special media for isolation that is not available in most clinical laboratories in the United States. Gram stain of exudates is only 50% sensitive for *H. ducreyi* and thus is not recommended.[59]

Nucleic acid–based assays have been developed for *H. ducreyi* that target a variety of genes (see Table 12.4). Amplification of 16S rRNA along with the use of two probes for amplicon detection has been shown to be 100% sensitive in detecting multiple strains of *H. ducreyi*.[63] In addition, the assay has a sensitivity of 83%

to 98% and a specificity of 51% to 67% (depending on the number of amplification cycles) in detecting *H. ducreyi* in clinical specimens. Another PCR assay targeting an intergenic spacer region between the *rrs* and *rrl* ribosomal RNA genes of *H. ducreyi* is 96% sensitive for *H. ducreyi* in genital ulcer swabs compared with a sensitivity of 56% for culture.[64]

Mycoplasma and Ureaplasma spp.

Mycoplasma hominis, *Mycoplasma genitalium*, and *Ureaplasma urealyticum* cause nongonococcal urethritis. The mycoplasmas, as discussed above for *M. pneumoniae*, are the smallest free-living, self-replicating organisms known. *M. genitalium* has the smallest genome and thus was one of the first organisms to have its genome fully sequenced.[65] *M. genitalium* was identified in 1981,[66] and culture methods described in 1996[67] are still labor-intensive and not widely available. *U. urealyticum* is related to the *Mycoplasma* spp. and is also a member of the *Mollicutes* class.

PCR assays have been developed that amplify the adhesion gene (*MgPa*)[68,69] or the rDNA gene of *M. genitalium*.[70,71] Urethral or endocervical swabs or first-pass urine samples are all acceptable and yield positive PCR results. *M. genitalium* has been detected by PCR in all specimen types. Studies have shown that by PCR more symptomatic men were positive for *M. genitalium* (20%), but asymptomatic men still had detectable *M. genitalium* (9%).[66] PCR has been vital in establishing *M. genitalium* as an important genital tract pathogen, and laboratory-developed PCR with hybridization is currently used for clinical detection of *M. genitalium*. PCR assays for *M. hominis* and *U. urealyticum* have been developed and are used in clinical laboratories for the diagnosis of these organisms. Assay development has been hindered due to the absence of a reliable gold standard assay for comparison and especially in the absence of clinical symptoms. Thus the clinical significance of PCR-positive specimens has been difficult to interpret.[23] Laboratory-developed PCR and PCR-hybridization assays are currently in use.

Genital tract specimens have been the target for the development of multiplex assays in which the presence of nucleic acid of multiple organisms can be determined from one specimen in a single tube. The organisms causing genital tract infections either overlap in their symptoms, making diagnosis difficult without specific laboratory testing, or infections can be caused by the presence of multiple organisms at the same time. One published report of multiplex PCR for genital tract specimens have indicated that when simultaneous detection of *T. pallidum*, *H. ducreyi*, and herpes simplex virus (HSV) types 1 and 2 in genital ulcers was performed by multiplex PCR, the sensitivity of the PCR assay for HSV was 100% (culture sensitivity was 71.8%), for *H. ducreyi* it was 98.4% (culture was 74.2%), and for *T. pallidum* it was 91% (dark-field sensitivity was 81%).[72] Since this first description of the multiplex assay, other groups have used the method to confirm the sensitivity of the assay for the targeted organisms and to examine the prevalence of these organisms in various geographic areas in different years.[59,73]

Viruses

The laboratory diagnosis of viruses has benefited probably more than the diagnosis of any other organism from molecular-based methods. In general, viruses are diagnosed by testing for antibodies against the virus, by measuring the presence or absence of viral antigens, or by detecting the growth of a virus in a culture system. Although some of these methods are well established for certain viruses, they all have major disadvantages.

Even though laboratory testing is available for antibodies against most viruses, the detection of antibodies against a virus is an indirect method of diagnosis. The host immune response has to be stimulated by the virus to produce antibodies. In the case of an immunodeficient patient, the lack of antibodies is due to host factors and not due to the lack of the virus, yet the lack of antibodies is often interpreted as a lack of the virus. Furthermore, using antibodies to diagnose an infection is often a retrospective indication of the infection. To interpret antibody testing with the most confidence, paired sera should be collected, one sample collected during the acute phase of the infection and the other collected as the patient is recovering. The titers of antibodies are measured in both samples. A fourfold or greater rise in titer level from the acute sample to the convalescent sample indicates the presence of the virus during the acute stage. Detecting IgM antibodies, in particular, during an acute infection is the best evidence for the presence of virus. But even detecting IgM, the first isotype of antibody produced in an acute infection, is not without problems. If the patient is in the very early stages of infection, IgM titers may be below detection limits and would be interpreted as negative. When the patient is infected with a virus and the antibodies are not detectable, they are in the "window" period. During this time, the patient is infected and infectious.

Antigen detection testing is available in the clinical laboratory only for some viruses. Assays that measure viral antigens are available more often for respiratory syncytial virus, influenza virus, rotavirus, HSV, cytomegalovirus (CMV), and hepatitis B virus (HBV). Viral antigens are detected by enzyme immunoassays or direct immunofluorescent assays.

The classical method for detection and identification of viruses in body fluids is tissue or cell culture. Monolayers of host cells are grown in vitro, the patient's specimen is inoculated onto the cells, and changes in the cells due to viral infection, called **cytopathic effect**, are observed microscopically by the technologist. The identity of the virus is confirmed using fluorescently labeled monoclonal antibodies. Culture has been the gold standard for many viruses, in particular, adenovirus, enteroviruses, CMV, influenza, and HSV, but it is not applicable to other viruses, such as the hepatitis viruses, because these viruses do not grow well in culture systems. Another disadvantage to viral culture is the amount of time required before viral growth is detectable. Although the shell vial system, where the sample is centrifuged onto a cell monolayer and tested with antiviral antibodies, has decreased detection time,[74,75] several days to weeks, depending on the virus, can pass before detection of cytopathic effect. Furthermore, some viruses do not produce a cytopathic effect on infecting cells, or the cytopathic effect that is produced is subtle and easily missed. In these cases, the cultures will be reported as a false-negative result. Another disadvantage of using viral cultures to detect and identify viral infections is that the specimen must be collected in the acute phase of the disease, that is, in the first 5 days of the illness, after which the amount of virus in body fluids decreases significantly and may result in false-negative cultures.

The many disadvantages of these diagnostic methods present a tremendous opportunity for molecular-based assays. Nucleic acid amplification assays have quickly become indispensable in the clinical virology laboratory. Molecular methods are well suited to targeting the various configurations of nucleic acids found in human pathogenic viruses (Table 12.5). Target amplification assays such as PCR, reverse transcriptase PCR (RT-PCR),

Table 12.5 **Genomes of Human Viruses**	
Double-Stranded DNA Viruses	Adenovirus
	BK virus
	Cytomegalovirus
	Epstein-Barr virus
	Hepatitis B virus
	Herpes simplex virus 1
	Herpes simplex virus 2
	Human papillomavirus
	JC virus
	Molluscum virus
	Rotavirus
	Vaccinia virus
	Varicella-zoster virus
Single-Stranded DNA Virus	Parvovirus
Double-Stranded RNA Virus	Rotavirus
Single-Stranded RNA Viruses	Colorado tick fever virus
	Coronavirus*
	Coxsackie virus*
	Dengue virus*
	Ebola virus†
	Echovirus*
	Hepatitis A virus*
	Hepatitis C virus
	Hepatitis D virus
	Hepatitis E virus
	Human T-cell leukemia virus‡
	Human immunodeficiency virus‡
	Influenza virus
	Measles virus†
	Mumps virus†
	Norwalk virus, norovirus
	Parainfluenza virus
	Poliovirus*
	Rabies virus
	Respiratory syncytial virus
	Rhinovirus*
	Rubella virus*
	Yellow fever virus*

*Positive RNA; directly translated.
†Negative RNA; complementary to the translated strand.
‡Retroviral replication requires a DNA intermediate.

quantitative (or real-time) PCR (qPCR), and transcription-mediated amplification (TMA) as well as signal amplification assays such as branched DNA (bDNA) amplification and hybrid capture are used in the clinical virology laboratory to diagnose or monitor viral infections. Table 12.6 summarizes the viruses for which nucleic acid amplification assays are available (either commercially or performed in-house) along with the type of amplification procedure, the targeted genes, and clinical utility. Molecular-based tests for HIV, EBV, HPV, HCV, and BK/JC viruses are frequently used in clinical laboratories and are discussed in more detail below.

Table 12.6 **Nucleic Acid Amplification Tests for Viruses**[8,125–127]

Virus	NAA Methodology	Amplified Target	Dynamic Range/ Sensitivity	Clinical Utility
Human immunodeficiency virus	PCR:	*gag* gene; 155 bp (HIV-1 group M (subtypes A-H), not HIV-2 or HIV-1 group O)	400–750,000 copies/mL (standard)	Viral quantitation
	HIV-1 DNA (Roche)		50–100,000 copies/mL (ultra-sensitive)	Disease prognosis Treatment monitoring
	RT-PCR (Amplicor and COBAS; Roche)			
	NASBA	*gag* (similar to Amplicor)	176,000–3,470,000 copies/mL	
	NucliSense (bio Merieux)	HIV-1 groups M, O, and N		
	bDNA: Versant HIV-1 (Bayer)	*pol;* subtypes of group M (subtypes A–G, but not group O)	75–500,000 copies/mL	
Cytomegalovirus (CMV)	Hybrid capture (Digene)	Immediate-early antigen 1	1400–600,000 copies/mL	Detect CMV DNA in organ transplant and AIDS patients and congenitally infected infants
	PCR	Major immediate-early antigen	400–50,000 copies/mL	
	NASBA qPCR	Glycoproteins B and H		Viral load determinations
	Major capsid protein	Detect HSV when asymptomatic or when cultures are negative		
Herpes simplex virus-1 and -2 (HSV)	PCR	Thymidine kinase		
	qPCR	DNA polymerase		

continued

Table 12.6 **Nucleic Acid Amplification Tests for Viruses**[8,125–127]**—cont'd**

Virus	NAA Methodology	Amplified Target	Dynamic Range/ Sensitivity	Clinical Utility
		DNA-binding protein		Diagnosis of HSV encephalitis and neonatal infections
		Glycoproteins gb, gc, gd, and gg		
Epstein-Barr virus (EBV)	PCR	EBNA1		EBV-associated malignancies
	qPCR	LMP-1	100–10^{10} copies/mL	Detect EBV in asymptomatic immunocompro-mised hosts
Human papillomavirus (HPV)	Hybrid capture (FDA-approved)	L1 or E1 open reading frames	10^5 copies/mL	Detection of HPV in endocervical swabs
	PCR			Differentiation of low-risk and high-risk types
	qPCR			Monitoring women with abnormal Pap smears
Hepatitis B virus	PCR		1000–40,000 copies/mL	Prognosis and moni-toring of antiviral treatment response
	bDNA		0.7–5000 meq/mL	
	Hybrid capture		142,000–1,700,000,000 copies/mL (standard) 4700–56,000,000 copies/mL (ultrasensitive)	
Parvovirus B19	PCR			Diagnosis of infections
Respiratory syncytial virus (RSV)	RT-PCR	Fusion glycoprotein (F) gene		Detection of RSV
		Nucleoprotein (N) gene		Differentiate between subgroups A and B
Parainfluenza viruses	RT-PCR	Hemagglutinin-neuraminidase con-served regions 5' noncoding region of F gene		Epidemiology

Table 12.6 **Nucleic Acid Amplification Tests for Viruses[8,125–127]—cont'd**

Virus	NAA Methodology	Amplified Target	Dynamic Range/ Sensitivity	Clinical Utility
Influenza viruses	RT-PCR	Conserved matrix (M) genes (influenza A and B)		Diagnose infections
		Nucleocapsid protein (influenza A)		Characterize isolates
		NS1 gene (influenza B)		Can be type- and subtype-specific
Metapneumovirus	RT-PCR	Fusion (F) gene RNA polymerase (L) gene		
Coronavirus	RT-PCR	RNA polymerase gene		Used to detect and characterize the SARS virus
		Nucleoprotein gene		
Norwalk virus	RT-PCR	RNA polymerase gene		
Rotavirus	RT-PCR	VP7 gene		
		VP4 gene		
Hepatitis C virus	RT-PCR	5' untranslated region (UTR)	600–800,000 IU/mL	
	bDNA	5' UTR and core protein gene	3200–40,000,000 copies/mL	
West Nile virus	RT-PCR			
	NASBA	Variety of gene targets based on genome of type strain NY99 0.01 PFU	0.1–1 PFU	Used for diagnosis and surveillance
Rubella virus	RT-PCR	Surface glycoprotein, E1, gene	Variable; sensitivity of 3–10 copies is best	Primarily for fetal diagnosis
				Used for diagnosis when serum is not available
				May be used to confirm positive serological results
Mumps virus	RT-PCR	Hemagglutinin, neuraminidase, P, SH, and F genes		Differentiate strains
Measles virus	RT-PCR	M, H, F, N		When culture is not practical or genotyping is required for diagnosis of MIBE or SSPE

continued

Table 12.6 **Nucleic Acid Amplification Tests for Viruses[8,125–127]—cont'd**

Virus	NAA Methodology	Amplified Target	Dynamic Range/ Sensitivity	Clinical Utility
				Differentiation of vaccine and wild-type strains
Enteroviruses (group A and B Cox- sackieviruses, echoviruses, and others)	RT-PCR	Conserved 5' nontrans- lated region		Performed on CSF to rule out enteroviral meningitis
BK Virus (polyomavirus)	PCR	Large T protein		Diagnosis of BK virus nephritis

MIBE = Measles inclusion body encephalitis
SSPE = Subacute sclerosing panencephalitis
PFU = Plaque-forming units

Human Immunodeficiency Virus

Human immunodeficiency virus (HIV) is unique among the RNA viruses in that it is a retrovirus that makes a DNA copy of genomic RNA using virally encoded reverse transcriptase. There are two types of HIV: HIV type 1, or HIV-1, and HIV type 2, or HIV-2. HIV-2 is a minor isolate found mainly in West Africa and is less pathogenic than HIV-1, causing more latent infections.[16] New strains continue to evolve.

HIV rapidly mutates and recombines so that multiple groups then divide into "clades," or subtypes, of the virus that are found in different locations in the world.[23] HIV group M causes 95% of the infections due to HIV around the world. Group M is further divided into eight clades (A, B, C, D, F, G, H, and J). Group M, clade B, is found most often in the United States and Europe. Group O HIV is found primarily in West Africa, and group N is found in Cameroon.[76]

To infect host cells, the HIV surface molecules gp120 and gp41 interact with CD4, a molecule that is expressed primarily on the surface of helper T lymphocytes and is also found on macrophages, dendritic cells, and other antigen-presenting cells. Chemokine receptors, in particular CCR5, on dendritic/Langerhans' cells and macrophages/ monocytes, and CXCR4 on CD4+ T cells form a complex with CD4 on the cell surface and also engage gp120.

After attachment to host cells via CD4-gp120 binding, the virus enters the cell, where reverse transcriptase makes cDNA from viral RNA. The cDNA integrates into the host DNA where it either persists in a stage of latency as the provirus or is replicated actively. Transcription and translation of viral peptides as well as production of viral RNA are performed by cellular components under the direction of virally encoded regulatory proteins (i.e., *tat*, *rev*, *nef*, and *vpr*).[76]

HIV infection is diagnosed by detecting antibodies specific for HIV in an EIA and confirming the specificity of detected antibodies for HIV products in a western blot or the APTIMA HIV-1 RNA Qualitative Assay (GenProbe), which has been approved by the FDA as an aid in the diagnosis of HIV-1 infection. The antigens used in the western blot tests may differ depending on the country of origin. For infants who have maternal IgG and for patients suspected of incubating HIV in whom antibody tests are negative, antigen detection tests measure the amount of HIV p24 antigen. Nucleic acid amplification assays, such as the COBAS® AmpliPrep/COBAS® TaqMan® HIV-1 Test (Roche Diagnostics), and the APTIMA® HIV-1 RNA Qualitative Assay (Abbott), are performed after an HIV diagnosis to determine how actively the virus is replicating (viral load), when to start antiretroviral therapy, and when to monitor efficacy of treatment. Rapid, noninvasive conjugated antigen tests such as the Rapidtest HIV® Lateral Flow Test (Health-Chem Diagnostics, LLC) may increase compliance with screening.[16]

Determining HIV Viral Load

The amount of HIV or viral load is used as a marker for disease prognosis as well as to track the timing and efficacy of antiretroviral therapy. Patients are 10 times more likely to progress to AIDS within 5 years if they have viral loads above 100,000 copies/mL within 6 months of seroconversion.[76] The goal of antiretroviral therapy is a viral load below 50 copies/mL of blood. Patients who maintain viral levels at fewer than 10,000 copies/mL in the early stages of the infection are at decreased risk of progression to AIDS.[77]

Patients who are effectively treated with antiretroviral therapy will have a significant reduction in viral load 1 week after the initiation of therapy. The lack of significant decrease in viral load during this time indicates the lack of efficacy. Highly active antiretroviral therapy (HAART), consisting of two reverse transcriptase inhibitors combined with a protease inhibitor or a nonnucleoside reverse transcriptase inhibitor, has reduced viral loads below the detection limits of even ultrasensitive assays for more than 3 years.[78] In patients receiving HAART, 2 $\log_{10}$ decreases in viral load have been documented. Viral load testing should be performed in conjunction with determining CD4 counts. In general, but not always, viral load and CD4 counts are inversely proportional; that is, the higher the viral load, the lower the CD4 count.[79]

Molecular-based methods used to quantify HIV in patient samples include PCR for integrated DNA, RT-PCR for viral RNA, nucleic acid sequence–based amplification (NASBA), and bDNA (see Table 12.6).

Table 12.7 compares the advantages and disadvantages of each of these assays for determining HIV viral load. Viral load should be determined before therapy is started, 2 to 8 weeks after therapy initiation to see the initial response, and then every 3 to 4 months to assess therapeutic effectiveness.

Because nucleic acid amplification assays use different amplification techniques, and sometimes different standards for quantifying, results from one method may not be comparable with those of another. In general, viral loads determined by the Amplicor RT-PCR (version 1.0) are about twofold higher than loads determined either by bDNA (version 2.0) or by NASBA.[130,131] On the other hand, viral loads determined by the bDNA (version 3.0) and Amplicor RT-PCR (version 1.5) are similar.[80] Even though results obtained by different methods are becoming more and more comparable, it is still recommended that laboratory professionals use the same method to determine viral loads when monitoring patients over time. Results should be expressed consistently as integers (copies/mL or IU/mL), log-transformed results (log IU/mL) or scientific notation ($a \times 10^b$ IU/mL), or a combination of these. CDC guidelines recommend reporting in integers and log-transformed copies. The Clinical and Laboratory Standards Institute subcommittee also recommends that the integers be rounded from units to the nearest tens to two significant figures.

Quantitative HIV-1 RNA testing in plasma has been the standard for monitoring drug therapy and HIV disease progression. The Multicenter AIDS Cohort Study, an ongoing project monitoring the clinical histories of treated and untreated HIV-infected men, has described laboratory measurements of viral load and clinical disease. The U.S. Department of Health and Human Services (DHHS) recommends an objective of maximal

Table 12.7 Advantages and Disadvantages of the Nucleic Acid Amplification Methods for HIV Viral Loads

Test	Advantages	Disadvantages
bDNA	High throughput	No internal control
	Broad dynamic range	
	Applicable for group M subtypes A–G	False-positive results reported
Amplicor RT-PCR	Internal control	Limited dynamic range
	Good specificity	
NASBA	Broad dynamic range	Does not detect all non-B subtypes
	Performed on many specimen types and volumes	

suppression of viral replication down to undetectable levels by sensitive analysis.

The first commercially produced tests could detect viral loads down to 400 to 500 copies/mL plasma; however, suppression to fewer than 20 copies/mL plasma was associated with longer response to therapy than suppression below 500 copies/mL,[81] which emphasizes the importance of a highly sensitive assay with a very low limit of detection for optimal treatment strategy and patient care. The lower **limit of detection** is defined as the lowest viral concentration that can be detected over background or a negative control in the test assay. Currently available FDA-approved HIV tests include the Bayer VERSANT HIV-1 RNA 3.0 Assay (bDNA), the Roche Amplicor MONITOR Test (RTPCR), and the bio-Merieux NucliSens HIV-1 QT Test (NASBA), with lower limits of detection of 75, 50, and 176 viral copies/mL plasma, respectively. The Abbott RealTime™ HIV-1 (qPCR) assay, a more automated method, has a limit of detection of 40 viral copies/mL.

In addition to sensitivity, all test methods, including HIV tests, should have certain characteristics (Table 12.8). Accuracy is an important requirement for viral load testing. It is established by the calibration of assays to a common standard. Tests must also have quantitative as well as qualitative accuracy that is a true measure of the viral level over a range of values. The viral load levels established by the DHHS and the International AIDS Society for the initiation of therapy must be consistently identified in independent laboratories as accurately as possible.

Real-time PCR methods offer linear measurement over a wider range than other methods, which precludes the requirement for dilution of high-titer specimens before analysis. The precision or reproducibility of the test used is also important for establishing statistically significant differences in the viral load over a serial testing period. The DHHS defines a minimally significant change as a threefold increase or decrease in viral load/mL plasma. And the high specificity of a test gives confidence that a positive result is truly positive. All subtypes of virus should be detected with equal efficiency to avoid under- or overestimating viral loads of certain subgroups.

No matter the method used, not much variability in viral loads will be distinguished among repeated samples; for example, quantifying RNA in the same patient will not change much over time (approximately $0.3 \log_{10}$ unit) as long as the patient is clinically stable and antiretroviral therapy has not begun or changed.[82] In order to be clinically relevant, viral load changes from one determination to another must vary by threefold ($0.5 \log_{10}$ unit). HIV-positive patients may experience transient increases in viral loads when they have other infections or receive vaccinations, but levels will return to baseline within a month.[83–85] Proficiency testing is available from the College of American Pathologists (CAP; Northfield, IL) and the CDC. The World Health Organization (WHO) has an HIV-1 RNA reference standard. Acrometrix (Benicia, CA), Boston Biomedica, Inc. (West Bridgewater, MA), and IMPATH-BCP, Inc. (Franklin, MA) have external standards and verification panels for HIV-1 viral load testing.

HIV Genotyping

Genotyping is used to monitor the development of antiretroviral drug resistance in HIV. Most of the antiretroviral drugs target the reverse transcriptase and protease enzymes, so these are the genes that are most often examined in genotyping procedures. Thus far, more than 100 mutations associated with drug resistance have been identified in HIV-1.[86,87]

To perform genotyping, viral RNA is extracted and PCR is used to amplify the whole protease gene and part of the reverse transcriptase gene. The products are analyzed for the presence of mutations by sequencing, hybridization onto high-density microarrays (GeneChip; Affymetrix, Santa Clara, CA), or reverse hybridization using the line probe assay (VERSANT HIV-1 Protease

Table 12.8 **Test Performance Features for Viral Load Measurement**

Characteristic	Description
Sensitivity	Lowest level detected at least 95% of the time
Accuracy	Ability to determine true value
Precision	Reproducibility of independently determined test results
Specificity	Negative samples are always negative and positive results are true positives
Linearity	A serial dilution of standard curve closely approximates a straight line
Flexibility	Accuracy of measurement of virus regardless of sequence variations

and RT Resistance Assays, LiPA; Bayer Corporation). Sequencing is performed most often, and there are currently two commercially available kits for this purpose: Trugene HIV-I genotyping kit and OpenGene DNA-sequencing system (Bayer) and ViroSeq HIV-1 genotyping system (Applied Biosystems). Once the sequence of the patient's virus is known, it is compared with a wild-type reference sequence to identify the mutations present in the patient's isolate, if any.

After the mutations have been identified, their significance in terms of the impact on antiretroviral therapy must be assessed, and this is generally accomplished through analysis by computer algorithms. The interpretation of genotyping results for the effect of a mutation on the development of resistance is very complicated. Resistance mutations have been well characterized for individual agents, but HIV-positive patients are more often on cocktails of drugs rather than one drug. Therefore, the impact of a mutation on multiple drugs must be considered. In addition, if HIV has multiple mutations, the interpretation of more than one mutation with respect to multiple drugs becomes more complex. The computer algorithm that is used to analyze genotypes takes into account primary and secondary mutations, cross-resistance, and the interactions between mutations that can affect resistance.[88]

Mutations found by genotyping are generally divided into two groups: **primary resistance mutations** and **secondary resistance mutations**. Primary resistance mutations are those that are specific for a particular drug, reduce the susceptibility of the virus to that drug, and appear in the viral genome shortly after treatment with that agent has begun. The mutated enzyme is generally not as active as the normal enzyme, so viral replication is decreased, but it still occurs. As treatment with the drug continues, secondary or compensatory mutations occur that try to recover the ability of the virus to replicate at a normal rate. The secondary mutations do not affect the susceptibility of the virus to the drug, but rather help the

virus replicate in the presence of the drug when one of its replication enzymes is not 100% functional.[76] Once a resistance genotype has been identified, the drug therapy of the patient should be changed as soon as possible to avoid the development of secondary mutations in the virus.

The results of genotyping procedures are reported by listing the mutations that have been identified in the protease and reverse transcriptase genes and the impact those mutations will have on each drug: no evidence of resistance, possible resistance, resistance, or insufficient evidence. The mutations are indicated by reporting a change in the amino acid that is coded by the changed codon, where the wild-type amino acid is written, followed by the position of the codon that is changed, followed by the new amino acid. For example, a mutation in codon 184 of the reverse transcriptase gene from ATG to GTG results in an amino acid change from methionine to valine, or M184V. This particular mutation makes the virus resistant to the cytidine analog, lamivudine.[88]

As with all other molecular-based assays, HIV genotyping procedures should employ adequate quality and contamination controls.[89] The sensitivity of the methods to detecting a minority of virions that contain mutations in the midst of a majority of wild-type virions is an important consideration. The sensitivity of the automated sequencing methods has been reported to be 20%, and the LiPA has a reported sensitivity of 4% (i.e., it can detect as few as 4/100 mutants in the presence of 96/100 wild types). Proficiency testing is available from CAP and Acrometrix. Acrometrix and Boston Biomedica Inc. provide independent control materials for use in genotyping assays.

Herpes Viruses

At least 25 viruses comprise the family *Herpesviridae*. Several herpes virus types frequently infect humans, including herpes simplex virus (HSV), cytomegalovirus (CMV), Epstein-Barr virus (EBV), and varicella zoster virus (VZV). In addition to causing overt disease, herpes viruses may remain silent and be reactivated many years after infection.

Herpes Simplex Virus
HSV has a relatively large viral genome encoding at least 80 protein products. About half of these proteins are

---

Advanced Concepts

For more information about specific mutations and the interactions of mutations, see http://www.iasusa.org and references 84 and 85.

involved in the interaction with the host cell or immune system. The other half control viral structure and replication. There are two types of HSV, HSV type 1 (HSV-1) and HSV type 2 (HSV-2). HSV-1 mainly causes cold sores or fever blisters; HSV-2 mainly causes genital sores, but can also cause mouth sores. HSV tests are usually done for genital sores, although body fluids, including blood, urine, tears, amniotic fluid, lavages, and spinal fluid, may also be tested.

HSV is detected by viral culture, antigen, and antibody tests. In viral culture, a swab from a sore is incubated in culture medium. Viral cultures may have to be performed more than once, as the virus may not be detected at all times of infection. The HSV antigen test is performed on a slide smear of material from the sore. Viral antigens are detected with labeled antibodies. The antibody test is done on blood to detect antibodies to the viral antigens. Antibodies may not be detectable 2 weeks to 3 months after initial infection; however, once the infection occurs, antibodies remain in the person for life. Western blot tests such as HerpeSelect® (Focus Diagnostics) can distinguish HSV-1 and HSV-2 using type-specific antigens gG1 and gG2 to detect the corresponding type-specific antibodies. Type-specific testing is important for prognosis and patient counseling.

Molecular tests for HSV are performed on sores and body fluids. PCR tests also offer the advantage of distinguishing HSV-1 from HSV-2. Methods include standard PCR and quantitative PCR targeting type-specific HSV genes (Table 12.6). The *MultiCode-RTx* qPCR Test (Era-Gen Biosciences, Inc.) has been cleared by the FDA for vaginal legion specimens and will distinguish between HSV-1 and HSV-2.

Epstein-Barr Virus

One of the most common human viruses is the Epstein-Barr virus (EBV), a member of the herpes virus family. Most people become infected with EBV sometime during their lives. Children can become infected with EBV once they lose maternal antibody protection, and according to the CDC, 95% of adults in the United States between ages 35 and 40 have likely been infected with EBV. First infection during adolescence or young adulthood causes infectious mononucleosis.

EBV establishes a permanent dormant infection in cells of the throat, blood, and immune system. Latent infection is characterized by the presence of EBV-encoded RNA (EBER). The virus can reactivate and is commonly found in the saliva of infected persons. EBV infection is associated with a variety of benign and malignant lesions, including oral hairy leukoplakia, inflammatory pseudotumor, Hodgkin disease, non-Hodgkin lymphoma, Burkitt lymphoma, gastric carcinoma, and nasopharyngeal carcinoma. Although EBV is present in these conditions, it is likely not the sole cause of disease.

Laboratory diagnosis of EBV infection has been performed by immunohistochemistry for EBV proteins in tissue and testing serum for antibodies to EBV-associated antigens, including the viral capsid antigen, the early antigen, and the EBV nuclear antigen (EBNA). Confirmation may be done by differentiation of IgG and IgM subclasses to the viral capsid antigen. The gold standard for tissue analysis is in situ hybridization of the EBER transcripts.[90] Repeated or unique sequences in EBV DNA may also be targets of in situ hybridization; however, the sensitivity of DNA probes is lower than those for EBER, due to the abundant presence of the EBER transcripts.

Southern blot analysis of EBV DNA, first described in 1986,[91] was based on variable numbers of terminal repeat sequences at the ends of each EBV DNA molecule. Each infecting genome can contain up to 20 terminal repeat sequences. When EBV DNA is cut with *Bam*H1, the resulting fragments vary in size, depending on the number of repeat sequences. The fragments were visualized with a probe complementary to the variable repeat.

Amplification methods are now used for detecting EBV in blood, body fluid, or tissue samples. EBV DNA can be amplified using primers complementary to conserved EBV sequences, and strain typing can be achieved by amplification of polymorphic regions of the viral genome. Quantitative PCR is used to determine EBV viral load in blood using a reference internal control.[92] A reported quantitative range of analysis is 100 to 10^{10} copies/mL (EBV R-gene™; Argene). As with other such tests, virus may still be present below the level of detection.

Cytomegalovirus

Most people have been infected with CMV without obvious illness. Like other herpes viruses, CMV can go dormant and reactivate. If symptoms occur, they are mild, except in immunocompromised individuals. The virus is shed in blood, urine, saliva, and other body fluids but dies quickly outside of the host.

Molecular detection of CMV is performed on cell-free plasma or other fluids. DNA is extracted and amplified by PCR using primers targeting the CMV polymerase (UL54) or glycoprotein B (gB) gene in regions that do not share sequence homology with other herpes viruses. Internal controls are included to avoid false-negative interpretation due to PCR inhibition. The level of detection of standard laboratory assays is such that no PCR product will be produced from normal plasma, even from people previously exposed to CMV. Automated amplification and detection of CMV with the COBAS Amplicor® (Roche) has an analytical sensitivity of one viral copy per microliter. Quantitative PCR using LightCycler or TaqMan technology reportedly shows better accuracy than COBAS with high viral titers and can detect 40 genome copies of virus per microliter of blood.[93,94] These assays may be affected by the presence of mutations in the target genes that interfere with primer hybridization. These mutations may confer resistance to antiviral therapy.

Varicella Zoster Virus

Varicella zoster virus (VZV, HHV3) is the causative agent of chickenpox and shingles (also called herpes zoster). The virus has a large genome containing over 70 open reading frames (ORFs). Polymorphisms in the ORF are used to determine the strain variations and genotype of viruses from different geographical areas. An attenuated live virus, VZV Oka, developed by selection in cell cultures, is the parental strain source of a VZV vaccine, which contains a mixture of genotypically distinct viral variants.

VZV is neurotropic, remaining latent in nerve cells and possibly reactivating years after primary infections to result in shingles, or palsy. It is found in more than 90% of young people living in temperate climates. There is no animal reservoir for VZV. Clinical tests include enzyme-linked immunosorbent assays and PCR methods for detection of antibodies to VZV in serum. Qualitative PCR methods include PCR with hybridization or direct gel electrophoresis. Quantitative PCR kits such as the VZV PCR Kit (Abbott Molecular) include internal controls to detect amplification inhibition.

Hepatitis C Virus

HCV is an enveloped RNA virus that causes viral hepatitis and cirrhosis and is also associated with causing hepatocellular carcinoma. The virus is transmitted parenterally like HIV. Acute infections are often asymptomatic and are rarely associated with jaundice; thus patients with acute HCV infections are usually not diagnosed at this stage. Among HCV-positive patients, 85% will develop chronic hepatitis, and even most of these patients will be asymptomatic. The development of chronic infections is due to the antigenic envelope proteins that elicit the production of antibodies. These proteins are encoded by hypervariable regions much like antibody genes themselves, resulting in extensive variation in the envelope proteins and the escape of the virus from antibodies.

The approach to diagnosing HCV infections is similar to that used for HIV. Serology is used to detect the presence of antibodies against HCV. If the patient has HCV antibodies, the specificity of the antibodies for HCV antigens is measured by Western blot, where the presence of antibodies with multiple HCV specificities confirms the diagnosis.

A variety of nucleic acid amplification assays for the qualitative detection and quantitation of HCV are available, including RT-PCR (Amplicor HCV; Roche), transcription-mediated amplification (VERSANT HCV RNA qualitative assay; Bayer) and branched DNA (VERSANT HCV RNA 3.0; Bayer). The qualitative HCV RNA assays are performed on patients with positive HCV antibody results to confirm active infection or on immunocompromised patients (who are often coinfected with HIV) in whom HCV infection is suspected but antibody tests are negative. The quantitative HCV RNA assays are used as for HIV to determine the viral load and to monitor viral replication in response to antiviral therapy. The viral load and the HCV genotype are used to determine the therapeutic protocol, both type of drug(s) as well as duration.[95]

Six genotypes (1a, 1b, 2, 3, 4, 5, and 6) and 80 subtypes of HCV have been identified. The genotype of HCV present in a given patient determines the treatment protocol used on that patient, as particular genotypes are associated with certain antiviral resistance patterns.[95] The HCV genotype is determined by analyzing the core and/or 5' untranslated regions of the genome.[96] Laboratory methods available for HCV genotyping are PCR with RFLP analysis and reverse hybridization (Inno-LiPA; Bayer) and direct DNA sequencing (HCV DupliType, Quest, TRUGENE®, Bayer; and ViroSeq™,

Celera). Inno-LiPA and TRUGENE are comparable in the identification of HCV genotypes, with direct comparison studies demonstrating 91% to 99% concordance between the methods.[97] A melt curve method comparable to Inno-LiPA has also been described.[98]

The National Institutes of Health consensus guidelines for managing HCV recommends evaluation of chronic infection in newly diagnosed seropositive individuals with testing down to 50 copies/mL. Patients who have viral loads greater than 2,000,000 copies/mL of plasma will not respond as well to conventional interferon-ribavirin therapy compared to patients who have fewer than 2,000,000 copies/mL. Determining the genotype of the virus is more critical to predicting treatment outcomes because genotypes 2 and 3 will respond better to treatment than genotype 1.[79] It has been observed that patients who have a 2 $\log_{10}$ decrease in HCV RNA 12 weeks after treatment begins have a 65% chance of responding, defined by the lack of detection of HCV RNA in qualitative assays where the detection limit is 50 to 100 copies of virus/mL of plasma. Patients who do not have a 2 $\log_{10}$ decrease in HCV RNA 12 weeks after treatment begins have only a 3% chance of responding.[99]

Human Papillomavirus

Human papillomavirus (HPV) is a double-stranded DNA virus recognized as oncogenic in several human cancers. There are over 200 HPV types; approximately 40 are transmitted sexually and are associated with cervical cancer. Of the sexually transmitted types of HPV, 12 to 15 oncogenic genotypes have strong association with cervical cancers and are considered high-risk (HR) HPV types.[100,101] HPV types 16, 18, 31, 33, 35, 39, 45, 51, 52, 56, 58, 59, 66, 68, and 73 are responsible for over 95% of cervical squamous carcinoma. HPV 66 has recently been identified as carcinogenic and HPV 72 and HPV 83 are borderline carcinogenic. HPV 6 and HPV 11, which cause genital warts, are not carcinogenic. The presence of high-risk HPV DNA in conjunction with an equivocal or ambiguous cytology result (atypical squamous cells of unknown significance, or ASC-US) indicates an increased risk for having an underlying cervical neoplasm. Persistent infection with high-risk HPV may be the main risk factor for development of high-grade cervical neoplasia and cancer. Women with normal cervical cytology who are negative for the high-risk HPV types are at low risk for having or developing cervical precancerous lesions.[102]

It is difficult to culture HPV in the laboratory, so detection relies on molecular testing. Two approaches to molecular detection of HPV are hybridization methods, such as the Hologic Cervista™ HPV HR and HPV 16/18 tests based on the Invader® technology (see Chapter 9, "Gene Mutations") or in situ hybridization[103,104] and amplification methods. The latter methods include target amplification, such as PCR, and signal amplification, such as the Qiagen/Digene Hybrid Capture HCII assay (see Chapter 7, "Nucleic Acid Amplification"). Both the Cervista tests and HCII can detect a minimum of 4000 to 5000 viral genomes. In addition, the Cervista test includes an internal detection/inhibition control to avoid false-negative results. Cervista also has the capacity for subtyping. Qiagen offers an ASR (Analyte Specific Reagent) for genotyping HPV subtypes 16, 18, and 41. Another method that is, to date, classified as RUO (Research Use Only) is the HPV Oncotect flow cytometry test (Invirion Diagnostics).

HPV expresses its early genes, E1 through E8, shortly after host infection. The E6 and E7 genes are overexpressed after integration of oncogenic genotypes of the HPV genome in the host genome. E6 and E7 gene products are involved in cellular transformation to cervical cancer. The HPV OncoTect test detects mRNA expression of oncogenes E6 and E7 in specific cell types identified by flow cytometry.[105] The PCR-based Roche Linear Array Genotyping test detects 37 high- and low-risk HPV types by hybridization of PCR products to immobilized probes for each of the mutations. Direct sequencing may also be used to detect more HPV types.

Methods may differ, not only in sensitivity to target viruses but with the ability to detect concurrent infection with different HPV types.[106,107] In all cases, patient management decisions reflect patients' overall cytology history and other risk factors in addition to the presence or absence of high-risk HPV types.

Respiratory Viruses

Viral infections are a major cause of hospitalizations in young children and elderly people and represent the seventh leading cause of death in the United States.[108] Over a dozen respiratory pathogens (viral and bacterial) are commonly encountered in the medical laboratory.

Advanced Concepts

Amplification methods that target the HPV L1 gene may not detect virus that has integrated into the host DNA, as that gene region may be lost, causing false-negative results. Coinfection with two or more HPV types will lower overall PCR efficiency for each type or selectively amplify only one type, also resulting in false-negative results.

Treatment and control of the spread of infection will depend on which of these are infecting a patient. For viral infections, molecular methods have been designed to detect multiple species in single analyses. For example the ProFlu-1 assay (Prodesse) is a real-time PCR method that detects influenza A, influenza B, and respiratory syncitial virus (RSV). Influenza A subtyping by melt curve analysis has been used as a screening method to detect the 2009 influenza A (H1N1) virus.[109] The ProParaflu Plus assay identifies parainfluenza 1, 2, and 3 viruses from nasal swabs.

RSV is detected using several assays. The NucliSens EasyQ® RSV Assay (BioMirieux) is an ASR for RSV A + B RNA that uses NASBA technology. The Luminex xTAG® RVP system (formerly known as ID-Tag™ from Tm Bioscience Corporation) is a bead array technology (see Chapter 9) for simultaneous detection of RSV A and B, influenza A, nonspecific influenza A, H1, H3, influenza B, parainfluenza 1, parainfluenza 2, parainfluenza 3, metapneumovirus, rhinovirus, and adenovirus. The test includes an MS-2 bacteriophage internal control and a lambda bacteriophage positive control. It aided in the detection of 2009 influenza A/HIN1 (swine flu) but could not identify the hemagglutinin gene of the 2009 influenza A/H1N1 directly.[110] Fluorescent antibody testing also fails to detect H1N1.[111] To address the swine flu incidence, the CDC published a real-time PCR protocol on the World Health Organization website to provide the method, primer, and probe sequences to laboratories that wished to validate a direct test for the H1N1 virus.

Seasonal and H1N1 flu viruses develop resistance to antiviral agents such as TamiFlu through sequence alterations. These mutations can be detected by direct sequencing. Real-time PCR methods have also been developed to detect the frequently occurring alteration H275Y in the neuraminidase gene (H274Y in N2 nomenclature).[112]

BK/JC Viruses

BK and JC viruses are human polyomaviruses, the primate counterpart of which is SV40. BK, JC, and SV40 share sequence and antigenic homology. They are double-stranded DNA viruses with 5000 bp genomes encoding 5 transcripts. Most polyomavirus infections are subclinical in adults. Infected children develop respiratory symptoms and some have cystitis. Several reagent sets are available for detection of BK or JC viruses in the clinical laboratory, including quantitative PCR tests made by Nanogen (ASR), TIB MOLBIOL (RUO), EraGen (RUO), Artus/Qiagen (RUO), Focus Diagnostics (RUO), and IntelligentMDx (RUO). Many laboratories have developed home-brew tests as well.

Fungi

Fungi are among the most ubiquitous microorganisms causing clinical infection. Traditional methods of identification by phenotype are becoming more difficult with the expanding diversity of organisms. Molecular methods, particularly sequencing and **PCR**, have allowed for detection and typing of fungi with greater sensitivity, specificity, and speed. Fungi are important causes of human disease, especially in immunocompromised patients. In addition, laboratory-acquired infections from fungi are a major risk for laboratory personnel. Fungal infections are most often diagnosed by direct staining methods and isolation of the causative agent in culture. As for other organisms, traditional smears and cultures are affected by sensitivity, organism viability, and the length of time required for the organism to grow. Despite these problems, direct smears and isolation of fungi are still the major methods for detecting fungi in clinical samples.

Fungi growing in culture are typically identified by their microscopic and macroscopic morphologies or by using fluorescent antibodies.[113] For some fungi, however, gene probes have been developed to confirm the identity of the organism growing in culture. The AccuProbe assays (GenProbe) are available for *Histoplasma*, *Blastomyces*, *Coccidioides*, and *Cryptococcus neoformans*. Using DNA probes for these organisms is faster and less hazardous than determining the microscopic morphology.

Broad-range PCR and subsequent analysis are often used for clinical analysis of fungi. In these approaches, primers anneal to DNA sequences that are common to most of the clinically relevant fungi, such as *Candida*, *Aspergillus*, *Rhizopus* and other zygomycetes, and *Histoplasma* and other dimorphic fungi.[114] Once the sequences are amplified, hybridization to species-specific probes or sequencing is used to identify the fungus to the genus or genus and species level. In-house developed, real-time PCR methods are also used for direct identification of *Aspergillis* and *Pneumocystis carinii*. *Blastomycetes*, *Coccidioides immitis*, and *Histoplasma capsulatum* are detected with direct probe hybridization assays (GenProbe). The probe methods can also be multiplexed.[115] Pulsed field gel electrophoresis is used in laboratory-developed methods for molecular typing of yeasts.

Molds are typed by PCR and sequencing of Internal Transcribed Spacer (ITS) regions or 28S rRNA. ITS sequences of DNA extracted from 24 to 48 mold cultures are compared with those of reference strains. This method is used in industrial and environmental settings to positively identify *Paecilomyces* species, which are saprophytic filamentous fungi found in soil and as air and water contaminants. *Paecilomyces lilacinus* and *Paecilomyces varioti* are an increasing cause of opportunistic human infections generally associated with the use of immunosuppression therapy, saline breast implants, or ocular surgery. Although these two species present differences in their in vitro susceptibility to antifungal agents, requiring identification before treatment, molecular testing in the clinical laboratory is not well developed.

Parasites

Parasites are typically detected and identified by morphology directly in clinical specimens, a method of diagnosis subject to false-negative results in cases of low organism concentrations and depending greatly on appropriately trained personnel. Molecular-based testing for parasites has been limited mainly because parasites are not a major cause of disease in developed countries. Increasingly, however, travelers from parasite-endemic countries bring parasites to developed countries and serve as a reservoir for transmission. In the laboratory, nucleic acid template preparation from oocysts and

spores of protozoan parasites is complicated by the nature of the organism and its resistance to disruption and lysis. Parasites found in complex matrices such as stool samples present a further difficulty due to inhibition of PCR and other enzymatic assays. However, expertise in identifying parasites by morphology is declining, demanding alternative methods of surveillance and detection of these organisms.

Recognition of these issues has made the development of molecular-based assays for parasite detection and identification more practical. Nucleic acid isolation for molecular testing has been addressed by using several methods, including extraction and extraction-free, filter-based protocols for preparation of DNA templates from oocysts and microsporidia spores. PCR methods are modified to accommodate sequence content, for example, low GC content in malaria.

PCR assays have been developed for the following parasites:[116]

- *Trypanosomacruzi* in patients with chronic Chagas disease
- *Trypanosomabrucei* subspecies *gambiense* and *rhodiense*
- *Plasmodium falciparum*, *P. malariae*, and *P. vivax* in blood and speciation
- *Leishmania* and differentiation to the species level
- *Toxoplasmagondii* in suspected congenital and central nervous system infections
- *Entamoeba histolytica*
- *Cryptosporidium* in water
- Microsporidial detection in stool and small intestine biopsies

In-house developed, real-time PCR methods are used in clinical laboratories for identification of *Babesia*, *Trichomonas microti* in blood and from ticks, *Encephalitozoon* species microsporidia, and *Trichomonas vaginalis*. Multiplex PCR methods have been designed to simultaneously detect multiple parasites, for example, multiplex real-time PCR assays for detection of *E. histolytica*, *G. lamblia*, and *C. parvum* simultaneously or *E. histolytica*, *G. intestinalis*, and *Cryptosporidium* spp. simultaneously in stool samples. The multiplex PCR methods also include an internal control to determine efficiency of the PCR and detect inhibition in the sample, which is likely in stool samples. The development of multiplex PCR assays to detect multiple parasites in stool samples is extremely useful. First, multiple parasites can cause diarrhea, and morphology is the only way to differentiate between causative agents. Second, patients can have multiple intestinal parasites at the same time, and laboratory detection of the presence of all parasites is important. Finally, multiple parasites are transmitted through the same source; thus, detection of all parasites and appropriate control measures will reduce large-scale outbreaks.

Antimicrobial Agents

Antimicrobial agents are of two types, those that inhibit microbial growth (-static, e.g., **bacteriostatic**, **fungistatic**) and those that kill organisms outright (-cidal, e.g., **bactericidal**, **fungicidal**). Antimicrobial agents for use in clinical applications are designed to be selective for the target organism with minimal effect on mammalian cells. These agents are also intended to distribute well in the host and remain active for as long as possible (long half-life). Ideally, the agents should have -cidal (rather than -static) activity against a broad spectrum of microorganisms.

Another way to classify antimicrobial agents is by their mode of action (Table 12.9). The ultimate effect of these agents is to inhibit essential functions in the target organism (Fig. 12-5). A third way to group antimicrobial agents is by their chemical structure. For example, there are two major types of agents that inhibit cell wall synthesis, the β-lactams with substituted ring structures and the glycopeptides.

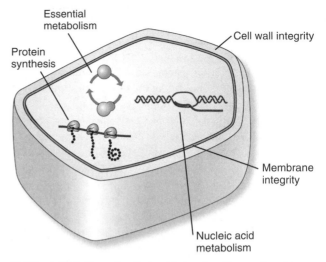

■ **Figure 12-5** Sites of antimicrobial action. Depending on the type of organism, several structures can be affected by antimicrobial agents. All of these are essential for cell growth and survival.

Resistance to Antimicrobial Agents

Microorganisms naturally develop defenses to antimicrobial agents. Resistant *Staphylococcus*, *Pseudomonas*, and *Klebsiella* spp. are becoming commonplace in healthcare institutions. Long-term therapy with antibiotics such as vancomycin can lead to the development of resistant clones of organisms. These clones may persist in low numbers below the detection levels of routine laboratory sensitivity testing methods.

Table 12.9 **Mode of Action of Antimicrobial Agents**

Mode of Action	Examples
Disrupts cell wall synthesis or integrity	Beta-lactams (penicillins and cephalosporins)
	Glycopeptides (vancomycin)
Disrupts cell membrane structure or function	Polymyxins (polymyxin B)
	Bacitracin
Inhibits protein synthesis	Aminoglycosides (gentamicin)
	Tetracyclines
	Macrolides (erythromycin)
	Lincosamides (clindamycin)
Inhibits nucleic acid synthesis or integrity	Quinolones (ciprofloxacin)
	Metronidazole
Inhibits metabolite synthesis	Sulfamethoxazole
	Trimethoprim

Advanced Concepts

The first antibiotics isolated were natural secretions from fungi and other organisms. Synthetic modifications of these natural agents were designed to increase the spectrum of activity (ability to kill more organisms) and to overcome resistance. For example, cephalosporins include such first-generation agents as cephalothin and cefazolin that are active against *Staphylococcus, Streptococcus,* and some Enterobacteriaceae. A second generation of cephalosporins—cefamondole, cefoxitin, and cefuroxime—is active against more Enterobacteriaceae and organisms resistant to β-lactam antibiotics. A third generation— cefotaxime, ceftriaxone, and ceftazidime—is active against *P. aeruginosa* as well as many Enterobacteriaceae and organisms resistant to β-lactam antibiotics. The fourth generation, cefepime, is active against an extended spectrum of organisms resistant to β-lactam antibiotics.

There are several ways in which microorganisms develop resistance (Table 12.10). First, bacteria can produce enzymes that inactivate the agent. Examples of this resistance mechanism are seen in *S. aureus* and *N. gonorrhoeae* that produce β-lactamase, an enzyme that cleaves the β-lactam ring of the β-lactam antimicrobials such as the penicillins. Cleavage of the β-lactam ring destroys the activity of penicillin, rendering the organism resistant to its antimicrobial action. Second, organisms produce altered targets for the antimicrobial agent. Mutations in the gene encoding a penicillin-binding protein, for example, a change in the structure of the protein,

render penicillin unable to bind to its target. Finally, bacteria exhibit changes in the transport of the antimicrobial agent either into or out of the cell. An example of this mechanism is seen in gram-negative bacteria that change their outer membrane proteins (porins) in order to decrease the influx of the antimicrobial agent. If the agent cannot get into the cell and bind to its target, then it is not effective in inhibiting or killing the bacterium.

All these resistance mechanisms involve a genetic change in the microorganism (Table 12.11). These genetic changes are most commonly brought about by mutation and selection processes. If a mutation results in a survival or growth advantage, cells with the mutation will eventually take the place of those without the mutation, which are less able to survive and procreate. This process is stimulated by antibiotic exposure, especially if the levels of antibiotics are less than optimal. For example, *S. aureus* developed resistance to antibiotics that target its penicillin-binding protein (PBP1) by replacing PBP1 with PBP2a encoded by the *mec*A gene. PBP2a found in **methicillin-resistant *S. aureus* (MRSA)** has a low binding affinity for methicillin.

Another genetic resistance mechanism is the acquisition of genetic factors from other resistant organisms through transformation with plasmids carrying resistance genes or transduction with viruses carrying resistance genes. Genetic factors can also be transferred from one bacterium to another by conjugation (see Chapter 1, "DNA," for a discussion of these processes). Genetically directed resistance can pass between organisms of different species. For example, MRSA (vancomycin-sensitive *S. aureus*) can gain vancomycin resistance from vancomycin-resistant *E. faecalis*. Vancomycin and other glycopeptides act by preventing the cross-linking of the peptidoglycan, thereby inhibiting cell wall production. Several genes have been found in enterococci that encode

Table 12.10 **Resistance Mechanisms**

Mechanism	Example	Examples of Agents Affected
Destruction of agent	β-lactamases	β-lactams
Elimination of agent	Multidrug efflux systems	β-lactams, fluoroquinolones, macrolides, chloramphenicol, trimethoprim
Altered cell wall structure	Thick cell walls that exclude agent	Vancomycin
	Altered agent binding sites	β-lactams
Alternate metabolic pathways	Altered enzymes	Sulfonamides, trimethoprim

Table 12.11 **Genes Conferring Resistance to Antimicrobial Agents in Particular Organisms[78]**

Organism	Antimicrobial Agent	Gene(s) Conferring Resistance
Staphylococcus aureus	Oxacillin	*mecA*
Streptococcus pneumoniae	Penicillin	*pbp1a* and *pbp1b*
Gram-negatives	β-lactams	*tem*, *shv*, *oxa*, *ctx-m*
Enterococcus	Vancomycin	*vanA*, *vanB*, *vanC*, *vanD*, *vanE*, *vanG*
Salmonella	Quinolones	*gyrA*, *gyrB*, *parC*, *parE*
Mycobacterium tuberculosis	Isoniazid	*katG*, *inhA*
	Rifampin	*rpoB*

altered binding proteins: *vanA*, *vanB*, *vanC*, *vanD*, *vanE,* and *vanG*. The expression of *vanA* and *vanB* is inducible and transferred from cell to cell by plasmids carrying vancomycin resistance genes on a **transposon**[117] (Fig. 12-6). The resulting vancomycin-resistant *S. aureus* (VRSA) uses lactic acid instead of alanine to build its cell wall. The VRSA cell wall, then, does not contain the target structure (D-ala-D-ala) for vancomycin. Development of resistance to particular drugs occurs with particular mutations: *rpoB* mutation is associated with rifampin resistance, and mutations in *katG*, *inhA*, *ahpC*, and *ndh* genes are associated with resistance to isoniazid.[118]

Molecular Detection of Resistance

Susceptibility to antimicrobial agents is determined by phenotypic or genotypic methods. The phenotypic development of resistance is detected by performing in vitro **susceptibility testing**. Testing for altered sensitivity to antimicrobial agents is of clinical significance especially when organisms persist in patients being treated with antimicrobial agents that are generally considered effective against the particular isolate or when large numbers of organisms are observed in normally sterile fluids, such as blood, cerebrospinal fluid, or urine. Phenotypic methods are generally used for aerobic bacteria, some mycobacteria, and yeast. For other organisms, such as viruses and filamentous fungi, phenotypic methods are not well standardized. Phenotypic methodologies include disk diffusion, broth dilution, and direct detection of resistance factors such as β-lactamase.

Susceptibility testing measures the **minimum inhibitory concentration (MIC)** of an antimicrobial agent, or the least amount of antimicrobial agent that inhibits the growth of an organism. Established guidelines define the MICs interpreted as indications of susceptibility or resistance for a given organism and antimicrobial agent pair. The determination of MICs to detect antimicrobial resistance is a phenotypic method. Although MIC methods are well established, and the results are generally reliable with regard to in vivo effectiveness of an agent for an organism, the results are sometimes difficult to interpret and the procedures are time-consuming, taking at least 48 hours after the specimen is collected.

Molecular methods that detect genes directly involved in the resistance of an organism to a particular agent

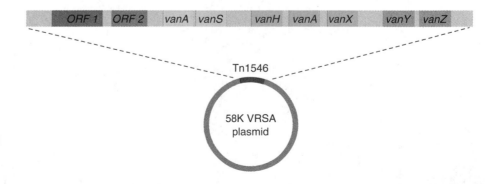

■ **Figure 12-6** Vancomycin-resistant *S. aureus* (VRSA) plasmid carrying transposon Tn1546 with vancomycin resistance genes.

offer a more straightforward prediction of antibiotic resistance. There are four reasons for using molecular-based methodologies. First, when an organism has an MIC at or near the breakpoint of resistance, detection of mutated genes contributing to resistance would be irrefutable evidence of the potential ineffectiveness of the agent. Second, genes involved in the resistance of organisms to antimicrobial agents can be detected directly in the clinical specimen closer to the time of collection and save the time required to isolate the organism and perform phenotypic MIC determinations on isolated colonies. With no requirement for culturing potentially dangerous microorganisms, there is less chance of hazardous exposure for the technologist as well. Third, monitoring the spread of a resistance gene in multiple isolates of the same organism is more useful in epidemiological investigations than following the trend in the MIC. Finally, molecular methods are considered the gold standard when new phenotypic assays are being developed.[118]

Beta-Lactam Antibiotic Resistance

One of the most effective antibiotics, penicillin, was first used therapeutically in the early 1940s (Fig. 12-7). Soon after that, resistance to penicillin through the production of β-lactamases (Fig. 12-8) was first recorded. *Streptococcuspyogenes* is one of very few organisms that are still predictably susceptible to penicillin. Penicillin and other β-lactam antimicrobials inhibit bacteria by interfering with an enzyme that is involved in the synthesis of the bacterial cell wall. In the laboratory, penicillin was modified to make it resistant to the bacterial β-lactamases (also known as penicillinases). Penicillinase-resistant penicillins, for example, methicillin or oxacillin (Fig. 12-9), were the products of that research. Before the emergence of resistance to these agents was first observed in 1965,

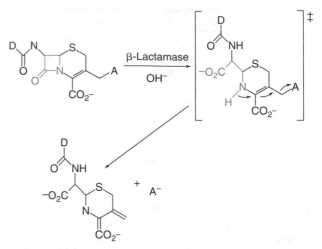

■ **Figure 12-8** The reaction catalyzed by beta-lactamase results in cleavage of the beta-lactam ring through an intermediate product (bracketed).

staphylococcal infections were treated successfully with methicillin/oxacillin for years.[119] MRSA and methicillin-resistant coagulase-negative staphylococci are a major cause of infections acquired in the hospital as well as in the community. As described above, expression of an altered penicillin-binding protein (PBP2' or PBP 2a encoded by the *mecA* gene) is the mechanism by which these organisms have become resistant. Oxacillin cannot bind to the altered target, and therefore it has no effect on the bacterial cells.

Rapid identification of MRSA isolates in clinical specimens by direct detection of *mecA* is critical for effective patient management and prevention of infections occurring in hospitals due to MRSA. PCR and other amplification assays have been developed for direct testing of clinical samples, and many assays have been tested for sensitivity and specificity.[119]

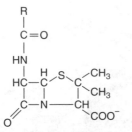

■ **Figure 12-7** Structure of penicillin, showing the carbon-nitrogen (CCCN) **beta-lactam** ring.

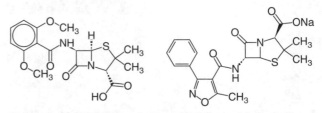

■ **Figure 12-9** Penicillin substitutes include methicillin (left) and oxacillin (right).

Glycopeptide Antibiotic Resistance

Glycopeptide antibiotics were originally isolated from plant and soil bacteria. Their structures contain either a glycosylated cyclic or polycyclic peptide. These antibiotics inhibit peptidoglycan synthesis in the cell wall of susceptible organisms (principally Gram-positive cocci). Glycopeptide antibiotics include vancomycin (Fig. 12-10), teicoplanin, and ramoplanin; oritavancin, dalbavancin, and telavancinare are semi-synthetic glycopeptide antibiotics. *Enterococcus* was the first organism in which glycopeptide resistance was reported.[120] Since then, vancomycin resistance has been observed in other organisms. Of most concern is emerging resistance to vancomycin in the staphylococci.[121]

The mechanism of vancomycin resistance can be acquired or intrinsic to the organism. The antibiotic binds and weakens cell wall structures of susceptible bacteria, ultimately causing cell lysis. Either the presence of the antibiotic itself or the weakening of the cell wall activates a set of *van* genes whose products modify the cell wall structure such that the antibiotic no longer binds. The *van* genes are carried on a cassette localized to a plasmid or on the bacterial chromosome.

PCR was used to detect the *vanA*, *vanB*, *vanC1*, and *vanC2* resistance genes in fecal samples as a way to screen for vancomycin-resistant enterococci (VRE).[11] The specificity of the *vanA* primers was 99.6% when compared with isolation of VRE in culture. The use of four primers allowed for the detection of VRE in 85.1% of the samples. Real-time PCR has also been used to detect VRE in fecal surveillance specimens. Whereas PCR of *vanA* and *vanB* was more sensitive when performed on enrichment broths rather than directly from fecal swabs, 88% of specimens that were culture-positive for VRE were PCR-positive.[122] Because PCR is faster than traditional culture methods and has comparable sensitivity and specificity to culture, it is an attractive method for screening large numbers of samples for a particular target.

Antimicrobial Resistance in M. tuberculosis

The use of molecular methods to detect antimicrobial resistance in *M. tuberculosis* is particularly attractive because traditional methods of determining antimicrobial susceptibility takes days, if not weeks, for this organism. The longer a patient with TB is inadequately treated, the more likely the development of resistance. Multidrug-resistant *M. tuberculosis* is a major problem around the world.[123] One group reported on the evolution of drug resistance of *M. tuberculosis* in a patient who was noncompliant with the treatment protocol. In over 12 years of poorly treated TB, subpopulations of the organism emerged due to the acquisition and accumulation of gene mutations that rendered the organism resistant to isoniazid, rifampin, and streptomycin.[124] Many nucleic acid amplification protocols have been developed to directly detect mutations in the genes associated with resistance to isoniazid and rifampin.[125–130] In general, these assays have demonstrated excellent sensitivity and specificity and provide rapid determination of drug susceptibility either directly from sputum or from cultures.

Thus, the advantages of using nucleic acid amplification assays for the determination of drug resistance include the rapid and specific detection of mutations in genes

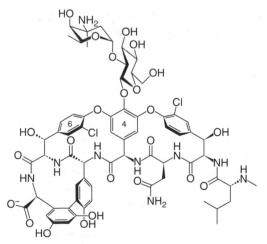

■ Figure 12-10 Structure of vancomycin.

associated with resistance to particular antimicrobial agents that provides irrefutable evidence of resistance in a short period.

Molecular Epidemiology

An **epidemic** is a disease or condition that affects many unrelated individuals at the same time; a rapidly spreading outbreak of an infectious disease is an epidemic. A **pandemic** is a disease that sweeps across wide geographical areas. Epidemiology includes collection and analysis of environmental, microbiological, and clinical data. In microbiology, studies are performed to follow the spread of pathogenic organisms within a hospital (**nosocomial** infections), from the actions of a physician (**iatrogenic** infections), and in a community. Molecular epidemiology is the study of causative genetic and environmental factors at the molecular level to ascertain the origin, distribution, and best strategies for prevention of disease. In infectious disease, these efforts are facilitated by the ability to determine the genetic similarities and differences among microbiological isolates.

In the laboratory, molecular methods are very useful for identifying and typing infectious agents.[131] In a single patient, this is informative for therapeutic efficacy; in groups of patients, it provides information for infection control. Typing systems are based on the premise that clonally related isolates share molecular characteristics distinct from unrelated isolates. Molecular technology provides analytical alternatives from the chromosomal to the nucleotide sequence level. These genotypic methods, in addition to established phenotypic methods, enhance the capability to identify and type microorganisms. While phenotypic methods are based on a range of biological characteristics, such as antigenic type or growth requirements, genotypic procedures target genomic or plasmid DNA (Table 12.12). Genome scanning methods, such as restriction enzyme analysis followed by PFGE, are used to find genetic similarities and differences, as are amplification and sequencing methods. The ability to discern genetic differences with increasing detail enhances the capability to type organisms regardless of their complexity. All methods, however, have benefits and limitations with regard to instrumentation, methodology, and interpretation.

Molecular methods are based on DNA sequence. DNA sequences range from highly conserved across species and genera to unique to each organism. Some of these

Table 12.12 **Epidemiological Typing Methods**

Class	Methods
Phenotypic	Biotyping, growth on selective media
	Antimicrobial susceptibility
	Serotyping, immunoblotting
	Bacteriophage typing
	Protein, enzyme typing by electrophoresis
Genotypic	Plasmid analysis
	Restriction endonuclease mapping
	Pulsed field gel electrophoresis
	Ribotyping
	Arbitrarily primed PCR, RAPD PCR
	Melt curve analysis
	REP-PCR, ERIC PCR, ITS, spa typing

sequences are strain- or species-specific but are still used for epidemiological testing since DNA analysis is highly reproducible and, depending on the target sequences, can discriminate between even closely related organisms. Most (but not all) molecular methods offer definitive results in the form of DNA sequences or gel band and peak patterns that can be interpreted objectively, which is less difficult than phenotypic determinations that often require experienced judgment. With commercial systems, the performance has become relatively simple for some molecular epidemiology tests, whereas others require a higher level of laboratory expertise.

Molecular Strain Typing Methods for Epidemiological Studies

In community or clinical settings, when the same organism is isolated multiple times, whether in the same patient or from different patients, the physician wats to know if the isolates were independently acquired, that is, came from different sources, or if they came from the same source. With this knowledge, the physician can act to control the transmission of the organism, especially if it is being transmitted from a common source and that source has been identified. Most of the time, these analyses are performed on organisms that have been transmitted nosocomially, but sometimes procedures to determine relatedness are performed on isolates from community outbreak situations.[132]

Many laboratory methods can be used to determine the relatedness of multiple isolates, both phenotypic (e.g., by serology and antimicrobial susceptibility patterns) and genotypic (e.g., pulsed field gel electrophoresis and ribo-typing).[133] The phenotypic methods suffer from a lack of reproducibility and their ability to discriminate between isolates is not very good. Genotypic methods are used almost exclusively to type bacterial strains to determine the relatedness of multiple isolates; these will be summarized in this section.

Plasmid Analysis

Plasmid analysis, or **plasmid fingerprinting**,[134] as it was known in the past, involves isolation and restriction mapping of bacterial plasmids. The same bacterial strain can have different plasmids carrying different phenotypes or resistance patterns. For this analysis, plasmid DNA is isolated from the specimen or culture and then digested with restriction enzymes. Plasmids are distinguished by the pattern of fragments generated when cut with the appropriate enzymes. Restriction analysis can also be performed on chromosomal DNA of organisms with small genomes. For organisms with larger genomes, whole genome analysis with restriction enzymes that cut frequently enough to identify plasmids will yield complex patterns that are more difficult to interpret.

Pulsed Field Gel Electrophoresis

Most molecular epidemiological tests are performed using **pulsed field gel electrophoresis (PFGE)**, which can identify organisms with larger genomes or multiple chromosomes. For PFGE analysis, the DNA is digested with restriction enzymes that cut infrequently within the genomic sequences. The resulting large fragments (hundreds of thousands of base pairs) are resolved by PFGE (see Chapter 5, "Resolution and Detection of Nucleic Acids," for a more detailed description of this system). Banding patterns will differ depending on the chromosomal DNA sequence of the organisms (Fig. 12-11). Tenover and colleagues devised a system to interpret the banding pattern of a test organism compared to that of the strain of organism known to be involved in an outbreak.[135] The interpretation of PFGE results follows the "rule of three" (Table 12.13), a method that has been used for typing numerous species, including strains of *Pseudomonas aeruginosa*, *Mycobacterium avium*, *Escherichia coli*, *N. gonorrhoeae*, VRE, and MRSA. Intralaboratory and inter-laboratory computerized databases of band patterns can be stored for reference. A national PFGE database is stored at the CDC (www.cdc.gov/pulsenet/index.htm). One disadvantage of using PFGE to type strains is the

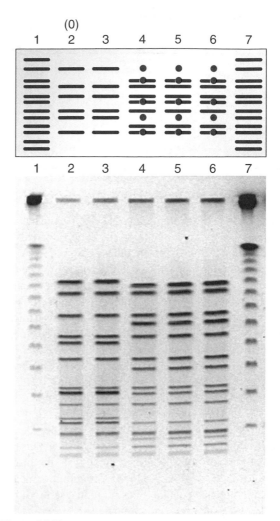

■ **Figure 12-11** PFGE of coagulase-negative *Staphylococcus* showing the outbreak (O) and four test strains (top panel). The gel image is shown in the bottom panel. The fragment shifts are marked in the top panel. Strains in lanes 4, 5 and 6 are the same but different from the outbreak strain (lane 2). The strain in lane 3 is the same as the outbreak strain. The s trains in lanes 4, 5, and 6 have at least five genetic differences and are not related to the outbreak. Lanes 1 and 7, molecular-weight markers. (Courtesy of Mary Hayden, MD, Rush Medical Laboratories, Rush University Medical Center, Chicago, IL.)

time involved to perform the assay, which can take 2 to 3 days to complete one analysis.

Restriction Fragment Length Polymorphism Analysis

Restriction fragment length polymorphism (RFLP) analysis by Southern blot is the same technique first used to

Table 12.13 Criteria for PFGE Pattern Interpretation

Category	Genetic Differences*	Fragment Differences*	Epidemiological Interpretation
Indistinguishable	0	0	Test isolate is the same strain as the outbreak strain
Closely related	1	2–3	Test isolate is closely related to the outbreak strain
Possibly related	2	4–6	Test isolate is possibly related to the outbreak strain
Different	≥3	≥6	Test isolate unrelated to the outbreak

*Compared with the outbreak strain

identify and investigate human genes (see Chapter 6, "Analysis and Characterization of Nucleic Acids and Proteins"). This method involves cutting DNA with restriction enzymes, resolving the resulting fragments by gel electrophoresis, and then transferring the separated fragments to a membrane for probing with a specific probe. Gene-specific probes are used to identify or subtype microorganisms such as *P. aeruginosa* in patients with cystic fibrosis and nosocomial *L. pneumophila* infections.[136,137]

Insertion elements are segments of DNA that move independently throughout the genome and insert themselves in multiple locations. Strains are typed based on how many insertions are present and where they are located. Isolates from the same strain will have the same number and location of elements. For strain typing of *M. tuberculosis* by this method, the probe is complementary to the insertion element, IS*6110*, and will bind to restriction fragments on the membrane that contain it, resulting in a series of bands that are easily analyzed and compared.[138,139]

The gene targets selected for RFLP depend on the organism under investigation and which genes will be most informative. Ribosomal RNA genes are highly informative over a range of microorganisms, which is the basis for a modification of the RFLP procedure called **ribotyping**. For this method, probes target the 16S and 23S rRNA genes. RFLP and ribotyping have been applied in industrial as well as clinical microbiology.[140,141]

RFLP can be done more rapidly using PCR amplification with gene-specific primers (**locus-specific RFLP**, or **PCR-RFLP**). This method requires amplification of specific regions by PCR (see Chapters 7, "Nucleic Acid Amplification," and 9, "Gene Mutations," for more details). The amplicons are then cut with restriction enzymes, yielding bands of informative size. An advantage of this procedure, in addition to its speed, is the simple banding pattern,

which is much easier to interpret. Although the method is limited by the sequences that can be amplified and differentiated through restriction enzyme digestion, proper gene selection provides a highly reproducible and discriminatory test.[142] In one study, an 820-bp amplified fragment of the *ureC* gene from *Helicobacter pylori* digested with *Sau*3A and *Hha*I yielded 14 different *Sau*3A patterns and 15 different *Hha*I patterns. These patterns were informative as to antibiotic sensitivity of the various types to clarithromycin or clarithromycin-omeprazole dual therapy.[143]

Arbitrarily Primed PCR

Arbitrarily primed PCR, or random amplified polymorphic DNA (RAPD) assay, is a modified PCR using 10-base-long oligonucleotides of random sequences to prime DNA amplification all over the genome.[144,145] The gel pattern of amplicons produced is characteristic of a given organism. If two organisms have the same pattern, they are considered the same type; if the patterns differ, they are different types. The RAPD assay is relatively fast and inexpensive; however, producing consistent results may be technically demanding. Accurate interpretation of RAPD raw data requires that the procedure conditions be followed strictly so that pattern differences (not necessarily patterns) are reproducible (Fig. 12-12).

Amplified Fragment Length Polymorphism (AFLP) Assay

AFLP is a name, rather than an acronym, chosen by the inventors of this assay due to its resemblance to RFLP.[146] The AFLP assay is based on the amplification of DNA fragments generated by cutting the test genome with restriction enzymes.[147] DNA isolated from the test strain is digested with *Hind*III or other restriction enzyme (Fig. 12-13). Short DNA fragments

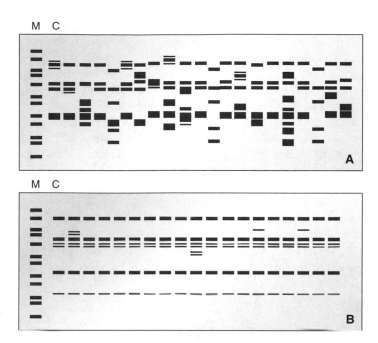

■ **Figure 12-12** RAPD gel results. An unacceptable gel pattern is represented in panel A. The bands are smeared, and variable producing patterns are too complex for positive identification of unrelated strains. The gel pattern represented in panel B is acceptable. Strain differences can be clearly identified by variations from the known strain (C). Molecular-weight markers are shown in lane M.

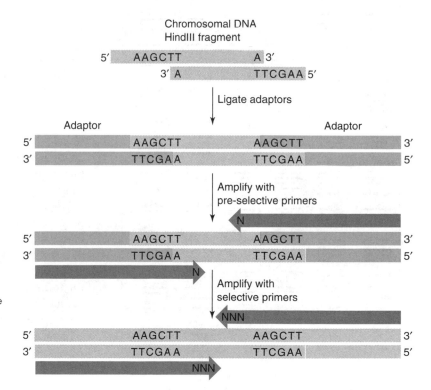

■ **Figure 12-13** AFLP analysis begins with restriction digestion of chromosomal DNA. The resulting fragments (top) are ligated with adaptors compatible with the restriction enzyme ends and complementary to primers used to amplify them. The first amplification is performed with preselective primers that end in a 3' base (N) selected by the user. Selective primers with three added 3' bases are used for a second round of PCR. This selection results in a characteristic pattern; only a fraction of the original fragments will be represented in the gel pattern.

or adaptors are ligated to the ends of the cut DNA. The adaptor-ligated fragments are then amplified in two steps with primers complementary to the adaptor sequences. Nucleotides located at the 3' end of the primers select for specific sequences in the restriction fragments. The amplicons are then resolved by gel or capillary electrophoresis (fluorescently labeled primers are used for capillary electrophoresis). The pattern will be characteristic of the strain or type of organism. This assay can be performed with one or two enzymes (e.g., *Eco*R1/*Mse*I or *Bam*H1/*Pst*I).

AFLP may detect more polymorphisms than RAPD analysis and is faster than PFGE. The procedure is more technically demanding, however, than a similar method, **REP-PCR** (next section). Gel patterns may also be complex (Fig. 12-14). Both high and low reproducibility for the method have been reported.[146,148]

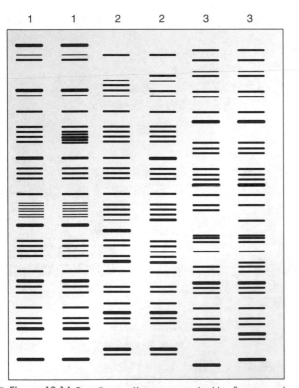

1   1   2   2   3   3

■ Figure 12-14 Banding patterns generated by fluorescent AFLP analysis. Note that duplicate specimens (1, 2, and 3) do not produce the exact pattern because of band shifts and different band intensities.

Interspersed Repetitive Elements

Copies of conserved sequences are found throughout the genomes of most organisms. These sequences may have arisen from viral integration or movement of transposable elements (stretches of DNA that move from one location to another in a non-Mendelian fashion, also called jumping genes). The genomic locations of these structures are related to species type and can be used to distinguish between bacterial isolates.

Enterobacterial repetitive intergenic consensus (ERIC) sequences are 126-bp-long genomic sequences found in some bacterial species that are highly conserved, even though they are not in coding regions.[149] These sequences are located between genes in operons or upstream or downstream of single open reading frames. ERIC sequences are flanked by inverted repeats that could form stem-loop or cruciform structures in DNA and are found only in gram-negative organisms, such as *Bartonella, Shigella, Pseudomonas, Salmonella, Enterobacter,* and others.

A related type of repetitive element, the repetitive extragenic palindromic (REP) sequence, is similar to the ERIC sequence in that it occurs in noncoding regions and contains an inverted repeat. REP sequences differ from ERIC sequences in size (REP sequences are only 38 bp long), in being more numerous in the genome, and in being present in multiple copies at a single location (Fig. 12-15).[150] PCR primed from these elements yields a series of products that can be resolved by gel, capillary electrophoresis, or microfluidics[151] into characteristic patterns (Fig. 12-16). These elements have been used for typing of clinically important organisms, such as *Clostridium difficile*[152] and fungal pathogens.[153]

Another repetitive element, **BOX**, was discovered in *S. pneumoniae*. BOX elements consist of different combinations of subunits: boxA, boxB, and boxC, 59, 45, and 50 bp long, respectively. Although these elements are not related to ERIC and REP sequences, they do form stem-loop structures, as do ERIC and REP. About 25 of these elements are present in the *S. pneumoniae* genome, where they may be involved in regulation of gene expression.[154]

Internal Transcribed Spacer Elements

The ribosomal RNA genes comprise the most conserved region in the genome. These genes are arranged as an

ERIC sequence

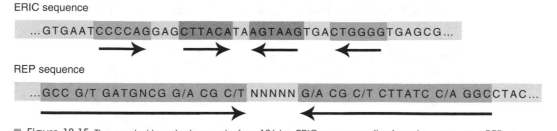

REP sequence

■ **Figure 12-15** The central inverted repeat of an 126-bp ERIC sequence (top) and a consensus REP sequence (bottom). ERIC sequences contain multiple inverted repeats (arrows) that can generate a secondary structure consisting of several stems and loops. REP sequences contain a conserved inverted repeat that forms a stem with a loop that includes 5 bp of variable sequence (N).

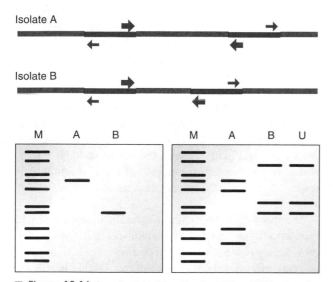

■ **Figure 12-16** Species identification by REP or ERIC primed amplification. REP and ERIC sequences are present in different chromosomal locations in bacterial subtypes A and B. PCR, which extends outward-oriented primers hybridized to the repeated sequences, generates amplicons of different sizes based on the placement of the element, as in the gel depicted in the bottom left panel where only one amplicon is shown. Multiple REPs and ERICs throughout the bacterial chromosome generate multiple amplicons with characteristic gel patterns (bottom right). An unknown isolate (U) is identified as the same strain as isolate B. M, molecular-weight markers.

operon, including a small subunit, 18S rRNA, 5.8S rRNA, and a large subunit, 28S rRNA. The **internal transcribed spacer (ITS)** 1 and 2 elements (**ITS1** and **ITS2**) are found in regions separating the 18S and the 28S rRNA genes. ITS1 is located between the 18S and the 5.8S gene, and ITS2 is located between the 5.8S and the 28S rRNA genes. Two additional elements, intergenic spacer (IGS) regions, IGSI and IGSII, are located between the rDNA repeat units (Fig. 12-17). Used for the identification and typing of yeast and molds, ITS sequences are conserved within species but polymorphic between species.[155,156] The ITS sequences are amplified using primers directed to the unique 17S and 26S gene sequences. The resulting amplicons are analyzed by sequencing, single-strand conformation polymorphism, density gradient gel electrophoresis, restriction enzyme analysis, or sequence-specific PCR.[157–159]

spa Typing

MRSA contains a variable number tandem repeat (VNTR) element in the 3' coding region of the protein A gene (*spa*).[160] The element consists of repeat units of 21 or 24 bp in length. Repeat units also vary by sequence of at least one position, with 38 sequence types so far described. The *spa* element can have 2 to 16 repeat units. Analysis of these elements by PFGE or sequencing and

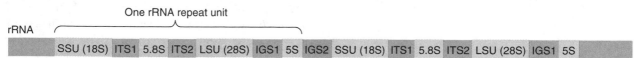

■ **Figure 12-17** Ribosomal RNA genes are arranged in multiple tandem units that include the major rRNA transcript (18S-28S) and the 5S gene. ITSs are located within the major transcript template area and IGSs in the region between the repeat units surrounding the 5S rRNA gene.

comparison to known isolates (*spa* **typing**) is used to identify MRSA. Almost 400 repeat profiles or *spa* types have been defined.

A similar sequence structure in the coagulase gene (*coa*) has also been used for *S. aureus* typing (*coa* **typing**).[161] The *coa* VNTR units are 81 bp in length, and fewer than 70 repeat profiles have been described. PCR amplification and sequence analysis are used to analyze *coa* types. The discriminatory power of this method is increased by analysis of other repeated sequences elsewhere in the MRSA genome. The combination of *spa* and VNTR typing has a discriminatory power equal to that of PFGE, with a more rapid turnaround time.

Multilocus Sequence Typing

Multilocus sequence typing (MLST) characterizes bacterial isolates by using sequences of internal fragments of housekeeping genes.[162,163] Six or seven genes are sequenced over 450 to 500 bases, and the sequences are assigned as alleles. Examples of housekeeping genes used in *S. aureus* MLST are shown in Table 12.14. Distinct alleles are defined as single base-pair differences or multiple changes resulting from recombination or other genetic events. An isolate type or the allelic profile is the collection of all seven alleles, also called the sequence type. Bacteria have enough variation so that there are multiple alleles of each housekeeping gene (30 alleles/locus), making up billions of allelic profiles.[164,165] Because the data generated by MLST is text sequence, the results can be compared with those in large databases, for example, pubmlst.org.

Table 12.14 **Example of Housekeeping Genes Sequenced in an MLST Test**

Gene	Gene Product	Number of Alleles
ArcC	Carbamate kinase	52
AroE	Shikimate dehydrogenase	88
GlpF	Glycerol kinase	55
Gmk	Guanylate kinase	51
Pta	Phosphate acetyltransferase	57
tpi	Triosephosphate isomerase	74
YqiL	Acetyl coenzyme A acetyltransferase	66

Comparison of Typing Methods

Genotypic methods used for strain typing are evaluated and compared based on five criteria. First, the target organism must be typable by the method used to detect it (**typing capacity**). A test that detects a genotypic or phenotypic characteristic that is not expressed in all members of a species will not accurately detect the target organisms at all times. A molecular assay must target a reasonably polymorphic DNA sequence, alleles of which are unambiguously associated with a given strain. Second, the method must be **reproducible**. A reproducible method yields the same result on repeated testing of the same organism or strain. Variations in cell characteristics, such as antigens or receptor expression, decrease reproducibility (precision). Third, the method must clearly distinguish between unrelated strains (**discriminatory power**). Reproducibility and discriminatory power are important for establishment of databases that can be used by independent laboratories. Fourth, ease of interpretation of results is important. Unclear or complex results will lower reproducibility and discriminatory power. Finally, ease of test performance is important in order to minimize chance of error or ambiguous results. A rating of representative methods is shown in Table 12.15.

The most desirable typing method is the one that will type all strains and have excellent reproducibility, discriminatory power, and ease of performance and interpretation. Unfortunately, no such method fits this profile, so the laboratory professionals performing these types of analyses may have to sacrifice ease of performance, for example, in order to get excellent discriminatory power when they are choosing which molecular typing method to use.

In conclusion, molecular-based methods are available for the detection, identification, and characterization of a number of microorganisms. For some, assays are used almost exclusively, such as for *N. gonorrhoeae*, *C. trachomatis*, and *B. pertussis*. For others, molecular-based tests are used to provide rapid results and supplement traditional testing, such as for *M. tuberculosis*. Finally, molecular-based methods are undergoing continuous development and experiencing increasing use compared to traditional culture and phenotypic methods.

Table 12.15 **Performance Comparison of Representative Molecular Epidemiology Methods***

Method	Typing Capacity	Discriminatory Power	Reproducibility[†]	Ease of Use	Ease of Interpretation[‡]
Plasmid analysis	Good	Good	Good	High	Good
PFGE	High	High	High	Moderate	Good–moderate
Chromosomal RFLP	High	Good	Good	High	Moderate–poor
Ribotyping	High	High	High	Good	High
PCR-RFLP	Good	Moderate	Good	High	High
RAPD	High	High	Poor	High	Good–High
AFLP	High	High	Good	Moderate	High
Repetitive elements	Good	Good	High	High	High
Sequencing	High	High	High	Moderate	Good–High

*From Olive and Bean.[89]

[†]Intralaboratory

[‡]Interpretation is influenced by the quality of the data.

CASE STUDY 12 • 1

During a holiday weekend at a luxury hotel, guests began to complain of stomach flu with nausea and vomiting. In all, more than 100 of the 200 guests who had dined at the hotel the previous evening described the same symptoms. Eight people had symptoms severe enough to warrant hospitalization. Most, however, recovered within 24 to 48 hours of the onset of symptoms. Health officials were notified. Interviews and epidemiological analyses pointed to a Norwalk-like virus infection, or norovirus, probably foodborne. Stool specimens (1 to 5 mL) from hospitalized patients and samples of the suspected food sources (500 mg) were sent for laboratory analysis by RT-PCR. RNA extracted with 1,1,2 trichloro-1,2,2, trifluoroethane was mixed with a guanidium thiocyanate buffer and isolated by organic (phenolchloroform) procedures. cDNA was synthesized using primers specific to the viral RNA polymerase gene, and strain-specific PCR primers were used to amplify the viral gene. The amplicons, resolved by agarose gel electrophoresis, are shown in the figure below.

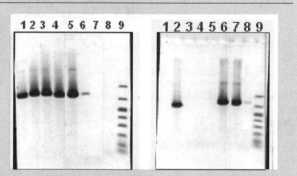

■ RT-PCR products were resolved on separate gels. Amplicons from four affected individuals (lanes 1–4, left). Lane 5, positive control; lane 6, sensitivity control; lane 7, negative control; lane 8, reagent blank. Specimens from suspected food sources (lanes 1–4, right). Lane 5, salad lettuce from the distributor; lanes 6–8, specimens from three hotel employees working the day of the outbreak; lane 9, molecular-weight marker.

QUESTIONS:

1. *Do these patients have norovirus?*
2. *What is the source of the organism?*
3. *When did the source get contaminated? Did the source come into the hotel infected, or was it infected inside the hotel?*

CASE STUDY 12 • 2

Five students from different local community high schools suffered recurrent skin infections with chronic wounds. Nasal swabs and skin specimens from the students were screened for MRSA by inoculation onto Mueller-Hinton agar supplemented with NaCl (0.68 mol/L) containing 6 µg/mL of oxacillin. The cultured organisms exhibited an MIC of more than 32 µg/mL vancomycin and a zone of inhibition of less than 14 mm in diameter. Isolates were sent to the CDC and referred for molecular testing. DNA isolated from the five cases and a control strain were embedded in agarose plugs and digested with *Sma*I for PFGE analysis. A depiction of the gel pattern is shown in the figure below.

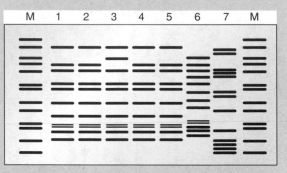

PFGE patterns of isolated strains. M, molecular-weight markers. Lanes 1–5, isolates from the community infections; lanes 6 and 7, unrelated hospital isolates.

Further PCR testing was performed on the isolates for virulence factors, particularly for *mecA* gene sequencing and detection of the Panton-Valentine leukocidin (PVL) genes, *lukS-PV* and *lukF-PV*. The results from these tests revealed that all five isolates contained the PVL genes and the type IV *mecA* element.

QUESTIONS:
1. Are all or some of the five isolates the same or different? Which isolates are the same, and which are different? What is the evidence to support your answer?
2. Was there a single source for these organisms or multiple sources?

CASE STUDY 12 • 3

A 39-year-old HIV-positive male has been monitored closely since his diagnosis as HIV-positive 5 years ago. The man was on HAART and compliant. He was relatively healthy and had not even had a cold in the last 4 years. The man had HIV viral loads as determined by Amplicor RT-PCR that were consistently close to 10,000 copies/mL, never varying more than 0.2 $\log_{10}$ unit, until the last 6 months, when his viral loads were trending up to 25,500, then 48,900, with his most recent result being 55,000 copies/mL. Genotyping performed on virus isolated from the patient revealed a mutation in the reverse transcriptase gene of M41L that is associated with resistance to zidovudine (AZT).

QUESTIONS:
1. What is the significance of the viral load results over the last 6 months?
2. What is the implication of the genotyping result for the patient's therapy?
3. How should this patient be monitored in the future?

• STUDY QUESTIONS •

1. Which of the following genes would be analyzed to determine whether an isolate of *Staphylococcus aureus* is resistant to oxacillin?
   a. *mecA*
   b. *gyrA*
   c. *inhA*
   d. *vanA*

2. Which of the following is a genotypic method used to compare two isolates in an epidemiological investigation?
   a. Biotyping
   b. Serotyping
   c. Ribotyping
   d. Bacteriophage typing

3. For which of the following organisms must caution be exercised when evaluating positive PCR results because the organism can be found as normal flora in some patient populations?
   a. *Neisseria gonorrhoeae*
   b. HIV
   c. *Chlamydophila pneumoniae*
   d. *Streptococcus pneumoniae*

4. Which of the following controls are critical for ensuring that amplification is occurring in a patient sample and that the lack of PCR product is not due to the presence of polymerase inhibitors?
   a. Reagent blank
   b. Sensitivity control
   c. Negative control
   d. Amplification control

5. A PCR assay was performed to detect *Bordetella pertussis* on sputum obtained from a 14-year-old girl who has had a chronic cough. The results revealed two bands, one consistent with the internal control and the other consistent with the size expected for amplification of the *B. pertussis* target. How should these results be interpreted?
   a. False-positive for *B. pertussis*.
   b. The girl has clinically significant *B. pertussis* infection.
   c. *B. pertussis* detection is more likely due to colonization.
   d. Invalid because two bands were present.

6. Which of the following is an advantage of molecular-based testing?
   a. Results stay positive long after successful treatment.
   b. Results are available within hours.
   c. Only viable cells yield positive results.
   d. Several milliliters of specimen must be submitted for analysis.

7. A molecular-based typing method that has high typing capacity, reproducibility and discriminatory power, moderate ease of performance, and good-to-moderate ease of interpretation is
   a. Repetitive elements
   b. PFGE

   c. Plasmid analysis
   d. PCR-RFLP

8. A patient has antibodies against HCV and a viral load of 100,000 copies/mL. What is the next test that should be performed on this patient's isolate?
   a. Ribotyping
   b. PCR-RFLP
   c. Hybrid capture

9. A positive result for HPV type 16 indicates
   a. High risk for antibiotic resistance
   b. Low risk for cervical cancer
   c. High risk for cervical cancer

10. Which of the following is used to type molds?
    a. Sequence-specific PCR
    b. Microarray
    c. ITS sequencing
    d. Flow cytometry

References

1. Brisson-Noel A, Gicquel B, Lecossier D, et al. Rapid diagnosis of tuberculosis by amplification of mycobacterial DNA in clinical samples. *Lancet* 1989;2: 1069–1071.
2. De Wit D, Steyn L, Shoemaker S, et al. Direct detection of *Mycobacterium tuberculosis* in clinical specimens by DNA amplification. *Journal of Clinical Microbiology* 1990;28:2437–2441.
3. Eisenach KD, Cave MD, Bates JH, et al. Polymerase chain reaction amplification of a repetitive DNA sequence specific for *Mycobacterium tuberculosis*. *Journal of Infectious Disease* 1990;161:977–981.
4. Bracca A, Tosello ME, Girardini JE, et al. Molecular detection of *Histoplasmacapsulatum* var. *capsulatum* in human clinical samples. *Journal of Clinical Microbiology* 2003;41:1753–1755.
5. Martagon-Villamil J, Shrestha N, Sholtis M, et al. Identification of *Histoplasmacapsulatum* from culture extracts by real-time PCR. *Journal of Clinical Microbiology* 2003;41:1295–1298.
6. Bialek R, Gonzalez GM, Begerow D, et al. Coccidioidomycosis and blastomycosis: Advances in molecular diagnostics. *FEMS Immunology & Medical Microbiology* 2005;45:355–360.

7. Johnson SM, Simmons KA, Pappagianis D. Amplification of coccidioidal DNA in clinical specimens by PCR. *Journal of Clinical Microbiology* 2004;42: 1982–1985.

8. Fiebelkorn KR, Nolte FS. RNA virus detection. In Persing DH, Tenover FC, Versalovic J, et al, eds. Molecular Microbiology. Diagnostic Principles and Practice. Washington, DC: ASM Press, 2004.

9. Hall GS. Molecular diagnostic methods for the detection of *Neisseriagonorrhoeae* and *Chlamydiatrachomatis. Reviews in Medical Microbiology* 2005;16:69–78.

10. Geha DJ, Uhl JR, Gustaferro CA, et al. Multiplex PCR for identification of methicillin-resistant staphylococci in the clinical laboratory. *Journal of Clinical Microbiology* 1994;32:1768–1772.

11. Satake S, Clark N, Rimland D, et al. Detection of vancomycin-resistant enterococci in fecal samples by PCR. *Journal of Clinical Microbiology* 1997; 35:2325–2330.

12. Hunt JM, Roberts GD, Stockman L, et al. Detection of a genetic locus encoding resistance to rifampin in mycobacterial cultures and in clinical specimens. *Diagnostic Microbiology and Infectious Disease* 1994;18:219–227.

13. Cockerill, III, FR, Uhl JR, Temesgen Z, et al. Rapid identification of a point mutation of the *Mycobacterium tuberculosis* catase-peroxidase (*katG*) gene associated with isoniazid resistance. *Journal of Infectious Disease* 1995;171:240–245.

14. Relman DA, Schmidt TM, MacDermott RP, et al. Identification of the uncultured bacillus of Whipple's disease. *New England Journal of Medicine* 1992;327:293–301.

15. Sefers S, Pei Z, Tang Y-W. False positives and false negatives encountered in diagnostic molecular microbiology. *Reviews in Medical Microbiology* 2005;16:59–67.

16. Wadowsky R, Laus S, Libert T, et al. Inhibition of PCR-Based Assay for Bordetella pertussis by using calcium alginate fiber and aluminum shaft components of a nasopharyngeal swab. *Journal of Clinical Microbiology* 1994;32:1054–1057.

17. Nolte FS, Caliendo AM. Molecular detection and identification of microorganisms. In Murray PR, Baron EJ, Jorgensen JH, et al., eds. Manual of Clinical Microbiology, 8th ed. Washington, DC: ASM Press, 2003.

18. National Committee for Clinical Laboratory Standards. Molecular diagnostic methods for infectious diseases; Approved guideline. (MM3-A). Wayne, PA: NCCLS, 1995.

19. Association for Molecular Pathology statement. Recommendations for in-house development and operation of molecular diagnostic tests. *American Journal of Clinical Pathology* 1999;111: 449–463.

20. Espy M, Uhl JR, Sloan LM, et al. Real-time PCR in clinical microbiology: Applications for routine laboratory testing. *Clinical Microbiology Reviews* 2006;19:165–256.

21. Kolbert CP, Rys PN, Hopkins M, et al. 16S ribosomal DNA sequence analysis for identification of bacteria in a clinical microbiology laboratory. In Persing DH, Tenover FC, Versalovic J, et al, eds. Molecular Microbiology: Diagnostic Principles and Practice. Washington, DC: ASM Press, 2004.

22. Kerr JR, Matthews RC. *Bordetella pertussis* infection: Pathogenesis, diagnosis, management, and the role of protective immunity. *European Journal of Clinical Microbiology and Infectious Diseases* 2000;19:77–88.

23. Winn WC, Allen S, Janda W, et al. Koneman's Color Atlas and Textbook of Diagnostic Microbiology, 6th ed. Baltimore: Lippincott Williams & Wilkins, 2006.

24. Chan EL, Antonishyn N, McDonald R, et al. The use of TaqMan PCR assay for detection of *Bordetella pertussis* infection from clinical specimens. *Archives of Pathology and Laboratory Medicine* 2002;126:173–176.

25. Yih W, Silva E, Ida J, et al. *Bordetella holmesii*–like organisms isolated from Massachusetts patients with pertussis-like symptoms. *Emerging Infectious Diseases* 1999;5:441–443.

26. Templeton KE, Scheltinga SA, van der Zee A, et al. Evaluation of real-time PCR for detection of and discrimination between *Bordetella pertussis*, *Bordetella parapertussis*, and *Bordetella holmesii* for clinical diagnosis. *Journal of Clinical Microbiology* 2003;41:4121–4126.

27. Caro V, Guiso N, Alberti C, et al. Proficiency program for real-time PCR diagnosis of *Bordetella pertussis* infections in French hospital laboratories and at the French National Reference Center for

Whooping Cough and other Bordetelloses. *Journal of Clinical Microbiology* 2009;47:3197–3203.

28. Knutsen E, Johnsborg O, Quentin Y, et al. BOX elements modulate gene expression in *Streptococcus pneumoniae*: Impact on the fine-tuning of competence development. *Journal of Bacteriology* 2006;188:8307–8312.

29. Fang GD, Fine M, Orloff J, et al. New and emerging etiologies for community-acquired pneumonia with implications for therapy: A prospective multicenter study of 359 cases. *Medicine* 1990;69:307–316.

30. Stout JE, Rihs JD, Yu VL. *Legionella*. In Murray PR, Baron EJ, Jorgensen JH, et al., eds. Manual of Clinical Microbiology, 8th ed. Washington, DC: ASM Press, 2003.

31. Rantakokko-Jalava K, Jalava J. Development of conventional and real-time PCR assays for detection of *Legionella* DNA in respiratory specimens. *Journal of Clinical Microbiology* 2001;39:2904–2910.

32. Reischl U, Linde H-J, Lehn N, et al. Direct detection and differentiation of *Legionella* spp. and *Legionella pneumophila* in clinical specimens by dual-color real-time PCR and melting curve analysis. *Journal of Clinical Microbiology* 2002;40: 3814–3817.

33. Cole ST, Brosch R, Parkhill J, et al. Deciphering the biology of *Mycobacterium tuberculosis* from the complete genome sequence. *Nature* 1998;393: 537–544.

34. Brosch R, Gordon SV, Eiglmeier K, et al. Genomics, biology, and evolution of the *Mycobacterium tuberculosis* complex. In Hatfull GF, Jacobs WR, eds. Molecular Genetics of Mycobacteria. Washington, DC: ASM Press, 2000.

35. Lipsky BA, Gates J, Tenover FC, et al. Factors affecting the clinical value of microscopy for acid-fast bacilli. *Reviews of Infectious Diseases* 1984;6:214–222.

36. European Society of Mycobacteriology. Decontamination, microscopy, and isolation. In Yates MD, Groothuis DG, eds. Diagnostic Public Health Mycobacteriology. London: Bureau of Hygiene and Tropical Disease, 1991.

37. Jost KCJ, Dunbar DF, Barth SS, et al. Identification of *Mycobacterium tuberculosis* and *M. avium* complex directly from smear-positive sputum specimens and BACTEC 12B cultures by high-performance liquid chromatography with fluorescence detection and computer-driven pattern recognition models. *Journal of Clinical Microbiology* 1995;35:907–914.

38. Chapin-Robertson K, Dahlberg S, Waycott S, et al. Detection and identification of *Mycobacterium* directly from BACTEC bottles by using a DNA-rRNA probe. *Diagnostic Microbiology & Infectious Disease* 1993;17:203–207.

39. Gamboa F, Fernandez G, Padilla E, et al. Comparative evaluation of initial and new versions of the Gen-Probe Amplified *Mycobacterium tuberculosis* direct test for direct detection of *Mycobacterium tuberculosis* in respiratory and nonrespiratory specimens. *Journal of Clinical Microbiology* 1998;36: 684–689.

40. D'Amato RF, Wallman AA, Hochstein LH, et al. Rapid diagnosis of pulmonary tuberculosis by using Roche AMPLICOR *Mycobacterium tuberculosis* PCR test. *Journal of Clinical Microbiology* 1995; 33:1832–1834.

41. Eisenach K, Sifford MD, Cave MD, Bates JH, Crawford JT. Detection of *Mycobacterium tuberculosis* in sputum samples using a polymerase chain reaction. *Pediatrics* 1991;144:1160–1163.

42. Miller N, Cleary T, Kraus G, Young AK, Spruill G, Hnatyszyn HJ. Rapid and specific detection of *Mycobacterium tuberculosis* from acid-fast bacillus smear-positive respiratory specimens and BacT/ALERT MP culture bottles by using fluorogenic probes and real-time PCR. *Journal of Clinical Microbiology* 2002;40:4143–4147.

43. Grayston JT. Background and current knowledge of *Chlamydia pneumoniae* and atherosclerosis. *Journal of Infectious Disease* 2000;181:S402–S410.

44. Everett KD, Bush RM, Anderson AA. Amended description of the order *Chlamydiales*, proposal of *Parachlamydiaceae* fam. nov. and *Simkaniaceae* fam. nov., each containing one monotypic genus, revised taxonomy of the family Chlamydiaceae, including a new genus and five new species and standards for the identification of organisms. *International Journal of Systematic Bacteriology* 1999;49:415–440.

45. Loens K, Ursi D, Goossens H, et al. Molecular diagnosis of *Mycoplasma pneumoniae* respiratory tract infections. *Journal of Clinical Microbiology* 2003;41:4915–4923.

46. Ieven M, Loens K, Goossens H. Detection and characterization of bacterial pathogens by nucleic acid amplification: State of the art review. In Persing DH, Tenover FC, Versalovic J, et al, eds. Molecular Microbiology: Diagnostic Principles and Practice. Washington, DC: ASM Press, 2004.

47. Boman J, Gaydos CA, Quinn TC. Molecular diagnosis of *Chlamydia pneumoniae* infection. *Journal of Clinical Microbiology* 1999;37:3791–3799.

48. de Barbeyrac B, Berner-Poggi C, Febrer F, et al. Detection of *Mycoplasma pneumoniae* and *Mycoplasma genitalium* in clinical samples by polymerase chain reaction. *Clinical Infectious Disease* 1993;17:83–89.

49. Falguera M, Nogues A, Ruiz-Gonzalez A, et al. Detection of *Mycoplasma pneumoniae* by polymerase chain reaction in lung aspirates from patients with community-acquired pneumonia. *Chest* 1996;110:972–976.

50. Ieven M, Usrsi D, Van Bever H, et al. Detection of *Mycoplasma pneumoniae* by two polymerase chain reactions and role of *M. pneumoniae* in acute respiratory tract infections in pediatric patients. *Journal of Infectious Disease* 1996;173:1445–1452.

51. Grondahl B, Puppe W, Hoppe A, et al. Rapid identification of nine microorganisms causing acute respiratory tract infections by single-tube multiplex reverse transcription-PCR: Feasibility study. *Journal of Clinical Microbiology* 1999;37:1–7.

52. Khanna M, Fan J, Pehler-Harrington K, et al. The pneumoplex assays, a multiplex PCR-enzyme hybridization assay that allows simultaneous detection of five organisms, *Mycoplasma pneumoniae*, *Chlamydia* (*Chlamydophila*) *pneumoniae*, *Legionella pneumophila*, *Legionella micdadei*, and *Bordetella pertussis*, and its real-time counterpart. *Journal of Clinical Microbiology* 2005;43:565–571.

53. McDonough EA, Barrozo CP, Russell KL, et al. A multiplex PCR for detection of *Mycoplasma pneumoniae*, *Chlamydophila pneumoniae*, *Legionella pneumophila*, and *Bordetella pertussis* in clinical specimens. *Molecular and Cellular Probes* 2005; 19:314–322.

54. Messmer TO, Sampson JS, Stinson A, et al. Comparison of four polymerase chain reaction assays for specificity in the identification of *Streptococcus pneumoniae*. *Diagnostic Microbiology and Infectious Disease* 2004;49:249–254.

55. Murdoch DR, Anderson TP, Beynon KA, et al. Evaluation of a PCR assay for detection of *Streptococcus pneumoniae* in respiratory and nonrespiratory samples from adults with community-acquired pneumonia. *Journal of Clinical Microbiology* 2003;41:63–66.

56. Dragovic B, Greaves K, Vashisht A, et al. Chlamydial co-infections among patients with gonorrhea. *International Journal of STD and AIDS* 2002;13: 261–263.

57. Janda WM, Knapp JS. *Neisseria* and *Moraxella catarrhalis*. In Murray PR, Baron EJ, Jorgensen JH, et al., eds. Manual of Clinical Microbiology, 8th ed. Washington, DC: ASM Press, 2003.

58. Norris SJ, Pope V, Johnson RE, et al. *Treponema* and other human host-associated spirochetes. In Murray PR, Baron EJ, Jorgensen JH, et al., eds. Manual of Clinical Microbiology, 8th ed. Washington, DC: ASM Press, 2003.

59. Totten PA, Manhart LE, Centurion-Lara A. PCR detection of *Haemophilus ducreyi*, *Treponema pallidum*, and *Mycoplasma genitalium*. In Persing DH, Tenover FC, Versalovic J, et al, eds. Molecular Microbiology: Diagnostic Principles and Practice. Washington, DC: ASM Press, 2004.

60. Liu H, Rodes B, Chen C-Y, et al. New tests for syphilis: Rational design of a PCR method for detection of *Treponema pallidum* in clinical specimens using unique regions of the DNA polymerase I gene. *Journal of Clinical Microbiology* 2001;39: 1941–1946.

61. Palmer HM, Higgins SP, Herring AJ, et al. Use of PCR in the diagnosis of early syphilis in the United Kingdom. *Sexually Transmitted Diseases* 2003;79:479–483.

62. Leslie DE, Azzato F, Karapanagiotidis T, et al. Development of a real-time PCR assay to detect *Treponema pallidum* in clinical specimens and assessment of the assay's performance by comparison with serological testing. *Journal of Clinical Microbiology* 2007;45:93–96.

63. Chui L, Albritton W, Paster B, et al. Development of polymerase chain reaction for diagnosis of chancroid. *Journal of Clinical Microbiology* 1993;31: 659–664.

64. Gu XX, Rossau R, Jannes G, et al. The rrs (16S)-rrl (23S) ribosomal intergenic spacer region as a target for the detection of *Haemophilus ducreyi* by a

hemi-nested-PCR assay. *Microbiology* 1998;144: 1013–1019.

65. Fraser CM, Gocayne JD, White O, et al. The minimal gene complement of *Mycoplasma genitalium*. *Science* 1995;270:397–403.

66. Tully JG, Taylor-Robinson D, Cole RM, et al. A newly discovered mycoplasma in the human urogenital tract. *Lancet* 1981;1:1288–1291.

67. Jensen JS, Hansen HT, Lind K. Isolation of *Mycoplasma genitalium* strains from the male urethra. *Journal of Clinical Microbiology* 1996;34: 286–291.

68. Jensen JS, Uldum SA, Sondergard-Andersen J, et al. Polymerase chain reaction for detection of *Mycoplasma genitalium* in clinical samples. *Journal of Clinical Microbiology* 1991;29:46–50.

69. Palmer HM, Gilroy CB, Furr PM, et al. Development and evaluation of the polymerase chain reaction to detect *Mycoplasma genitalium*. *FEMS Microbiology Letters* 1991;61:199–203.

70. Jensen JS, Borre MB, Dohn B. Detection of *Mycoplasma genitalium* by PCR amplification of the 16S rDNA gene. *Journal of Clinical Microbiology* 2003;41:261–266.

71. Yoshida T, Deguchi T, Ito M, et al. Quantitative detection of *Mycoplasma genitalium* from first-pass urine of men with urethritis and asymptomatic men by real-time PCR. *Journal of Clinical Microbiology* 2002;40:1451–1455.

72. Orle KA, Gates CA, Martin DH, et al. Simultaneous PCR detection of *Haemophilus ducreyi*, *Treponema pallidum* and herpes simplex virus types 1 and 2 from genital ulcers. *Journal of Clinical Microbiology* 1996;34:49–54.

73. McIver CJ, Rismanto N, Smith C, et al. Multiplex PCR testing detection of higher-than-expected rates of cervical *Mycoplasma*, *Ureaplasma*, and *Trichomonas* and viral agent infections in sexually active Australian women. *Journal of Clinical Microbiology* 2009;47:1358–1363.

74. Lipson SM, Costello P, Forlenza S, et al. Enhanced detection of cytomegalovirus in shell vial cell culture monolayers by preinoculation treatment of urine with low-speed centrifugation. *Current Microbiology* 1990;20:39–42.

75. LaSala P, Bufton K, Ismail N, et al. Prospective comparison of R-mix(tm) shell vial system with direct antigen tests and conventional cell culture for respiratory virus detection. *Journal of Clinical Virology* 2007;38:210–216.

76. Lathey JL, Hughes MD, Fiscus SA, et al. Variability and prognostic values of virologic and CD4 cell measures in human immunodeficiency virus type 1-infectd patients with 200-500 CD4 cells/mm^3 (ACTG 175). *Journal of Infectious Disease* 1998;177:617–624.

77. Leligdowicz A, Feldmann J, Jaye A, et al. Direct relationship between virus load and systemic immune activation in HIV-2 infection. *Journal of Infectious Diseases* 2010;20:114–122.

78. Hill CE, Caliendo AM. Viral load testing. In Persing DH, Tenover FC, Versalovic J, et al, eds. Molecular Microbiology: Diagnostic Principles and Practice. Washington, DC: ASM Press, 2004.

79. Schupbach J. Human immunodeficiency viruses. In Murray PR, Baron EJ, Jorgensen JH, Pfaller MA, Yolken RH. Manual of Clinical Microbiology, 8th ed. Washington, DC: ASM Press, 2003.

80. Elbeik T, Charlebois E, Nassos P, et al. Quantitative and cost comparison of ultrasensitive human immunodeficiency virus type 1 RNA viral load assays: Bayer bDNA quantiplex versions 3.0 and 2.0 and Roche PCR Amplicor Monitor version 1.5. *Journal of Clinical Microbiology* 2000;38: 1113–1120.

81. Raboud J, Montaner JS, Conway B, et al. Suppression of plasma viral load below 20 copies/ml is required to achieve a long-term response to therapy. *AIDS* 1998;12:1619–1624.

82. Saag MS, Holodniy M, Kuritzkes DR, et al. HIV viral load markers in clinical practice. *Nature Medicine* 1996;2:625–629.

83. Donovan RM, Bush CE, Markowitz NP, et al. Changes in virus load markers during AIDS-associated opportunistic diseases in human immunodeficiency virus–infected persons. *Journal of Infectious Disease* 1996;174:401–403.

84. O'Brien WA, Grovit-Ferbas K, Namazi A, et al. Human immunodeficiency virus–type 1 replication can be increased in peripheral blood of seropositive patients after influenza vaccination. *Blood* 1995;86:1082–1089.

85. Staprans SI, Hamilton BL, Follansbee SE, et al. Activation of virus replication after vaccination of HIV-1-infected individuals. *Journal of Experimental Medicine* 1995;182:1727–1737.

86. Hanna GJ, D'Aquila RT. Clinical use of genotypic and phenotypic drug resistance testing to monitor anti-retroviral chemotherapy. *Clinical Infectious Disease.* 2001;32:774–782.

87. Hirsch MS, Conway B, D'Aquila RT, et al. Anti-retroviral drug resistance testing in adults with HIV-1 infection. *Journal of the American Medical Association* 2001;283:2417–2426.

88. Caliendo AM, Yen-Lieberman B. Viral genotyping. In Persing DH, Tenover FC, Versalovic J, et al, eds. Molecular Microbiology: Diagnostic Principles and Practice. Washington, DC: ASM Press, 2004.

89. Parisi M, Soldini L, Di Perri G, et al. Offer of rapid testing and alternative biological samples as practical tools to implement HIV screening programs. *New Microbiology* 2009;32:391–396.

90. Ambinder R, Mann RB. Epstein-Barr-encoded RNA in situ hybridization: Diagnostic applications. *Human Pathology* 1994;25:602–605.

91. Raab-Traub N, Flynn K. The structure of the termini of the Epstein-Barr virus as a marker of clonal cellular proliferation. *Cell* 1986;47:883–889.

92. Fan H, Gulley ML. Molecular methods for detecting Epstein-Barr virus. Molecular Pathology Protocols. Totowa, NJ: Humana Press, 2001.

93. Schaade L, Kockelkorn P, Ritter K, et al. Detection of cytomegalovirus DNA in human specimens by LightCycler PCR. *Journal of Clinical Microbiology* 2000;38:4006–4009.

94. Guiver M, Fox AJ, Mutton K, et al. Evaluation of CMV viral load using TaqMan CMV quantitative PCR and comparison with CMV antigenemia in heart and lung transplant recipients. *Transplantation* 2001;71:1609–1615.

95. Shuhart MC, Gretch DR. Hepatitis C and G viruses. In Murray PR, Baron EJ, Jorgensen JH, et al., eds. Manual of Clinical Microbiology, 8th ed. Washington, DC: ASM Press, 2003.

96. Gorrin, G, Friesenhahn M, Lin P, et al. Performance evaluation of the VERSANT HCV RNA qualitative assay by using transcription-mediated amplification. *Journal of Clinical Microbiology* 2003;41:310–317.

97. Sherman KE, Rouster SD, Horn PS. Comparison of methodologies for quantification of hepatitis C virus (HCV) RNA in patients coinfected with HCV and human immunodeficiency virus. *Clinical Infectious Diseases* 2002;35:482–487.

98. Bullock G, Bruns DE, Haverstick DM. Hepatitis C genotype determination by melting curve analysis with a single set of fluorescence resonance energy transfer probes. *Clinical Chemistry* 2002;48:2147–2154.

99. Lee SS, Heathcote EJ, Reddy KR, et al. Prognostic factors and early predictability of sustained viral response with peginterferon alfa-2a (40KD). *Journal of Hepatology* 2002;37:500–506.

100. Meijer C, Snijders PJ, Castle PE. Clinical utility of HPV genotyping. *Gynecologic Oncology* 2006;103:12–17.

101. Stoler M, Castle PE, Solomon D, Schiffman M. The expanded use of HPV testing in gynecologic practice per ASCCP-guided management requires the use of well-validated assays. *American Journal of Clinical Pathology* 2007;127:335–337.

102. Kjaer S, Hogdall E, Frederiksen K, et al. The absolute risk of cervical abnormalities in high risk human papilloma virus-positive, cytologically normal women over a 10-year period. *Cancer Research* 2006;66:10630–10636.

103. De Marchi Triglia R, Metze K, et al. HPV in situ hybridization signal patterns as a marker for cervical intraepithelial neoplasia progression. *Gynecologic Oncology* 2009;112:114–118.

104. Lee W, Tubbs RR, Teker AM, et al. Use of in situ hybridization to detect human papillomavirus in head and neck squamous cell carcinoma patients without a history of alcohol or tobacco use. *Archives of Pathology & Laboratory Medicine* 2008;132:1653–1656.

105. Narimatsu R, Patterson BK. High-throughput cervical cancer screening using intracellular human papillomavirus E6 and E7 mRNA quantification by flow cytometry. *American Journal of Clinical Pathology* 2005;123:716–723.

106. Vaccarella S, Franceschi S, Snijders PJF, et al. Concurrent infection with multiple human papillomavirus types: Pooled analysis of the IARC HPV Prevalence Surveys. *Cancer Epidemiology Biomarkers and Prevention*, 2010;19:503–510.

107. Kurtycz DF, Smith M, He R, et al. Comparison of methods trial for high-risk HPV. *Diagnostic Cytopathology* 2010;38:104–108.

108. http://www.cdc.gov/flu/about/disease.htm About the Flu; Influenza: The Disease, Centers for Disease Control, 2004.

109. Stone B, Burrows J, Schepetiuk S, et al. Rapid detection and simultaneous subtype differentiation of influenza A viruses by real time PCR. *Journal of Virological Methods* 2004;117:103–112.

110. Ginocchio C, St. George K. Likelihood that an unsubtypeable Influenza A result in the Luminex xTAG Respiratory Virus Panel is indicative of novel A/H1N1 (swine-like) influenza. *Journal of Clinical Microbiology* 2009;47:1027–1029.

111. Kapelusznik L, Patel R, Jao J, et al. Severe pandemic (H1N1) 2009 influenza with false negative direct fluorescent antibody assay: Case series. *Journal of Clinical Virology* 2009; 46:279–281.

112. Bolotin S, Robertson AV, Eshaghi A, et al. Development of a novel real-time reverse-transcriptase PCR method for the detection of H275Y positive influenza A H1N1 isolates. *Journal of Virological Methods*2009;158:190–194.

113. Kaufman L, Standard PG, Jalbert M, et al. Immunohistologic identification of *Aspergillus* spp. and other hyaline fungi by using polyclonal fluorescent antibodies. *Journal of Clinical Microbiology* 1997;35:2206–2209.

114. Van Burik JA, Myerson D, Schreckhise RW, et al. Panfungal PCR for detection of fungal infection in human blood specimens. *Journal of Clinical Microbiology* 1998;36:1169–1175.

115. Pounder JI, Hansen D, Woods GL. Identification of Histoplasma capsulatum, Blastomyces dermatitidis, and Coccidioides species by Repetitive-Sequence-Based PCR. *Journal of Clinical Microbiology* 2006;44:2977–2982.

116. Petri, Jr, WA. Overview of the development, utility, and future of molecular diagnostics for parasitic disease. In Persing DH, Tenover FC, Versalovic J, et al, eds. Molecular Microbiology: Diagnostic Principles and Practice. Washington, DC: ASM Press, 2004.

117. Weigel L, Clewell DB, Gill SR, et al. Genetic analysis of a high-level vancomycin-resistant isolate of *Staphylococcus aureus*. *Science* 2003;302:1569–1571.

118. Tenover FC, Rasheed JK. Detection of antimicrobial resistance genes and mutations associated with antimicrobial resistance in microorganisms. In Persing DH, Tenover FC, Versalovic J, et al, eds.

Molecular Microbiology: Diagnostic Principles and Practice. Washington, DC: ASM Press, 2004.

119. Metan G, Zarakolu P, Unal S. Rapid detection of antibacterial resistance in emerging gram-positive cocci. *Journal of Hospital Infection* 2005;61:93–99.

120. Leclercq R, Derlot E, Duval J, et al. Plasmid-mediated resistance to vancomycin and teicoplanin in *Enterococcus faecium*. *New England Journal of Medicine* 1988;319:157–161.

121. Centers for Disease Control and Prevention. *Staphylococcus aureus* resistant to vancomycin-United States, 2002. *Morbidity and Mortality Weekly Report* 2002;51;565–567.

122. Palladino S, Kay ID, Flexman JP, et al. Rapid detection of *vanA* and *vanB* genes directly from clinical specimens and enrichment broths by real-time multiplex PCR assay. *Journal of Clinical Microbiology* 2003;41:2483–2486.

123. Espinal MA, Laszlo A, Simonsen L, et al. Global trends in resistance to antituberculosis drugs. *New England Journal of Medicine* 2001;344: 1294–1303.

124. Meacci F, Orru G, Iona E, et al. Drug resistance evolution of a *Mycobacterium tuberculosis* strain from a noncompliant patient. *Journal of Clinical Microbiology* 2005;43(7):3114–3120.

125. Grace Lin S-Y, Probert W, Lo M, et al. Rapid detection of isoniazid and rifampin resistance mutations in *Mycobacterium tuberculosis* complex from cultures or smear-positive sputa by use of molecular beacons. *Journal of Clinical Microbiology*. 2004; 42:4204–4208.

126. Mokrousov I, Otten T, Filipenko M, et al. Detection of isoniazid-resistant *Mycobacterium tuberculosis* strains by a multiplex allele-specific PCR assay targeting katG codon 315 variation. *Journal of Clinical Microbiology* 2002:40:2509–2512.

127. de Viedma DG, del Sol Diaz Infantes M, Lasala F, et al. New real-timer PCR able to detect in a single tube multiple rifampin resistance mutations in *Mycobacterium tuberculosis*. *Journal of Clinical Microbiology* 2002:40:988–995.

128. Cavusoglu C, Turhan A, Akinci P, et al. Evaluation of the genotype MTBDR assay for rapid detection of rifampin and isoniazid resistance in *Mycobacterium tuberculosis* isolates. *Journal of Clinical Microbiology* 2006:44:2338–2342.

129. Bang D, Andersen AB, Thomsen VO. Rapid genotypic detection of rifampin- and isoniazid-resistant *Mycobacterium tuberculosis* directly in clinical specimens. *Journal of Clinical Microbiology* 2006; 44:2605–2608.

130. Ruiz M, Torres MJ, Llanos AC, et al. Direct detection of rifampin- and isoniazid-resistant *Mycobacterium tuberculosis* in auramine-rhodamine–positive sputum specimens by real-time PCR. *Journal of Clinical Microbiology* 2004;42:1585–1589.

131. Olive DM, Bean P. Principles and applications of methods for DNA-based typing of microbial organisms. *Journal of Clinical Microbiology* 1999;37:1661–1669.

132. Tenover FC. Bacterial strain typing through the decades: A personal reflection. In Persing DH, Tenover FC, Versalovic J, et al, eds. Molecular Microbiology: Diagnostic Principles and Practice. Washington, DC: ASM Press, 2004.

133. Tenover FC, Arbeit RD, Goering RV. How to select and interpret molecular strain typing methods for epidemiological studies of bacterial infections: A review for healthcare epidemiologists. *Infection Control and Hospital Epidemiology* 1997;18: 426–439.

134. Schaberg DR, Tompkins LS, Falkow S. Use of agarose gel electrophoresis of plasmid deoxyribonucleic acid to fingerprint gram-negative bacilli. *Journal of Clinical Microbiology* 1981;13: 1105–1110.

135. Tenover F, Arbeit RD, Goering RV, et al. Interpreting chromosomal DNA restriction patterns produced by pulsed-field gel electrophoresis: Criteria for bacterial strain typing. *Journal of Clinical Microbiology* 1995;33:2233–2239.

136. Loutit J, Tompkins S. Restriction enzyme and Southern hybridization analyses of *Pseudomonas aeruginosa* strains from patients with cystic fibrosis. *Journal of Clinical Microbiology* 1991;29: 2897–2900.

137. Tram C, Simonet M, Nicolas MH, et al. Molecular typing of nosocomial isolates of *Legionella pneumophila* serogroup 3. *Journal of Clinical Microbiology* 1990;28:242–245.

138. Riley LW. Molecular Epidemiology of Infectious Diseases: Principles and Practices. Washington, DC: ASM Press, 2004.

139. Van Embden JDA, Cave MD, Crawford JT, et al. Strain identification of *Mycobacterium tuberculosis* by DNA fingerprinting: Recommendations for a standardized methodology. *Journal of Clinical Microbiology* 1993;31:406–409.

140. Lima P, Correia AM. Genetic fingerprinting of *Brevibacterium linens* by pulsed-field gel electrophoresis and ribotyping. *Current Microbiology* 2000;41:50–55.

141. Pignato S, Giammanco G, Grimont F, et al. Molecular typing of *Salmonella enterica* subsp. *enterica* serovar *Wien* by rRNA gene restriction patterns. *Research in Microbiology* 1992;143:703–709.

142. Al Dahouk S, Tomaso H, Prenger-Berninghoff E, et al. Identification of *Brucella* species and biotypes using polymerase chain reaction-restriction fragment length polymorphism (PCR-RFLP). *Critical Reviews in Microbiology* 2005;31:191–196.

143. Stone G, Shortridge D, Flamm RK, et al. PCR-RFLP typing of *ureC* from *Helicobacter pylori* isolated from gastric biopsies during a European multi-country clinical trial. *Journal of Antimicrobial Chemotherapy* 1997;40:251–256.

144. Lowe A, Hanotte O, Guarino L. Standardization of molecular genetic techniques for the characterization of germ plasma collections: The case of random amplified polymorphic DNA (RAPD). *Plant Genetic Resources Newsletter* 1996;107:50–54.

145. Munthali M, Ford-Lloyd B-V, Newbury HJ. The random amplification of polymorphic DNA for fingerprinting plants. *PCR Methods and Applications* 1992;1:274–276.

146. Dijkshoorn L, Aucken H, Gerner-Smidt P, et al. Comparison of outbreak and nonoutbreak *Acinetobacter baumannii* strains by genotypic and phenotypic methods. *Journal of Clinical Microbiology* 1996;34:1519–1525.

147. Gibson R, Slater E, Xerry J, et al. Use of an amplified–fragment length polymorphism technique to fingerprint and differentiate isolates of *Helicobacter pylori*. *Journal of Clinical Microbiology* 1998;36:2580–2585.

148. Kremer K, Arnold C, Cataldi A, et al. Discriminatory power and reproducibility of novel DNA typing methods for *Mycobacterium tuberculosis* complex strains. *Journal of Clinical Microbiology* 2005;43:5628–5638.

149. Hulton C, Higgins CF, Sharp PM. ERIC sequences: A novel family of repetitive elements in the genomes of *Escherichia coli, Salmonella typhimurium* and other enterobacteria. *Molecular Microbiology* 1991;5:825–834.

150. Versalovic J, Koeuth T, Lupski JR. Distribution of repetitive DNA sequences in eubacteria and application to fingerprinting of bacterial genomes. *Nucleic Acids Research* 1991;19:6823–6831.

151. Healy M, Reece K, Walton D, et al. Identification to the species level and differentiation between strains of *Aspergillus* clinical isolates by automated repetitive sequence–based PCR. *Journal of Clinical Microbiology* 2004;42:4016–4024.

152. Spigaglia P, Mastrantonio P. Evaluation of repetitive element sequence–based PCR as a molecular typing method for *Clostridium difficile*. *Journal of Clinical Microbiology* 2003;41:2454–2457.

153. Hierro N, González A, Mas A, et al. New PCR-based methods for yeast identification. *Journal of Applied Microbiology* 2004;97:792–801.

154. Knutsen E, Johnsborg O, Quentin Y, et al. BOX elements modulate gene expression in *Streptococcus pneumoniae*: Impact on the fine-tuning of competence development. *Journal of Bacteriology* 2006;188;8307–8312.

155. Bruns T, White TJ, Taylor JW. Fungal molecular systematics. *Annual Review of Ecology* 1991;22: 525–564.

156. Hillis D, Dixon M. Ribosomal DNA: Molecular evolution and phylogenetic inference. *Quarterly Review of Biology* 1991;66:411–453.

157. Kumar M, Shukla PK. Use of PCR targeting of internal transcribed spacer regions and single-stranded conformation polymorphism analysis of sequence variation in different regions of rRNA genes in fungi for rapid diagnosis of mycotic keratitis. *Journal of Clinical Microbiology* 2005;43:662–668.

158. Lebuhn M, Bathe S, Achouak W, et al. Comparative sequence analysis of the internal transcribed spacer 1 of *Ochrobactrum* species. *Systematic and Applied Microbiology* 2005;29:265–275.

159. Sugita C, Makimura K, Uchida K, et al. PCR identification system for the genus *Aspergillus* and three major pathogenic species: *Aspergillus fumigatus, Aspergillus flavus* and *Aspergillus niger*. *Medical Mycology* 2004;42:433–437.

160. Shopsin B, Gomez M, Montgomery SO, et al. Evaluation of protein A gene polymorphic region DNA sequencing for typing of *Staphylococcus aureus* strains. *Journal of Clinical Microbiology* 1999;37:3556–3563.

161. Shopsin B, Gomez M, Waddington M, et al. Use of coagulase gene (*coa*) repeat region nucleotide sequences for typing of methicillin-resistant *Staphylococcus aureus* strains. *Journal of Clinical Microbiology* 2000;38:3453–3456.

162. Birtles A, Hardy K, Gray SJ, et al. Multilocus sequence typing of *Neisseria meningitidis* directly from clinical samples and application of the method to the investigation of meningococcal disease case clusters. *Journal of Clinical Microbiology* 2005;43:6007–6014.

163. Rakeman J, Bui U, Lafe K, et al. Multilocus DNA sequence comparisons rapidly identify pathogenic molds. *Journal of Clinical Microbiology* 2005;43:3324–3333.

164. Maiden M, Bygraves JA, Feil E, et al. Multilocus sequence typing: A portable approach to the identification of clones within populations of pathogenic microorganisms. *Proceedings of the National Academy of Sciences* 1998;95:3140–3145.

165. Urwin R, Maiden MC. Multilocus sequence typing: A tool for global epidemiology. *Trends in Microbiology* 2003;11:479–487.

Chapter **13**

Molecular Detection of Inherited Diseases

OUTLINE

OBJECTIVES

- Describe Mendelian patterns of inheritance as exhibited by family pedigrees.

- Give examples of laboratory methods designed to detect single-gene disorders.

- Discuss non-Mendelian inheritance, and give examples of these types of inheritance, such as mitochondrial disorders and trinucleotide repeat expansion diseases.

- Show how genomic imprinting can affect disease phenotype.

Molecular and cytogenetic analyses are a critical component of diagnostic testing, especially for diseases that arise from known genetic events. The identification of a molecular or chromosomal abnormality is a direct observation of the source of some diseases. Methods to detect gene and chromosomal mutations are discussed in Chapter 8, "Chromosomal Structure and Chromosomal Mutations," and Chapter 9, "Gene Mutations." This chapter will present examples of clinical laboratory tests commonly performed in molecular genetics using these techniques.

The Molecular Basis of Inherited Diseases

Mutations are heritable changes in DNA nucleotide sequences. These changes range from single base-pair or point mutations of various types to chromosomal aneuploidy (see Chapter 8). Not all mutations lead to disease.

Polymorphisms are proportionately represented genotypes in a given population (see Chapter 11, "DNA Polymorphisms and Human Identification"). Changes in the DNA sequence among groups of individuals (sequence polymorphisms) are located within genes or outside of genes. Benign polymorphisms, those that do not lead to adverse phenotypes, are useful for mapping disease genes, determining parentage, and identity testing. Balanced polymorphisms have offsetting phenotypes caused by the same sequence change.

Epigenetic alterations do not change the primary DNA sequence, yet are heritable. Three forms of epigenetic changes in DNA are DNA methylation, usually alterations of cytosine in CpG islands; **genomic imprinting**, and chromatin remodeling. DNA methylation shuts down RNA transcription of individual genes. Genomic imprinting selectively inactivates gene expression in chromosomal regions, for example, X-chromosome inactivation. Chromatin remodeling sequesters large regions of chromosomal DNA through protein binding and histone modification. Histone modification controls the availability of DNA for RNA transcription.

Mutations in germ cells result in inherited disease. Mutations in somatic cells result in cancer and some congenital malformations. Diseases with genetic components are often referred to as **congenital** ("born with") diseases. Congenital disorders are not necessarily heritable, however. Congenital disorders are those present in individuals at birth. Specifically, congenital disorders result when some factor, such as a drug, a chemical, an infection, or an injury, upsets the developmental process. Thus, an infant can have a heritable disease, such as hemophilia, that can be passed on to future generations or a congenital condition, such as spina bifida, that cannot be passed on.

Advanced Concepts

According to the **Lyon hypothesis** (or Lyon's hypothesis) first stated by Mary Lyon in 1961, only one X chromosome remains genetically active in females.[1,2] In humans, one X chromosome is inactivated at random about the 16th day of embryonic development. The inactive X can be seen as a **Barr body** (X chromatin) in the interphase nucleus. Not all X genes are shut off in the inactivated X chromosome. Furthermore, reactivation of genes on the inactivated X occurs in germ cells before the first meiotic division for production of eggs.

Chromosomal Abnormalities

Genome mutations (abnormalities in chromosome number) can be detected by karyotyping, ploidy studies using flow cytometry, and fluorescent in situ hybridization (FISH) studies (see Chapter 8). Humans have 44 **autosomes** (non-sex chromosomes) and 2 sex chromosomes. Humans are normally diploid, having two of each chromosome (except for the one X chromosome and one Y chromosome in males). **Polyploidy** (more than two of any autosome) in animals results in infertility and abnormal appearance. Aneuploidy (gain or loss of any autosome) occurs with 0.5% frequency in term pregnancies and 50% in spontaneous abortions. Aneuploidy is usually caused by erroneous separation of chromosomes during egg or sperm production (chromosomal nondisjunction). Autosomal trisomy/monosomy (three copies/one copy of a chromosome instead of two) results from fertilization of gametes containing an extra chromosome or missing a chromosome ($n + 1$ or $n - 1$ gametes, respectively). Autosomal monosomy is generally, but not always, incompatible with life. Sex chromosome aneuploidy is more frequently tolerated, although associated with phenotypic abnormalities.

Mosaicism, two or more genetically distinct populations of cells from one zygote in an individual (in contrast to **chimerism**: two or more genetically distinct cell populations from different zygotes in an individual), results from mutation events affecting somatic or germ cells. Early segregation errors during fertilized egg division occasionally give rise to mosaicism. Mosaicism is relatively common with sex chromosomes, for example, 45,X/47,XXX (normal female chromosome complement is 46, XX). In this case, later nondisjunction will yield additional populations. Rarely, autosomal haploids will be lost with the retention of the **triploid** lineage, for example, 45,XY,–21, 46,XY/47,XY,+21→46,XY/47,XY,+21. Examples of genome mutations are shown in Table 13.1.

Chromosome mutations (abnormalities in chromosome structure) larger than 4 million bp can be seen by karyotyping; smaller irregularities can be seen with the higher resolution of FISH (see Chapter 8). Structural alterations include translocations (reciprocal, nonreciprocal), inversions (paracentric, pericentric), deletions (terminal, interstitial, ring), duplications (isochromosomes), **marker chromosomes**, and derivative chromosomes.

Structural mutations require breakage and reunion of DNA. Chromosomal breakage is caused by chemicals and radiation. Chromosomal breakage also results from chromosome breakage syndromes, for example, Fanconi anemia, Bloom syndrome, and ataxia telangiectasia. Some aberrations have no immediate phenotypic effect

Table 13.1 Examples of Genome Mutations

Disorder	Genetic Abnormality	Incidence	Clinical Features
Down syndrome	Trisomy 21, 47,XY,+21	1/700 live births	Flat facial profile, mental retardation, cardiac problems, risk of acute leukemia, eventual neuropathological disorders, abnormal immune system
Edward syndrome	Trisomy 18, 47,XY,+18	1/3000 live births	Severe, clenched fist; survival less than 1 year
Patau syndrome	Trisomy 13, 47,XY,+13	1/5000 live births	Cleft palate, heart damage, mental retardation, survival usually less than 6 mo
Klinefelter syndrome	47,XXY	1/850 live births	Male hypogonadism, long legs, gynecomastia (male breast enlargement), low testosterone level
XYY syndrome	47,XYY	1/1000 live births	Excessive height, acne, 1% to 2% behavioral disorders
Turner syndrome	45,X and variants	1/2000 live births	Bilateral neck webbing, heart disease, failure to develop secondary sex characteristics, hypothyroidism
Multi X females	47,XXX; 48,XXXX	1/1200 newborn females	Mental retardation increases with increasing X

(reciprocal translocations, inversions, some deletions, some insertions). Approximately 7.4% of conceptions have chromosome mutations. Chromosome mutations are observed in 50% of spontaneous abortions and 5% of still-births. Examples of diseases arising from inherited chromosome structure abnormalities are shown in Table 13.2.

Chromosome translocations are another type of frequently observed structural abnormality. Translocations are usually somatic events (not inherited) and are most commonly seen in cancer (see Chapter 14, "Molecular Oncology").

Patterns of Inheritance in Single-Gene Disorders

Most phenotypes result from the interaction of multiple genetic and environmental factors. Some phenotypes, however, are caused by alteration of a single gene. The genetic change may be a **loss-of-function** mutation, for example deletion of a gene with loss of the gene product. Alternatively, the gene alteration may be a gain-of-function mutation, for example, a mutation that activates a gene, causes its overexpression, or alters its protein function, resulting in a new phenotype.

The phenotype of a loss-of-function mutation depends on the type of protein affected. Even though only one of the two homologous copies of a gene is mutated, the mutated protein can interfere with the function of the normal protein produced from the unmutated chromosome. Complex metabolic pathways are susceptible to loss-of-function mutations because of extensive interactions between and among proteins. Key structural proteins, especially multimeric complexes, risk dominant negative

phenotypes (Fig. 13-1). Gain-of-function mutations are less common than loss-of-function mutations. In this case, new properties of the mutant allele are responsible for the disease phenotype. Gain-of-function mutations include gene expression/stability defects that generate gene products at inappropriate sites or times.

If the phenotype occurs as predicted by Mendelian genetics, patterns of inheritance can be established. Patterns of inheritance (**transmission patterns**) are determined

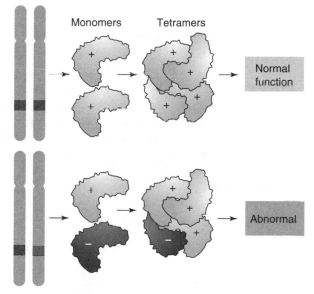

Chromosomes

Monomers   Tetramers

Normal function

Abnormal

■ Figure 13-1 Dominant negative mutations affect multimeric proteins. In this illustration, a single mutant monomer affects the function of the assembled tetramer.

Table 13.2 **Examples of Chromosomal Mutations**

Disorder	Genetic Abnormality	Incidence	Clinical Features
DiGeorges syndrome and velocardiofacial syndrome	del(22q)	1/4000 live births	CATCH 22 (cardiac abnormality/abnormal facies, T-cell deficit, cleft palate, hypercalcemia)
Cri du chat syndrome	del(5p)	1/20,000–1/50,000 live births	Growth deficiency, catlike cry in infancy, small head, mental retardation
Contiguous gene syndrome; Wilms tumor, aniridia, genitourinary anomalies, mental retardation syndrome	del(11p)	1/15,000 live births	Aniridia (absence of iris), hemihypertrophy (one side of the body seems to grow faster than the other), and other congenital anomalie

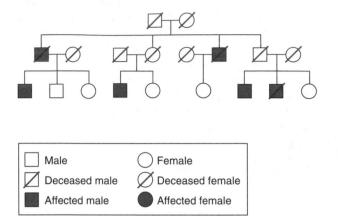

■ **Figure 13-2** A pedigree is a diagram of family phenotype or genotype. The pedigree will display the transmission pattern of a disease.

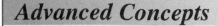

Advanced Concepts

Autosomal-dominant mutations can originate from **new mutations** in germ cells, that is, DNA changes that arise in cells that produce eggs or sperm. Establishment of a new mutation as a dominant mutation in a family or in a population is influenced by its effect on reproductive fitness.

by examination of family histories. A **pedigree** is a diagram of the inheritance pattern of a phenotype of family members (Fig 13-2). There are three main transmission patterns: autosomal-dominant, autosomal-recessive, and **X-linked** or sex-linked recessive. These patterns refer to the disease phenotype.

In **autosomal-dominant** transmission, the disease phenotype will be present in individuals with one or both chromosomes mutated. Therefore, a child of an affected parent and an unaffected parent has a 50% to 100% likelihood of expressing the disease phenotype (Fig. 13-3). Dominant mutations can be either gain-of-function or loss-of-function.

Autosomal-recessive is the largest category of Mendelian disorders. The likelihood of the disease phenotype in offspring is 25%, indicating the presence of the recessive mutation in at least one chromosome in each of the parents. Autosomal-recessive diseases are more often observed as a result of inbreeding where two individuals

heterozygous for the same mutation produce offspring (Fig. 13-4). New mutations are rarely detected in autosomal-recessive transmission patterns. Almost all inborn errors of metabolism are autosomal-recessive.[1] Risk factors for neoplastic diseases, tumor suppressor gene mutations (see Chapter 14, "Molecular Oncology"), fall in this category.

Most **sex-linked** disorders are X-linked because relatively few genes are carried on the Y chromosome. X-linked mutations are almost always recessive. X-linked dominant diseases are rare, for example, vitamin D–resistant rickets. Even though one X chromosome is inactivated in females, the inactivation is reversible so that a second copy of X-linked genes is available. In contrast, males are **hemizygous** for X-linked genes, having only one copy on the X chromosome. Males, therefore, are more likely to manifest the disease phenotype (Fig. 13-5).

Transmission patterns are complicated by biological factors such as **penetrance** and **variable expressivity** that will influence the expression of the phenotype in the

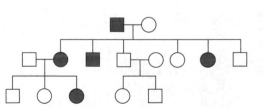

■ **Figure 13-3** In an autosomal-dominant transmission pattern, heterozygous individuals express the affected phenotype (filled symbols).

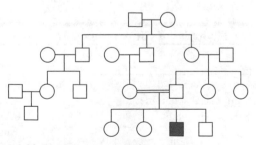

■ **Figure 13-4** Autosomal-recessive mutations are not expressed in heterozygotes. The phenotype is displayed only in a homozygous individual; in this illustration, produced by the inbreeding of two cousins (double horizontal line).

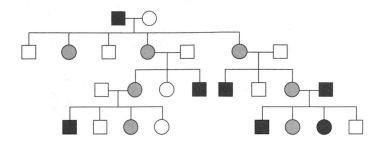

■ Figure 13-5 X-linked recessive diseases are carried by females but manifested most often in males.

presence of a mutation. Penetrance is the frequency of expression of disease phenotype in individuals with a gene lesion. A mutation with incomplete penetrance will not always result in the disease phenotype. Complete penetrance is expression of the disease phenotype in every individual with the mutated gene. Variable expressivity is a range of phenotypes in individuals with the same gene lesion. Variable expressivity reflects the interaction of other gene products and the environment on the disease phenotype.

Molecular Basis of Single-Gene Disorders

Single-gene disorders affect structural proteins, cell surface receptor proteins, growth regulators, and enzymes. Examples of diseases resulting from such disorders are shown in Table 13.3, as well as molecular methods that have been or could be used to detect these gene lesions. (See Chapters 9 and 10 for more detailed explanations of the methodologies.) Note that not all of these methods are in common use in molecular diagnostics. Some diseases are effectively analyzed by morphological studies or biochemistry. For instance, hemoglobin S is classically detected by protein electrophoresis. As with all abnormalities, final diagnosis requires physiological, morphological, and laboratory results.

Lysosomal Storage Diseases

Lysosomes are cellular organelles in which cellular products of ingestion are degraded by acid hydrolase enzymes (Fig. 13-6). These enzymes work in an acid environment. Substrates come from intracellular turnover (**autophagy**) or outside the cell through phagocytosis or endocytosis (**heterophagy**). Lysosomal storage disorders result from incompletely digested macromolecules due to loss of enzyme function. Storage disorders include defects in any proteins required for normal lysosomal function, giving rise to physical abnormalities. The organs affected depend on the location and site of degradation of substrate material. Table 13.4 lists examples of storage diseases, which are screened by gene product testing, that is, by measuring the ability of serum enzymes to digest test substrates. With the discovery of genes that code for the enzymes and their subunits, molecular testing has been used to some extent. Mutations can be detected by direct sequencing, usually after an initial biochemical screening test for loss of enzyme activity.

Molecular Diagnosis of Single-Gene Disorders

Genetic lesions in single-gene disorders are detected by a variety of hybridization/amplification methods and nucleotide sequencing. Examples of some frequently tested genes are given below.

Factor V Leiden

The Leiden mutation in the factor V coagulation gene (F5 located at 1q23) was discovered in 1994 at the University of Leiden in the Netherlands. The Leiden mutation (1691 A→G, R506Q) in exon 10 of the F5 gene causes a hypercoagulable (thrombophilic) phenotype. The genotype is present in heterozygous form in 4%–7% of the general population, and 0.06% to 0.25% of the population is homozygous for this mutation. Overall, the annual occurrence of the phenotype of deep venous thrombosis is 1 per every 1000 persons. The disorder is treated with anticoagulants. The risk of thrombosis increases with contraceptive use in women (Table 13.5).

Table 13.3 Single-Gene Disorders and Molecular Methods

Type of Protein	Type of Disease	Example	Gene (Location)	Type of Mutation	Examples of Molecular Methods
Structural	Hemoglobinopathies	Sickle cell anemia	Hemoglobin beta (11p15.5)	Missense	Sequencing, PCR-RFLP
	Connective tissue disorders	Marfan syndrome	Fibrillin (15q21.1)	Missense	Sequencing, linkage analysis[36]
	Cell membrane–associated protein dysfunction	Muscular dystrophy	Dystrophin, DMD (Xp12.2)	Deletion	Southern blot RFLP,[37] multiplex PCR, linkage analysis
Cell surface receptor proteins	Hypercholesteremia	Familial hypercholesteremia	Low-density lipoprotein receptor (19p13.2)	Deletions, point mutations	Probe amplification,[38] sequencing
	Nutritional disorders	Vitamin D–resistant rickets	Vitamin D receptor (12q12-q14)	Point mutations	Southern blot RFLP, sequencing
Cell growth regulators	Fibromas	Neurofibromatosis type 1 (von Recklinghausen disease)	Neurofibromin tumor suppressor (17q11.2)	Missense, frameshift, splice site mutations	Sequencing, linkage analysis
	Fibromas	Neurofibromatosis type 2 (von Recklinghausen disease)	Merlin tumor suppressor, NF-2 (22q12)	Nonsense, frameshift, splice site mutations	Linkage analysis
	Cancer predisposition	Li-Fraumeni syndrome*	p53 tumor suppressor gene, TP53 (17p13)	Missense mutations	Sequencing, SSCP, DGGE
Enzymes	Metabolic diseases	Alkaptonuria (ochronosis)	Homogentisic acid oxidase (3q21-q23)	Missense, frameshift, splice site mutations	cDNA sequencing,[39] SSCP[40]
	Phenylketonuria	Phenylalanine hydroxylase, PAH or PKU1 (12q24.1)	Splice site, missense mutations, deletions	Ligase chain reaction,[41,42] direct sequencing	
	Immunodeficiencies	Severe combined immunodeficiency	Adenosine deaminase (20q13.11)	Point mutations	Direct sequencing, capillary electrophoresis[43]

*A significant proportion of LFS and LFL (Li-Fraumeni–like) kindred do not have demonstrable *TP53* mutations.

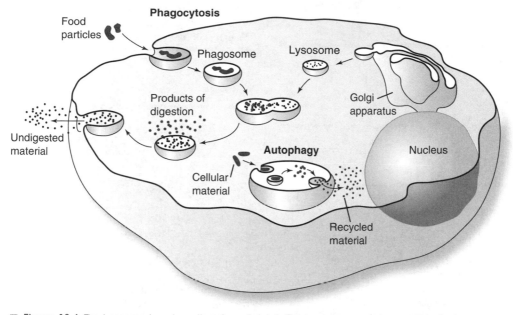

■ **Figure 13-6** The lysosome is a depository for cell debris. The lysosome contains enzymes that are active in its acid environment to digest proteins delivered from phagocytosis of foreign bodies, endocytosis, and autophagy of internal cellular components.

Several approaches have been taken to test for the Leiden mutation. Polymerase chain reaction (PCR) methods include the use of PCR-RFLP (restriction fragment length polymorphism), SSP-PCR (PCR with sequence-specific primers; Figs. 13-7 and 13-8), real-time PCR, and melt curve and Luminex technology. Nonamplification methods, such as Invader technology, have also been developed to test for this gene mutation.

Prothrombin is the precursor to thrombin in the coagulation cascade and is required for the conversion of fibrinogen to fibrin. A mutation in the 3′ untranslated region of the gene that codes for prothrombin or coagulation factor II, F2 (11p11-q12), results in an autosomal-dominant increased risk of thrombosis (see Table 13.5). Laboratories often test for both F2 and F5 mutations at the same time. Both may be present in the same individual, in

Table 13.4 **Storage Diseases**

Substrate Accumulated	Disease
Sphingolipids	Tay-Sachs disease
Glycogen	Von Gierke, McArdle, and Pompe disease
Mucopolysaccharides	Hurler, Sheie (MPS I), Hunter (MPS II), Sanfilipo (MPS III), Morquio (MPS IV), Maroteauz-Lamy (MPS VI), Sly (MPS VII)
Mucolipids	Pseudo-Hurler polydystrophy
Sulfatides	Niemann-Pick disease
Glucocerebrosides	Gaucher disease

Table 13.5 **Risk of Thrombosis Relative to Normal (1) Under the Indicated Genetic (F5, Prothrombin) and Environmental (OCP) Influences**

Status	Risk of Thrombosis
Normal	1
Oral contraceptive (OCP) use	4
Prothrombin mutation, heterozygous	3
Prothrombin mutation + OCP	16
R506Q heterozygous	5–7
R506Q heterozygous + OCP	30–35
R506Q homozygous	80
R506Q homozygous + OCP	100+

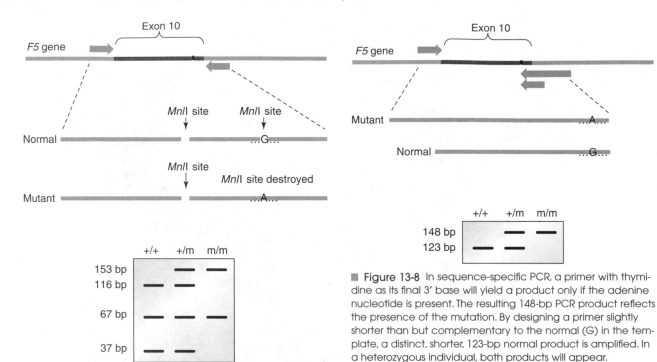

■ **Figure 13-7** PCR-RFLP for the factor V Leiden mutation. The R506Q amino acid substitution is caused by a G to A change in exon 10 of the F5 gene. This DNA mutation destroys an *Mnl*I restriction enzyme site. An amplicon including the site of the mutation, when cut with *Mnl*I, will yield three fragments in normal DNA (+/+) and two products in homozygous mutant DNA (m/m). A heterozygous specimen (+/m) will yield a combination of the normal and mutant pattern.

■ **Figure 13-8** In sequence-specific PCR, a primer with thymidine as its final 3' base will yield a product only if the adenine nucleotide is present. The resulting 148-bp PCR product reflects the presence of the mutation. By designing a primer slightly shorter than but complementary to the normal (G) in the template, a distinct, shorter, 123-bp normal product is amplified. In a heterozygous individual, both products will appear.

which case the risk of thrombosis is greater than with one of the mutations alone. An example of a multiplex PCR-RFLP method to simultaneously test for both mutations was described previously (see Fig. 9-28). In this method, primers that amplify prothrombin and factor V are designed to destroy or produce *Hind*III restriction sites in the presence of the F5 or F2 mutation, respectively. The sizes of the amplicons and their restriction fragments allow resolution of both simultaneously by agarose gel electrophoresis.[2] Automated methods are especially amenable to the detection of multiple single-gene mutations. The Luminex COAG panel on the Luminex XMAP200 detects Factor V Leiden, prothrombin and methylenetetrahydrofolate reductase gene (*MTHFR*), and C677T and A1298C polymorphisms.

Hemachromatosis

Hemachromatosis is an autosomal-recessive condition that causes overabsorption of iron from food. Iron accumulation subsequently causes pancreas, liver, and skin damage, heart disease, and diabetes. Classically, diagnosis is made through measurement of blood iron levels, transferrin saturation, or liver biopsy. This condition is easily treated by phlebotomy.

At the molecular level, hemachromatosis is caused by dysfunction of the hemachromatosis type I gene, HFE or HLA-H (6p21.3). HFE codes for a membrane-bound protein that binds with β_2 microglobulin and transferrin on the membrane of cells in the small intestine and also on the placenta. The protein directs iron absorption based on cellular iron loads. In the absence of HFE function, intestinal cells do not sense iron stores, and iron absorption continues into overload.

The most frequently observed mutation in hemachromatosis is C282Y, present in approximately 10% of the Caucasian population, with disease frequency of 2 to 3 per 1000 people. Other mutations most frequently detected in the HFE protein are H63D and S65C (Fig. 13-9). The

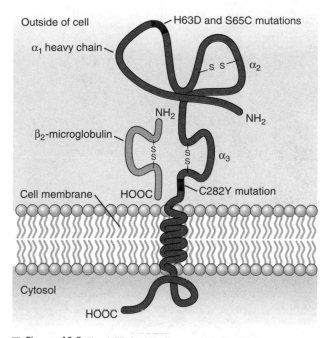

Figure 13-9 The HFE protein is associated with β$_2$-microglobulin in the cell membrane. The location of the frequently occurring mutations is shown.

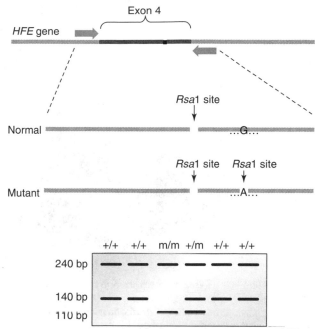

Figure 13-10 Detection of the C282Y mutation by PCR-RFLP. The G→A mutation in exon 4 of the HFE gene produces a site for the restriction enzyme, *Rsa*1. This region is first amplified using primers flanking exon 4 of the gene (arrows). In a normal specimen, the enzyme will produce two fragments, 240 bp and 140 bp. If the mutation is present, the 140 bp normal fragment is cut to a 110-bp and a 30-bp fragment (the 30-bp fragment is not shown). Heterozygous individuals will have both the 140-bp and the 110-bp fragments.

C282Y mutation is detectable using a variety of methods, including PCR-RFLP (Fig. 13-10).

Cystic Fibrosis

Cystic fibrosis (CF) is an autosomal-recessive, life-threatening disorder that causes severe lung damage and nutritional deficiencies. Earlier detection by genetic analysis and improved treatment strategies have improved survival to beyond the fourth decade of life for some CF patients. CF affects the cells that produce mucus, sweat, saliva, and digestive juices. Normally, these secretions are thin, but in CF a defective gene causes the secretions to become thick and sticky. Respiratory failure is the most dangerous consequence of CF. About 30,000 American adults and children are living with this disorder. Gene therapy may some day help correct lung problems in people with CF.

CF is caused by loss of function of the cystic fibrosis transmembrane conductance regulator gene (*CFTR*,

7q31.2). The gene codes for a chloride channel membrane protein (Fig. 13-11). The first and most frequently observed mutation in *CFTR* is a 3-bp deletion that removes a phenylalanine residue from position 508 of the protein (1521_1523delCTT or F508del).[3] More than 1300 other mutations and variations have been reported in and around the *CFTR* gene in diverse populations. A list of mutations, their locations, and references is available through the Human Genome Variation Society at www.genet.sickkids.on.ca.

Genetic testing for CF is important for diagnosis and genetic counseling, as early intervention is most effective in relieving symptoms of the disease. Molecular tests designed to detect a variety of mutations in *CFTR*[4] include RFLP, PCR-RFLP, heteroduplex analysis, temporal temperature gradient gel electrophoresis,

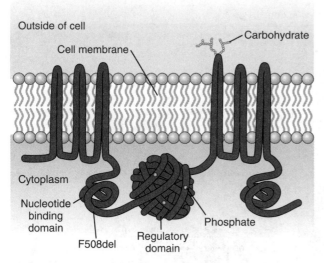

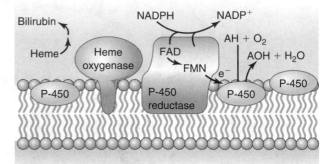

Figure 13-11 The cystic fibrosis transmembrane conductance regulator forms a channel in the cell membrane. The F508del and other mutations that affect its function are responsible for the phenotype of cystic fibrosis.

Figure 13-12 Cytochrome P-450 proteins are expressed in the liver and other organs. NAPDH cytochrome P-450 reductase catalyzes the reduction of NADPH and transfers electrons to flavin adenine dinucleotide (FAD). Electrons flow through FAD and flavin mononucleotide (FMN) to the cytochromes. The cytochromes then oxidize a variety of substrates (AH). NAPDH cytochrome P-450 reductase also works with heme oxygenase for metabolism of heme to biliverdin and eventually to bilirubin.

single-strand conformation polymorphism (SSCP), SSP-PCR, Invader, bead array technology (Tag-It, TM Bioscience), and direct sequencing. These tests use panels of 23 (American College of Medical Genetics or ACMG 23) up to 44 mutations. The decisions as to which mutations and how many mutations to test are influenced by population differences and the variable expressivity of the mutations.

Cytochrome P-450

Cytochrome P-450 comprises a group of enzymes localized to the endoplasmic reticulum of the cell (Fig. 13-12). These enzymes are mono-oxygenases; that is, they participate in enzymatic hydroxylation reactions and also transfer electrons to oxygen:

$$A\text{—}H + B\text{—}H_2 + O_2 \rightarrow A\text{—}OH + B + H_2O$$

where A is the substrate and B is the hydrogen donor. These enzymes influence steroid, amino acid, and drug metabolism using NADH or NADPH as hydrogen donors. Oxygenation of lipophilic drugs renders them more easily excreted (Fig. 13-13).

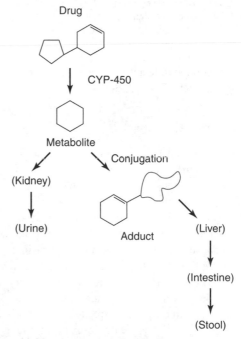

Figure 13-13 The oxidation activities of cytochrome P-450 proteins metabolize a variety of structurally diverse chemicals, including clinically used drugs.

The cytochrome P-450 system is present in high concentrations in the liver and small intestine where the enzymes metabolize and detoxify compounds taken in orally. The P-450 system varies from one person to another. This may in part account for the different effects of drugs on different people. Hormones, caffeine, chemotherapeutic drugs, antidepressants, and oral contraceptives are examples of compounds affected by these polymorphisms.[5,6] CYP-450 polymorphisms may also compound interactions of multiple drugs taken simultaneously.[7,8]

There are over 30 reported variations of CYP-450 enzymes. Enzymes are classified according to families and subfamilies. For example, CYP2A6 is cytochrome P-450, subfamily IIA, polypeptide 6. CYP1A2 and the enzymes in the CYP2 and CYP3 families are considered to be most important in drug metabolism. Some of the enzymes reported to inhibit or induce drug metabolism include CYP1A2, CYP2A6, CYP2B6, CYP2C8, CYP2C9, CYP2C18, CYP2C19, CYP2D6, CYP2E1, CYP3A4, and CYP3A5-7. The genes coding for these enzymes are located throughout the genome.

Genetic polymorphisms of cytochrome P-450 genes are unequally distributed geographically and in different ethnic populations. Testing for these polymorphisms is used to predict the response to drugs sensitive to metabolism by this enzyme system. In the laboratory, testing for CYP-450 polymorphisms is performed by allele-specific PCR for particular polymorphisms. Multiple CYP-450 genetic variants may be screened by microarray,[9] bead array technology,[10] or mass spectrometry.[11] The Autogenomics Infiniti Analyzer is an RUO automated array system with the capacity to detect multiple CYP mutations.

Methylenetetrahydrofolate Reductase

The *MTHFR* gene product catalyzes the conversion of 5,10-methylenetetrahydrofolate to 5-methyltetrahydrofolate, which is required for conversion of homocysteine to methionine (Fig. 13-14). Mutations in the methylenetetrahydrofolate reductase gene (*MTHFR*) can lead to cardiovascular disease and complications in pregnancy. At least 24 mutations in *MTHFR* have been identified in symptomatic people. The resulting single amino acid

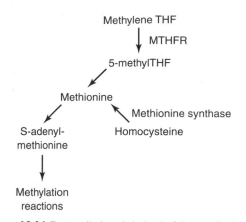

■ **Figure 13-14** The methylenetetrahydrofolate reductase enzyme catalyzes the conversion of 5,10-methylenetetrahydrofolate (methylene THF) to 5-methyltetrahydrofolate (5-methylTHF), which is required for remethylation of homocysteine to methionine and other methylation reactions.

substitutions in the protein affect the structure and/or the function of the enzyme. When homocysteine cannot be converted to methionine, homocysteine builds up in the bloodstream and is excreted in the urine (homocystinuria). In addition, methionine is depleted. *MTHFR* variants, 677C>T (A222V) and 1298A>C (E429A), are relatively common in many populations.[12] Both substitutions produce defective forms of the *MTHFR* protein, with the A222V variant being thermolabile.

The common *MTHFR* variants can be detected using PCR-RFLP and real-time PCR, although care must be taken to avoid sequences giving false-positive restriction patterns using RFLP.[13] Direct sequencing is the most definitive method of variant detection. Melt curve analysis methods have been reported that can be multiplexed with other markers.[14,15]

Single-Gene Disorders with Nonclassical Patterns of Inheritance

Mitochondrial mutations, genomic imprinting, and **gonadal mosaicism** do not follow Mendelian rules of inheritance. Mitochondrial mutations are inherited maternally (Fig. 13-15). Genomic imprinting is methylation

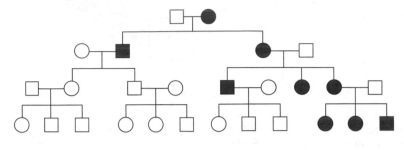

■ **Figure 13-15** Mitochondrial mutations are maternally inherited.

of DNA (and associated histone modifications) responsible for specific expression of genes in different cells and tissues. Imprinting is reset at meiosis and fertilization and is different in egg and sperm production. Gonadal mosaicism is the generation of new mutations in germ line cells. The mutated cells give rise to eggs or sperm carrying the mutation, which then becomes a heritable phenotype. Unusual pedigrees result (Fig. 13-16). Gonadal mosaicism is expected when phenotypically normal parents have more than one affected child, for example, in osteogenesis imperfecta, an autosomal-dominant phenotype in a child from unaffected parents.

Mutations in Mitochondrial Genes

Mitochondria are cellular organelles responsible for energy production. They contain their own genome, a circular DNA molecule 16,569 base pairs in length (Fig. 13-17). The mitochondrial genome contains 37 genes, including a 12S and 16S rRNA, 22 tRNAs, and 13 genes required for oxidative phosphorylation. In addition, the mitochondrial DNA (mtDNA) contains a 1000-nt control region that encompasses transcription and replication regulatory elements (see Chapter 9, "DNA Polymorphisms and Human Identification"). A database of mitochondrial genes and mutations is available at www.MITOMAP.org.[16]

> ## *Advanced Concepts*
>
> An example of the nature of imprinting is illustrated by comparing mules and hinnies. A mule is the product of a male horse and a female donkey. A hinny is the product of a female horse and a male donkey. These animals are quite different in phenotype, even though they contain essentially the same genotype. The differences are due to different patterns of methylation (imprinting) in egg and sperm cells. Another illustration of the effects of imprinting is seen in animals cloned by nuclear transfer. Because this process bypasses the generation of eggs and sperm and fertilization, imprinting is not reset from the mature methylation patterns, and cloned animals display unexpected phenotypes, such as larger size or early onset of age-related diseases.

Mutations in mitochondrial genes affect energy production and are therefore manifested as diseases in the most energy-demanding organs, muscles, and the nervous system.[17,18] Mutations in several genes in the mitochondrial genome result in a number of disease

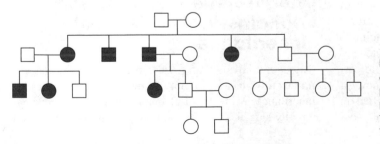

■ **Figure 13-16** Gonadal mosaicism arises as a result of a new mutation. In this example, a dominant disease phenotype has been inherited from two unaffected parents. The mutation is present only in the germ cells of the first-generation parents but is inherited in all cells of the offspring.

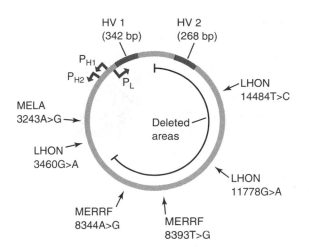

Figure 13-17 Mutations and deletions throughout the mitochondrial genome are associated with muscular and neurological disorders.

are frequently analyzed by PCR-RFLP (Fig. 13-19) and a variety of other methods used for detection of nuclear chromosomal mutations. Interpretation of mitochondrial mutation analysis is complicated by the extent of heteroplasmy (mutated mitochondria and normal mitochondria in the same cell) and the nature of the mutation.[20] A range of phenotypes may be present, even in the same family.

Genes that control mitochondrial functions are also found on the nuclear genome (Table 13.7). Unlike mitochondrial mutations that display maternal inheritance, these disorders have autosomal patterns of inheritance. Although the causative gene mutation is located on a nuclear gene, analysis of mitochondria may still show deletions or other mutations caused by the loss of the nuclear gene function.

Trinucleotide Repeat Expansion Disorders

Triplet repeats are short tandem repeats (STRs) with 3-bp repeating units (see Chapter 9 for more detailed explanation of STRs). During DNA replication and meiosis, these STRs can expand (or contract) in length due to slippage of the replisome on the template. Triplet-repeat mutations may occur in coding and noncoding sequences of genes. The

syndromes involving muscular and neurological disorders (Table 13.6).

Mitochondrial mutations are easily detected by a variety of molecular methods. Southern blot has been used for detecting large deletions (Fig. 13-18). Deletions are also detectable using PCR methods.[19] Point mutations

Table 13.6 **Diseases Resulting from Mutations in Mitochondrial Genes**

Disorder	Gene Affected	Molecular Methodology
Kearnes-Sayre syndrome	2–7 kb deletions[44]	Southern blot, PCR, PCR-RFLP
Pearson syndrome	Deletions	Southern blot analysis of leukocytes, PCR-RFLP[45]
Pigmentary retinopathy, chronic progressive external ophthalmoplegia	tRNA (tyr) deletion,[46] deletions	PCR-RFLP, Southern blot analysis of muscle biopsy[47]
Leber hereditary optic neuropathy	Cyt6 and URF* point mutations	PCR-RFLP
Mitochondrial myopathy, encephalopathy, lactic acidosis, and strokelike episodes	tRNA (leu) point mutations	PCR-RFLP, sequencing
Myoclonic epilepsy with ragged red fibers	tRNA (lys) point mutations	PCR-RFLP
Diabetes, deafness	tRNA (leu) point mutation	PCR-RFLP
Neuropathy, ataxia, retinitis pigmentosa (NARP)	ATPase VI point mutation	PCR-RFLP
Subacute necrotizing encephalomyelopathy with neurogenic muscle weakness, ataxia, retinitis pigmentosa (Leigh's with NARP)	ATPase VI, NADH:ubiquinone oxidoreductase subunit mutations	PCR-RFLP
Mitochondrial DNA depletion syndrome	Thymidine kinase gene mutations	PCR, sequencing

*Unknown reading frame

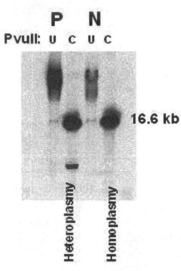

■ **Figure 13-18** A mitochondrial deletion as revealed by Southern blot. DNA was cut with *Pvu*II, a restriction enzyme that cuts once in the mitochondrial genome. The membrane was probed for mitochondrial sequences. Normal mitochondria (N) yield one band at 16.6 kb when cut with *Pvu*II (C). Supercoiled, nicked, and a few linearized mitochondrial DNA circles can be seen in the uncut DNA (U). DNA from a patient with Kearnes-Sayres syndrome (P) yields two mitochondrial populations, one of which has about 5 kb of the mitochondrial genome–deleted sequences. Because both normal and mutant mitochondria are present, this is a state of heteroplasmy. (Photo courtesy of Dr. Elizabeth Berry-Kravis, Rush University Medical Center.)

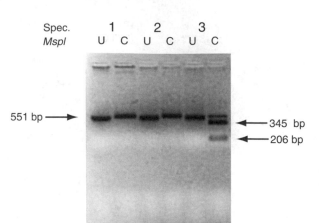

■ **Figure 13-19** Detection of the NARP mitochondrial point mutation (ATPase VI 8993T>C or T>G) by PCR-RFLP. The PCR product was digested with the enzyme *Msp*I (C) or undigested (U). If the mutation is present, the enzyme will cut the PCR product into two pieces, as seen is specimen 3. (Photo courtesy of Dr. Elizabeth Berry-Kravis, Rush University Medical Center.)

most well-known examples of triplet repeat expansion diseases are fragile X syndrome and Huntington disease.

Fragile X Syndrome

Fragile X syndrome is associated with a triplet repeat (CGG) expansion in the noncoding region 5' to the fragile X mental retardation gene, *FMR*-1 (Fig. 13-20). The expansion becomes so large in full fragile X syndrome (more than 2000 CGG repeats) that chromosomal compaction is disrupted and the region is microscopically visible (Fig. 13-21). The CGG repeat expansion 5' to the *FMR*-1 gene also results in methylation of the DNA in the repeat region and transcriptional shutdown of *FMR*-1.

Symptoms of fragile X syndrome include learning disorders and mental retardation (IQ approximately 20), long face, large ears, and macro-orchidism (large genitalia). Symptoms are more apparent at puberty and increase in severity with each generation in a fragile X family, a phenomenon called **anticipation** (Fig. 13-22).

Table 13.7 **Some Mitochondrial Disorders Caused by Nuclear Gene Mutations**

Disorder	Gene Affected (Location)	Molecular Methodology
Mitochondrial DNA depletion syndrome	Succinate-CoA ligase, ADP-forming, beta subunit, SUCLA 2 (13q12.2-q13)	Southern blot
Mitochondrial neurogastrointestinal encephalomyopathy	Platelet-derived endothelial cell growth factor, ECGF (22q13-qter)	Sequencing
Progressive external ophthalmoplegia	Chromosome 10 open reading frame 2, C10ORF2 (10q24); polymerase, DNA, gamma, POLG (15q25); solute carrier family 25 (mitochondrial carrier), member 4, SLC25A4/ANT1, (4q25)	Southern blot, SSCP, sequencing[48]

Advanced Concepts

In addition to family history, clinical tests including electroencephalography, neuroimaging, cardiac electrocardiography, echocardiography, magnetic resonance spectroscopy, and exercise testing are important for accurate diagnosis of mitochondrial disorders. High blood or cerebrospinal fluid lactate concentrations as well as high blood glucose levels are observed in patients with some mitochondrial diseases. More direct tests, such as histological examination of muscle biopsies and respiratory chain complex studies on skeletal muscle and skin fibroblasts, are more specific for mitochondrial dysfunction.

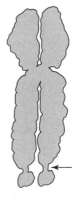

Fragile X chromosome
(in metaphase)

■ **Figure 13-21** The fragile X chromosome is characterized by a threadlike process just at the telomere of the long arm of the X chromosome (arrow). This is the site of disorganization of chromatin structure by the GC-rich repeat expansions.

In addition to observation of the fragile X chromosome by karyotyping, the state of the repeat expansion is also analyzed using PCR and by Southern blot. Although premutations in fragile X carriers are easily detected by PCR, Southern blot has been required to detect the full fragile X expansion covering thousands of base pairs. Southern blot also reveals cases of mosaicism where both premutations and full fragile X chromosomes are present in separate cell populations from the same patient (Fig. 13-23). PCR methods of analysis with resolution by capillary electrophoresis are based on primers that bind

inside the CGG triplet-repeat region.[21] Using touchdown PCR, the resulting triplet-repeat primed amplicon resolves as a ladder pattern detectable by capillary electrophoresis or smear by agarose gel electrophoresis[22] (Fig. 13-24).

Huntington Disease

Huntington disease, first described by George Huntington in 1872, is associated with expansion within the huntingtin

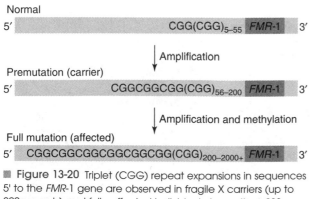

Normal

5′ ▬▬▬▬▬▬▬▬ CGG(CGG)_{5–55} FMR-1 3′

↓ Amplification

Premutation (carrier)

5′ ▬▬▬▬▬▬ CGGCGGCGG(CGG)_{56–200} FMR-1 3′

↓ Amplification and methylation

Full mutation (affected)

5′ ▬ CGGCGGCGGCGGCGGCGG(CGG)_{200–2000+} FMR-1 3′

■ **Figure 13-20** Triplet (CGG) repeat expansions in sequences 5′ to the FMR-1 gene are observed in fragile X carriers (up to 200 repeats) and fully affected individuals (more than 200 repeats). Normally, there are fewer than 60 repeats. Expansion results from amplification of the triplet sequences during meiotic recombination events. The very large repeats (more than 200 repeats) are methylated on the C residues. This methylation turns off FMR-1 transcription.

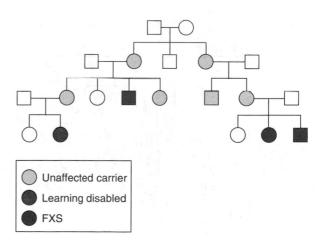

○ Unaffected carrier
● Learning disabled
● FXS

■ **Figure 13-22** The symptoms of fragile X syndrome (FXS) become more severe with each generation. The fragile X chromosome cannot be transmitted from fathers to sons but can be transmitted from grandfathers to grandsons through their daughters.

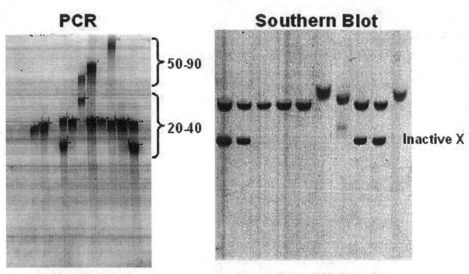

PCR   **Southern Blot**

50-90

20-40

Inactive X

Premutations   **Full Mutations**

■ Figure 13-23 Detection of premutations by PCR (left) and full fragile X mutations by Southern blot (right). Primers (one of which is labeled with ^{32}P) flanking the repeat region are used to generate labeled PCR products. Premutations appear as large amplicons in the 50 to 90 repeat range on the autoradiogram at left. Normal samples fall in the 20 to 40 repeat range. Full fragile X repeats are too large and GC-rich to detect by standard PCR. Southern blots reveal full mutations in three of the samples shown. The inactive (methylated) X chromosome in four female patients is detected by cutting the DNA with a methylation-specific restriction enzyme. (Photos courtesy of Dr. Elizabeth Berry-Kravis, Rush University Medical Center.)

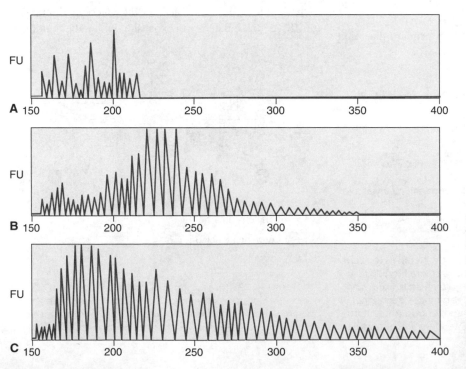

■ Figure 13-24 Fragile X permutations and full mutations appear as altered peak patterns in an electropherogram. PCR products of the *FMR*-1 CGG region in the normal X chromosome (a) are detected as peaks of less than 250 bases, while the premutation (b) and full fragile X mutation (c) are visible as regular peaks extending up to 400 bases. (FU, fluorescence units.)

structural gene (*HD* or *HTT*, 4p16.3). In this repeat expansion, the sequence CAG expands from 9 to 37 repeats to 38 to 86 repeats. The clinical symptoms of Huntington disease include impaired judgment, slurred speech, difficulty in swallowing, abnormal body movements (chorea), personality changes, depression, mood swings, unsteady gait, and an intoxicated appearance. With an onset in the 30s or 40s, these symptoms do not become obvious until the fourth or fifth decade of life, usually after family planning. The child of a person with Huntington disease has a 50% chance of inheriting the disorder. Genetic counseling, therefore, is important for younger persons with family histories of this disease, especially with regard to having children.

In contrast to fragile X, where the repeat expansion takes place 5' to the coding sequences of *FMR-1*, the Huntington expansion occurs within the coding region of the *HD* gene. The triplet expansion inserts multiple glutamine residues in the 5' end of the huntingtin protein. This causes the protein to aggregate in plaques, especially in nervous tissue, causing the neurological symptoms seen in this disease.[25] The expansion does not reach the size of the fragile X expansion and is detectable by standard PCR methods (Fig. 13-25).

Idiopathic Congenital Central Hypoventilation Syndrome

Idiopathic congenital central hypoventilation syndrome (CCHS) is a rare pediatric disorder characterized by inadequate breathing while asleep. Affected children may also experience hypoventilation while awake. CCHS occurs in association with an intestinal disorder called Hirschsprung disease and symptoms of diffuse autonomic nervous system dysregulation/dysfunction. A number of gene mutations have been observed in CCHS, including a polyalanine expansion of the paired-like homeobox (*PHOX*2b) gene (4p12)13.[26] The Phox2b protein is a transcription factor containing a domain (homeobox) similar to other proteins that bind DNA.

In CCHS, an imperfect triplet-repeat (GCN) expansion occurs inside of the *PHOX*2b gene, resulting in the insertion of multiple alanine residues into the protein. The severity of the disease increases with increasing numbers of repeats. The expansion is detected by PCR (Fig. 13-26).[27] CCHS is usually apparent at birth. In some children, a

---

Advanced Concepts

The function of the *FMR-1* gene product is not fully understood. The FMR protein has domains similar to those of RNA binding proteins. Based on these observations, FMR may control expression of other genes by binding to certain RNA structures and preventing translation.[23,24]

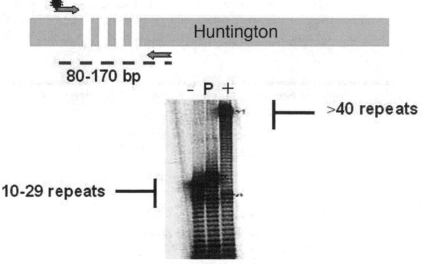

■ Figure 13-25 The huntingtin repeat expansion occurs within the coding region of the huntingtin gene. The expansion is detected directly by PCR using primers flanking the expanded region (top). A ^{32}P-labeled primer is used, and the bands are detected by autoradiography of the polyacrylamide gel (bottom). In this example, PCR products from the patient (P) fall within the normal range with the negative control (–). The positive control (+) displays the band sizes expected in Huntington's disease. (Photos courtesy of Dr. Elizabeth Berry-Kravis, Rush University Medical Center.)

gcagcagcagcggcggcggccgcggcagcggcggcggcggcagcggcagcggcggcagct

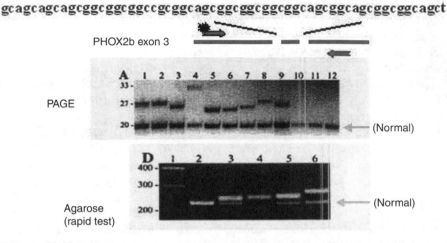

PHOX2b exon 3

PAGE

Agarose
(rapid test)

■ **Figure 13-26** The triplet repeat expansion of *PHOX*2b includes triplets that code for alanine (top). The expansion is detected by PCR with a ^{32}P-labeled primer and polyacrylamide gel electrophoresis (center) or by standard PCR and agarose gel electrophoresis (bottom). Normal specimens yield a single PCR product. CCHS specimens yield another, larger product in addition to the normal product. The standard PCR test can rapidly show the presence of the expansion, and the PAGE test allows determination of the exact number of alanine codons that are present in the expansion. (Photos courtesy of Dr. Elizabeth Berry-Kravis, Rush University Medical Center.)

late onset of the disease occurs at 2 to 4 years of age. An estimated 62% to 98% of patients with CCHS have the *PHOX*2b gene mutation.[27]

Other Triplet Expansion Disorders

Fragile X, Huntington disease, and CCHS are three of a group of diseases caused by **trinucleotide repeat** disorders. This category of diseases is subclassified into polyglutamine expansion disorders, which include Huntington disease and nonpolyglutamine expansion disorders, examples of which are listed in Table 13.8.

Genomic Imprinting

Genomic imprinting is transcriptional silencing through histone or DNA modification. Imprinting occurs during egg and sperm production and is therefore different in the DNA brought in by the egg from that brought in by the sperm upon fertilization (Fig. 13-27). The difference is exhibited in genetic disorders in which one or the other allele of a gene is lost.

All or part of chromosomes are lost through a variety of mechanisms. Chromosomal nondisjunction produces gametes with more or less than one copy of each

Table 13.8 **Examples of Nonpolyglutamine Expansion Disorders**

Disorder	Gene	Repeat	Expansion, (Normal) – (Symptomatic)*
Fragile XE	Fragile X mental retardation 2 (Xq28)	GCC	(6–35) – (over 200)
Friedreich ataxia	Frataxin, FRDA or X25 (9q13)	GAA	(7–34) – (over 100)
Myotonic dystrophy	Dystrophia myotonica protein kinase (9q13.2–13.3)	CTG	(5–37) – (over 50)
Spinocerebellar ataxia type 8	Spinocerebellar ataxia type 8 (13q21)	CTG	(16–37) – (110–250)
Spinocerebellar ataxia type 12[†]	Spinocerebellar ataxia type 12 (5q31–33)	CAG	(7–28) – (66–78)

*The phenotypic effects of intermediate numbers of repeats is not known.
[†]Although CAG codes for glutamine, this expansion occurs outside of the coding region of this gene and is not translated.

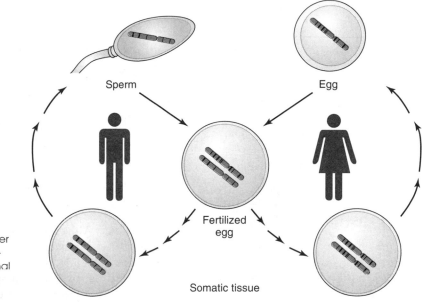

Figure 13-27 Sperm and egg cells have different imprinting patterns, which are further modified at fertilization and during development in somatic tissue. Maternal and paternal imprinting is maintained in spermatogenesis and oogenesis.

chromosome (Fig. 13-28). The resulting zygote will have genetic information carried on the affected chromosome from only one parent (**uniparental disomy**). Loss of a chromosome or deletion of part of one of the two homologous chromosomes also removes genetic information from one parent. Uniparental disomy/deletion demonstrates the nature of imprinting on chromosome 15. A deletion in the paternal chromosome 15, del(15)(q11q13), causes Prader-Willi syndrome. Symptoms of this disorder include mental retardation, short stature, obesity, and hypogonadism. Loss of the same region from the maternal chromosome 15 results

in Angelman syndrome, a disorder with very different symptoms, including ataxia, seizures, and inappropriate laughter. Both syndromes can occur in four ways: a deletion on the paternal or maternal chromosome 15, a mutation on the paternal or maternal chromosome 15, a translocation with loss of the critical region from one chromosome, and maternal or paternal uniparental disomy in which both chromosomes 15 are inherited from the mother and none from the father or vice versa.

Cytogenetic methods are still used to test for these genetic lesions. Translocations and some deletions are detectable by standard karyotyping. High-resolution

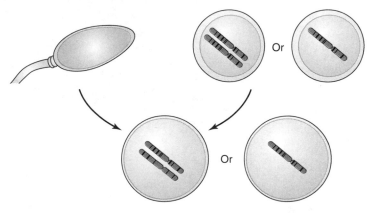

Figure 13-28 Uniparental disomy results from the inheritance of two hologous chromosomes from one parent, instead of one from each parent. This occurs when aberrant gametes carry two or no copies of a given chromosome.

karyotyping can detect smaller deletions; however, other cases are not detectable microscopically. Newer methods, such as FISH, with labeled probes to the deleted region[29] can detect over 99% of cases. PCR, RFLP, or STR analysis has been used to demonstrate uniparental disomy.[30] As imprinting (DNA methylation) is different on maternal and paternal chromosomes, methylation-specific PCR,[31] methylation-sensitive restriction enzymes,[32] melt curve analysis,[33] and Southern blot using methylation-specific restriction enzymes[34] have also been proposed as methods to aid in the diagnosis of these disorders.

Array CGH Technology

The implementation of array technology in cytogenetics permits simultaneous testing of multiple genetic lesions in a single test. Comparative genome hybridization (CGH) is especially useful in this application (see Chapter 6, "Analysis and Characterization of Nucleic Acids"). Prenatal chromosome abnormalities are routinely screened by cytogenetics. Prenatal testing by array CGH (aCGH) offers a higher detection rate than standard FISH and karyotyping. For example, the SignatureChipOS™ and the Signature PrenatalChipOS® (Signature Genomics, Perkin Elmer) tests for copy number abnormalities in over 500 gene regions responsible for over 200 known genetic syndromes.[35] The 135,000 probes include unique **pseudoautosomal** probes to detect abnormalities involving the X and Y chromosomes and probes to pericentromeric regions (surrounding centromeres) to test for marker chromosomes and aneuploidy. Abnormalities found with aCGH may be confirmed by FISH testing, if single FISH probes are available for the abnormal region.

Multifactorial Inheritance

Most disorders (and normal conditions) are controlled by multiple genetic and environmental factors. Multifactorial inheritance is displayed as a continuous variation in populations with normal distribution, rather than as a specific inheritance pattern. Nutritional or chemical exposures alter this distribution. Phenotypic expression is conditioned by the number of controlling genes inherited.

Limitations to Molecular Testing

Although molecular testing for inherited diseases is extremely useful for early diagnosis and genetic counseling, there are circumstances in which genetic testing may not be the optimal methodology. To date, most therapeutic targets are phenotypic, so treatment is better directed to the phenotype. In genes with variable expressivity, finding a gene mutation may not predict the severity of the phenotype. For instance, clotting time and transferrin saturation are better guides for anticoagulant treatment than the demonstration of the causative gene mutations.

Molecular testing may discover genetic lesions in the absence of symptoms. This raises a possible problem as to whether treatment is indicated. Finally, most diseases are caused by dysfunction of multicomponent systems, so several genetic lesions may be present or polymorphic states of other normal genes may influence the disease state. As array technology and haplotype mapping designed to scan at the genomic level are further developed, these methods may contribute to better diagnosis of complex diseases.

CASE STUDY 13 • 1

A young mother was worried about her son. Having observed others, she was very aware of how her baby was expected to grow and acquire basic skills. As the child grew, however, he showed signs of slow development. His protruding ears and long face were becoming more noticeable as well. The pediatrician recommended chromosomal analysis for the mother and child. A constriction at the end of the X chromosome was found in the son's karyotype. The mother's karyotype was normal 46,XX. A Southern blot analysis for fragile X was performed on a blood specimen from the mother but showed no obvious abnormality. PCR analysis produced the following results:

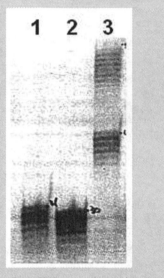

■ PCR analysis of the FMR promoter region showing two normal patterns (lanes 1 and 2) and the mother's pattern.

QUESTIONS:

1. What do the PCR results in lane 3 indicate?
2. Why were there no abnormalities detected by Southern blot?
3. How would this result be depicted using triplet-primed PCR and capillary electrophoresis?

CASE STUDY 13 • 2

A 14-year-old girl with muscle weakness and vision difficulties (retinopathy) was referred for clinical tests. A muscle biopsy was performed, and aberrant mitochondria were observed in thin sections. Histochemical analysis of the muscle tissue revealed cytochrome oxidase deficiency in the muscle cells. A skeletal muscle biopsy specimen was sent to the molecular genetics laboratory for analysis of mitochondrial DNA. Southern blot analysis of PvuII cut mitochondrial DNA exhibited a band at 11,500 bp in addition to the normal mitochondrial band at 16,500 bp as shown below:

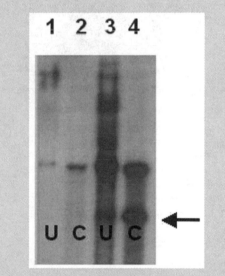

■ Southern blot of mitochondrial DNA uncut (U) and cut with PvuII (C). Lanes 1 and 2, normal control; lanes 3 and 4, patient. Arrow points to a 16,000-kb band.

QUESTIONS:

1. What is the 16,000 bp product? What is the 11,500 bp product?
2. What condition is associated with a 5-kb mitochondrial deletion?
3. Is this a case of homoplasmy or heteroplasmy?

CASE STUDY 13 • 3

A 40-year-old man was experiencing increasing joint pain, fatigue, and loss of appetite. He became alarmed when he suffered heart problems and consulted his physician. Routine blood tests revealed high serum iron (900 μg/dL) and 80% transferrin saturation. Total iron binding capacity was low (100 μg/dL). The man denied any extensive alcohol intake. A blood specimen was sent to the molecular genetics laboratory for detection of mutations in the hemachromatosis gene. The results are shown below.

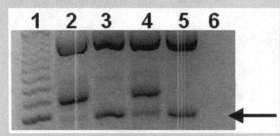

▓ PCR-RFLP analysis of exon 4 of the HFE gene. The PCR product contains 1 recognition site for the restriction enzyme, *Rsal.* An additional *Rsal* site is created by the C282Y (G→A) mutation, the most common inherited mutation in hemochromatosis. This extra site results in fragments of 240 bp, 110 bp (arrow) and 30 bp (not shown) instead of the 240 bp and 140 bp normal fragments. Lane 1, molecular-weight markers; lane 2, normal control; lane 3, homozygous C282Y; lane 4, heterozygous C282Y; lane 5, patient specimen; lane 6, reagent blank.

QUESTIONS:

1. *Does this patient have the C282Y mutation?*
2. *Is this mutation heterozygous or homozygous?*
3. *Based on these results, what is the likely explanation for the patient's symptoms?*

CASE STUDY 13 • 4

A 30-year-old woman was brought to the emergency room with a painfully swollen left leg. She informed the nurses that she was taking contraceptives. Deep vein thrombosis was suspected, and compression ultrasound was ordered to look for pulmonary embolism. A clotting test for APC resistance resulted in a 1.5 ratio of clotting time with and without APC. An ELISA test for D-dimer was positive. The patient was immediately treated with heparin, and blood samples were taken. A blood sample was sent to the molecular genetics laboratory to test for the factor V Leiden 1691 G→A mutation and prothrombin 20210 G→A mutations. The results are shown below.

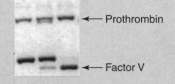

▓ Agarose gel electrophoresis showing the band pattern for prothrombin 20210/factor V Leiden mutation detection by multiplex SSP-PCR-RFLP. Specimens with mutations have *Hind*III recognition sites and are cut to smaller fragments with *Hind*III. Lane 1, normal control (prothrombin, 407 bp, factor V, 241 bp); lane 2, heterozygous controls, prothrombin (407, 384 bp)/factor V Leiden (241, 209bp); lane 3, patient specimen.

QUESTIONS:

1. *Does this patient have a clotting disorder?*
2. *Is there a Factor V mutation? Is there a prothrombin mutation?*
3. *If present, is either mutation homozygous or heterozygous?*

• STUDY QUESTIONS •

1. Which of the following is not a triplet-repeat expansion disorder?
   a. Fragile X syndrome
   b. Huntington disease
   c. Factor V Leiden
   d. Congenital central hypoventilation syndrome

2. A gene was mapped to region 3, band 1, subband 1, of the long arm of chromosome 2. How would you express this location from an idiogram?

3. Which of the following can be detected by PCR?
   a. Complex chromosomal abnormalities
   b. Full fragile X disorder
   c. Mitochondrial point mutations

4. A patient was tested for Huntington disease. PCR followed by PAGE revealed 25 CAG units.
   a. This patient has Huntington disease
   b. This patient has a 1/25 chance of contracting Huntington disease.
   c. This patient is normal at the Huntington locus.
   d. The test is inconclusive.

5. The factor V Leiden mutation can be detected by:
   a. PCR-RFLP
   b. SSP-PCR
   c. Invader technology
   d. All of the above methods

6. The most frequently occurring mutation in the HFE gene results in the replacement of cysteine (C) with tyrosine (Y) at position 282. How is this expressed according to the recommended nomenclature?

7. MELAS is a disease condition that results from an A to G mutation at position 3243 of the mitochondrial genome. This change creates a single *Apa*I restriction site in a PCR product that includes the mutation site. What would you expect from a PCR-RFLP analysis for this mutation on a patient with MELAS?
   a. A single PCR product resistant to digestion with *Apa*I
   b. A single PCR product that cuts into two fragments upon digestion with *Apa*I
   c. A single PCR product only if the mutation is present
   d. Two PCR products

8. A father affected with a single-gene disorder and an unaffected mother have four children (three boys and a girl), two of whom (one boy and the girl) are affected. Draw the pedigree diagram for this family.

9. D16S539, an STR, was analyzed in the family described in Question 8. The results showed that the father had the 6,8 alleles and the mother had the 5,7 alleles. The affected children had the 5,6 and 6,7 alleles, and the unaffected children had the 5,8 and 7,8 alleles.
   a. If D16S539 is located on chromosome 16, where is the gene for this disorder likely to be located?
   b. To which allele of D16S539 is the gene linked?

   How might one perform a DNA analysis for the presence of the disorder?
   c. Analyze D16S539 for the 6 allele by PCR
   d. Sequence the entire region of the chromosome where D16S539 was located
   e. Test as many STRs as possible by PCR
   f. Use Invader technology to detect the unknown gene mutation.

10. Exon 4 of the HFE gene from a patient suspected of having hereditary hemachromatosis was amplified by PCR. The G to A mutation, frequently found in hemachromatosis, creates an *Rsa*1 site in exon 4. When the PCR products are digested with *Rsa*1, which of the following results would you expect to see if the patient has the mutation?
    a. None of the PCR products will be cut by *Rsa*1.
    b. There will be no PCR product amplified from the patient DNA.
    c. The patient's PCR product will yield extra bands upon *Rsa*1 digestion.
    d. The normal control PCR products will yield extra *Rsa*1 bands compared with the patient sample.

11. Almost all people with the C282Y or H63D HFE gene mutations develop hemachromatosis symptoms. This is a result of:
    a. Iron loss
    b. Excessive drinking
    c. High penetrance
    d. Healthy lifestyle
    e. Glycogen accumulation

12. The majority of disease-associated mutations in the human population are:
    a. Autosomal dominant
    b. Autosomal recessive
    c. X-linked
    d. Found on the Y chromosome

13. Luminex bead array technology is most appropriate for which of the following?
    a. Cystic fibrosis mutation detection
    b. Chromosomal translocation detections
    c. STR linkage analysis
    d. Restriction fragment length polymorphisms

14. What chemical change in DNA is associated with imprinting?

15. What accounts for the different phenotypes of Prader-Willi syndrome, del(15)(q11q13), and Angelman syndrome, del(15)(q11q13)?

References

1. Anderson J. The Lyon hypothesis. *British Medical Journal* 1963;5367:1215–1216.
2. Davidson R. The Lyon hypothesis. *Journal of Pediatrics* 1964;65:765–775.
3. Kerem B, Buchanan JA, Durie P, et al. DNA marker haplotype association with pancreatic sufficiency in cystic fibrosis. *American Journal of Human Genetics* 1989;44:827–834.
4. McGinniss M, Chen C, Redman JB, et al. Extensive sequencing of the CFTR gene: Lessons learned from the first 157 patient samples. *Human Genetics* 2005;118:331–338.
5. Orlando R, Piccoli P, De Martin S, et al. Effect of the CYP3A4 inhibitor erythromycin on the pharmacokinetics of lignocaine and its pharmacologically active metabolites in subjects with normal and impaired liver function. *British Journal of Clinical Pharmacology* 2003;55:86–93.
6. Orlando R, Piccoli P, De Martin S, et al. Cytochrome P450 1A2 is a major determinant of lidocaine metabolism in vivo: Effects of liver function. *Clinical Pharmacology and Therapeutics* 2004;75:80–88.
7. Jin Y, Desta Z, Stearns V, et al. CYP2D6 genotype, antidepressant use, and tamoxifen metabolism during adjuvant breast cancer treatment. *Journal of the National Cancer Institute* 2005;97:30–39.
8. Granfors M, Backman JT, Laitila J, et al. Oral contraceptives containing ethinyl estradiol and gestodene markedly increase plasma concentrations and effects of tizanidine by inhibiting cytochrome P450 1A2. *Clinical Pharmacology and Therapeutics* 2005;78:400–411.
9. de Leon J, Susce MT, Murray-Carmichael E. The AmpliChip CYP450 genotyping test: Integrating a new clinical tool. *Molecular Diagnosis & Therapy* 2006;10:135–151.
10. de Leon J, Arranz MJ, Ruano G. Pharmacogenetic testing in psychiatry: A review of features and clinical realities. *Clinical Laboratory Medicine* 2008;28:599–617.
11. Falzoi M, Mossa A, Congeddu E, et al. Multiplex genotyping of CYP3A4, CYP3A5, CYP2C9 and CYP2C19 SNPs using MALDI-TOF mass spectrometry. *Pharmacogenomics* 2010;11:559–571.

12. Ogino S, Wilson RB. Genotype and haplotype distributions of MTHFR677C>T and 1298A>C single nucleotide polymorphisms: A meta-analysis. *Journal of Human Genetics* 2003;48:1–7.

13. Allen R, Gatalica Z, Knezetic J, et al. A common 1317TC polymorphism in MTHFR can lead to erroneous 1298AC genotyping by PCR-RE and TaqMan® probe assays. *Genetic Testing* 2007;11: 167–173.

14. Seipp M, Durtschi JD, Liew MA, et al. Unlabeled oligonucleotides as internal temperature controls for genotyping by amplicon melting. *Journal of Molecular Diagnostics* 2007;9:284–289.

15. Seipp M, Pattison D, Durtschi JD, et al. Quadruplex genotyping of F5, F2, and MTHFR variants in a single closed tube by high-resolution amplicon melting. *Clinical Chemistry* 2008;54:108–115.

16. Brandon M, Lott MT, Nguyen KC, et al. MITOMAP: A human mitochondrial genome database—2004 update. *Nucleic Acids Research* 2005;33: D611–D13.

17. Leonard J, Schapira AH. Mitochondrial respiratory chain disorders I: Mitochondrial DNA defects. *Lancet* 2000;355:299–304.

18. Leonard J, Schapira AH. Mitochondrial respiratory chain disorders II: Neurodegenerative disorders and nuclear gene defects. *Lancet* 2000;355: 389–394.

19. Mkaouar-Rebai E, Chamkha I, Kammoun T, et al. A case of Kearns-Sayre syndrome with two novel deletions (9.768 and 7.253kb) of the mtDNA associated with the common deletion in blood leukocytes, buccal mucosa and hair follicles. *Mitochondrion* 2010;10:449-455.

20. Moraes C, Atencio DP, Oca-Cossio J, et al. Techniques and pitfalls in the detection of pathogenic mitochondrial DNA mutations. *Journal of Molecular Diagnostics* 2003;5:197–208.

21. Yu P, Sinitsyna I, Lyon E. A precise sizing method for Fragile X (CGG)n repeats. *Journal of Molecular Diagnostics* 2006;8:627.

22. Lyon E, Laver T, Yu P, et al. A simple, high-throughput assay for Fragile X expanded alleles using triple repeat primed PCR and capillary electrophoresis. *Journal of Molecular Diagnostics* 2010;12:505–511.

23. Sohn E. Fragile X's missing partners identified. *Science* 2001;294:1809.

24. Moine H, Mandel J-L. Do G quartets orchestrate fragile X pathology? *Science* 2001;294:2487–2488.

25. Marx J. Huntington's research points to possible new therapies. *Science* 2005;310:43–45.

26. Amiel J, Laudier B, Attié-Bitach T, et al. Polyalanine expansion and frameshift mutations of the paired-like homeobox gene *PHOX*2b in congenital central hypoventilation syndrome. *Nature Genetics* 2003;33:459–461.

27. Weese-Mayer D, Berry-Kravis EM, Zhou L, et al. Idiopathic congenital central hypoventilation syndrome: Analysis of genes pertinent to early autonomic nervous system embryologic development and identification of mutations in *PHOX*2b. *American Journal of Medical Genetics* 2003; 123A:267–278.

28. D'Alessandro V, Mason TBA, II, Pallone MN, et al. Late-onset hypoventilation without *PHOX*2b mutation or hypothalamic abnormalities. *Journal of Clinical Sleep Medicine* 2005;1:169–172.

29. Nieuwint A, Van Hagen JM, Heins YM, et al. Rapid detection of microdeletions using fluorescence in situ hybridisation (FISH) on buccal smears. *Journal of Medical Genetics* 2000;37:e4.

30. Mutirangura A, Greenberg F, Butler MG, et al. Multiplex PCR of three dinucleotide repeats in the Prader-Willi/Angelman critical region (15q11-q13): Molecular diagnosis and mechanism of uniparental disomy. *Human Molecular Genetics* 1993;2: 143–151.

31. Chotai K, Payne SJ. A rapid, PCR-based test for differential molecular diagnosis of Prader-Willi and Angelman syndromes. *Journal of Medical Genetics* 1998;35:472–475.

32. Hung C, Lin SY, Lin SP, et al. Identification of CpG methylation of the SNRPN gene by methylation-specific multiplex PCR. *Journal of Electrophoresis* 2009;30:410–416.

33. Wang W, Law HY, Chong SS. Detection and discrimination between deletional and non-deletional Prader-Willi and Angelman syndromes by methylation-specific PCR and quantitative melting curve analysis. *Journal of Molecular Diagnostics* 2009;11:446–449.

34. Glenn C, Saitoh S, Jong MT, et al. Gene structure, DNA methylation, and imprinted expression of the human SNRPN gene. *American Journal of Human Genetics* 1996;58:335–346.

35. Shaffer L, Coppinger J, Alliman S, et al. Comparison of microarray-based detection rates for cytogenetic abnormalities in prenatal and neonatal specimens. *Prenatal Diagnosis* 2008;28:789–795.

36. Toudjarska I, Kilpatrick MW, Lembessis P, et al. Novel approach to the molecular diagnosis of Marfan syndrome: Application to sporadic cases and in prenatal diagnosis. *American Journal of Medical Genetics* 2001;99:294–302.

37. Upadhyaya M, Maynard J, Rogers MT, et al. Improved molecular diagnosis of facioscapulohumeral muscular dystrophy (FSHD): Validation of the differential double digestion for FSHD. *Journal of Medical Genetics* 1997;34:476–479.

38. Wang J, Ban MR, Hegele RA. Multiplex ligation-dependent probe amplification of LDLR enhances molecular diagnosis of familial hypercholesterolemia. *Journal of Lipid Research* 2005;46: 366–372.

39. Ramos S, Hernandez M, Roces A, et al. Molecular diagnosis of alkaptonuria mutation by analysis of homogentisate 1,2 dioxygenase mRNA from urine and blood. *American Journal of Medical Genetics* 1998;78:192–194.

40. Felbor U, Mutsch Y, Grehn F, et al. Ocular ochronosis in alkaptonuria patients carrying mutations in the homogentisate 1,2-dioxygenase gene. *British Journal of Ophthalmology* 1999; 83:680–683.

41. Landegren U, Kaiser R, Sanders J, et al. A ligase-mediated gene detection technique. *Science* 1988; 24:1077–1080.

42. Tuchman M. Molecular diagnosis of medium-chain acyl-coA dehydrogenase deficiency by oligonucleotide ligation assay. *Clinical Chemistry* 1998;44:10–11.

43. Carlucci F, Tabucchi A, Aiuti A, et al. Capillary electrophoresis in diagnosis and monitoring of adenosine deaminase deficiency. *Clinical Chemistry* 2003;49:1830–1838.

44. Zeviani M, Moraes CT, DiMauro S, et al. Deletions of mitochondrial DNA in Kearnes-Sayre syndrome. *Neurology* 1988;38:1339–1346.

45. De Coo I, Gussinklo T, Arts PJ, et al. A PCR test for progressive external ophthalmoplegia and Kearns-Sayre syndrome on DNA from blood samples. *Journal of Neurological Science* 1997;149:37–40.

46. Raffelsberger T, Rossmanith W, Thaller-Antlanger H, et al. CPEO associated with a single nucleotide deletion in the mitochondrial tRNATyr gene. *Neurology* 2001;57:2298–2301.

47. Moraes C, DiMauro S, Zeviani M, et al. Mitochondrial DNA deletions in progressive external ophthalmoplegia and Kearns-Sayre syndrome. *New England Journal of Medicine* 1989;320:1293–1299.

48. Kiechl S, Horváth R, Luoma P, et al. Two families with autosomal-dominant progressive external ophthalmoplegia. *Journal of Neurology Neurosurgery and Psychiatry* 2004;75:1125–1128.

Molecular Oncology

OBJECTIVES

- Identify checkpoints in the cell division cycle that are critical for regulated cell proliferation.
- List molecular targets that are useful for diagnosis and monitoring of solid tumors.
- Explain how microsatellite instability is detected.
- Describe loss of heterozygosity and its detection.
- Contrast cell-specific and tumor-specific molecular targets.
- Show how clonality is detected using antibody and T-cell receptor gene rearrangements.
- Describe translocations associated with hematological malignancies that can be used for molecular testing.
- Interpret data obtained from the molecular analysis of patients' cells, and determine if a tumor population is present.

Oncology is the study of tumors. A tumor, or **neoplasm**, is a growth of tissue that exceeds and is not coordinated with normal tissue. Tumors are either benign (not recurrent) or malignant (invasive and tending to recur at multiple sites). **Cancer** is a term that includes all malignant tumors. Molecular oncology is the study of cancer at the molecular level, using techniques that allow direct detection of genetic alterations, down to single base-pair changes.

Classification of Neoplasms

Cancer is generally divided into two broad groups, solid tumors and hematological malignancies. Solid tumors are designated according to the tissue of origin as **carcinomas** (epithelial) or **sarcomas** (bone, cartilage, muscle, blood vessels, fat). **Teratocarcinomas** consist of multiple cell types. Benign tumors are named by adding the suffix "-oma" directly to the tissue of origin. For example, an adenoma is a benign glandular growth; an adenocarcinoma is malignant.

Metastasis is the movement of dislodged tumor cells from the original (primary) site to other locations. Only malignant tumors are metastatic. No one characteristic of the primary tumor predicts the likelihood of metastasis. Factors affecting both tumor and surrounding normal tissue are likely involved in the metastatic process. The presence of metastasis increases the difficulty of treatment. Clinical analysis may be performed to detect the presence of relocated or circulating metastasized cells to aid in treatment strategy.

With regard to hematological malignancies, tumors arising from white blood cells are referred to as leukemias and lymphomas. **Leukemia** is a neoplastic disease of blood-forming tissue in which large numbers of white blood cells populate the bone marrow and peripheral blood. **Lymphoma** is a neoplasm of lymphocytes that forms discrete tissue masses. The difference between these diseases is not clear, as lymphocytic leukemias and lymphomas can display bone marrow and blood symptoms similar to those of leukemias. Furthermore, chronic lymphomas can progress to leukemia. Conversely, leukemias can display lymphomatous masses without overpopulation of cells in the bone marrow.

Within lymphomas, *Hodgkin disease* or *Hodgkin's lymphoma* includes a group of disorders that are histologically and clinically different from all other types of lymphoma, termed *non-Hodgkin's lymphoma (NHL)*. **Plasma cell** neoplasms, which arise from terminally differentiated B cells, are also classified in a separate category. Some of the physiological symptoms of plasma cell tumors are related to the secretion of immunoglobulin fragments by these tumors.

Molecular Basis of Cancer

Normally cells divide, arrest, differentiate, or expire in response to intracellular and extracellular signals controlling the **cell division cycle** (Fig. 14-1). Cancer is caused by non-lethal mutations in DNA that disrupt the signaling process such that proliferation and survival are favored and not regulated by normal signaling. Affected genes are classified as gatekeeper genes and caretaker genes.

Gatekeeper genes include **oncogenes** and **tumor suppressor genes**. These genes control the cell division cycle and cell survival. Oncogenes promote cell division and cell survival and include cell membrane receptors that are bound by growth factors, hormones, and other

Advanced Concepts

As imaging technology advanced, classification of NHL evolved. The earliest was the Rappaport classification in 1966, developed at the Armed Forces Institute of Pathology. The Keil classification, used in Europe, and the Lukes and Collins classification, used in the United States, were proposed in 1974. In 1982, an international group of hematopathologists proposed the Working Formulation for Clinical Usage for classification of NHL.[1] The Working Formulation was revised in 1994 by the International Lymphoma Study Group, which proposed the World Health Organization/Revised European-American Classification of Lymphoid Neoplasms (REAL). The REAL classification included genetic characteristics in addition to morphological tissue architecture. The latest classification is an update of the 2001 version approved by the World Health Organization. With increasing ability to detect molecular characteristics of cells, including patterns of gene expression, classification will continue to be refined.

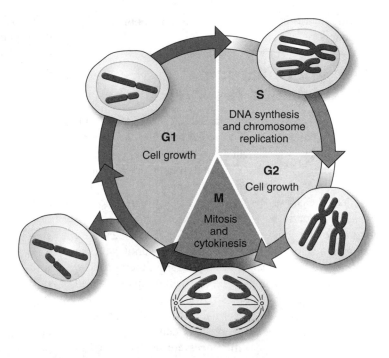

■ **Figure 14-1** The cell division cycle. After mitosis (M), there are two haploid (one diploid) complements of chromosomes (46 chromosomes) in the G1 phase of the cell division cycle. DNA is replicated during the S phase, resulting in four haploid (two diploid) complements in the G2 phase. The chromosomes are distributed to two daughter cells at mitosis, each receiving 46 chromosomes. Cancer results when the cell division cycle proceeds from the G1 to S or G2 to M phase inappropriately.

extracellular signals. These receptors transduce signals through the cell membrane into the cytoplasm through a series of protein modifications that ultimately reach the nucleus and activate factors that initiate DNA synthesis (move the cell from G1 to S phase of the cell cycle) or mitosis (move from G2 to M). Oncogenes also support cell survival by inhibiting **apoptosis**, or self-directed cell death. More than 100 oncogenes have been identified in the human genome.

Tumor suppressor gene products slow down or stop cell division. Tumor suppressors include factors that control transcription, or translation of genes required for cell division. Tumor suppressors also participate in repairing DNA damage and in promoting apoptosis. Tumor suppressors counteract the movement of the cell from G1 to S or G2 to M phase. These two points are therefore referred to as the G1 checkpoint and G2 checkpoint in the cell division cycle. More than 100 tumor suppressor genes have been identified.

Particular tumor suppressor genes might also be classified as caretaker genes. Caretaker genes maintain genetic stability through DNA repair and maintenance of chromosomal organization. Loss of caretaker functions results in unrepaired DNA damage and chromosomal structural mutations.

In cancer cells, mutations in oncogenes are usually **gain-of-function** mutations, resulting from amplification or translocation of DNA regions containing the genes or activating mutations that cause aberrant activity of the proteins. Mutations in tumor suppressor genes are usually **loss-of-function** mutations, resulting in inactivation of the tumor suppressor gene products. These mutations may occur through deletion, translocation, or mutation of the genes. Molecular laboratory testing aids in the diagnosis and treatment strategies for tumors by

Advanced Concepts

A third category of cancer genes, landscapers, has also been proposed. Landscapers affect the environment of a potential tumor rather than the tumor cells directly. Mutations in these genes establish a stromal environment that may be more conducive than normal tissue to tumor growth. For example, juvenile polyposis syndrome and ulcerative colitis are nonmalignant conditions with molecular abnormalities that result in increased risk of colon cancer.

detecting abnormalities in specific tumor suppressors or oncogenes.

Analytical Targets of Molecular Testing

Although not yet completely standardized, several tests are performed in almost every molecular pathology laboratory. These include tests that target *tissue-specific* or *tumor-specific* genes. Tissue-specific targets are molecular characteristics of the type of tissue from which a tumor arose. The presence of DNA or RNA from these targets in abnormal amounts or locations is used to detect and monitor the presence of the tumor. For example, molecular tests are designed to detect DNA or RNA from cytokeritin genes in gastric cancer, carcinoembryonic antigen in breast cancer, and rearranged immunoglobulin or T-cell receptor genes in lymphoma. Although tissue-specific markers are useful, they are also expressed by normal cells, and their presence does not always prove the presence of cancer.

In contrast, tumor-specific genes are not expressed in normal cells and are, therefore, more definitive with respect to the presence of tumor. Tumor-specific genetic structures result from genome, chromosomal, or gene abnormalities in oncogenes and tumor suppressor genes that are associated with the development of the tumor. Gene mutations and chromosomal translocations are found in solid tumors, leukemias, and lymphomas. Genome mutations, or **aneuploidy**, result in part from the loss of coordinated DNA synthesis and cell division that occurs when tumor suppressors or oncogenes are dysfunctional. Research is ongoing to find more of these tumor-specific markers to improve molecular oncology testing.

The following sections describe procedures most commonly performed in molecular pathology laboratories; however, due to the rapid advances in this area, the descriptions cannot be all-inclusive. The discussion is divided into solid tumor testing and testing for hematological malignancies. As will be apparent, however, some tests are applicable to both types of malignancies.

Gene and Chromosomal Mutations in Solid Tumors

A number of tests are routinely performed to aid in the diagnosis, characterization, and monitoring of solid tumors. Some of these tests have been part of molecular pathology for many years. Others are relatively new to the clinical laboratory. The methods applied to detect molecular characteristics of tumors are described in Section II of this text.

Human Epidermal Growth Factor Receptor 2, HER2/neu/erb-b2 1 (17q21.1)

HER2/neu was discovered in rat neuro/glioblastoma cell lines in 1985.[2] Later it was found to be the same gene as the avian erythroblastic leukemia viral oncogene homolog 2, or *ERBB2,* which codes for a 185-kd cell membrane protein that adds phosphate groups to tyrosines on itself and other proteins (tyrosine kinase activity). This receptor is one of several **transmembrane** proteins with tyrosine kinase activity (Fig. 14-2). It is very similar to a family of epidermal growth factor receptors that are overexpressed in some cancers (Fig. 14-3).

In normal cells, this protein is required for cells to grow and divide. *HER2/neu* is overexpressed in 25% to 30% of human breast cancers, in which overexpression of *HER2/neu* is a predictor of a more aggressive growth and metastasis of the tumor cells. It is also an indication for use of the anti-*HER2/neu* antibody drug Herceptin (trastuzumab) therapy, which works best on tumors overexpressing *HER2/neu*. Herceptin therapy is currently indicated for women with *HER2/neu*-positive (*HER2/neu* overexpressed) breast cancer that has spread to lymph nodes or other organs.

Testing for the overexpression of the *HER2/neu* oncogene is often performed by immunohistochemistry (IHC) using monoclonal and polyclonal antibodies to detect the HER2/neu protein. The Hercep Test was developed by Dako and Genentech as a method to define conditions for performance and interpretation of the IHC test. The IHC test, which is cheaper and more readily available in most institutions, works best on fresh or frozen tissue. Fluorescent in situ hybridization (FISH), which measures DNA and RNA of *HER2/neu*, is more reliable than IHC, especially in older, fixed tissue.[3,4]

Chromogenic in situ hybridization (CISH) is another method that has been used to detect *HER2/neu* gene amplification.[6,7] CISH is a less expensive method that uses a standard bright field microscope. In addition to gene amplification, CISH technology also detects deletions, translocations, or change in the number of chromosomes. CISH slide images are permanent, facilitating

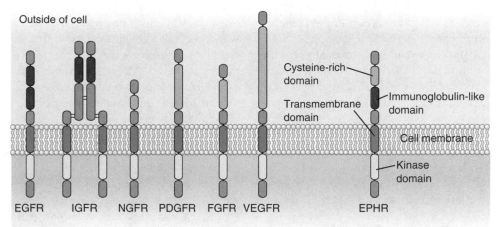

Outside of cell

Cysteine-rich domain

Transmembrane domain

Immunoglobulin-like domain

Cell membrane

Kinase domain

EGFR   IGFR   NGFR   PDGFR   FGFR   VEGFR   EPHR

Cytoplasm

■ **Figure 14-2** Receptor tyrosine kinases include epidermal growth factor receptor (EGFR), insulin growth factor receptor (IGFR), nerve growth factor receptor (NGFR), platelet-derived growth factor receptor (PDGFR), fibroblast growth factor receptor (FGFR), vascular endothelial growth factor receptor (VEGFR), and ephrin receptor (EPHR). These molecules share similarities in that they include a kinase domain, transmembrane domain, cysteine-rich domain, and immunoglobulin-like domain.

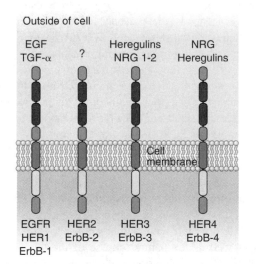

Outside of cell

EGF TGF-α   ?   Heregulins NRG 1-2   NRG Heregulins

Cell membrane

EGFR HER1 ErbB-1   HER2 ErbB-2   HER3 ErbB-3   HER4 ErbB-4

Cytoplasm

■ **Figure 14-3** The ErbB family of growth factor receptors includes the *HER2* receptor and EGFR. The factors that bind to these receptors on the cell surface begin a cascade of events, including autophosphorylation and phosphorylation of other proteins by the receptors. These factors include the epidermal growth factor (EGF), human transforming growth factor alpha (TGF-α), heregulins, and neuregulins (NRG). EGF and NRG heregulins are small peptides that are active in the development of various cell types such as gastric mucosa, the heart, and the nervous system.

Advanced Concepts

Southern, Northern, and Western studies have shown that *HER2/neu* gene amplification is highly correlated with the presence of increased *HER2/neu* RNA and protein.[5] In contrast to IHC, which measures increased amounts of HER2/neu protein, FISH directly detects increased copy numbers of the *HER2/neu* gene in DNA. *HER2/neu* gene amplification occurs as a result of tandem duplication of the gene or other genetic events as the tumor cells continue to divide. FISH testing for *HER2/neu* gene amplification requires a labeled probe for the *HER2/neu* gene and a differently labeled control probe for the centromere of chromosome 17. For instance, the PathVysion reagent set (Vysis) includes the *HER-2* probe that spans the entire *HER2/neu* gene labeled in Spectrum Orange and a CEP 17 probe that binds to the centromere of chromosome 17 labeled in Spectrum Green. The copy number of *HER2/neu* relative to the copy number of CEP 17 indicates whether *HER2/neu* is amplified (present in multiple copies on the same chromosome). Data are reported as a ratio of the number of *HER2* signals to chromosome 17 centromere signals. A ratio of more than 2 is considered positive or amplified. The number of signals is enumerated in 50 to 100 cells.

documentation and consultations. Probes with repetitive sequences removed, such as Subtraction Probe Technology™ (Invitrogen), were designed to address these limitations. CISH has shown 86% to 96% concordance with FISH in comparison studies of *HER2/neu* amplification.[8]

Although FISH and CISH are more accurate and less subjective methods than IHC, IHC is faster, less expensive, and allows the pathologist to assess target gene expression along with other visible landmarks on the slide. Furthermore, protein overexpression (detectable by IHC) can occur without gene amplification (detectable by ISH). Some laboratories use IHC as an initial screening method and then confirm results with FISH or CISH.

Epidermal Growth Factor Receptor, EGFR (7p12)

The epidermal growth factor receptor gene (*EGFR, ERBB1*) is another member of the *ERBB* family of growth factor receptors that also includes *ERB3/HER3* and *ERB4/HER4* (see Fig. 14-3). All of these proteins are located in the cell membrane and form dimers with one another upon binding of growth factor from outside the cell (Fig. 14-4). Binding of specific ligands such as growth factors evoke the tyrosine kinase activity of the receptors and initiates proliferation signals through the cell cytoplasm.

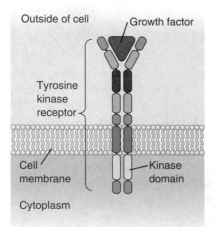

■ **Figure 14-4** Upon binding by epidermal growth factor (EGF), the EGFR receptor in the cell membrane forms a dimer with itself or with other members of the ERBB family of receptors. The dimerization initiates a cascade of events, starting with phosphorylation of the receptor itself catalyzed by the kinase domain.

EGFR is frequently overexpressed in solid tumors. In research studies, overexpression has been correlated with poor clinical outcome. For this reason the EGF receptor has been an attractive target for the design of therapeutic drugs. Monoclonal antibodies such as cetuximab (Erbitux) block ligand binding to the receptor and may also elicit an immune response against the tumor cells. Other agents inhibit the kinase activity of the receptor. Of these tyrosine kinase inhibitors, erlotinib (Tarceva), gefitinib (Iressa), and sunitinib malate (Sutent) have been studied in clinical trials.

Based on the association of *HER2/neu* overexpression with Herceptin effectiveness, IHC analysis of *EGFR* expression was considered a way to predict response to monoclonal antibody drugs.[9] The Dako Cytomation EGFR PharmDx test kit was approved by the United States Food and Drug Administration for this application. Interpretation of the results of *EGFR* expression testing and the predictive value of the test are not always straightforward, however.[10] Quantitative real-time polymerase chain reaction (PCR) and FISH analysis have also been proposed as methods to assess the number of *EGFR* gene copies[11]

One possible predictor of response to tyrosine kinase inhibiting agents is the presence of specific mutations found in the kinase domain of *EGFR*.[12–15] *EGFR* exon 19 deletions and the exon 21 point mutation comprise the majority of activation or sensitizing mutations. Tumors with activating mutations are more sensitive to *EGFR* kinase inhibitors than those without mutations. A number of methods are used to detect *EGFR* mutations, including sequence-specific PCR, single-strand conformational polymorphism (SSCP), and direct sequencing.[12,16,17] Detection of mutations in the *EGFR* kinase region is now performed to guide treatment strategy using *EGFR* inhibitors.

Testing for predictors of response to *EGFR* inhibitors or prognosis is complex because several clinical and genetic factors contribute to the response to targeted therapies as well as the natural course of the tumor. These include intronic polymorphisms in the *EGFR* gene,[18] expression of other components of the signal transduction pathway,[19,20] or other tumor suppressors such as p53.[21]

Kirsten Rat Sarcoma Viral Oncogene Homolog, K-ras (12p12), Neuroblastoma ras, N-ras (1p13), Harvey Rat Sarcoma Viral Oncogene Homolog, H-ras (11p15)

Signals from extracellular stimuli, such as growth factors or hormones, are transmitted through the cell cytoplasm to the nucleus, resulting in cell proliferation or differentiation (Fig. 14-5). The mitogen-activated protein kinase (MAPK) pathway is a cascade of phosphorylation events that transmit growth signals from the cell membrane to the nucleus. Critical components of this pathway are small proteins that bind to GTP in order to become active. These small GTP binding proteins include the *ras* genes that receive signals from the cell surface proteins and activate the initial steps of the MAPK cascade (Fig. 14-6). Mutations in *ras* **proto-oncogenes** occur in many types of cancers.

Mammals have three different *ras* genes that produce four similar proteins, K-ras4A, K-ras4B, N-ras, and H-ras. The Ras proteins differ in their carboxy termini, the end of the proteins that anchors them to the inner surface of the cell membrane (Table 14.1, Fig. 14-7). Because they bind and hydrolyze GTP for energy, the *ras* genes are members of a family of G-proteins. The GTP hydrolysis is regulated by GTPase activating proteins (GAPs).

Mutations in *K-ras* are the most common oncogene mutations in human cancers. The most frequently occurring mutations are located in codons 12, 13, 22, and 61 of

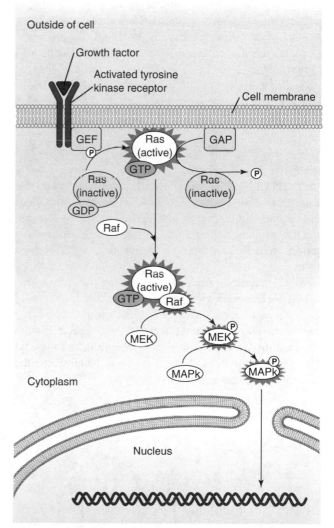

■ **Figure 14-6** Activation of membrane-bound K-ras is initiated by activated receptors bound to mitogens (growth factors or hormones). Active K-ras bound to GTP then initiates a cascade of phosphorylation events that end in the nucleus, where transcription factors modulate gene expression. GDP/GTP exchange on K-ras is modulated by GTPase activating proteins (GAPs), guanosine nucleotide exchange factors (GEFs), and guanosine nucleotide dissociation inhibitors (GDIs).

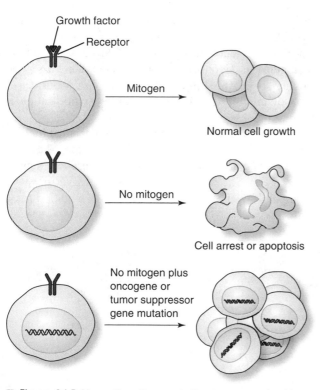

■ **Figure 14-5** Normally cells grow in the presence of nutrients and factors that stimulate cell division (mitogens). Lack of mitogen stimulation results in cell arrest, or apoptosis. If oncogene or tumor suppressor gene mutations stimulate aberrant growth signals, cells grow in the absence of controlled stimulation.

Advanced Concepts

Regulation of ras GTPase activity is controlled by rasGAP. Several other GAP proteins besides rasGAP are important in signal transduction. Two clinically important proteins of the GAP family of proteins are the gene product of the neurofibromatosis type-1 (*NF1*) locus and the gene product of the breakpoint cluster region (*BCR*) gene. The *NF1* gene is a tumor suppressor gene, and the protein encoded is called neurofibromin. The *BCR* locus is rearranged in the Philadelphia+ chromosome (Ph+) observed in chronic myelogenous leukemias and acute lymphocytic leukemias.

Table 14.1 **Four ras Proteins Synthesized from Three Genes, *K-ras*, *N-ras*, and *H-ras****

Protein	Modification	Location
K-ras4A	Farnesylation + palmitoylation	?
K-ras4B	Farnesylation + polybasic amino acids	Plasma membrane
N-ras	Farnesylation + palmitoylation	Golgi
H-ras	Farnesylation + palmitoylation	Golgi

*K-ras4A and K-ras4B arise from alternate splicing of transcripts of the same gene.

the *K-ras* gene. These mutations affect sequences coding for the GTP-binding domain of the protein and throw the Ras protein into a permanently active state that does not require stimulation from GTP hydrolysis. As a result, the Ras proteins harboring these single nucleotide substitutions remain constitutively active in the GTP-bound form.

K-ras mutations are highly correlated with tumor histology and may predict the progress of tumorigenesis in early-stage tumors. Furthermore, the presence of *K-ras* mutations may affect treatment strategy, especially with targeted therapies such as kinase inhibitors and farnesyl transferase inhibitors (K-ras protein is localized to the cell membrane through a farnesyl group).

K-ras mutations are detected and identified by SSCP screening and direct sequencing. Although comprehensive with regard to the possible constellation of activating mutations, detection of mutations by direct sequencing is limited to 10% to 20%. Microdissection of tumor tissue from thin sections can increase sensitivity as well as pre-sequencing methods such as co-amplification at lower denaturation temperature PCR (COLD-PCR).[22] Pyrosequencing has also been applied to *K-ras* mutation analysis. The PyroMark KRAS kit (Qiagen) can be used to specifically genotype codons 12 and 13. In addition, mutations in codon 61 can be analyzed using a second primer set provided in the test. A biochip test for detection of multiple specific mutations by hybridization is also available.[23,24]

K-ras mutation analysis may be accompanied by testing for the V600E mutation in the *B-raf* gene. The *B-raf* gene product is a kinase enzyme that transduces signals from *K-ras*. Since they are on the same signal transduction pathway, the presence of the V600E mutation has a

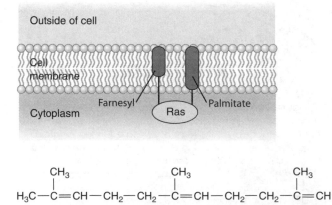

■ **Figure 14-7** Ras proteins are anchored to the cell membrane through farnesyl groups (chemical structure at bottom) and palmitoyl groups on the ras proteins. K-ras has only farnesyl groups, whereas N-ras and H-ras have both farnesyl and palmitoyl groups.

similar effect as the presence of the *K-ras* activating mutations. Furthermore, mutations in *K-ras* and *B-raf* are mutually exclusive, that is, they are not observed together in the same tumor. The *B-raf* V600E mutation occurs almost exclusively in tumors located in the proximal colon and with promoter hypermethylation of *MLH1*, the gene involved in the initial steps of tumor development. Conversely, *B-raf* mutations are not detected in those cases with or presumed to have a germline mutation in either *MLH1* or *MSH2*.[25] *B-raf* mutation detection has been achieved using several methods, including restriction fragment length polymorphism analysis, allele-specific PCR, qPCR, single-strand conformation analysis, direct sequencing, and allelic discrimination.[26] As of 2010, the National Comprehensive Cancer Network recommends *B-raf* testing when *K-ras* mutations are not found.

Ewing Sarcoma, EWS (22q12)

A group of tumors arising from primitive neuroectodermal tissue (PNET)/Ewing sarcomas comprise a family of childhood neoplasms referred to as the Ewing family. Although immunohistochemical staining for the cell surface glycoprotein, p30/p32MIC2, using the HBA71 antibody is helpful in diagnosis of these tumors, no unique characteristics distinguish the different types of tumors that make up this group.

Detection of specific translocations involving the *EWS* gene at 22q12 (also called *EWSR1* for *EWS* breakpoint region 1) by cytogenetic or molecular methods is useful for diagnostic and prognostic accuracy (Table 14.2). Translocations of *EWS* with the *FLI-1* gene at 11q24, t(11;22)(q24;q12) are present in 85% of Ewing sarcomas. Another translocation between *EWS* and the *ERG* gene at 21q22 is present in 5% to 10% of Ewing sarcomas. Other

Table 14.2 **EWS Translocation Partners**

Translocation	Tumor
EWS-FLI-1	Ewing sarcoma, peripheral PNET (72%)
EWS-ERG	Ewing sarcoma, peripheral PNET (11%)
*EWS-WT1**	Desmoplastic small round cell tumor
EWS-ATF1	Clear cell sarcoma

*The *WT1* gene is also associated with Wilms' tumor (WT), one of the common solid tumors of childhood, accounting for 8% of childhood cancers. Several genes or chromosomal areas affect the development of WT: *WT1* at 11p13, *WT2* at 11p15.5, *WT3* at 16q, *WT5* at 7p15-p11.2, and *WT4* at 17q12-q21.

partners for the *EWS* gene, such as *ETV1* at 7p22, *E1AF* at 17q12, and *FEV* at 2q33, are present in fewer than 1% of cases.[27,28] The occurrence of these rearrangements was first revealed by cytogenetics[29,30] and then by PCR methods.[31]

Current laboratory testing at the molecular level involves detection of the tumor-specific translocations by reverse transcriptase polymerase chain reaction (RT-PCR) (Fig. 14-8). Positive results are revealed by the presence of a 120-190–bp PCR product. Negative specimens will not yield a product. As with all assays of this type, an amplification control, such as GAPDH or 18S RNA (see Chapter 7, Nucleic Acid Amplification), must accompany all samples to avoid false-negative results. These tests are performed on fresh, frozen, or paraffin-embedded tissue.[28,32,33] Primers to additional *EWS* translocation partners are used to detect related PNET tumors.

Synovial Sarcoma Translocation, Chromosome 18—Synovial Sarcoma Breakpoint 1 and 2, SYT-SSX1, SYT-SSX2 t(X;18)(p11.2;q11.2)

A recurrent reciprocal translocation between chromosome 18 and the X chromosome is found in synovial sarcoma, a rare type of cancer of the muscle, fat, fibrous tissue, blood vessels, or other supporting tissue of the body. Synovial sarcoma accounts for 8% to 10% of all sarcomas and occurs mostly in young adults. About 80% of cases have the t(X;18) translocation.

The t(X;18) translocation fuses the synovial sarcoma translocation, chromosome 18 gene (*SS18* or *SYT*) with

---

Advanced Concepts

K-ras must be associated with cellular membranes in order to act. The membrane association is driven by the hydrophobic farnesyl group covalently attached to the ras protein by the enzyme farnesyl transferase. In the absence of farnesyl modification, even mutated ras proteins are not active. Therefore, therapies have been designed to inhibit the farnesylation of ras. These are farnesyl transferase inhibitors.

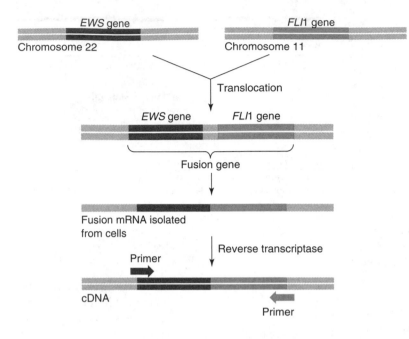

Fusion mRNA isolated
from cells

Figure 14-8 RT-PCR is used to detect the t(11:22) mutation in Ewing's sarcoma. One primer is designed to hybridize to the *EWS* gene on chromosome 22 and one primer to the *FLI1* gene on chromosome 11. If the translocation has occurred, the resulting fusion transcript isolated from the tumor cells will yield cDNA that is amplifiable with the *EWS* and *FLI1* primers.

either of two related genes on the X chromosome, synovial sarcoma translocated to X (*SSX1* and *SSX2*). The latter genes are two of five variants, *SSX1*, *SSX2*, *SSX3*, *SSX4*, and *SSX5*. With rare exceptions, only *SSX1* and *SSX2* are fused to *SYT* in the t(X;18) translocation.[34] The fusion gene acts as an aberrant transcription factor, with both activation and repression functions from the *SYT* and *SSX* portions, respectively.

The t(X;18) translocation is detected by FISH or RT-PCR.[34,35] In the RT-PCR, total RNA reverse-transcribed to cDNA is amplified with primers specific for *SSX* and *SYT* genes. In a semi-nested version of this procedure, the *SSX* primer used in the first round is a consensus primer for both *SYT-SSX1* and *SYT-SSX2*. After the first amplification, *SSX1*- and *SSX2*-specific primers discriminate between the two translocation types. The PCR products are detected by agarose gel electrophoresis and ethidium bromide staining. This method can be performed on fresh, frozen, or fixed tissue, depending on the condition of the specimen RNA.

Paired Box-Forkhead in Rhabdomyosarcoma, PAX3-FKHR, PAX7-FKHR, *t(1;13), t(2;13)*

Rhabdomyosarcoma (RMS) is the most common soft-tissue sarcoma of childhood, accounting for 10% of all solid tumors in children. In addition to alveolar rhabdomyosarcoma (ARMS), there are two additional histological forms

of RMS: embryonal (RMS-E) and primitive (RMS-P). Although histological classification of RMS is sometimes difficult, accurate diagnosis is important for management and treatment of this malignancy because ARMS has a worse prognosis than other subtypes.

Translocations involving the Forkhead in the Rhabdomyosarcoma gene (*FKHR*, also called *FOXO1A*) and the paired box genes (*PAX3* and *PAX7*) are frequently found in ARMS.[36] The chimeric genes resulting from the translocations encode transcriptional activators with DNA-binding motifs homologous to the Forkhead transcription factor first discovered in the fruit fly, *Drosophila*. *PAX-FKHR* translocations have been observed in all subtypes of RMS but are more characteristic of ARMS. Furthermore, *PAX7-FKHR*, t(2;13), is associated with better outcome than *PAX3-FKHR*, t(1;13). Mutations in the *PAX3* gene are also found in Waardenburg syndrome, a congenital auditory pigmentary syndrome.[37]

The majority of ARMS displays the t(2;13) translocation, with the t(1;13) variant present with one-third the frequency of t(2;13).[38] Both translocations are detected by FISH, RT-PCR, and real-time PCR.[39-41]

Tumor Protein 53, TP53 *(17p13)*

Mutations in *TP53* are found in all types of cancer, and about 50% of all cancers have *TP53* mutations. The gene product of *TP53*, p53, is a 53,000-dalton, DNA-binding protein that controls expression of other genes. Normally, p53 participates in the arrest of cell division in the event of DNA damage. The arrest in the G1 phase of the cell cycle allows repair enzymes to correct the DNA damage before DNA synthesis begins. Once the damage is repaired, p53 protein is removed by binding to another protein, MDM2, and degradation. If the damage persists, p53 promotes apoptosis of the abnormal cell. When p53 is not functional, replication proceeds on damaged templates, resulting in the potential for further genetic abnormalities and survival of the abnormal cells. Also, the mutant protein does not degrade properly and accumulates in the cell nucleus and cytoplasm. Reactivation of mutant p53 is a strategy for the design of novel anticancer therapies.[42]

Several studies have shown that mutated *TP53* in tumor tissue is an indicator of poor prognosis in breast, lung, colon, and other types of cancers. The significance of *TP53* status as a predictor of decreased survival time or tumor relapse is, however, controversial.[43] Part of the controversy arises from the different methods used to detect *TP53* mutations. The most common method is detection of the stabilized mutant protein by IHC. Several monoclonal antibodies directed at different epitopes in the p53 protein have been used for this purpose. Because normal p53 protein is transient, significant staining (+2 or above on a scale of 0 to +4) of p53 is considered positive for the mutation.

SSCP (see Chapter 9, "Gene Mutations") and direct sequencing (see Chapter 10, "DNA Sequencing") of microdissected tumor tissue are other methods often used to detect *TP53* mutations. Sequencing and SSCP methods cover at least exons 5 to 8 or 4 to 9 of the *TP53* gene, because these exons encode the regions involved in DNA binding and protein-protein interactive functions of the p53 protein. Screening is routinely performed on frozen or fixed paraffin-embedded tumor tissue.

Both protein and DNA analyses are used to screen for somatic p53 mutations. A number of studies, however, have shown that mutations detected on the protein level by immunohistochemistry do not correlate with mutations found by direct DNA analysis.[44–46] There are several explanations for these discrepancies (Table 14.3). Use of microarray technology to screen expression of multiple genes along with *TP53* has been proposed as a more accurate method for predicting survival than either IHC or mutation analysis of *TP53* alone.[47] Methods that include sequencing of the entire *TP53* coding region on cDNA, in combination with IHC, is another accurate approach.[45,48]

In addition to screening for somatic alterations, mutation analysis of *TP53* is also performed to aid in the diagnosis of Li-Fraumeni syndrome, a cancer-prone condition caused by inherited mutations in the p53 gene. In this case, normal tissue will be heterozygous for the mutation, removing the challenge of isolating pure samples of tumor tissue. Once an inherited mutation is detected, further analysis of relatives requires targeting only that mutation.

Ataxia Telangiectasia Mutated Gene, ATM (11q22)

Predisposition to cancer is one symptom of the neurological disease ataxia telangiectasia (AT). AT occurs in at least 1/40,000 live births. This disease is caused by mutations in the *ATM* (A-T mutated) gene on chromosome 11. *ATM* mutations are also present in some types of leukemias and lymphomas. Carriers of the autosomal-recessive mutations in *ATM* are at increased risk for developing leukemia, lymphoma, or other types of cancers.

The *ATM* gene product is a member of the phosphatidylinositol-3 kinase family of proteins that respond

Table 14.3 **Sources of Potential Inaccuracies of p53 Mutation Analysis**

Method	False Positive	False Negative
IHC	Staining of normal p53 protein	Deletions or mutations in p53 that remove Ab binding epitopes; promoter mutations
SSCP	Alternate conformers; silent DNA polymorphisms	Less than 5% mutant cells in specimen; mutations outside of the exons screened
Sequencing	PCR mutagenesis; high background	Less than 10% mutant cells in specimen; mutations outside of sequenced area

to DNA damage by phosphorylating other proteins involved in DNA repair and/or control of the cell cycle. The ATM protein participates in pausing the cell cycle at the G1 or G2 phase to allow completion of DNA repair.

Direct DNA sequencing is the method of choice for detection of *ATM* mutations, especially in family members of carriers of previously identified mutations. Another method used is SSCP.[49,50] A functional test for repair of double-strand breaks induced by irradiation is also performed for *ATM*. For this assay, exponentially growing cells are irradiated (1.5 Gy/min), and after 2 hours Colcemid (0.06 µg/mL) is added to inhibit spindle formation. The cells are harvested 2 hours later for Giemsa staining, and the karyotypes are examined for structural chromosome abnormalities. The ratio of aberrations/cell is calculated from the number of chromatid and chromosome breaks (counted as one breakage event) in addition to dicentric chromosomes, translocations, ring chromosomes, and chromatid exchange figures (counted as two breakage events).[51]

If a mutation is identified in a patient with ataxia telangiectasia, other family members may be tested for the presence of the same mutation. Presence of a mutation in family members identifies those with increased risk of AT. Heterozygous carriers of an *ATM* mutation may also be at increased risk for mantle cell lymphoma, B-cell lymphocytic leukemia, or T-cell prolymphocytic leukemia.

Breast Cancer 1 Gene, BRCA1 (17q21), and Breast Cancer 2 Gene, BRCA2 (13q12)

Approximately 5% of breast cancers result from inherited gene mutations, mostly in the breast cancer genes *BRCA1*[52,53] and *BRCA2*.[54,55] Women who carry a mutation in *BRCA1* have a 60%–80% lifetime risk of breast or ovarian cancer. Men carrying a mutation, especially in *BRCA2*, have a 100-fold increased risk of breast cancer compared with men without a mutation, as well as increased risk of colon and prostate cancer. Both men and women can transmit the mutation to subsequent generations. The *BRCA1* gene product has a role in embryonic development, and both *BRCA1* and *BRCA2* gene products may also be involved in DNA repair. *BRCA1* and *BRCA2* interact with the RAD51 protein, possibly as a complex to repair damaged DNA.[56]

SSCP, PTT, ddF (see Chapter 9), and other procedures have been used to screen for mutations in these genes.

The screening method used for clinical applications, however, is direct sequencing. Three mutations, 187delAG (also called 185delAG) and 5382insC (also called 5385insC) in *BRCA1* and 6174delT in *BRCA2*, occur frequently in particular ethnic populations.[57,58] These known mutations can be easily detected by a number of targeted assays, including sequence-specific PCR and allele-specific oligomer hybridization. The BRACAnalysis® test (Myriad Genetics) is performed by bidirectional sequencing of *BRCA1* and *BRCA2*. Single Site and Multisite 3 BRACAnalysis are sequencing tests directed to a specified site and the frequently occurring 187del, 5385insC, and 6174delT mutations, respectively.

Just as with any genetic analysis, testing for *BRCA1* and *BRCA2* mutations requires thorough patient counseling and education.[59-61] The significance of a *BRCA* mutation will depend on several factors, including penetrance of the gene mutations.[62] If a mutation is not detected in the coding sequences of the genes, the possibility of mutations in the noncoding regions cannot be ruled out.

Von Hippel-Lindau Gene, VHL (3p26)

Benign blood vessel tumors in the retina were first reported by Eugen von Hippel, a German ophthalmologist, in 1895. In 1926, Arvid Lindau, a Swedish pathologist, further noted that these retinal tumors were linked to tumors in the blood vessels in other parts of the central nervous system, sometimes accompanied by cysts in the kidneys and other internal organs, and that the condition was heritable. The Von Hippel-Lindau syndrome (VHL) is now recognized as a genetic condition involving the abnormal growth of blood vessels in organs, especially those that are particularly rich in blood vessels. It is caused by mutations in the *VHL* gene, which is located on the short arm of chromosome 3. Normally, *VHL* functions as a tumor suppressor gene, promoting cell differentiation. *VHL* may also play a role in sensing hypoxia (low oxygen levels in tissues).[63] VHL syndrome is a predisposition for renal cell carcinoma and other cancers.[64]

Deletions, point mutations, and splice site mutations have been described in patients with VHL. In addition, cases of renal cell carcinoma and tumors of the adrenal gland are accompanied by varied somatic mutations in the *VHL* gene.[65,66] Mutations in the *VHL* gene are detectable by SSCP, and linkage studies have been reported as a method for detecting inherited mutations in family members.[67] Direct sequencing, however, is the preferred method of testing for *VHL* gene mutations.

V-myc Avian Myelocytomatosis Viral-Related Oncogene, Neuroblastoma-Derived, MYCN or n-myc (2p24)

The *n-myc* gene on the short arm of chromosome 2 (2p24) is amplified in cases of neuroblastoma and retinoblastoma. *n-myc* is an oncogene that is counteracted by the tumor suppressor gene, neurofibromatosis type 1 (*NF1*). The *n-myc* gene product is a member of the MYC family of proteins (see *c-myc*). *n-myc* gene amplification is detectable by FISH or dot blot analysis.[68–70] Transcription of *n-myc* may also be measured using real-time PCR.[71]

Rearranged During Transfection (RET) Proto-oncogene, (10q11)

The *RET* proto-oncogene is located on the long arm of chromosome 10 (10q11). The *RET* gene product is a membrane tyrosine kinase that participates in sending cell growth and proliferation signals to the nucleus.[72] The *RET* gene is 55 kb in length. The first intron in the gene covers about 24 kb, with exons 2 to 20 contained in the remaining 31 kb. This general structure of a large first intron with small exons is characteristic of tyrosine kinase receptors, such as the *KIT*, *EGFR*, and platelet derived growth factor (*PDGF*) receptor genes.

The *RET* gene is an example of how different mutations in the same gene result in different diseases. Translocations that result in overexpression of *RET* are found in thyroid papillary carcinomas. Point mutations that activate *RET* (also called *MEN2A*) are found in inherited multiple endocrine neoplasia (MEN) syndromes, a group of diseases resulting in abnormal growth and function of the pituitary, thyroid, parathyroid, and adrenal glands. In contrast, loss of function mutations in the *RET* gene are found in Hirschsprung disease, a rare congenital lack of development of nerve cells in the colon that results in colonic obstruction. Mutations have been

reported in about 50% of congenital cases and 20% of sporadic cases of this disorder. Because about 16% of children with congenital central hypoventilation syndrome (CCHS) have Hirschsprung disease, *RET* mutations were also sought in CCHS. Most of the mutations detected were determined as polymorphic variants, however.[73]

Detection of *RET* gene mutations can aid in diagnosis of MEN diseases.[74,75] Clinical testing targets mainly exons 10, 11, and 16, where most reported mutations have been found. Screening for *RET* gene mutations has been performed by PCR-RFLP, direct sequencing, SSCP, and denaturing gradient gel electrophoresis (DGGE).[75–77]

Isocitrate Dehydrogenase 1 (IDH1, 2q33.3) and Isocitrase Dehydrogenase 2 (IDH2, 15q26.1)

The *IDH* genes code for a dimeric cytosolic NADP-dependent isocitrate dehydrogenase that catalyzes decarboxylation of isocitrate into alpha-ketoglutarate. Mutations in the arginine codon at position 132,R132, of *IDH1*was reported in more than 70% of grade II and III astrocytomas and oligodendrogliomas and in glioblastomas that developed from them. Tumors without mutations in *IDH1* often have mutations affecting the analogous amino acid (R172) of the *IDH2* gene.[78]

PCR methods. including real-time and fluorscent melt curve analyses, have been developed for detection of the clinically important mutations in *IDH1* and *IDH2*.[79] Since this test requires tumor tissue from brain, the test is most often performed on paraffin-embedded tissue.[80] Tumors containing *IDH* mutations showed a less aggressive course in patients than those without. *IDH* mutations have also been reported in acute myelogenous leukemia, where they are associated with a worse outcome.[81,82]

Other Molecular Abnormalities

Increasing numbers of molecular abnormalities are being used to aid in the diagnosis and monitoring of solid tumors. Some examples of potential diagnostic targets are shown in Table 14.4. As molecular aberrations in oncogenes and tumor suppressor genes are identified, molecular analysis becomes more important in their rapid and accurate detection.

Microsatellite Instability

Lynch syndrome, or hereditary nonpolyposis colorectal cancer (HNPCC), is an inherited form of colon carcinoma,

---

Advanced Concepts

The *n-myc* gene encodes a nuclear protein with a basic helix-loop-helix (bHLH) domain that dimerizes with another bHLH protein in order to bind DNA.

Table 14.4 **Molecular Abnormalities in Some Solid Tumors**

Gene	Location	Mutation	Detection Method	Associated Disease
Adenomatous polyposis of the colon	5q21	5q deletion, t(5;10)	Southern blot, FISH, sequencing, SSCP	Familial adenomatous polyposis of the colon
Retinoblastoma (Rb, RB1)	13q14.1	13q deletion, t(X;13)	Southern blot, FISH, sequencing	Retinal neoplasm, osteosarcoma
MET proto-oncogene, hepatocyte growth factor receptor	7q31	Missense mutations	Sequencing	Renal carcinoma
KIT proto-oncogene, stem cell factor receptor (SCFR)	4q12	Missense mutations	Sequencing	Gastrointestinal stromal tumors
Folliculin (FLCL, BHD)	17p11.2	Insertions, deletions in a C8 tract in exon 11	Sequencing	Birt-Hogg-Dube syndrome (hair follicle hamartomas, kidney tumors)
Fumarate hydratase	1q42.1	Frameshift mutations	Sequencing	Hereditary leiomyomatosis, renal cell cancer
Activin A Receptor (ALK4)	12q13	Gene fusion		Pancreatic carcinoma, lung cancer
Epidermal Growth Factor Receptor (EGFR)	7p12	Missense mutations, deletions	SSP-PCR, SSCP, Sequencing	Lung cancer, glioblastoma
Avian Erythroblastic Leukemia Viral Oncogene Homolog (ERBB-2, HER2)	17q21	Amplification	Immunohistochemistry, FISH	Breast cancer
Platelet Derived Growth Factor Alpha (PDGFRa)	4q12	Deletion	Immunohistochemistry, FISH, CISH	Idiopathic hypereosinophilic syndrome
Methylguanine DNA Methyl Transferase (MGMT)	10q26	Promoter methylation	MSP-PCR, Real Time PCR	Glioblastoma treated with temozolomide
Phosphatase and Tensin Homolog (PTEN)	10q23.31	Deletion	FISH	Glioblastoma

accounting for about 5% of all colon cancers.[83–86] Predisposition to cancer in this syndrome is caused by mutations in the *MSH2* and *MLH1* genes. Mutations in the *MSH6* and *hPMS2* genes have also been found. These genes are responsible for correcting replicative errors and mismatched bases in DNA, a process called **mismatch repair (MMR)**. The MMR system was originally discovered in bacteria (*Escherichia coli*) and further studied in yeast (*Saccharomyces cerevisiae*). Similar (homologous) genes were subsequently identified in humans and named after the bacterial and yeast genes (Table 14.5). Their gene products form a protein complex that binds to mismatched bases in the DNA

double helix or loops formed by replicative errors. At the end of S phase (DNA replication), the system recognizes errors in the newly synthesized daughter strand and uses the template strand, which is methylated, as a guide for repair (Fig. 14-9).

Included in the types of DNA lesions that are repaired by this system are replication errors (RERs) caused by slippage between the replication apparatus and the DNA template (Fig. 14-10). RERs occur especially in microsatellites where 1–3 nucleotides are repeated in the DNA sequence (see Chapter 11, "DNA Polymorphisms and Human Identification"). If the errors remain in the DNA until the next round of replication, new alleles will

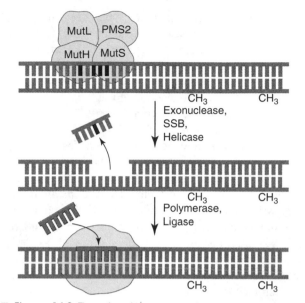

■ Figure 14-9 The mismatch repair system recognizes a mismatch (top) in the newly synthesized unmethylated strand of DNA. The complex of proteins recruits exonucleases, single-strand DNA binding proteins (SSB), and helicases to remove the erroneous base (center). Polymerases and DNA ligase then replace the missing bases and restore the final phosphodiester bond.

Table 14.5 **Genes of the MMR System**

Human Gene	Bacterial Gene	Function
MSH2	MutS	Single mismatch, loop repair
MSH3	MutS	Loop repair
MSH4	MutS	Meiosis
MSH5	MutS	Meiosis
MSH6/GTBP	MutS	Single mismatch repair
MLH1	MutL	Mismatch repair
hPMS2	MutL	Mismatch repair (postmeiotic segregation in yeast)
hPMS1	MutL	Mismatch repair (postmeiotic segregation in yeast)

arise, generating increasing numbers of alleles for the locus, or **microsatellite instability (MSI)**. In contrast, a stable locus will retain the same alleles through many rounds of replication. Microsatellite slippage occurs about every 1000 to 10,000 normal cell divisions, most of which are repaired in normal cells. Dysfunction of one or more components of the MMR system will result in MSI, an increase in the number of alleles due to lack of repair. The majority of MMR mutations in HNPCC are found in the *MSH2* and *MLH1* genes. Mutations in *hPMS2* account for fewer than 1%, and mutations in *hPMS1* and *MSH3* are rare. Although direct sequencing of the affected genes is definitive and identifies the specific mutation in a family, the test may miss mutations outside of the structural gene sequences or in other genes.[87,88]

About 90% of HNPCC cases display MSI. Because loss of MMR gene function causes MSI, MSI can be used to screen indirectly for mutations in the MMR genes. If a person has inherited a mutation in one copy of an MMR gene, somatic mutation of the remaining copy will result in the MSI phenotype in the tumor cells. MSI, therefore, will be apparent in the tumor where both functional copies of the gene have been lost but not in normal tissue that retains one normal copy of the gene. To perform this test, therefore, normal and tumor tissue from the patient must be compared. MSI is apparent from the increased number of alleles in the tumor tissue compared with that in the normal tissue. MSI is detected by PCR amplification of microsatellite loci and gel electrophoresis (Fig. 14-11) or **capillary gel electrophoresis** (Fig. 14-12). The detection of instability (more bands or peaks in the tumor tissue compared with the normal tissue) is strong evidence for HNPCC.

The National Cancer Institute has recommended that the screening of two mononucleotide repeat loci, BAT25 and BAT26, and three dinucleotide repeat loci, D5S346, D2S123, and D17S250, is sufficient for determination

■ **Figure 14-10** Replication errors result from slippage during DNA replication. If the error is not repaired, the next round of replication will create a new allele (top, right) of the original locus. Additional uncorrected errors will produce more alleles.

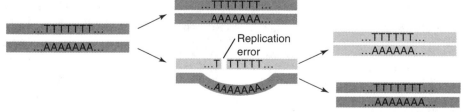

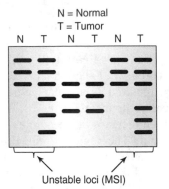

N = Normal
T = Tumor

Unstable loci (MSI)

■ **Figure 14-11** Microsatellite instability (MSI) as detected by gel electrophoresis results in increased alleles in tumor cells (T) compared with normal cells (N), as shown in the first and last pair of lanes. Stability is indicated by identical patterns in both tumor and normal cells (middle two lanes).

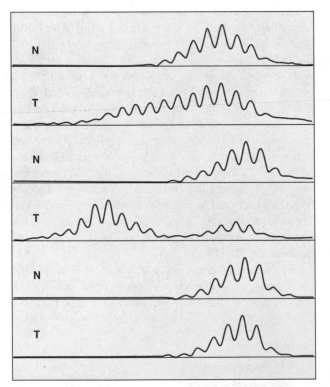

■ **Figure 14-12** MSI detected by capillary gel electrophoresis. DNA from tumor (T) is compared with DNA from normal cells from the same patient (N). Increased alleles in the tumor scans reveal instability at those loci (top four scans). Stable loci look the same in normal and tumor tissue (bottom two scans).

of MSI.[89] Alternative markers have been proposed, and some laboratories test additional loci to ensure amplification of at least five loci.[90,91] Furthermore, mononucleotide repeat structures may be more sensitive markers for MSI than dinucleotide repeats, so some laboratories prefer mononucleotide repeat loci.

If at least two of the five or at least 40% of loci show instability, the specimen is classified as high instability (MSI-H). Tumors showing MSI in one or less than 40% of loci tested are classified as low instability (MSI-L). If no MSI is detected in the loci tested, the tumor is stable (MSS). With the present state of clinical correlation, MSI-L and MSS tumors are interpreted as microsatellite-stable, and MSI-H tumors are considered microsatellite-unstable. MSI-H is reported as MSI-unstable with an increased likelihood that the patient has HNPCC.[89] If MSI is discovered, the inherited mutation can be confirmed by immunohistochemistry and/or direct sequencing of the *MLH1, MSH2,* and/or *MSH6* genes.[92]

Loss of Heterozygosity

Once a gene mutation is identified in a family, targeted resequencing is used to test for the mutation in other family members. In an inherited condition such as HNPCC or inherited breast and ovarian cancer, blood samples are sufficient for mutation analysis in unaffected individuals. In tumor cells, further testing for **loss of heterozygosity (LOH)** may be performed. LOH reveals the loss of the "good allele" at a locus, uncovering the homologous locus with a recessive mutation. LOH can be detected by PCR amplification of heterozygous STR or variable number tandem repeat (VNTR) loci closely linked to the disease gene. Amplification of loci in tumor cells with LOH will reveal a loss of the allele linked to the normal allele of the gene when compared with the mutant allele (Fig. 14-13). Comparing peak heights in normal (N) and tumor (T) tissues, the formula for LOH is:

$$\frac{\text{(peak height of normal allele in N/peak height of normal allele in T)}}{\text{(peak height of mutant allele in T/peak height of mutant allele in N)}}$$

A ratio of less than 0.5 or more than 2 indicates LOH. Alternately, LOH is assumed if the peak height of the

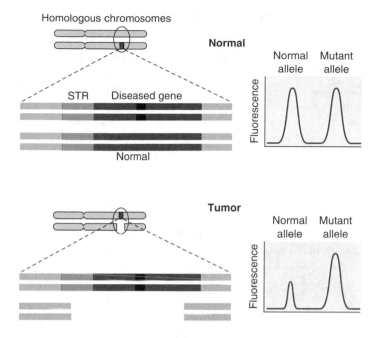

Figure 14-13 Loss of heterozygosity (LOH) is detected by PCR and capillary electrophoresis of heterozygous STR loci linked to disease genes. A deletion or loss of the normal allele uncovering a recessive mutant allele is identified by the loss of the STR linked to the normal gene (right).

normal allele in the tumor is less than 40% of the height of the normal allele in the normal DNA. Care must be taken not to mistake technical artifacts, such as allelic dropout or PCR bias, for LOH. When analyzing tumor tissue, it may be necessary to test more than one area of tumor to confirm LOH.

Gene Expression Patterns

Advances in array technology have led to applications of genomic studies to clinical testing. There is great potential in the area of molecular oncology, as subtle differences in tumor biology can affect the efficacy of chosen treatments. Targeted therapies have proven to be effective, but not in all cases due to molecular variation in tumors. For example, as described above, the drug Herceptin has been used effectively to treat *HER2/neu* positive tumors. Alternative therapies are used for *HER2/neu* negative tumors. Estrogen and progesterone expression are used in the selection of patients for endocrine therapies. Array technology has made possible the use of multigene panels, such as Oncotype DX® (Genomic Health; 21 genes) and MammaPrint® (Agendia; 70 genes), to assess gene expression patterns for prognostic predictions in patients with *HER2/neu* negative, estrogen receptor (ER), progesterone receptor (PR) positive tumors.[93] Additional arrays are being investigated to predict response to specific therapeutic agents.[94]

Tissue of Origin

Cancer cells can move from the site of the original tumor to other tissues in a process called metastasis. When malignant cells are found at a given site, they may have originated there, or, alternatively, they may have migrated there from another site or tissue. The tissue of origin of the tumor cells is important for proper treatment. There are several diagnostic tests for tumors of unknown origin. The Pathwork® Tissue of Origin Test (Pathwork Diagnostics) is a gene expression array comparison of 1500 genes in excised tumor cells to expression patterns of a panel of 15 known tissue types, representing 90% of all solid tumors. Theros CancerTYPE ID® (Bio-Theranostics) measures expression of 92 genes by qPCR to distinguish 39 different tumor types and 64 subtypes.[95] The miRview™ test (Rosetta Genomics) is based on tissue-specific microRNA (miR) expression.[96]

Molecular Targets in Hematological Malignancies

Gene Rearrangements in Leukemia and Lymphoma

Gene rearrangements analyzed for hematological malignancies include **V(D)J recombination**, the normal intrachromosomal rearrangements in B and T lymphocytes as well as the abnormal interchromosomal translocations that can occur in any cell type.

V(D)J Recombination

To develop antibody diversity, lymphocytes undergo normal genetic rearrangement of immunoglobulin (Ig) heavy and light chain genes and T-cell receptor genes (Fig. 14-14). The **gene rearrangement** process is a series of intrachromosomal recombination events mediated by recombinase enzymes that recognize specific sequences flanking the gene segments. This process occurs independently in each lymphocyte, so a repertoire of antibodies is available to match any random invading antigen.

Immunoglobulin Heavy Chain Gene Rearrangement in B Cells

Each antibody consists of two heavy chains and two light chains. The locus coding for the immunoglobulin heavy chain is located on chromosome 14. The unrearranged, or **germline**, configuration of the immunoglobulin heavy chain locus consists of a series of gene segments or repeated exons coding for the functional parts of the antibody protein (Fig. 14-15). These include 123 to 129 variable (V_H) regions (38 to 46 functional gene segments) and 9 joining (J_H) regions (6 functional), one of which will connect one variable region with a constant (C_H) region of the antibody or receptor. There are 11 constant regions (9 functional). The immunoglobulin heavy chain gene also contains 27 diversity (D_H) regions

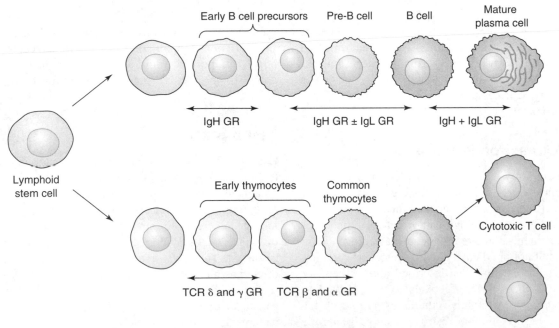

■ **Figure 14-14** Gene rearrangements (GR) are normal processes that occur in B and T lymphocytes as they mature from lymphoid stem cells. The genes coding for immunoglobulin heavy and light chains (IgH and IgL, respectively) begin the rearrangement process in early B cells and pre–B cells. The T-cell receptor (TCR) genes rearrange in the order δ, γ, β, and α chains.

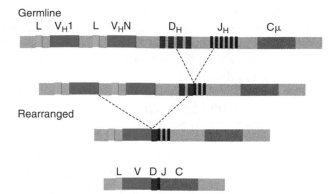

Germline

L V_H1 L V_HN D_H J_H $C\mu$

Rearranged

L V D J C

■ **Figure 14-15** The immunoglobulin heavy chain gene on chromosome 14 consists of a series of variable (V), diversity (D), and joining (J) gene segments (germline configuration). The V segments are accompanied by a short leader region (L), coding for amino acids that will direct secretion or localization of the protein. One of each type of segment V, D, and J is selected and combined by an intrachromosomal recombination event, first D and J, and then V and D. The C (constant) segments are joined through splicing or a secondary recombination event, class switching.

genes. After the V(D)J rearrangement occurs, the gene is transcribed, and one of the constant regions is joined to the final messenger RNA by splicing or, alternatively, by a secondary recombination event (class switching). The maintenance of the constant regions in the DNA allows for antibody-type switching during the immune response.

(23 functional), one of which will connect the variable and joining regions. The V segments are each preceded by a leader region (L). The leader region codes for a short sequence of amino acids found on the amino terminus of the protein that mark the antibody for secretion or membrane insertion.

As B lymphocytes mature, selected gene segments are joined together so that the rearranged gene contains only one of each V_H, D_H, and J_H segment (see Fig. 14-15). Initially, one D_H and one J_H segment are joined together. The DNA between the two segments is looped out and lost. The D_H-J_H rearrangement occurs in both alleles of the heavy chain gene locus on both chromosomes. Then a V_H segment is chosen in only one allele and joined to the D_H segment. The completion of the gene rearrangement process and expression of the rearranged gene of only one of the two homologous immunoglobulin heavy chain gene alleles is an example of **allelic exclusion**. The rearrangement on the other chromosome will proceed if the first rearrangement fails or is not productive.

When the DNA is cut in the process of the gene rearrangement, terminal deoxynucleotidyl transferase may add nucleotides at the V-D-J junctions, further diversifying the coding sequences of individual antibody

Antibody diversity is ensured by three separate events during and after the gene rearrangement process. The first is the selection of gene segments. The second is the imprecise joining of the segments together with addition of nucleotide bases at the junction.[98] Third, after the gene rearrangement process has finished and the B cell has encountered antigen, **somatic hypermutation** occurs in the variable regions of the rearranged heavy and light chain genes. This mutation process requires the action of an enzyme called activation-induced cytidine deaminase, altering C residues to base pair with A instead of G residues, resulting in different amino acid substitutions in the antibody protein. Changing of the variable region sequences underlies the process of **affinity maturation**.

As the B cells replicate, those producing antibodies with greater affinity for the antigen are favored, generating subclones of cells that may replace the original reactive clone. Over the course of an infection, therefore, antibodies with increased affinity are produced.

Immunoglobulin Light Chain Gene Rearrangement in B Cells

Like the Ig heavy chain gene on chromosome 14, the Ig light chain genes consist of series of gene segments in the germline configuration (Fig. 14-16). Two separate genes code for the Ig light chains: the kappa locus on chromosome 2 and the lambda locus on chromosome 22. At the kappa locus, there is a single constant gene segment,

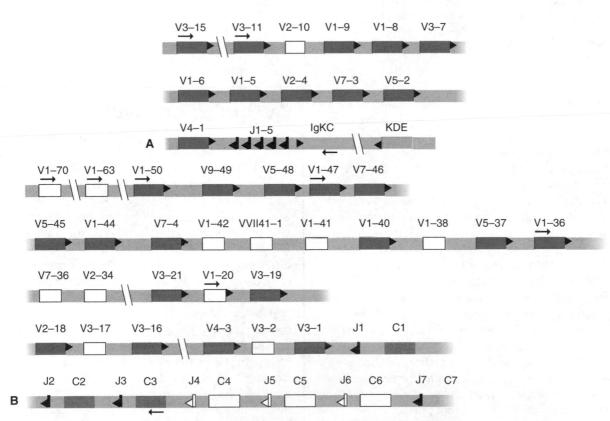

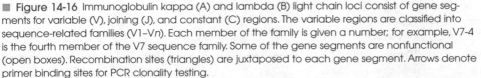

■ **Figure 14-16** Immunoglobulin kappa (A) and lambda (B) light chain loci consist of gene segments for variable (V), joining (J), and constant (C) regions. The variable regions are classified into sequence-related families (V1–V*n*). Each member of the family is given a number; for example, V7-4 is the fourth member of the V7 sequence family. Some of the gene segments are nonfunctional (open boxes). Recombination sites (triangles) are juxtaposed to each gene segment. Arrows denote primer binding sites for PCR clonality testing.

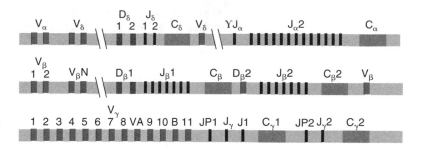

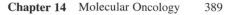

■ **Figure 14-17** *General structure of the T-cell receptor genes. The gene for the delta T-cell receptor chain is contained in the alpha locus (top). The beta and gamma chains are located at separate loci.*

5 joining (J_κ) gene segments, and at least 76 variable (V_κ) gene segments (30–35 functional) belonging to 7 sequence-related families.[99,100] In addition there is a **kappa deleting element (KDE)** located at 24 kbp 3' to the constant region. This element determines deletion of the Ig_κ constant region in cells producing Ig lambda light chains. The Ig lambda gene locus consists of 52 variable (V_λ) gene segments (29 to 33 functional) from 10 V_λ families and 7 J_λ (4 to 5 functional) and 7 to 11 C_λ gene segments (4 to 5 functional) occupying 1140-kb of DNA.[101]

The immunoglobulin light chain gene rearrangement process is similar to that of the immunoglobulin heavy chain gene rearrangement. Selected gene segments are joined together, with loss of the intervening DNA and possible insertion of nucleotides at the junction. The kappa locus rearranges first and then the lambda locus, if necessary. If the lambda locus rearranges, the kappa locus undergoes a secondary recombination through the KDE so that the cell does not produce both types of light chains.

During differentiation of the B cells from precursor stem cells, rearrangement, recombination, and mutation of the immunoglobulin V, D, and J regions ultimately result in functional VJ (light chain) and VDJ (heavy chain) genes.

T-Cell Receptor Gene Rearrangement

The T-cell receptor is composed of two of four chains—α, β, γ, and δ—with characteristic structures resembling

immunoglobulin V, J, and C regions (Fig. 14-17). The α and β chains are encoded on chromosome 14 (the δ gene is located inside of the α gene), and γ and β are located on chromosome 7. The four chains form pairs, making two types of receptors, $\alpha\beta$ and $\gamma\delta$. T-cell receptor genes have fewer variable gene segments than the immunoglobulin genes, and the genes for the γ and α chains have no diversity regions (Table 14.6). The V regions of the receptor chains undergo gene rearrangement by intrachromosomal recombination as described for the immunoglobulin genes (Fig. 14-18).

Rearrangement of the T-cell receptor chains proceeds in a manner similar to that of the immunoglobulin genes. The V, (D), and J segments are joined together with addition or deletion (**trimming**) of nucleotides at the junctions between the gene segments.

The extracellular domains of the T-cell receptor dimers are held in conformation by interchain disulfide bridges

---

Advanced Concepts

The T-cell receptor δ gene is flanked by TCRδ-deleting elements. Recombination between these elements or between Vα and Jα result in deletion of the TCRδ gene.

Table 14.6 **T-Cell Receptor Gene Segments**

T-Cell Receptor Chain	Variable Gene Segments*	Diversity Gene Segments	Joining Gene Segments*	Constant Gene Segments
α	54/45	0	60/50	1
β	67/47	2	14/13	2
δ	3	3	4	2
γ	14/6	0	5	2

*Total gene segments/functional gene segments

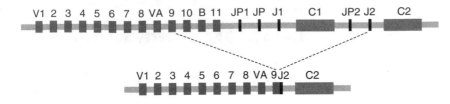

■ **Figure 14-18** T-cell receptor gamma gene rearrangement occurs through selection of variable (V) and joining (J) segments.

between cysteine residues in the T-cell receptor peptides. The T-cell receptor chains also have a hydrophobic transmembrane region and a short cytoplasmic region. Although most cells express the αβ receptor, γδ receptors can represent a predominant population in certain tissues, such as the intestinal tract.

Detection of Clonality

Gene rearrangements occur independently in each lymphocyte so that a normal population of lymphocytes is **polyclonal** with respect to their rearranged immunoglobulin or T-cell receptor genes. Overrepresentation of a single rearrangement in a specimen cell population can be an indication and characteristic of a lymphoma or leukemia. When over 1% of cells make the same gene rearrangement, the cell population is referred to as **monoclonal** with respect to the rearranged genes.

Immunoglobulin Heavy Chain Gene Rearrangements

Clonality can be detected by Southern blot.[102–104] Detection of clonality by Southern blot will be described using the immunoglobulin heavy chain gene as an example. Restriction sites have been mapped in the germline configuration of the immunoglobulin heavy chain gene on

chromosome 14 (*IGH*, 14q32). The enzymes *Bam*H1, *Eco*R1, and *Hind*III are commonly used for this procedure (Fig. 14-19). When the germline sequence is rearranged, the restriction sites are moved, created, or deleted, resulting in a unique restriction pattern for every gene rearrangement. DNA isolated from white blood cells is cut with the restriction enzymes, transferred to a nitrocellulose membrane, and hybridized with a probe to the joining region of the *IGH* gene. Normal results should reveal the expected fragments generated from the germline DNA; in the example, an 18-kbp *Eco*R1 fragment, an 18-kbp *Bam*H1 fragment, and an 11-kbp *Hind*III fragment. The normal fragments are visible for two reasons. First, a normal patient specimen contains cells other than lymphocytes that do not undergo gene rearrangement. The second reason for the presence of the germline bands is that only one chromosome in a lymphocyte undergoes gene rearrangement, leaving the homologous chromosome in the germline state. If the first rearrangement fails or is unproductive, then the

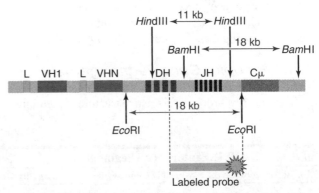

■ **Figure 14-19** Restriction map of the germline immunoglobulin heavy chain gene. The fragments indicated by the arrows will be detectable with the probe shown at the bottom. Gene rearrangement will affect the placement of the restriction sites such that fragments of different sizes will be generated from a rearranged gene.

> ## *Advanced Concepts*
>
> It is important to distinguish a large monoclonal population of tumor cells from a reactive clone or **oligoclone** of cells responding to an antigen. Oligoclones are not only smaller than leukemic or lymphomatous populations but transient in nature, so they should not be consistently present in serial analyses.

second chromosome will rearrange, an event that occurs in fewer than 10% of lymphocytes for the heavy chain gene.

Also, in a normal specimen, there will be millions of immunoglobulin gene rearrangements, so no one rearrangement is present in high enough amounts to be visible as nongermline bands on the membrane or autoradiogram; thus, only the germline bands will be visible. If, however, 2% to 5% of the cells in the specimen consist of a clone of cells all with the same gene rearrangement, that clone will be detected by the presence of additional bands different from the germline bands (Fig. 14-20). The number and location of these bands is not predictable, as they depend on the nature of the gene rearrangement in the cell giving rise to the clonal population. They are, however, characteristic of that particular monoclonal population. Interpretation of the results, therefore, is positive if bands other than germline are present, and negative if only the germline bands are present.

Advanced Concepts

Three enzymes are used for this assay to avoid false-positive results due to cross-hybridization artifacts (see Chapter 6, "Analysis and Characterization of Nucleic Acids and Proteins"). The chance of true rearranged bands being identical to cross-hybridization patterns for all three enzymes is negligible. In addition, cross-hybridization patterns are constant with the same hybridization conditions, in contrast to true monoclonal gene rearrangement bands that differ for each monoclonal population.

Analysis of clonality by Southern blot affords the advantage of detecting all gene rearrangements, including incomplete rearrangements involving only the D and J regions of the gene. The Southern blot method is limited by the requirement for at least 20 to 30 μg of high-quality DNA from the specimen. This is not always available, either because the specimen is limiting with respect to cell number or it is in poor condition, as in paraffin-embedded specimens. Gene rearrangement monoclonality is most frequently analyzed by PCR. For this method, forward primers complementary to the variable region and reverse primers complementary to the variable, joining or constant regions of the B- or T-cell–rearranged genes are used.[105] The resulting amplicons are resolved by agarose, polyacrylamide, or capillary electrophoresis. A normal cell population will yield amplicons consisting of fragments of different lengths, yielding a cloud or

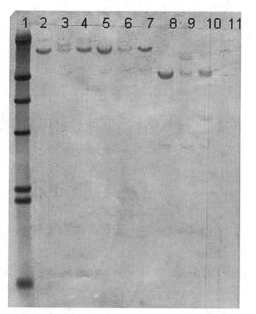

■ Figure 14-20 Results from an immunoglobulin heavy chain gene rearrangement test by Southern blot with colorimetric detection. Lane 1, molecular-weight markers. Lanes 2, 6, and 8 show the normal 18-kbp, 18-kbp, and 11-kbp bands expected from the germline gene in a normal specimen cut with EcoR1, BamH1, and HindIII, respectively. Lanes 3, 6, and 9 show patient DNA with no detectable monoclonality. Lanes 4, 7, and 10 show a patient with a monoclonal cell population.

Advanced Concepts

Other methods designed to increase detection rate for *IGH* gene rearrangements utilize primers to the leader region in addition to the FR primers.[106–108] Deletion of the *IgH* locus can occur in some lymphomas, however, precluding amplification with any primers. If the gene rearrangement cannot be amplified, clonality at the immunoglobulin heavy chain gene locus cannot be used for diagnosis or monitoring.

smear of bands. A monoclonal cell population will yield a predominant or single band or peak. The presence of the band or peak is interpreted as a positive result.

The major limitation of gene rearrangement studies by PCR is the inability to amplify all possible gene rearrangements, as primer binding sites are lost during recombination and somatic mutation. Different approaches to the variable-region primer binding sites have been taken to address this problem (Fig. 14-21). The immunoglobulin heavy chain gene variable region is divided into two types of domains. The **complementarity determining regions (CDRs)** code for the amino acids that will contact the antigen. The CDRs, therefore,

are the most variable, or unstable, in sequence. The **framework regions** (FRs) code for the amino acids that have more of a structural role in the antibody protein and are more stable in sequence. Standard methods for clonality utilize a forward **consensus primer** to the innermost framework region, FR3, and the reverse primer complementary to the joining region. Alternatively, framework 2 (FR2) or framework 1 (FR1) primers directed at the other two framework regions may be used. These primers detect those rearrangements that have lost or mutated the FR3 primer binding site.

The consensus primers have sequences that match the most frequently occurring sequences in the framework regions and may not be identical to any one sequence. Enough nucleotides will hydrogen bond, however, to match most rearrangements. Primers directed at the diversity region are useful for amplification of the germline configuration of the immunoglobulin heavy chain genes as well as D_H-J_H rearranged genes.[109] Primers complementary to the 7 family-specific sequences of the *IGH* diversity region and a primer to the 5'-most joining region (J_H1) are used to amplify the D_H-J_H junction. The primer complementary to the D_H7–27 segment, the sequences closest to the joining region, will yield a defined product from the Ig heavy chain gene in the germline configuration (Fig. 14-22). Diversity region primers are also useful for targeting incomplete rearrangements where the variable region primer binding sites are lost.[106,110]

In 2003, a primer set was designed by the European Commission BIOMED-2 group to amplify an increased number of possible immunoglobulin heavy chain

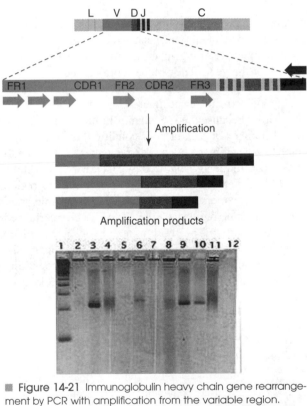

Figure 14-21 Immunoglobulin heavy chain gene rearrangement by PCR with amplification from the variable region. Forward primers complementary to the variable region and reverse primers complementary to the joining region are used to amplify the diversity region (top). In a polyclonal specimen, amplification products in a range of sizes will result. These products produce a dispersed pattern on an ethidium bromide–stained agarose gel (lanes 4, 8, 11). If at least 1% of the sample is representative of a monoclonal gene rearrangement, that product will be amplified preferentially and revealed as a sharp band by gel electrophoresis (lanes 3, 6, 9, and 10).

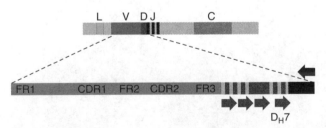

Figure 14-22 Immunoglobulin heavy chain gene rearrangement by PCR with amplification from the diversity region. Forward primers complementary to the diversity region and reverse primers complementary to the joining region yield a polyclonal pattern in normal samples. The D_H7 primer will yield a specific 350-bp product from the unrearranged (germline) gene due to the short distance between the D_H7 gene segment and the joining region primer.

gene rearrangements.[105,111,112] This set is comprised 107 primers multiplexed in 18 PCR reactions. In addition to immunoglobulin heavy chain, T-cell receptor gene rearrangements, these primers are directed at two translocations, t(14;18) and t(11;14) (see sections on translocations below).

Another approach to the detection of clonality is to make patient-specific primers. For this method, a consensus primer is used to amplify the rearranged gene from a positive specimen. The amplification product is then purified from the gel or from the PCR reaction mix and sequenced. Primers exactly matching the variable region sequence of that specimen are then manufactured for use on subsequent samples. The advantage of this method is that it is more sensitive, as fewer or none of the gene rearrangements from normal cells are amplified. Furthermore, the tumor load can be measured quantitatively by real-time PCR. The disadvantage of this approach is that the method is more time-consuming to perform and the primers used are patient-specific. Moreover, in a patient with a chronic condition, who is likely to undergo monitoring, tumors cells may undergo mutation in the variable region that will inactivate the specific primer binding, requiring manufacture of new primers.

Immunoglobulin Light Chain Gene Rearrangements

The immunoglobulin light chain genes are also targets for clonality detection.[113–115] In addition to Southern blot, PCR and RT-PCR have been used to detect light chain gene clonality. Targeting the immunoglobulin light chain genes is especially useful for tumors arising from terminally differentiated B cells (plasma cells) that have undergone extensive somatic hypermutation at the heavy chain gene locus. In these tumors, the rearranged heavy chain genes are frequently unamplifiable, yielding false-negative results because of accumulation of base changes in the variable region primer binding sites. Many of these tumor cell gene rearrangements are amplifiable, however, at the light chain genes.[116]

Gene rearrangements in the kappa light chain locus are amplified using primers complementary to the sequence families of the V_κ region or to the intron between the J_κ regions and C_κ. Opposing primers are complementary to C_κ and to one or more of the five joining regions. Alternatively, the KDE can be used for a primer binding site (Fig. 14-23). Using the KDE allows detection of lambda-expressing cells that have deleted J_κ or C_κ.[117]

Approximately one-third of B-cell malignancies have Ig_λ gene rearrangements.[118] Ig_λ gene rearrangements are also present in 5% to 10% of kappa-expressing B cell tumors. Therefore, detection of clonality at the Ig_κ locus on chromosome 22 is also useful for confirming or monitoring diagnosis of B-cell leukemias and lymphomas. Forward primers complementary to V_λ gene segments and reverse primers to the J_λ and C_λ gene segments are frequently used for these assays (Fig. 14-24).

T-Cell Receptor Gene Rearrangements

T-cell receptor gene rearrangements are performed in a manner similar to the immunoglobulin gene rearrangements by Southern blot and PCR.[119–121] For Southern

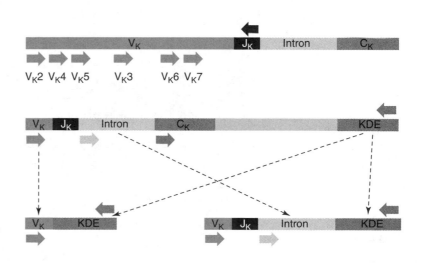

■ Figure 14-23 The immunoglobulin light chain kappa locus can be amplified by standard PCR procedures from the variable region, the intronic region, or the kappa deleting element.

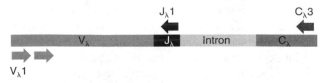

■ **Figure 14-24** The immunoglobulin light chain lambda locus can be amplified by standard PCR procedures from the variable region to the joining region or the constant region. Reverse transcriptase PCR is used with the constant region primers to eliminate the intron between the constant and joining regions.

blot studies, probes complementary to the variable, joining, and diversity regions of the T-cell receptor genes have been used to detect monoclonal populations. Just as with immunoglobulin gene rearrangements, no one gene rearrangement should be visible in a normal specimen. The presence of a large monoclonal population is revealed by the bands detectable in addition to the germline bands seen in the normal control (Fig. 14-25).

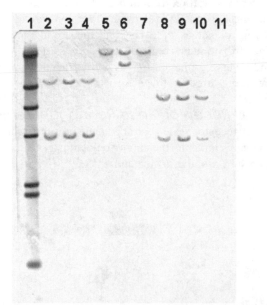

■ **Figure 14-25** T-cell receptor gene rearrangements detected by Southern blot using a probe mixture of sequences complementary to $J_\beta 1$ and $J_\beta 2$. Lane 1, molecular-weight markers. Lanes 2, 5, and 8, normal control cut with EcoR1, BamH1, and HindIII, respectively. Lanes 3, 6, and 9, a positive specimen cut with EcoR1, BamH1, and HindIII, respectively. Lanes 4, 7, and 10, negative specimen cut with EcoR1, BamH1, and HindIII, respectively. Note the additional bands in the positive specimen lanes.

The T-cell receptor gene rearrangement assays done by PCR target most often the TCRγ gene. Assays are also performed on the TCRβ and TCRδ genes. Detection of gene rearrangements in TCRα is difficult due to the 85-kb length of the Jα gene segments. TCRα gene rearrangements may be inferred from TCRδ gene deletions.[121] Primers are designed complementary to the rearranged gene segments (Fig. 14-26). Multiple primer sets are often used to ensure detection of the maximum potential gene rearrangement.[122] PCR will yield a product consistent with a single gene rearrangement in a positive sample, whereas a normal sample will yield a polyclonal pattern (Fig. 14-27). Due to the limited range of lengths of the population of rearranged T-cell receptor genes, heteroduplex analysis, SSCP, or DGGE may be used to improve resolution of the polyclonal and monoclonal patterns.[123]

PCR Amplicon Banding Patterns

Interpretation of clonality by PCR depends on gel banding patterns. As shown in Figures 14-21 and 14-27, amplification of a polyclonal cell population will yield a series of amplicons that resolve over a range of sizes (smear) after electrophoresis. If at least 1% of the cells in the sample have the same gene rearrangement, the product will resolve to a sharp (clonal) band on the gel. The size of the clonal product should be within the range of the smear; however, rare products may appear slightly outside this range.[124]

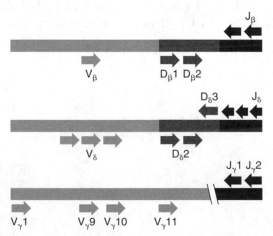

■ **Figure 14-26** T-cell receptor beta and delta gene rearrangements detected by PCR use primers to the variable, diversity, and joining regions of the rearranged genes. Some assays use multiple primers to the TCR gamma variable region.

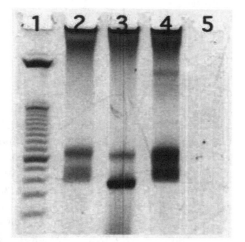

■ **Figure 14-27** T-cell receptor gene rearrangement by PCR and heteroduplex analysis. Bands were separated by polyacrylamide gel electrophoresis and stained with ethidium bromide. Lanes 2 and 4 show a polyclonal pattern. A positive result (monoclonal pattern) is shown in lane 3. Lane 1, molecular-weight marker; lane 5, reagent blank.

False-negative polyclonal patterns or the absence of bands may result from primers that do not match the gene rearrangement in the tumor. Another complication in interpretation of the banding patterns is the presence of artifactual single bands that are misinterpreted as true clonal bands. Patterns of multiple single bands may arise from specimens with low cell numbers, such as cerebrospinal fluids or paraffin sections. In this case, usually more than one or two single bands occur. The bands may not indicate monoclonality, rather that only a few cells are present. These cells may or may not be malignant. False-positive single band patterns may also occur within polyclonal smears detected on nondenaturing polyacrylamide gels (PAGE). Heteroduplex analysis is recommended if amplicons are resolved by nondenaturing PAGE.

Similar problems occur with resolution by capillary electrophoresis where peak heights and widths are compared to distinguish wide polyclonal peaks from narrow monoclonal spikes.[125] Pretreatments such as eosin staining may yield false single bands by capillary electrophoresis.[126]

Translocations in Hematological Malignancies

Gene rearrangements in immunoglobulin and T-cell receptor genes are normal and take place regardless of the presence of malignancy. The unique nature of the gene rearrangement system with cell-specific antibody and antibody receptor formation are exploited to find abnormal cell populations clonally derived from these cell-specific features. Targeting these gene rearrangements, however, can only be applied to tumors arising from lymphocytes. Other types of malignancies, such as myeloid tumors, cannot be analyzed using these targets.

Often, development of the cancer state results in DNA anomalies (translocations or other types of mutations) that can be applied to clinical discovery and monitoring of tumors. These abnormal genetic events aid in diagnosis of specific types of hematological tumors, such as the translocations that are highly associated with chronic myelogenous leukemia, promyelocytic leukemia, or follicular lymphoma. Furthermore, these mutations usually involve tumor suppressor genes and oncogenes and this has helped to determine the molecular events leading to the tumor phenotype.

Translocations are the exchange of DNA between chromosomes (see Chapter 8, "Chromosomal Structure and Chromosomal Mutations"). If the translocation disrupts activity or expression of oncogenes or tumor suppressor genes, a cancer phenotype can occur. Several translocations are frequently found in certain types of tumors.

t(14;18)(q32;q21)

The reciprocal translocation between the long arms of chromosomes 14 and 18 moves and disregulates the *BCL2* gene located on chromosome 18q21.3. *BCL2* (B-cell leukemia and lymphoma 2 or B-cell CLL/lymphoma 2) is an oncogene. The gene product of *BCL2* is a member of a group of related proteins that control apoptosis (cell death initiated by internal cellular signals). The Bcl2 protein inhibits apoptosis in B lymphocytes, that is, enhances survival of cells. Survival of genetically damaged cells that normally would die from apoptosis but are surviving due to overexpression of anti-apoptotic factors such as Bcl2 may contribute to the development of tumors. One of the most frequent hematological malignancies, follicular lymphoma, is associated with the t(14;18) translocation.

The partner of chromosome 18 in this translocation is chromosome 14. The breakpoint of chromosome 14 is in the vicinity of the immunoglobulin heavy chain gene. The translocation may occur through cryptic recognition sites on chromosome 18 for the gene rearrangement

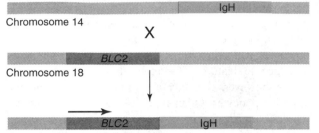

t(14;18) translocated chromosome

■ **Figure 14-28** The t(14;18) translocation moves the *BCL2* gene intact to the long arm of chromosome 14 next to the joining region of the immunoglobulin heavy chain gene (IgH). The translocation breakpoints on chromosome 18 are 3' to the *BCL2* gene (arrow indicating the direction of transcription).

recombinase enzymes that normally work on chromosome 14 during the gene rearrangement process. As a result, an abnormal interchromosomal exchange occurs, instead of the normal intrachromosomal exchange events of the gene rearrangement (Fig. 14-28). There are several breakpoints in the chromosome 18 region 3' to the *BCL2* gene, most of which occur in the major breakpoint region (MBR). About 10% to 20% of the breakpoints fall into a cluster closer to the *BCL2* gene, thousands of bases from the MBR, in the minor cluster region (MCR). An intermediate cluster region (ICR) and other breakpoints outside of MBR and MCR have also been reported.[127,128]

Molecular detection of the t(14;18) translocation is performed by cytogenetic procedures, including karyotyping and FISH, as well as Southern blot or PCR. Karyotyping and FISH methods are described in Chapter 8. The t(14;18) karyotype will have one abnormal chromosome 14 and one abnormal chromosome 18 due to the reciprocal translocation. The translocation is detected as a combining of probes for chromosome 14 and chromosome 18 (Fig. 14-29). Unlike genetic diseases, where all cells will have the mutation, all cells in the specimen do not necessarily have the translocation.

For Southern blot, a probe to the MBR region of chromosome 18 will reveal the translocation by the presence of bands different from those expected from normal chromosome 18 (Fig. 14-30). Although the Southern blot procedure has the advantage of detecting all breakpoints, the translocation is more easily and rapidly detected by PCR. Primers to chromosome 18 paired with primers complementary to the Ig heavy chain joining region will yield a product only if the two chromosomes have been joined by the translocation. The amplicons are visualized by gel electrophoresis, as shown in Figure 14-31, or by capillary electrophoresis, the latter method requiring fluorescent labeling of one of the PCR primers.

The t(14;18) translocation can also be detected using real-time PCR. Several methods are available for this analysis, and although laboratory methods differ, results are reasonably consistent in comparison testing.[129,130] Most methods include a standard curve for regression analysis of the test sample measurements (Fig. 14-32). Alternatively, internal controls, such as known amounts of plasmid DNA, may be added to the test specimens. In this method, the amount of translocated cells (or translocated chromosomes) is determined relative to the internal control. There are also several approaches to reporting final results. Most frequently, results are reported as percent translocated cells in the specimen tested. For instance, the raw number of translocated cells is determined by linear regression analysis. The raw number of

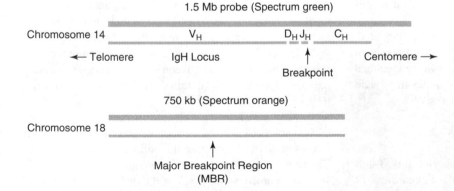

■ **Figure 14-29** Fluorogenic probes for detection of the t(14;18) translocation (Abbott Molecular). The chromosome 14 probe covering the region of the immunoglobulin heavy chain gene has a green signal. The chromosome 18 probe displays an orange signal. Normal cells will have two green and two orange signals. The translocation is revealed by a combination of one orange and one green signal in the nucleus.

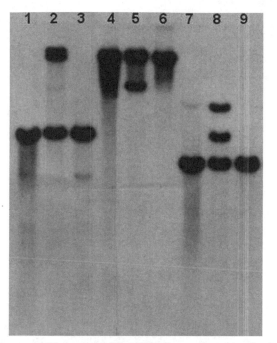

■ **Figure 14-30** Analysis of the t(14;18) gene translocation by Southern blot with chemiluminescent detection. Lanes 1, 4, and 7 are the normal control cut with *Eco*R1, *Bam*H1, and *Hin*dlll, respectively. Lanes 3, 6, and 9 show results from a normal patient specimen. Lanes 2, 5, and 8 are results from a specimen positive for the t(14;18) translocation. Note the extra bands in the positive specimen.

cells is then divided by the number of total cells represented in the PCR reaction.

For example, a dilution series ranging from 50 to 10,000 translocated cells in 1 million untranslocated cells generates a standard curve with the formula $y = 1.5631 \ln(x) + 42.396$, where y is the threshold cycle number (see Chapter 7, "Nucleic Acid Amplification") and x is the number of translocated cells (using 50 ng of DNA per sample). According to this formula, if a given sample crosses the fluorescent threshold at $y = 36$ cycles (average of duplicate measurements), the number of cells (x) is approximately 60. Assuming that 50 ng of DNA represents 7500 cells (1 ng of DNA = approximately 150 cells), $60/7500 = 0.008$. $0.008 \times 100 = 0.8\%$ translocated cells in the specimen. For the t(14;18) translocation, sensitivities of 0.0025% have been reported, with a linear range of 0.01% to 10%.[131] Data are accumulating to determine the clinical significance of the qualitative and quantitative results.[132–134]

The main limitation of any PCR procedure targeting the t(14;18) translocation is the inability of the primers to detect all of the possible breakpoints on chromosome 18. Several primer pairs and sets of primer pairs have been designed to address this problem.[105] Test reports should include an estimation of false-negative results expected due to breakpoints that remove the binding sites for the primers used. Unless a translocation has been previously observed by a given PCR method, a negative result may be reported with the disclaimer that a translocation may be present but undetectable with the primers used. Translocations with breakpoints not recognized by PCR primers may still be detected by FISH or karyotyping for diagnostic purposes.

t(9;22)(q34;q11)

The t(9;22) translocation is a reciprocal exchange between the long arms of chromosomes 9 and 22. The translocation generates the Philadelphia chromosome (Ph1), which is present in 95% of cases of chronic myelogenous leukemia (CML), 25% to 30% of adult acute lymphoblastic leukemia (ALL), and 2%–10% of pediatric ALL. The breakpoints of the t(9;22) translocation occur within two genes: the breakpoint cluster region (*BCR*) gene on chromosome 22 and the cellular counterpart of the Abelson leukemia virus tyrosine kinase (c-*abl*) on chromosome 9 (Fig. 14-33). The result of the translocation is a chimeric or fusion gene with the head of the *BCR* gene and the tail of the c-*abl* gene. Both *BCR* and c-*abl* genes are tyrosine kinases; that is, they phosphorylate other genes at tyrosine residues. The fusion gene is also a kinase but has aberrant kinase activity.

There are two major forms of the *BCR/ABL* fusion gene, joining either exon 13 or 14 (b2 or b3) of the *BCR* gene to c-*abl* exon 2 (a2; Figure 14-34). The b2a2 or b3a2 fusion genes code for a 210 kilodalton protein, p210. A third form of the fusion gene joins exon 1 of *BCR* with exon a2 of c-*abl*, resulting in expression of an e1a2 transcript, which codes for a p190 protein. Another, less common, fusion junction occurs at exon 19 of the *BCR* gene (c3). The c3a2 transcript encodes a p230 protein. All of the fusion proteins have been observed in CML; however, p190 occurs mostly in ALL.

Detection of the t(9;22) translocation can be performed by karyotyping, FISH, Southern blot and PCR as described above for detection of t(14;18). A t(9;22) karyotype will have the Philadelphia chromosome and one

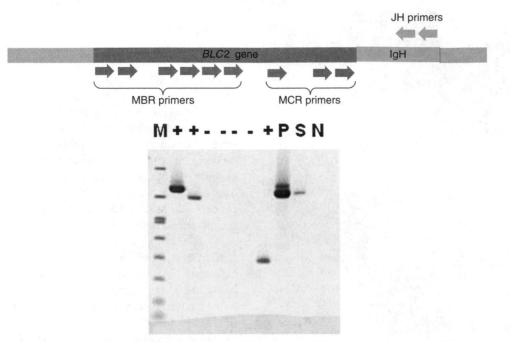

■ **Figure 14-31** Analysis of the t(14;18) gene translocation by PCR with agarose gel electrophoresis. Several primers are used for detection of the translocated chromosome (top). Because the forward primers are on chromosome 18 and the reverse primers are on chromosome 14, a PCR product will be generated only from the t(14;18) translocated chromosome (bottom). M, molecular-weight marker; +, positive specimen; –, negative specimen; P, positive control; S, sensitivity control; N, negative control.

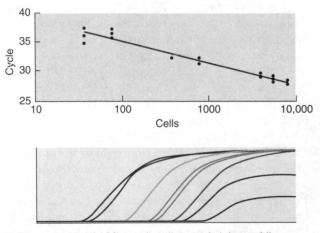

■ **Figure 14-32** t(14;18) translocation analysis by real-time PCR. A standard curve is established using cultured cells with the t(13;18) translocation (Dhl-6) counted and diluted into cultured cells without the translocation (HL-60). The results shown are from DNA isolated from each mixture of cells and analyzed by real-time PCR using a TaqMan probe.

abnormal chromosome 9. The translocation detected by FISH analysis with probes complementary to *BCR* and *abl* sequences is detected by the combining of the two probe colors.

Southern blot is performed using a probe to the breakpoint area, for instance, a 1.2-kb fragment complementary to the 3' end of the *BCR* gene. Restriction fragment patterns will differ in translocated cells (Fig. 14-35). Other probes to *BCR* may also be used to ensure detection of all breakpoints.

The rationale described above for t(14;18) translation detection by PCR is used for t(9;22); that is, forward primers are designed to hybridize to the *BCR* gene on chromosome 22 and reverse primers to chromosome 9 in the c-*abl* gene (Fig. 14-36). A product will result only if the two genes are joined by the translocation. Unlike the *BCL2* gene translocation break point, which is 3' to the intact gene, the breakpoints in the BCR and *abl* genes are within the genes, particularly in introns. The primer

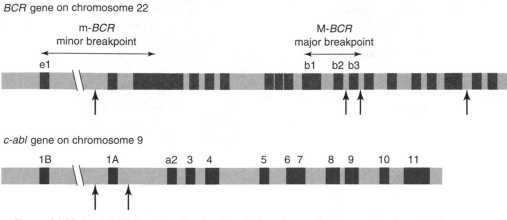

BCR gene on chromosome 22

m-BCR
minor breakpoint

M-BCR
major breakpoint

e1

b1 b2 b3

c-abl gene on chromosome 9

1B   1A   a2 3 4   5   6 7   8 9   10   11

■ Figure 14-33 The t(9;22) translocation begins with breakage of chromosomes 9 and 22 in introns of the BCR and c-abl genes (arrows). The breakpoints are located within introns of both genes.

binding sites are located in the exons closest to the breakpoints of the two genes. Due to the length of the introns that separate the primer binding sites, RT-PCR has been commonly utilized.[135,136] To minimize the risk of

false-positive results, this method may require confirmatory testing, especially for adult ALL.[137]

Several recommendations for optimal performance have been proposed, including the use of primers capable

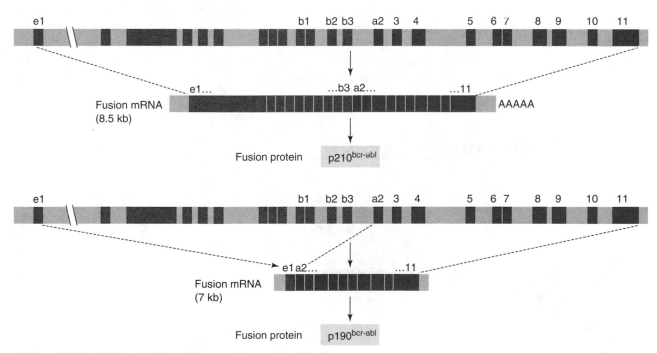

e1   b1 b2 b3 a2 3 4   5 6 7 8 9   10   11

Fusion mRNA
(8.5 kb)

e1...   ...b3 a2...   ...11   AAAAA

Fusion protein   p210bcr-abl

e1   b1 b2 b3 a2 3 4   5 6 7 8 9   10   11

e1 a2...   ...11

Fusion mRNA
(7 kb)

Fusion protein   p190bcr-abl

■ Figure 14-34 p210 and p190 are the two main fusion proteins produced by the t(9;22) translocation. They differ in the amount of the BCR gene that is attached to the c-abl gene.

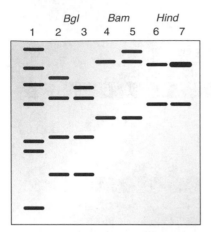

■ **Figure 14-35** Southern blot of a t(9;22) translocation with a probe to the 3′ end of the *BCR* gene. Lane 1, molecular-weight marker; lanes 2, 4, and 6, normal control cut with *Bgl*II, *Bam*H1, and *Hind*III, respectively; lanes 3, 5, and 7, a specimen positive for the translocation cut with *Bgl*II, *Bam*H1, and *Hind*III, respectively. Note the shift in the sizes of the bands in lanes 3 and 5 compared with lanes 2 and 4. (A doublet is not quite resolved from the larger band in lane 7.)

of detecting both major and minor breakpoints in the *BCR* gene and an internal **RNA integrity control** (or amplification control) to avoid false-negative results from poor RNA quality or inadequate cDNA synthesis.[138,139] Transcripts from the *abl* or *BCR* genes are used most frequently for RNA integrity control for the t(9;22) translocation, but any unique gene with constitutive

expression may be used. Target amplicons can be detected by agarose gel electrophoresis and ethidium bromide staining (Fig. 14-37) or by capillary gel electrophoresis. Fluorescent dye–labeled primers are required for the latter detection method.

Quantification by real-time PCR provides an estimation of treatment response, especially with imatinib and other targeted therapies for CML and ALL. Although cytogenetic methods, especially FISH and standard RT-PCR, are most practical for diagnosis and in the early stages of treatment, quantitative PCR provides a valuable estimation of tumor load over the course of treatment.[140,141] Several commercial reagent sets are available for t(9;22) detection by qRT-PCR. The Roche LightCycler® - t(9;22) Quantification Kit provides all reagents for cDNA and PCR in mixes requiring only addition of sample RNA. The Ipsogen FusionQuant® kits can be used on multiple instruments in addition to the Light Cycler.

Because transcript levels are being measured using qRT-PCR, it is important to stabilize the specimen RNA on receipt, for example by re-suspending the white blood cells in protective buffers (see Chapter 4, Nucleic Acid Extraction Methods). Another recommendation is to collect at least 10 mL of peripheral blood for analysis to avoid false-negative results.[142] A standard curve or a high and low positive control and negative control should accompany each run. Frequently used TaqMan methods report measurements as a ratio of the *BCR-abl* transcript

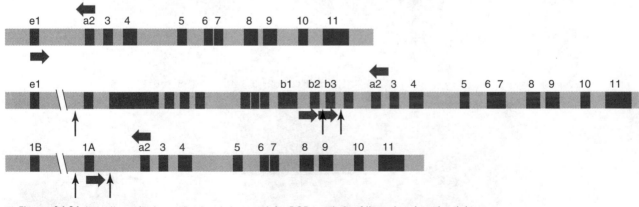

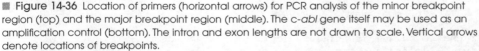

■ **Figure 14-36** Location of primers (horizontal arrows) for PCR analysis of the minor breakpoint region (top) and the major breakpoint region (middle). The c-*abl* gene itself may be used as an amplification control (bottom). The intron and exon lengths are not drawn to scale. Vertical arrows denote locations of breakpoints.

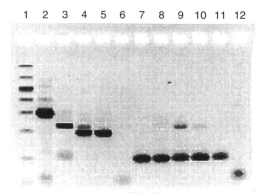

1 2 3 4 5 6 7 8 9 10 11 12

■ **Figure 14-37** Results of a standard RT-PCR test for the t(9;22) translocation. Lane 1, molecular-weight marker; lane 2, b3a2 breakpoints; lane 3, b2a2 breakpoints; lanes 4 and 5, e1a2 breakpoints; lane 6, negative specimen; lanes 7 to 11 are RNA integrity (amplification) controls for specimens in lanes 2 to 6; lane 12, reagent blank.

level to the RNA integrity control, usually the *abl* transcript, the *BCR* transcript, or the transcript of a housekeeping gene, such as *G6PDH*.[141,143-145] For example, a standard curve for transcript number generates the formula, $y = -1.7318\text{Ln}(x) + 48.627$, where y is the threshold cycle number and x is the number of transcripts. If quantitative PCR analysis of the patient specimen RNA yielded a threshold cycle number of 39 (average of duplicate samples) for *BCR-abl* transcripts and a threshold cycle number of 30 for the *abl* transcripts, then solving for x yields 300 *BCR-abl* transcripts and 50,000 *abl* transcripts in the sample. Thus, $(300/50,000) \times 100 = 0.6\%$. A three-log drop in transcript levels or a *BCR-abl/abl* × 100 level below 0.05% has been proposed as indicative of good prognosis.[146,147]

Imatinib response is affected by several resistance mechanisms, including overexpression of the *BCR-abl*

Advanced Concepts

A slightly different formula, $[BCR\text{-}abl/(abl \times BCR\text{-}abl)] \times 100$, for the transcript ratio is used if the *abl* primers also amplify the *BCR-abl* translocation.[148] In the calculation shown in the text, *BCR-abl/abl* × 100 yields 0.6%; $[BCR\text{-}abl/(abl - BCR\text{-}abl)] \times 100$ yields 0.85%.

kinase protein and decreased cellular uptake or increased cellular elimination of the drug. The most common mechanism of resistance to imatinib is the presence of resistance mutations in the *abl* kinase portion of the gene. Over 50 different *abl* kinase mutations have been found in patients showing resistance to imatinib. Second- and third-generation *abl* kinase inhibitors have been designed to be effective against these resistant tumors.[149] Direct sequencing is the recommended method for *abl* kinase mutation detection; however, other assays have been proposed, including allele-specific PCR[150] and Invader technology.[151]

t(15;17)(q22;q11.2-q12)

The reciprocal translocation between the long arms of chromosomes 15 and 17 results in fusion of the retinoic acid receptor alpha (*RARA*) gene on chromosome 15 with the myelocytic leukemia (*MYL*, or *PML*) gene on chromosome 17. Both genes contain zinc finger binding motifs and therefore bind DNA as transcription factors. The *PML/RARA* fusion is found in promyelocytic leukemia. The presence of this translocation is also a predictor of the response to retinoic acid therapy. The translocation forms a fusion gene with the first three (type A or S translocation) or six (type B or L translocation) exons of the *PML* gene joining to exons 2–6 of the *RARA* gene (Fig. 14-38).

Test methods similar to those described above for *BCR-abl* translocation are used to detect t(15;17), most frequently reverse transcriptase PCR and quantitative reverse transcriptase PCR. Primers complementary to sequences in exon 3 or 6 of the *PML* gene and exon 2 of *RARA* generate products only if the translocation has occurred. The presence of the translocation product, therefore, is interpreted as a positive result. As with any test of this type, an amplification control is required to avoid false-negative results. For quantitative PCR, results normalized to an internal control, using calculations as described above, yield the most consistent day-to-day results (lowest coefficient of variance).[152] The PML-RARA FusionQuant®Kits (Ipsogen) are premixed reagents designed to detect multiple breakpoints.

t(11;14)(q13;q32)

This translocation joins the immunoglobulin heavy chain gene region on chromosome 14 with part of the long arm of chromosome 11. The cyclin D1 (*CCND1*) gene, also called the parathyroid adenomatosis 1 gene

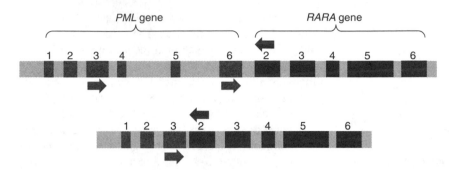

■ **Figure 14-38** Location of primers for PCR analysis of the long (top) and the short (bottom) translocated *PML* and *RARA* genes. The first three or six exons of the *PML* gene are fused to exon 2 of the *RARA* gene. The intron and exon lengths are not drawn to scale.

(*PRAD 1*) or *BCL1*, on chromosome 11 is attached to the long arm of chromosome 14 in the intron between the immunoglobulin heavy chain gene joining region and constant region. The translocation increases expression of *CCND1*, resulting in passage of the cell cycle from the G1 to the S phase of the cell cycle. This translocation is found primarily in mantle cell lymphoma (MCL) but may also be present in chronic lymphocytic leukemia, B-prolymphocytic leukemia, plasma cell leukemia, multiple myeloma, and splenic lymphoma. The t(11;14) translocation is thought to be a definite characteristic of MCL; however, only 50% to 70% of MCLs have a detectable t(11;14).

Methods for detection of t(11;14) are similar to those described above used for t(14;18) translocation. Cytogenetic karyotyping and FISH studies are useful for initial diagnosis and monitoring, respectively. Southern blot methods have been replaced mostly with PCR and RT-PCR methods.[156] In situ hybridization to detect an increase in *CCDN1* transcription has also been proposed.[157] Of the breakpoints on chromosome 11, 80% are in the major translocation cluster 5' to the *CCND1* gene (Fig. 14-39). The rest are dispersed in other areas 5' or 3' to the gene. PCR analysis detects 40% to 60% of the translocation breakpoints.[158] A PCR product will result only if the translocation has occurred (and the primer binding sites are maintained) and can be detected by gel or capillary electrophoresis.

t(8;14)(q24;q11)

The avian myelocytomatosis viral oncogene homolog (*c-myc*) gene on chromosome 8 is one member of a gene family that includes *n-myc* and *l-myc*. The *c-myc* gene codes for a helix-loop-helix/leucine zipper transcription factor that binds to another protein, Max, and activates transcription of other genes. The t(8;14) is

Advanced Concepts

In this translocation, the reciprocal fusion gene *RARA/PML* is also expressed in 70%–80% of cases of APL. Nonreciprocal events can produce either fusion alone as well.[153,154] Although the reciprocal fusion may participate in the tumorigenesis process, it does not predict response to all transretinoic acid therapy.[155] The presence of the reverse transcript may be used to confirm the translocation and could be useful in cases where the *PML/RARA* transcript is poorly expressed.

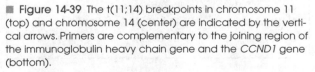

■ **Figure 14-39** The t(11;14) breakpoints in chromosome 11 (top) and chromosome 14 (center) are indicated by the vertical arrows. Primers are complementary to the joining region of the immunoglobulin heavy chain gene and the *CCND1* gene (bottom).

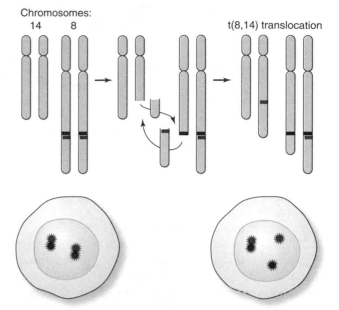

Figure 14-40 The t(8;14) breakpoint detected by CISH (Invitrogen). Two probes labeled with biotin or digoxigenin are complementary to sequences flanking the chromosome 14 breakpoint. In the absence of the translocation (left), the probes will appear next to one another in the nucleus. The translocation (right) will move one probe to chromosome 14, leaving the other behind on chromosome 8, resulting in separation of the signals in the nucleus.

associated with Burkitt lymphoma; in addition, translocations at (2;8) and t(8;22) are found in about 10% of Burkitt lymphomas.

In the t(8;14) translocation, the breakpoints on chromosome 8 are spread over a 190-kbp region 5' to and within the *c-myc* gene. As a result of the t(8;14) translocation, the *c-myc* gene is separated from its normal promoter and regulatory region and moved into the switch recombination region of the immunoglobulin heavy chain gene on chromosome 14. In the t(2;8) and the t(8;22) translocations, the chromosome 8 breakpoints are 3' to the gene, and *c-myc* is moved into the immunoglobulin kappa locus on chromosome 2 or lambda locus on chromosome 22. Translocations of *c-myc* into the T-cell receptor alpha gene have also been reported.[162]

In the laboratory, *c-myc* translocations have been commonly detected by Southern blot analysis with a probe complementary to exon 3 of the *c-myc* gene, for instance, a [32]P- or digoxigenin-labeled 1.4-kb *Cla*I-*Eco*RI restriction fragment. Interphase FISH and CISH (Invitrogen) can also be used to detect the t(8;14) translocation with separate probes to chromosomes 8 and 14 or with chromosome 14 probe pairs (Fig. 14-40).[163] Overexpression of *c-myc* is detectable by Northern blot.[164] Amplification of the gene can be detected by FISH using a 120-kb *c-myc* (8q24.12-q24.13) probe labeled with Spectrum Orange (Vysis).[165]

Gene Mutations in Hematological Malignancies

FMS-related Tyrosine Kinase 3 (FLT3), 13q12

Four classes of growth factor receptor tyrosine kinases have been categorized (see Figure 14-2).[166] One class,

represented by the ERBB family, was described in earlier sections. A second class includes dimeric receptors such as the insulin growth factor receptor as well as several proto-oncogenes. Members of the third class, including FMS, PDGF, FLT1, and KIT, display five immunoglobulin-like domains in the extracellular region, and the catalytic domain is interrupted by a hydrophilic "interkinase" sequence of variable length. The fibroblast growth factor receptors represent the fourth class, which differ from the third class by having only three immunoglobulin-like domains in the extracellular region and a short kinase insert in the intracellular domain. FLT3 is a member of the third class of tyrosine kinase receptors.[167]

Mutations in *FLT3* aberrantly activate the FLT3 kinase and predict poor prognosis in AML. *FLT3* mutations may also be prognostic in some cases of APL.[168] These mutations include internal tandem duplications (ITD) close to the transmembrane domain or point mutations affecting an aspartic acid residue in the kinase domain (D835 mutations). The ITD can easily be detected by PCR with primers flanking the potentially duplicated region. The size of the amplicon observed by agarose or capillary gel electrophoresis will increase in the event of an ITD.[169] D835 mutations can be detected by PCR-RFLP, where an *Eco*RV restriction site is destroyed by the presence of the mutation or by real-time PCR with FRET probes.[170] In performing these assays, it is important to have adequate representation of tumor cells in the specimen to avoid false-negative results from the presence of an excess of normal cells.

Nucleophosmin/Nucleoplasmin Family, Member 1 (NPM1), 5q35

Nucleophosmin is a nucleolar phosphoprotein that is likely involved with ribosomal assembly. It may also participate in centrosome duplication. *NPM1* mutations are found in 46% to 60% of cytogencially normal AML patients. *NPM1* mutations in patients that lack *FLT3*-ITD are associated with a significantly improved outcome. *NPM1* mutations are detected by direct sequencing or PCR and fragment analysis.

CCAAT/Enhancer-Binding Protein, Alpha (CEBPA), 19q13.1

Mutations in *CEBPA* are found in 15% to 18% of cases of cytogenetically normal AML and are associated with a favorable prognosis. *CEBPA* mutations define a category of "acute myeloid leukemia with mutated *CEBPA*" in the 2008 WHO Classification.[171] *CEBPA* mutations in leukemic cells are detected by a combination of PCR amplification, fragment analysis, and direct sequencing of the coding and junctional regions of the *CEBPA* gene. *CEBPA* gene mutations are prognostic in dual *FLT3*-ITD–negative, *NPM1*-negative specimens.

Janus Kinase 2 (JAK2), 9p24

The *JAK2* gene codes for a kinase enzyme that phosphorylates several Signal Transducer and Activator of Transcription (*STAT*) gene products, bringing about cellular responses. A high proportion of patients with polycythemia vera, essential thrombocythemia, or idiopathic myelofibrosis carry a dominant mutation causing a valine-to-phenylalamine amino acid substitution at position 617 of the Jak2 protein (V617F).[172,173] Detection of this mutation aids in the diagnosis of these myeloproliferative disorders. A convenient method of detection is multiplex sequence-specific PCR. This assay uses four primers, one forward and one reverse primer flanking the region of the mutation, one forward primer ending at the mutation site complementary to the normal base, and a fourth reverse primer also ending at the site of the mutation but complementary to the mutant base. The mutation is revealed as the product of the fourth reverse primer and the outer forward primer (see Chapter 9, Figure 9-12). This approach is also applied in real-time PCR methods that result in detection of the mutation by fluorescence. However, they may miss the V617F mutation when other abnormalities are present.[174]

In some laboratories, white blood cells are fractionated in order to perform JAK2 testing specifically on the granulocyte fraction in order to better assess the heterozygous state of the mutation. Heterozygosity is determined by a mutant band/normal band intensity ratio of approximately 1. The importance of the mutant/normal ratio is based on more recent data suggesting that the heterozygous/homozygous state of the V617F mutation has implications regarding which myeloproliferative disorder is present.[175] Furthermore, very low levels of V617F may be found in normal individuals.[176]

Four mutations affecting exon 12 of *JAK2* identified in some V617F-negative patients were originally reported:

Advanced Concepts

Targeted therapies are agents designed to eradicate tumor cells by recognizing unique aberrrations not present in normal cells. A drawback to the use of these agents is that patients may have tumors that lack particular abnormalities recognized by the therapeutic agent. The growing use of targeted therapies for cancer makes the mutation status of each individual an important factor in determining treatment. Array technology has been applied to mutational screening on a research basis but not yet in the medical laboratory. For example, the Sequenom OncoCarta™ Panel uses MassArray technology (see Chapter 9) to screen for 238 mutations in 19 genes known to affect outcome in various cancer types. This panel has been extended to cover additional genes and mutations in individual laboratories.

F537-K539delinsL, K539L, H538QK539L, N542E543del. These mutations are not located in the kinase domain of the Jak2 protein, but do promote higher signalling in the cell than does the V617F mutation. While the exon 12 mutations are not found in essential thrombocythemia, mutations in the myeloproliferative leukemia (*MPL*) gene may be present, suggesting a molecular differentiation between polycythemia and thrombocythemia.[177] These mutations are detected using direct sequencing, although other methods such as NIRCA have been reported for *JAK2*.[178]

Test Panels

As the number of diagnostically and prognostically important molecular abnormalities grows, testing for groups of mutations or panels, rather than singal abnormalities, becomes more practical. Furthermore, automated methods will facilitate such complex testing. Array technologies have already been applied to this type of test, for example the Oncotype DX and MammaPrint DX described above. The Autogenomics Infiniti Analyzer is a further automation of the microarray technology with multiple RUO applications, including cancer gene mutation testing.

Table 14.7 Chromosomal Abnormalities Associated with Leukemias and Lymphomas

Disease	Chromosomal Mutation
Pre-B acute lymphoblastic leukemia	t(1;19)
Acute lymphocytic leukemia	t(4;11), t(11;14), t(9,22), del(12)(p11) or (p11p13) or t(12)(p11), i(17q)
B-cell leukemia	t(2;8), t(8;14), t(8;22), t(11;14)
Acute T-lymphocytic leukemia	t(11;14), del(9)(p21 or 22)
Acute myeloid leukemia/myelodysplastic syndrome	t(11q23)-multiple partners
Acute myeloid leukemia (M2)	t(8;21), t(6;9)
Acute promyelocytic leukemia (M3)	t(15;17), 14q+
Acute myelomonocytic leukemia (M4)	t(11;21), inv(16)(p13q22)
Acute monocytic leukemia (M5)	t(9;11), del(11)(q23), t(11q23)-multiple partners
Chronic myelogenous leukemia	t(9;22), t(11;22), +8, +12, i(17q)
Acute lymphocytic leukemia	t(9;22), t(12;21), t(8;14), t(2;8), t(8;22), t(11q)
Acute nonlymphocytic leukemia	t(8;21), -Y
Chronic lymphocytic leukemia	14q+, +12, t(14;19), del(11)(q22), del(13q), del(17)(p13)
T-chronic lymphocytic leukemia	Inv(14)(q11q32) or t(14;14)(q11;q32)
Burkitt lymphoma	t(8;14), t(2;8), t(8;22)
Diffuse large B-cell lymphoma	t(3q27), t(14;18); t(8;14)
T-cell lymphoma	t(8;14)
Follicular lymphoma	t(14;18), t(8;14)
Mantle cell lymphoma	t(11;14)
Multiple myeloma	t(14q32), 14q+
Acute nonlymphocytic leukemia	inv(3q)(q21q26),dup(3q),t(3q;3q), -5 or inv5(p10)
Myeloproliferative/myelodysplastic disease	del(5)(q12q33), -7 or del(7)(q22), +8, +9
Myeloproliferative/myeloblastic disease	del(13)(q12 or q14), +21
Hairy cell leukemia	14q+
Waldenström macroglobinemia	14q+
Mucosa-associated lymphoid tissue lymphoma	t(11;18), t(14;18), t(1;14)
Polycythemia vera	del(20)(q11.2q13.3)

Additional Chromosomal Abnormalities

Tumor suppressor genes and oncogenes are disrupted by numerous genetic events. A number of specific abnormalities are associated with particular diseases (Table 14.7). These chromosome irregularities are targets for diagnosis of the associated diseases.

To date, many molecular oncology tests are developed by individual laboratories from published or original procedures rather than purchased as a set of reagents or in kit form from a commercial source. The final details of these procedures are often determined empirically, so, in detail, a test procedure can differ from one laboratory to another. Even after the test method is established, troubleshooting performed as it is put to use on a routine basis may further modify the procedure. Some reactions that work well for short-term research purposes may prove to be less consistent under the demands of the clinical laboratory setting.

Biotechnology is rapidly developing standard reagent sets for the most popular tests, but these may also differ from one supplier to another. Furthermore, due to market demands, test reagent kits may be modified or discontinued. If replacement reagents are available, they may not be identical to those previously used. Ongoing tests then have to be optimized. This can be a concern where turnaround times are critical. It then becomes the responsibility of the technologist to perform and monitor tests on a regular basis to maintain consistency and accuracy of results. The technologist who understands the biochemistry and molecular biology of these tests will be better able to respond to these problems. In addition, the current pace of evolution in the sciences makes it possible for a knowledgeable technologist to recognize significant discoveries that offer potential for improvements in testing.

CASE STUDY 14 • 1

A 40-year-old woman with a history of non-Hodgkin lymphoma reported to her physician for follow-up testing. Her complete blood cell count (CBC) was normal, including a white blood cell (WBC) count of 11,000/μL. Morphological studies on a bone marrow biopsy and a bone marrow aspirate revealed several small aggregates of mature and immature lymphocytes. Flow cytometry studies were difficult to interpret because there were too few B cells in the bone marrow aspirate specimen. No chromosomal abnormalities were detected by cytogenetics. A bone marrow aspirate tube was also sent for molecular analysis: immunoglobulin heavy chain gene rearrangement and t(14;18) gene translocation analysis by PCR. The patient's results are shown in lanes 2 of the gel images below.

■ Immunoglobulin heavy chain gene rearrangement results (left): lane 1, molecular-weight marker; lanes 2 to 4, patient specimens; lane 5, positive control; lane 6, sensitivity; lane 7, negative control; lane 8, reagent blank. t(14;18) gene translocation test (right): lane 1, molecular-weight marker; lanes 2 to 6, patient specimens; lane 7, positive control; lane 8, sensitivity; lane 9, negative control.

QUESTIONS:

1. Does this patient have an amplifiable gene rearrangement?
2. Are the translocation results on the right consistent with those of cytogenetics?
3. What control is missing from the translocation analysis?

CASE STUDY 14 • 2

A 54-year-old woman with thrombosis, a high platelet count (900,000/µL), and a decreased erythrocyte sedimentation rate was tested for polycythemia vera. Megakaryocyte clusters and pyknotic nuclear clusters were observed in a bone marrow biopsy. Overall cellularity was decreased. In the CBC, WBC and neutrophil counts were normal. Iron stores were also in the normal range. A blood sample was submitted to the molecular pathology laboratory for JAK2 V617F mutation analysis by multiplex sequence-specific PCR (See Chapter 9, Figure 9-12). The results are shown below.

QUESTIONS:

1. *What is the source of the two bands in the normal control in lane 4?*
2. *What is the source of the additional band in the positive control in lane 3?*
3. *Does this patient have the JAK2 V617F mutation?*

■ Agarose gel electrophoresis of SSP-PCR amplicons. Extension of a *JAK2* V617F-specific primer produces a 270-bp band in addition to the normal 500- and 230-bp bands. Lane 1, molecular-weight markers; lane 2, patient specimen; lane 3, V617F mutant control; lane 4, normal control; lane 5, reagent blank.

CASE STUDY 14 • 3

Paraffin-embedded sections were submitted to the molecular diagnostics laboratory for p53 mutation analysis. The specimen was a small tumor (intraductal carcinoma in situ) discovered in a 55-year-old woman. Lymph nodes were negative. Slides stained with hematoxylin and eosin were examined for confirmation of the location of tumor cells on the sections. These cells were dissected from the slide. DNA isolated from the microdissected tumor cells was screened by SSCP for mutations in exons 4 to 9 of the p53 gene. The results for exon 5 are shown below.

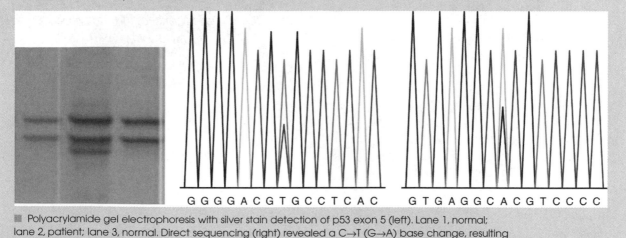

■ Polyacrylamide gel electrophoresis with silver stain detection of p53 exon 5 (left). Lane 1, normal; lane 2, patient; lane 3, normal. Direct sequencing (right) revealed a C→T (G→A) base change, resulting in a R→H amino acid change at position 175.

(case study continues on page 408)

CASE STUDY 14 • 3—cont'd

QUESTIONS:
1. What information is gained from the SSCP results?
2. What is the source of the additional band in the patient SSCP lane?
3. What further confirmation/information is gained from direct sequencing?

CASE STUDY 14 • 4

Colon carcinoma and three polyps were resected in a right hemicolectomy of a 33-year-old man. Although there was no family history, the man's age and the location of the tumor warranted testing for hereditary nonpolyposis colorectal carcinoma. Histological staining was negative for MSH2 protein. Paraffin sections and a blood sample were submitted to the molecular pathology laboratory for microsatellite instability testing. DNA was isolated from tumor cells dissected from four paraffin sections and from the patient's white blood cells. Both were amplified at the five microsatellite loci recommended by the National Cancer Institute. The results are shown below.

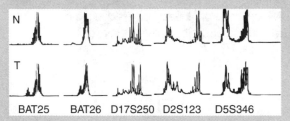

■ MSI analysis of normal cells (N, top row) and tumor cells (T, bottom row) at the five NCI loci.

QUESTIONS:
1. What are the indications for MSI analysis in this case?
2. What accounts for the difference in the peak patterns in the BAT25 and BAT26 loci?
3. How would you interpret the results of this analysis according to NCI recommendations?

CASE STUDY 14 • 5

A 23-year-old college student was sent to the student health office with a painful bruise that had persisted for several weeks. He was referred to the local hospital, where the physician ordered a bone marrow biopsy and a CBC. His WBC count was 28,000/μL; red blood cells, 2 million/μL; hemoglobin 8, hematocrit 20, platelets, 85,000/μL. Neutrophils were 7%, lymphocytes were 5%, and blasts were 95%. The pathologist who examined the bone marrow biopsy requested flow cytometry analysis of the aspirate. The cells expressed 84% CD20, 82% CD34, 92% HLA-DR, and 80% CD10/CD19. The results of these tests indicated a diagnosis of acute lymphoblastic leukemia. A blood specimen was sent to the cytogenetics laboratory for chromosomal analysis. Twenty metaphases examined had a normal 46,XY chromosomal complement. Interphase FISH was negative for t(9;22) in 500 nuclei.

QUESTIONS:
1. What is the significance of the cytogenetic test results?
2. What other molecular abnormalities might be present in this type of tumor?

• STUDY QUESTIONS •

1. What are the two important checkpoints in the cell division cycle that are crossed when the regulation of cell division is affected?

2. An *EWS-FLI-1* translocation was detected in a solid tumor by RT-PCR. Which of the following does this result support?
   a. Normal tissue
   b. Ewing sarcoma
   c. Inherited breast cancer
   d. Microsatellite instability

3. Mutation detection, even by sequencing, is not definitive with a negative result. Why?

4. Which of the following predict efficacy of *EGFR* tyrosine kinase inhibitors?
   a. Overexpression of EGFR protein
   b. Activating mutations in the *EGFR* gene

5. What is the advantage of microdissection of tumor tissue in testing for tumor-specific molecular markers?

6. Why are *K-ras* activating mutations and the *B-raf* V600E mutation mutually exclusive in colon cancer?

7. What mechanism is responsible for continued sequence changes in the immunoglobulin heavy chain gene variable regions after gene rearrangement has occurred?

8. Why are translocation-based PCR tests more sensitive than IgH, IgL, and T-cell receptor gene rearrangement tests?

9. A PCR test for the *BCL2* gene translocation is performed on a patient with suspected follicular lymphoma. The results show a bright band at 400 bp (amplification control) and another at about 300 bp for this patient. The negative control has only the 400 bp band. How would you interpret these results?

10. Which of the following misinterpretations would result from PCR contamination?
    a. False-positive for the t(15;17) translocation
    b. False-negative for the t(15;17) translocation
    c. False-negative for a gene rearrangement

11. After amplification of the t(12;21) breakpoint by RT-PCR, the PCR products were loaded and resolved on an agarose gel. What might be the explanation for each of the following observations when the gel is exposed to ultraviolet light? (Positive and amplification controls and a reagent blank control are included in the run.)
    a. The gel is blank (no bands, no molecular-weight standard).
    b. Only the molecular-weight standard is visible.
    c. The molecular-weight standard is visible; there are bands in every lane at 200 bp, even in the reagent blank lane.

12. What is observed on a Southern blot for gene rearrangement in the case of a positive result?
    a. No bands
    b. Germline bands plus rearranged bands
    c. Smears
    d. Germline bands only

13. Cyclin D1 promotes passage of cells through the G1 to S cell division cycle checkpoint. What test detects translocation of this gene to chromosome 14?
    a. t(14;18) translocation analysis (*BCL2, IGH*)
    b. t(15;17) translocation analysis (*PML/RARA*)
    c. t(11;14) translocation analysis (*BCL1/IGH*)
    d. t(8;14) translocation analysis (*MYC/IGH*)

14. What is one advantage of the Southern blot procedure over the PCR procedure for detecting clonal gene rearrangements?
    a. Southern blot requires less sample DNA than does PCR.
    b. The PCR procedure cannot detect certain gene rearrangements that are detectable by Southern blot.
    c. Southern blot results are easier to interpret than PCR results.
    d. PCR results are not accepted by the College of American Pathologists.

15. Interpret the following results from a translocation assay.

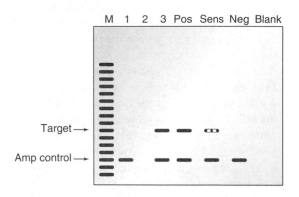

Are the samples positive, negative, or indeterminate?
Sample 1:
Sample 2:
Sample 3:

References

1. The Non-Hodgkin's Lymphoma Pathologic Classification Project. National Cancer Institute. Sponsored study of classification of non-Hodgkin's lymphomas: Summary and description of working formulation for clinical usage. *Cancer* 1982;49: 2112–2135.
2. Yang-Feng T, Schechter AL, Weinberg RA, et al. Oncogene from rat neuro/glioblastomas (human gene symbol NGL) is located on the proximal long arm of human chromosome 17 and EGFR is confirmed at 7p13-q11.3. *Cytogenetics and Cell Genetics* 1985;40:784.
3. Pauletti G, Godolphin W, Press MF, et al. Detection and quantitation of *HER-2/neu* gene amplification in human breast cancer archival material using fluorescence in situ hybridization. *Oncogene* 1996;13: 63–72.
4. Press M, Slamon DJ, Flom KJ, et al. Evaluation of *HER-2/neu* gene amplification and overexpression: Comparison of frequently used assay methods in a molecularly characterized cohort of breast cancer specimens. *Journal of Clinical Oncology* 2002;20: 3095–3105.
5. Slamon D, Godolphin W, Jones LA, et al. Studies of the *HER-2/neu* proto-oncogene in human breast and ovarian cancer. *Science* 1989;244:707–712.
6. Kounelis S, Kapranos N, Malamos N, et al. Evaluation of *HER-2* gene status in breast cancer by chromogenic in situ hybridization: Comparison with immunohistochemistry. *Anticancer Research* 2005;25:939–946.
7. Tanner M, Gancberg D, Di Leo A, et al. Chromogenic in situ hybridization: A practical alternative for fluorescence in situ hybridization to detect *HER-2/neu* oncogene amplification in archival breast cancer samples. *American Journal of Pathology* 2000;157:1467–1472.
8. Madrid M, Lo RW. Chromogenic in situ hybridization (CISH): A novel alternative in screening archival breast cancer tissue samples for *HER-2/neu* status. *Breast Cancer Research* 2004;6:R593–R600.
9. Spaulding D, Spaulding BO. Epidermal growth factor receptor expression and measurement in solid tumors. *Seminars in Oncology* 2002;29:45–54.
10. Younes M. Is immunohistochemistry for epidermal growth factor receptor expression a poor predictor of response to epidermal growth factor receptor–targeted therapy? *Journal of Clinical Oncology* 2005;23:923.
11. Murthy S, Magliocco AM, Demetrick DJ. Copy number analysis of *c-erb-B2* (*HER-2/neu*) and topoisomerase IIa genes in breast carcinoma by quantitative real-time polymerase chain reaction using hybridization probes and fluorescence in situ hybridization. *Archives of Pathology and Laboratory Medicine* 2005;129:39–46.
12. Paez J, Janne PA, Lee JC, et al. *EGFR* mutations in lung cancer: Correlation with clinical response to gefitinib therapy. *Science* 2004;304:1497–1500.
13. Lynch T, Bell DW, Sordella R, et al. Activating mutations in the epidermal growth factor receptor underlying responsiveness of non–small-cell lung cancer to gefitinib. *New England Journal of Medicine* 2004;350:2129–2139.
14. Tsao M-S, Sakurada A, Cutz J-C, et al. Erlotinib in lung cancer: Molecular and clinical predictors of outcome. *New England Journal of Medicine* 2005; 353:133–144.
15. Shepherd F, Pereira JR, Ciuleanu T, et al. Erlotinib in previously treated non–small-cell lung cancer. *New England Journal of Medicine* 2005;353:123–132.
16. Marchetti A, Martella C, Felicioni L, et al. *EGFR* mutations in non–small-cell lung cancer: Analysis

of a large series of cases and development of a rapid and sensitive method for diagnostic screening with potential implications on pharmacologic treatment. *Journal of Clinical Oncology* 2005;23:857–865.

17. Pan Q, Pao W, Ladanyi M. Rapid polymerase chain reaction–based detection of epidermal growth factor receptor gene mutations in lung adenocarcinomas. *Journal of Molecular Diagnostics* 2005;7:396–403.

18. Taron M, Ichinose Y, Rosell R, et al. Activating mutations in the tyrosine kinase domain of the epidermal growth factor receptor are associated with improved survival in gefitinib-treated chemorefractory lung adenocarcinomas. *Clinical Cancer Research* 2005;11:5878–5885.

19. Tonon G, Wong K-K, Maulik G, et al. High-resolution genomic profiles of human lung cancer. *Proceedings of the National Academy of Sciences* 2005;102:9625–9630.

20. Han S, Hwang PG, Chun DH, et al. Epidermal growth factor receptor (EGFR) downstream molecules as response predictive markers for gefitinib in chemotherapy-resistant non–small-cell lung cancer. *International Journal of Cancer* 2005;113: 109–115.

21. Jassem J, Jassem E, Jakobkiewicz-Banecka J, et al. *P53* and *K-ras* mutations are frequent events in microscopically negative surgical margins from patients with nonsmall cell lung carcinoma. *Cancer* 2004;100:1951–1960.

22. Zuo Z, Chen SS, Chandra PK, et al. Application of COLD-PCR for improved detection of *KRAS* mutations in clinical samples. *Modern Pathology* 2009;22:1023–1031.

23. Fabjani G, Kriegshaeuser G, Schuetz A, et al. Biochip for *K-ras* mutation screening in ovarian cancer. *Clinical Chemistry* 2005;51:784–87.

24. Maekawa M, Nagaoka T, Taniguchi T, et al. Three-dimensional microarray compared with PCR single-strand conformation polymorphism analysis/DNA sequencing for mutation analysis of K-ras codons 12 and 13. *Clinical Chemistry* 2004;50:1322–1327.

25. Domingo E, Laiho P, Ollikainen M, et al. *BRAF* screening as a low-cost effective strategy for simplifying HNPCC genetic testing. *Journal of Medical Genetics* 2004;41:664–668.

26. Benlloch S, Payá A, Alenda C, et al. Detection of BRAF V600E mutation in colorectal cancer:

Comparison of automatic sequencing and real-time chemistry methodology. *Journal of Molecular Diagnostics* 2006;8:540–543.

27. Navarro S, Noguera R, Pellan A, et al. Atypical pleomorphic extraosseous Ewing tumor/peripheral primitive neuroectodermal tumor with unusual phenotypic/genotypic profile. *Diagnostic Molecular Pathology* 2002;11:9–15.

28. Qian X, Jin, L, Shearer B, et al. Molecular diagnosis of Ewing's sarcoma/primitive neuroectodermal tumor in formalin-fixed paraffin-embedded tissues by RT-PCR and fluorescence in situ hybridization. *Diagnostic Molecular Pathology* 2005;14:23–28.

29. Noguera R. Cytogenetics and tissue culture of small round cell tumors of bone and soft tissue. *Seminars in Diagnostic Pathology* 1996;13:171–183.

30. Akerman M, Dreinhofer K, Rydholm A, et al. Cytogenetic studies on fine-needle aspiration samples from osteosarcoma and Ewing's sarcoma. *Diagnostic Cytopathology* 1996;15:17–22.

31. Takeuchi T, Iwasaki H, Ohjimi Y, et al. Renal primitive neuroectodermal tumor: A morphologic, cytogenetic, and molecular analysis with the establishment of two cultured cell lines. *Diagnostic Molecular Pathology* 1997;6:309–317.

32. Adams V, Hany MA, Schmid M, et al. Detection of t(11;22)(q24;q12) translocation breakpoint in paraffin-embedded tissue of the Ewing's sarcoma family by nested reverse transcription–polymerase chain reaction. *Diagnostic Molecular Pathology* 1996;5: 107–113.

33. Kelley T, Tubbs RR, Prayson RA. Molecular diagnostic techniques for the clinical evaluation of gliomas. *Diagnostic Molecular Pathology* 2005;14:1–8.

34. Panagopoulos I, Mertens F, Isaksson M, et al. Clinical impact of molecular and cytogenetic findings in synovial sarcoma. *Genes Chromosomes Cancer* 2001;31:362–372.

35. Nilsson G, Skytting B , Xie Y, et al. The SYT-SSX1 variant of synovial sarcoma is associated with a high rate of tumor cell proliferation and poor clinical outcome. *Cancer Research* 1999;59:3180–3184.

36. Barr F, Galili N, Holick J, et al. Rearrangement of the PAX3 paired box gene in the paediatric solid tumour alveolar rhabdomyosarcoma. *Nature Genetics* 1993;3:113–117.

37. Tassabehji M, Newton VE, Liu X-Z, et al. The mutational spectrum in Waardenburg syndrome. *Human Molecular Genetics* 1995;4:2131–2137.

38. Whang-Peng J, Knutsen T, Theil K, et al. Cytogenetic studies in subgroups of rhabdomyosarcoma. *Genes Chromosomes Cancer* 1992;5:299–310.

39. Jin L, Majerus J, Oliveira A, et al. Detection of fusion gene transcripts in fresh-frozen and formalin-fixed paraffin-embedded tissue sections of soft-tissue sarcomas after laser capture microdissection and RT-PCR. *Diagnostic Molecular Pathology* 2003;12:224–230.

40. Tiffin N, Williams RD, Shipley J, et al. *PAX7* expression in embryonal rhabdomyosarcoma suggests an origin in muscle satellite cells. *British Journal of Cancer* 2003;89:327–332.

41. Edwards R, Chatten J, Xiong Q-B, et al. Detection of gene fusions in rhabdomyosarcoma by reverse transcriptase–polymerase chain reaction assay of archival samples. *Diagnostic Molecular Pathology* 1997;6:91–97.

42. Farnebo M, Bykov VJ, Wiman KG. The p53 tumor suppressor: A master regulator of diverse cellular processes and therapeutic target in cancer. *Biochemical Biophysicial Research Communications* 2010;396:85–89.

43. Kyzas P, Loizou KT, Ioannidis JP. Selective reporting biases in cancer prognostic factor studies. *Journal of the National Cancer Institute* 2005;97:1043–1055.

44. Lohmann D, Ruhri C, Schmitt M, et al. Accumulation of p53 protein as an indicator for *p53* gene mutation in breast cancer: Occurrence of false-positives and false-negatives. *Diagnostic Molecular Pathology* 1993;2:36–41.

45. Casey G, Lopez ME, Ramos JC, et al. DNA sequence analysis of exons 2 through 11 and immunohistochemical staining are required to detect all known p53 alterations in human malignancies. *Oncogene* 1996;13:1971–1981.

46. Visscher D, Sarkar FH, Shimoyama RK, et al. Correlation between p53 immunostaining patterns and gene sequence mutations in breast carcinoma. *Diagnostic Molecular Pathology* 1996;5:187–193.

47. Miller L, Smeds J, George J, et al. An expression signature for p53 status in human breast cancer predicts mutation status, transcriptional effects, and patient survival. *Proceedings of the National Academy of Sciences* 2005;102:13550–13555.

48. Falette N, Paperin MP, Treilleux I, et al. Prognostic value of *p53* gene mutations in a large series of node-negative breast cancer patients. *Cancer Research* 1998;58:1451–1455.

49. Liu Q, Feng J, Buzin C, et al. Detection of virtually all mutations-SSCP (DOVAM-S): A rapid method for mutation scanning with virtually 100% sensitivity. *BioTechniques* 1999;26:932–942.

50. Buzin C, Wen CY, Nguyen VQ, et al. Scanning by DOVAM-S detects all unique sequence changes in blinded analyses: Evidence that the scanning conditions are generic. *BioTechniques* 2000;28:746–753.

51. Girard P-M, Foray N, Stumm M, et al. Radiosensitivity in Nijmegen breakage syndrome cells is attributable to a repair defect and not cell cycle checkpoint defects. *Cancer Research* 2000;60:4881–4888.

52. Castilla L, Couch FJ, Erdos MR, et al. Mutations in the *BRCA1* gene in families with early-onset breast and ovarian cancer. *Nature Genetics* 1994;8:387–391.

53. Smith S, DiCioccio RA, Struewing JP, et al. Localisation of the breast-ovarian cancer susceptibility gene (*BRCA1*) on 17q12–21 to an interval of < or = 1 cM. *Genes, Chromosomes Cancer* 1994;10:71–76.

54. Stratton M, Ford D, Neuhasen S, et al. Familial male breast cancer is not linked to the *BRCA1* locus on chromosome 17q. *Nature Genetics* 1994;7:103–107.

55. Wooster R, Bignell G, Lancaster J, et al. Identification of the breast cancer susceptibility gene *BRCA2*. *Nature* 1995;378:789–792.

56. Brugarolas J, Jacks T. Double indemnity: p53, BRCA and cancer. *Science* 1997;3:721–722.

57. Satagopan J, Offit K, Foulkes W, et al. The life-time risks of breast cancer in Ashkenazi Jewish carriers of *BRCA1* and *BRCA2* mutations. *Cancer Epidemiology Biomarkers and Prevention* 2001;10:467–473.

58. Tonin P, Weber B, Offit K, et al. Frequency of recurrent *BRCA1* and *BRCA2* mutations in Ashkenazi Jewish breast cancer families. *Nature Medicine* 1996;2:1179–1183.

59. Lerman C, Narod S, Schulman K, et al. *BRCA1* testing in families with hereditary breast-ovarian cancer. A prospective study of patient decision

making and outcomes. *Journal of the American Medical Association* 1996;275:1885–1892.

60. Botkin J, Croyle RT, Smith KR, et al. A model protocol for evaluating the behavioral and psychosocial effects of *BRCA1* testing. *Journal of the National Cancer Institute* 1996;88:872–882.

61. Roussi P, Sherman KA, Miller S, et al. Enhanced counseling for women undergoing *BRCA1/2* testing: Impact on knowledge and psychological distress results from a randomised clinical trial. *Psychology and Health* 2010;25:401–415.

62. Phelan C, Rebbeck TR, Weber BL, et al. Ovarian cancer risk in *BRCA1* carriers is modified by the *HRAS1* variable number of tandem repeat (VNTR) locus. *Nature Genetics* 1996;12:309–311.

63. Pastore Y, Jedlickova K, Guan Y, et al. Mutations of von Hippel-Lindau tumor-suppressor gene and congenital polycythemia. *American Journal of Human Genetics* 2003;73:412–419.

64. Wait S, Vortmeyer AO, Lonser RR, et al. Somatic mutations in *VHL* germline deletion kindred correlate with mild phenotype. *Annals of Neurology* 2004;55:236–240.

65. Foster K, Prowse A, van den Berg A, et al. Somatic mutations of the von Hippel-Lindau disease tumour suppressor gene in nonfamilial clear cell renal carcinoma. *Human Molecular Genetics* 1994;3:2169–2173.

66. Bender B, Gutsche M, Glasker S, et al. Differential genetic alterations in von Hippel-Lindau syndrome–associated and sporadic pheochromocytomas. *Journal of Clinical Endrocrinology and Metabolism* 2000;85:4568–4574.

67. Glenn G, Linehan WM, Hosoe S, et al. Screening for von Hippel-Lindau disease by DNA polymorphism analysis. *Journal of the American Medical Association* 1992;267:1226–1231.

68. de Cremoux P, Thioux M, Peter M, et al. Polymerase chain reaction compared with dot blotting for the determination of *N-myc* gene amplification in neuroblastoma. *International Journal of Cancer* 1997;72:518–521.

69. Shapiro D, Valentine MB, Rowe ST, et al. Detection of *N-myc* gene amplification by fluorescence in situ hybridization: Diagnostic utility for neuroblastoma. *American Journal of Pathology* 1993;142:1339–1346.

70. Grady-Leopardi E, Schwab M, Ablin AR, et al. Detection of *N-myc* oncogene expression in human neuroblastoma by in situ hybridization and blot analysis: Relationship to clinical outcome. *Cancer Research* 1986;46:3196–3199.

71. Layfield L, Willmore-Payne C, Shimada H, et al. Assessment of *N-myc* amplification: A comparison of FISH, quantitative PCR monoplexing, and traditional blotting methods used with formalin-fixed, paraffin-embedded neuroblastomas. *Analytical and Quantitative Cytology and Histology* 2005;27:5–14.

72. Takahashi M, Ritz J, Cooper GM. Activation of a novel human transforming gene, *ret,* by DNA rearrangement. *Cell* 1985;42(2):581–588.

73. Bolk G, Salomon R, Pelet A, et al. Segregation at three loci explains familial and population risk in Hirschsprung disease. *Nature Genetics* 2002;31:89–93.

74. Stratakis C. Clinical genetics of multiple endocrine neoplasias, Carney complex and related syndromes. *Journal of Endocrinology* 2001;24:370–383.

75. Sanso G, Domene HM, Garcia R, et al. Very early detection of RET proto-oncogene mutation is crucial for preventive thyroidectomy in multiple endocrine neoplasia type 2 children: Presence of C-cell malignant disease in asymptomatic carriers. *Cancer* 2002;94:323–330.

76. Attie T, Pelet A, Edery P, et al. Diversity of *RET* proto-oncogene mutations in familial and sporadic Hirschsprung disease. *Human Molecular Genetics* 1995;4:1381–1386.

77. Seri M, Yin L, Barone A, et al. Frequency of *RET* mutations in long- and short-segment Hirschsprung disease. *Human Mutation* 1997;9:243–249.

78. Yan H, Parsons DW, Jin G, et al. *IDH1* and *IDH2* mutations in gliomas. *New England Journal of Medicine* 2009;360:765–773.

79. Horbinski C, Kelly L, Nikiforov YE, et al. Detection of *IDH1* and *IDH2* mutations by fluorescence melting curve analysis as a diagnostic tool for brain biopsies. *Journal of Molecular Diagnostics* 2010;12:487–492.

80. Horbinski C, Kofler J, Kelly LM, et al. Diagnostic use of *IDH1/2* mutation analysis in routine clinical testing of formalin-fixed, paraffin-embedded glioma tissues. *Journal of Neuropathology & Experimental Neurology* 2009;68:1319–1325.

81. Marcucci G, Maharry K, Wu YZ, et al. *IDH1* and *IDH2* gene mutations identify novel molecular subsets within de novo cytogenetically normal acute myeloid leukemia: A Cancer and Leukemia Group B study. *Journal of Clinical Oncology* 2010;28: 2348–2355.

82. Wagner K, Damm F, Gehring G, et al. Impact of *IDH1* R132 mutations and an *IDH1* single nucleotide polymorphism in cytogenetically normal acute myeloid leukemia: SNP rs11554137 is an adverse prognostic factor. *Journal of Clinical Oncology* 2010;28:2356–2364.

83. Lynch H, Smyrk TC, Watson P, et al. Genetics, natural history, tumor spectrum and pathology of hereditary nonpolypoisis colorectal cancer: An updated review. *Gastroenterology* 1988;104: 1535–1549.

84. Lynch H, Smyrk TC, Lynch JF. Overview of natural history, pathology, molecular genetics and management of HNPCC (Lynch syndrome). *International Journal of Cancer* 1996;69:38–43.

85. Xia L, Shen W, Ritacca F, et al. A truncated *hMSH2* transcript occurs as a common variant in the population: Implications for genetic diagnosis. *Cancer Research* 1996;56:2289–2292.

86. Srivastava S, Rossi SC. Early detection research program at the NCI. *International Journal of Cancer* 1996;69:35–37.

87. Shin K-H, Shin J-H, Kim J-H, et al. Mutational analysis of promoters of mismatch repair genes *hMSH2* and *hMLH1* in hereditary nonpolyposis colorectal cancer and early onset colorectal cancer patients: Identification of three novel germline mutations in promoter of the *hMSH2* gene. *Cancer Research* 2002;62:38–42.

88. Sun X, Zheng L, Shen B. Functional alterations of human exonuclease 1 mutants identified in atypical hereditary nonpolyposis colorectal cancer syndrome. *Cancer Research* 2002;62:6026–6030.

89. Boland C, Thibodeau SN, Hamilton SR, et al. A National Cancer Institute workshop on microsatellite instability for cancer detection and familial predisposition: Development of international criteria for the determination of microsatellite instability in colorectal cancer. *Cancer Research* 1998;58:5248–5257.

90. Frazier M, Sinicrope FA, Amos CI, et al. Loci for efficient detection of microsatellite instability in hereditary nonpolyposis colorectal cancer. *Oncology Reports* 1999;6:497–505.

91. Watanabe T, Wu TT, Catalano PJ, et al. Molecular predictors of survival after adjuvant chemotherapy for colon cancer. *New England Journal of Medicine* 2001;344:1196–1206.

92. Halvarsson B, Lindblom A, Rambech E, et al. Microsatellite instability analysis and/or immunostaining for the diagnosis of hereditary nonpolyposis colorectal cancer? *Virchows Archiv* 2004;444: 135–141.

93. Dowsett M, Dunbier AK. Emerging biomarkers and new understanding of traditional markers in personalized therapy for breast cancer. *Clinical Cancer Research* 2008;14:8019–8026.

94. Desmedt C, Ruiz-Garcia E, Andre F. Gene expression predictors in breast cancer: Current status, limitations and perspectives. *European Journal of Cancer* 2008;44:2714–2720.

95. Ma X, Patel R, Wang X, et al. Molecular classification of human cancers using a 92-gene real-time quantitative polymerase chain reaction assay. *Archives of Pathology & Laboratory Medicine* 2006;130:465–473.

96. Rosenfeld N, Aharonov R, Meiri E, et al. MicroRNAs accurately identify cancer tissue origin. *Nature Biotechnology* 2008;26:462–469.

97. Zhang T, Franklin A, Boboila C, et al. Downstream class switching leads to IgE antibody production by B lymphocytes lacking IgM switch regions. *Proceedings of the National Academy of Sciences* 2010;107:3040–3045.

98. Meier J, Lewis SM. P nucleotides in V(D)J recombination: A fine-structure analysis. *Molecular and Cellular Biology* 1993;13:1078–1092.

99. Weichhold G, Ohnheiser R, Zachau HG. The human immunoglobulin kappa locus consists of two copies that are organized in opposite polarity. *Genomics* 1993;16:503–511.

100. Barbie V, Lefranc M-P. The human immunoglobulin kappa variable (*IGKV*) genes and joining (*IGKJ*) segments. *Experimental and Clinical Immunogenetics* 1998;15:171–183.

101. Frippiat J-P, Williams SC, Tomlinson IM, et al. Organization of the human immunoglobulin lambda light-chain locus on chromosome 22q11.2. *Human Molecular Genetics* 1995;4:983–991.

102. Yuen E, Brown RD. Southern blotting of IgH rearrangements in B-cell disorders. *Methods in Molecular Medicine* 2005;113:85–103.

103. Arber D. Molecular diagnostic approach to non-Hodgkin's lymphoma. *Journal of Molecular Diagnostics* 2000;2(4):178–190.

104. Beishuizen A, Verhoeven MA, Mol EJ, et al. Detection of immunoglobulin kappa light-chain gene rearrangement patterns by Southern blot analysis. *Leukemia* 1994;8:2228–2236.

105. van Dongen J, Langerak AW, Bruggemann M, et al. Design and standardization of PCR primers and protocols for detection of clonal immunoglobulin and T-cell receptor gene recombinations in suspect lymphoproliferations: Report of the BIOMED-2 Concerted Action BMH4-CT98-3936. *Leukemia* 2003;12:2257–2317.

106. Gonzalez D, Balanzategui A, Garcia-Sanz R, et al. Incomplete DJH gene rearrangements of the IgH gene are frequent in multiple myeloma patients: Immunobiological characteristics and clinical applications. *Leukemia* 2003;17:1398–1403.

107. Szczepaski T, Willemse MJ, van Wering ER, et al. Precursor-B-ALL with DH–JH gene rearrangements have an immature immunogenotype with a high frequency of oligoclonality and hyperdiploidy of chromosome 14. *Leukemia* 2001;15:1415–1423.

108. Campbell M, Zelenetz AD, Levy S, et al. Use of family-specific leader region primers for PCR amplification of the human heavy chain variable region gene repertoire. *Molecular Immunology* 1992;29:193–203.

109. Muschen M, Rajewsky K, Brauninger A, et al. Rare occurrence of classical Hodgkin's disease as a T-cell lymphoma. *Journal of Experimental Medicine* 2000;191:387–394.

110. Gonzalez D, Garcia-Sanz R. Incomplete DJH rearrangements. *Methods in Molecular Medicine* 2005;113:165–173.

111. Evans P, Pott C, Groenen PJ, et al. Significantly improved PCR-based clonality testing in B-cell malignancies by use of multiple immunoglobulin gene targets. Report of the BIOMED-2 Concerted Action BHM4-CT98-3936. *Leukemia* 2007;21:207–214.

112. Brüggemann M, White H, Gaulard P, et al. Powerful strategy for polymerase chain reaction-based clonality assessment in T-cell malignancies Report of the BIOMED-2 Concerted Action BHM4 CT98-3936. *Leukemia* 2007; 21:215–221.

113. Araujo M, Carvalhais A, Campos A, et al. Clonality detection in apheresis products from multiple myeloma and non-Hodgkin lymphoma patients. *Transplantation Proceedings* 2000;32:2676.

114. van der Velden V, Willemse MJ, van der Schoot CE, et al. Immunoglobulin kappa-deleting element rearrangements in precursor-B acute lymphoblastic leukemia are stable targets for detection of minimal residual disease by real-time PCR. *Leukemia* 2002;16:928–936.

115. Shiokawa S, Nishimura J, Ohshima K, et al. Establishment of a novel B-cell clonality analysis using single-strand conformation polymorphism of immunoglobulin light chain messenger signals. *American Journal of Pathology* 1998;153: 1393–1400.

116. Buckingham L, Vardouniotis A, Coon JS. Molecular detection of multiple myeloma at the immunoglobulin light chain locus. *Journal of Molecular Diagnostics* 2002;4:241.

117. Rosenquist R, Menestrina F, Lestani M, et al. Indications for peripheral light-chain revision and somatic hypermutation without a functional B-cell receptor in precursors of a composite diffuse large B-cell and Hodgkin's lymphoma. *Laboratory Investigation* 2004;84:253–262.

118. Tumkaya T, van der Burg M, Garcia-Sanz R, et al. Immunoglobulin lambda isotype gene rearrangements in B-cell malignancies. *Leukemia* 2001;15: 121–127.

119. Breit T, Wolvers-Tettero IL, Beishuizen AV, et al. Southern blot patterns, frequencies, and junctional diversity of T-cell receptor delta gene rearrangements in acute lymphoblastic leukemia. *Blood* 1993;82:3063–3074.

120. Miller J, Wilson SS, Jaye DL, et al. An automated semiquantitative B- and T-cell clonality assay. *Journal of Molecular Diagnostics* 1999;4:101–117.

121. Szczepanski T, Beishuizen A, Pongers-Willemse MJ, et al. Cross-lineage T-cell receptor gene rearrangements occur in more than ninety percent of childhood precursor-B acute lymphoblastic leukemias: Alternative PCR targets for detection of minimal residual disease. *Leukemia* 1999;13: 196–205.

122. Lawnicki L, Rubocki RJ, Chan WC, et al. The distribution of gene segments in T-cell receptor gene rearrangements demonstrates the need for multiple primer sets. *Journal of Molecular Diagnostics* 2003;5:82–87.

123. Theodorou I, Bigorgne C, Delfau MH, et al. VJ rearrangements of the TCR gamma locus in peripheral T-cell lymphomas: Analysis by polymerase chain reaction and denaturing gradient gel electrophoresis. *Journal of Pathology* 1996;178:303–310.

124. Langerak A. Undersized, oversized? It is not one-size-fits-all in lymphoid clonality detection. *Leukemia Research* 2008;32:203–204.

125. Lee S, Berg KD, Racke FK, et al. Pseudo-spikes are common in histologically benign lymphoid tissues. *Journal of Molecular Diagnostics* 2000;2:145–152.

126. Murphy K, Berg KD, Geiger T, et al. Capillary electrophoresis artifact due to eosin: Implications for the interpretation of molecular diagnostic assays. *Journal of Molecular Diagnostics* 2005; 7:143–148.

127. Batstone P, Goodlad JR. Efficacy of screening the intermediate cluster region of the *bcl2* gene in follicular lymphoma by PCR. *Journal of Clinical Pathology* 2004;58:81–82.

128. Albinger-Hegyi A, Hochreutener B, Abdou M-T, et al. High frequency of t(14;18)-translocation breakpoints outside of major breakpoint and minor cluster regions in follicular lymphomas: Improved polymerase chain reaction protocols for their detection. *American Journal of Pathology* 2002;160:823–832.

129. Gomez M, Wu X, Wang YL. Detection of bcl-2-IGH using single-round PCR assays. *Diagnostic Molecular Pathology* 2005;14:17–22.

130. Hsi E, Tubbs RR, Lovell MA, et al. Detection of bcl-2/J(H) translocation by polymerase chain reaction: A summary of the experience of the molecular oncology survey of the College of American Pathologists. *Archives of Pathology and Laboratory Medicine* 2002;126:902–908.

131. McGregor D, Keever-Taylor CA, Bredeson C, et al. The implication of follicular lymphoma patients receiving allogeneic stem cell transplantation from donors carrying t(14;18)-positive cells. *Bone Marrow Transplant* 2005;35:1049–1054.

132. Montoto S, Lopez-Guillermo A, Colomer D, et al. Incidence and clinical significance of bcl-2/IgH rearrangements in follicular lymphoma. *Leukemia and Lymphoma* 2003;44:71–76.

133. Ladetto M, Mantoan B, Ricca I, et al. Recurrence of bcl-2/IgH polymerase chain reaction positivity following a prolonged molecular remission can be unrelated to the original follicular lymphoma clone. *Experimental Hematology* 2003;31(9):784–788.

134. Colleoni G, Duarte LC, Kerbauy FR, et al. Possible influence of clinical stage and type of treatment in the persistence of residual circulating t(14;18)-positive cells in follicular lymphoma patients. *Leukemia and Lymphoma* 2004;45: 539–545.

135. Maurer J, Janssen JW, Thiel E, et al. Detection of chimeric bcr-abl genes in acute lymphoblastic leukaemia by the polymerase chain reaction. *Lancet* 1991;337:1055–1058.

136. Gleissner B, Gakbuget N, Bartram CR, et al. Leading prognostic relevance of the BCR-ABL translocation in adult acute B-lineage lymphoblastic leukemia: A prospective study of the German Multicenter Trial Group and confirmed polymerase chain reaction analysis. *Blood* 2002; 99:1536–1543.

137. Gleissner B, Rieder H, Thiel EF, et al. Prospective bcr-abl analysis by polymerase chain reaction in adult acute B-lineage lymphoblastic leukemia: Reliability of RT-nested PCR and comparison to cytogenetic data. *Leukemia* 2001;15:1834–1840.

138. Burmeister T, Maurer J, Aivado M, et al. Quality assurance in RT-PCR–based BCR/ABL diagnostics: Results of an interlaboratory test and a standardization approach. *Leukemia* 2000;14:1850–1856.

139. van der Velden V, Boeckx N, Gonzalez M, et al. Differential stability of control gene and fusion gene transcripts over time may hamper accurate quantification of minimal residual disease: A study within the Europe Against Cancer Program. *Leukemia* 2004;18:884–886.

140. Lion T, Gaiger A, Henn T, et al. Use of quantitative polymerase chain reaction to monitor residual disease in chronic myelogenous leukemia during treatment with interferon. *Leukemia* 1995;9: 1353–1360.

141. Branford S, Hughes TP, Rudzki Z. Monitoring chronic leukemia therapy by real-time quantitative

PCR in blood is a reliable alternative to bone marrow cytogenetics. *British Journal of Haematology* 1999;107:587–599.

142. Muller M, Hardt T, Paschka P, et al. Standardization of preanalytical factors for minimal residual disease analysis in chronic myelogenous leukemia. *Acta Haematologica* 2004;112:30–33.

143. Moravcova J, Regner J, Mouckova D, et al. Disease status in patients with chronic myeloid leukemia is better characterized by bcr-abl/bcr transcript ratio than by bcr-abl transcript level, which may suggest a role of normal bcr gene in the disease pathogenesis. *Neoplasma* 2005;52: 119–125.

144. Jones C, Yeung C, Zehnder JL. Comprehensive validation of a real-time quantitative bcr-abl assay for clinical laboratory use. *American Journal of Clinical Pathology* 2003;120(1):42–48.

145. Neumann F, Herold C, Hildebrandt B, et al. Quantitative real-time reverse-transcription polymerase chain reaction for diagnosis of bcr-abl positive leukemias and molecular monitoring following allogeneic stem cell transplantation. *European Journal of Haematology* 2003;70:1–10.

146. Hughes T, Kaeda J, Branford S, et al. International Randomised study of interferon versus STI571 study group: Frequency of major molecular responses to imatinib or interferon alfa plus cytarabine in newly diagnosed chronic myeloid leukemia. *New England Journal of Medicine* 2003;349:1423–1432.

147. Cortes J, Talpaz M, O'Brien S, et al. Molecular responses in patients with chronic myelogenous leukemia in chronic phase treated with imatinib mesylate. *Clinical Cancer Research* 2005;11(9): 3425–32.

148. Wang L, Pearson K, Pillitteri L, et al. Serial monitoring of bcr-abl by peripheral blood real-time polymerase chain reaction predicts the marrow cytogenetic response to imatinib mesylate in chronic myeloid leukaemia. *British Journal of Haematology* 2002;118:771–777.

149. Santos F, Ravandi F. Advances in treatment of chronic myelogenous leukemia—New treatment options with tyrosine kinase inhibitors. *Leukemia and Lymphoma* 2009;50:16–26.

150. Manrique Arechavaleta G, Scholl V, Perez V, et al. Rapid and sensitive allele-specific (AS)-RT-PCR assay for detection of T315I mutation in chronic myeloid leukemia patients treated with tyrosine-kinase inhibitors. *Clinical and Experimental Medicine*, 2011;11:55–59.

151. Yamamoto M, Kakihana K, Ohashi K, et al. Serial Monitoring of T315I BCR-ABL mutation by Invader assay combined with RT-PCR. *International Journal of Hematology* 2009;89:482–488.

152. Slack J, Bi WL, Livak KJ, et al. Preclinical validation of a novel, highly sensitive assay to detect PML-RARa mRNA using real-time reverse-transcription polymerase chain reaction. *Journal of Molecular Diagnostics* 2005;3:141–149.

153. Lafage-Pochitaloff M, Alcalay M, Brunel V, et al. Acute promyelocytic leukemia cases with nonreciprocal *PML/RARA* or *RARA/PML* fusion genes. *Blood* 1995;85:1169–1174.

154. Vizmanos J, Larráyoz MJ, Odero MD, et al. Two new molecular *PML-RARA* variants: Implications for the molecular diagnosis of APL. *Haematologica* 2002;87:ELT37.

155. Mozziconacci M, Liberatore C, Brunel V, et al. In vitro response to all-trans retinoic acid of acute promyelocytic leukemias with nonreciprocal PML/RARA or RARA/PML fusion genes. *Genes Chromosomes Cancer* 1998;22:241–250.

156. Fan H, Gulley ML, Gascoyne RD, et al. Molecular methods for detecting t(11;14) translocations in mantle-cell lymphomas. *Diagnostic Molecular Pathology* 1998;7:209–214.

157. Williams M, Nichols GE, Swerdlow SH, et al. In situ hybridization detection of cyclin D1 mRNA in centrocytic/mantle cell lymphoma. *Annals of Oncology* 1995;6:297–299.

158. Wijers-Koster P, Droese J, et al. t(11;14) with *BCL1-IGH* rearrangement. *Leukemia* 2003;17: 2296–2298.

159. Lacy J, Summers WP, Watson M, et al. Amplification and deregulation of myc following Epstein-Barr virus infection of a human B-cell line. *Proceedings of the National Academy of Sciences* 1987;84: 5838–5842.

160. Lazo P, DiPaolo JA, Popescu NC. Amplification of the integrated viral transforming genes of human papillomavirus 18 and its 5'-flanking cellular sequence located near the myc protooncogene in HeLa cells. *Cancer Research* 1989;49:4305–4310.

161. Morse B, Rotherg PG, South VJ, et al. Insertional mutagenesis of the myc locus by a LINE-1 sequence in a human breast carcinoma. *Nature* 1988;333:87–90.

162. Erikson J, Finger L, Sun L, et al. Deregulation of c-myc by translocation of the alpha-locus of the T-cell receptor in T-cell leukemias. *Science* 1986;232:884–886.

163. Siebert R, Matthiesen P, Harder S, et al. Application of interphase fluorescence in situ hybridization for the detection of the Burkitt translocation t(8;14)(q24;q32) in B-cell lymphomas. *Blood* 1998;91:984–990.

164. Choi J-Y, Hong Y-S, Park H-Y. Stimulation of c-myc proto-oncogene expression by transforming growth factor a in human ovarian cancer cells. *Experimental and Molecular Medicine* 1997;29: 203–208.

165. Blancato J, Singh B, Liu A, et al. Correlation of amplification and overexpression of the c-myc oncogene in high-grade breast cancer: FISH, in situ hybridisation and immunohistochemical analyses. *British Journal of Cancer* 2004;90: 1612–1619.

166. Ullrich A, Schlessinger J. Signal transduction by receptors with tyrosine kinase activity. *Cell* 1990;61:203–212.

167. Rosnet O, Mattei M-G, Marchetto S, et al. Isolation and chromosomal localization of a novel FMS-like tyrosine kinase gene. *Genomics* 1991;9: 380–385.

168. Chillón M, Santamaría C, García-Sanz R, et al. Long *FLT3* internal tandem duplications and reduced *PML-RAR* expression at diagnosis characterize a high-risk subgroup of acute promyelocytic leukemia patients. *Haematologica* 2010;95: 745–751.

169. Mills K, Gilkes AF, Walsh V, et al. Rapid and sensitive detection of internal tandem duplication and activating loop mutations of *FLT3*. *British Journal of Haematology* 2005; 130:203–208.

170. Scholl S, Krause C, Loncarevic IF, et al. Specific detection of Flt3 point mutations by highly sensitive real-time polymerase chain reaction in acute myeloid leukemia. *Journal of Laboratory and Clinical Medicine* 2005;145:295–304.

171. Vardiman J, Thiele J, Arber DA, et al. The 2008 revision of the World Health Organization (WHO) classification of myeloid neoplasms and acute leukemia: Rationale and important changes. *Blood* 2009;114:937–951.

172. Baxter E, Scott LM, Campbell PJ, et al. Acquired mutation of the tyrosine kinase *JAK2* in human myeloproliferative disorders. *Lancet* 2005;365: 1054–1061.

173. Kralovics RPF, Buser AS, Teo S-S, et al. A gain-of-function mutation of JAK2 in myeloproliferative disorders. *New England Journal of Medicine* 2005;352:1779–1790.

174. Warshawsky I, Mularo F, Hren C, et al. Failure of the Ipsogen MutaScreen kit to detect the *JAK2* 617V>F mutation in samples with additional rare exon 14 mutations: Implications for clinical testing and report of a novel 618C>F mutation in addition to 617V>F. *Blood* 2010;115:3175–3176.

175. Plo I, Vainchenker W. Molecular and genetic bases of myeloproliferative disorders: questions and perspectives. *Clinical Lymphoma Myeloma* 2009;9: S329–S339.

176. Sidon P, El Housni H, Dessars B, et al. The *JAK2* V617F mutation is detectable at very low level in peripheral blood of healthy donors. *Leukemia* 2006;20:1622.

177. Scott L, Tong W, Levine RL, et al. *JAK2* exon 12 mutations in polycythemia vera and idiopathic erythrocytosis. *New England Journal of Medicine* 2007;356:459–468.

178. Kambas K, Mitroulis I, Kourtzelis I, et al. Fast and reliable mutation detection of the complete exon 11-15 *JAK2* coding region using non-isotopic RNase cleavage assay (NIRCA). *European Journal of Haematology* 2009;83:215–219.

DNA-Based Tissue Typing

OBJECTIVES

- Describe the structure and function of the major histocompatibility (MHC) locus.

- List the human leukocyte antigens (HLAs) that are encoded by the MHC locus, and explain their role in tissue engraftment and rejection.

- Compare and contrast the levels of typing resolution that are achieved by different laboratory methods.

- Describe the laboratory methods used to identify HLAs by **serology** testing.

- Describe the DNA-based testing methods used for the identification of HLAs.

- Explain how combining different test methods to identify HLAs increases resolution and resolves ambiguities.

- Discuss factors, in addition to the HLAs, that affect engraftment.

- Relate the use of HLA typing for confirming disease diagnosis and predisposition.

The **major histocompatibility complex (MHC)** is a group of genes located on the short arm of chromosome 6. In humans, the MHC gene products are called **human leukocyte antigens (HLAs)**. The HLAs were named for their role in the rejection of transplanted organs. Kidney, heart, liver, lungs, skin, pancreas, corneas, blood, bone marrow, and hematopoietic stem cells can be transplanted from one human to another. Transplanted organs, except in the case of identical twins, are **allografts**, indicating genetic differences between the donor of the organ and the recipient. When a transplant is performed, compatibility (matching) of the HLA of the organ donor and the recipient increases the chance for a successful engraftment that will function for several years. If the donor and recipient are not HLA-matched, then the recipient's immune system (primarily mediated by T lymphocytes as well as B lymphocytes) will recognize the donor organ as nonself (foreign) and will mount an immune response against the organ, resulting in its destruction, loss of function, and rejection by the recipient.

The role of the clinical laboratory is to evaluate the HLAs of potential donors and recipients and to help predict successful organ engraftment while avoiding **graft versus host disease (GVHD)**. GVHD is the reciprocal of graft rejection whereby immunocompetent cells in the donor organ recognize recipient cells as foreign and attack and destroy the recipient cells, resulting in significant morbidity and potential mortality to the recipient. The process of HLA identification utilizes methods targeting cell-associated antigens as well as serum antibodies. Most **tissue typing**, as HLA identification is commonly called, is performed by serological methods using antibodies to the different HLAs found in the human population. Increasingly, however, DNA typing methods are being implemented for this purpose, increasing the sensitivity and specificity of the typing procedure.

The MHC Locus

The human MHC locus was discovered in the early 1950s. Investigators independently noted that blood from women who had borne children or from previously transfused persons contained antibodies that agglutinated leukocytes.[1,2] This discovery led to serological typing methods that originally identified two polymorphic gene loci, HLA-A and HLA-B, followed soon after by the identification of HLA-C and other genes. A test for typing these loci was designed

from the observation that large, immature, mononuclear cells proliferated if lymphocytes from unrelated individuals were mixed and cultured together.[3,4] Results from this **mixed lymphocyte culture (MLC)** reaction did not always agree with the results of serological typing, however. The discrepancy was partly resolved by the discovery of additional genes comprising the HLA-D locus.[5–7]

Human leukocyte antigens are divided into three classes (I, II, and III), all encoded by a gene complex located on chromosome 6p (Fig. 15-1). The MHC locus includes genes other than those that code for the HLA. Cytokine genes and genes encoding tumor necrosis factor α (TNF-α) and tumor necrosis factor β (TNF-β) are located inside of the main HLA complex.[11]

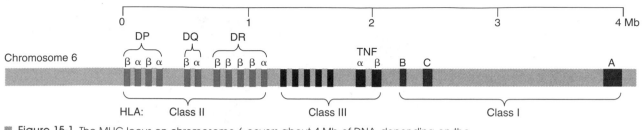

Figure 15-1 The MHC locus on chromosome 6 covers about 4 Mb of DNA, depending on the individual. Class I genes are 3 to 6 kb long, and class II genes are 4 to 11 kb in length. TNF-α and TNF-β are not part of the polymorphic HLA system.

In addition to the main MHC locus, gene regions extending beyond the HLA-DP genes toward the centromere and the HLA-F genes toward the telomere comprise the **extended MHC locus** (xMHC). The xMHC locus covers 8 Mb and includes the hemochromatosis gene *HLA-F* (also called *HFE*), the farthest telomeric gene in the complex.[14,15] The most centromeric locus of the extended MHC is the tapasin region. Tapasin is required for antigenic peptide processing.[16,17] Some genes that are associated with disease conditions, such as *HFE* linked to the MHC locus, are the basis for the association of particular disease states with HLA type (see Chapter 11, "DNA Polymorphisms and Human Identification"). The role of the immune system in other disease states, such as autoimmune diseases and susceptibility to infections, also links HLA type to disease.

The gene products of the MHC—class I, II, and III proteins—are present in different amounts on different tissues (Table 15.1). Classes I and II are the strongest antigens expressed on cells. Class I molecules (designated as A, B, or C) are expressed on all nucleated cells, whereas class II molecules (designated as D) are only expressed constitutively on "professional antigen-presenting cells," such as B lymphocytes, dendritic cells, and macrophages.

As illustrated in Figure 15-2, class I molecules consist of a long (heavy) chain of 346 amino acids (44 kD) associated with a smaller peptide, β-2 microglobulin, which is 99 amino acids (12 kD) in size and is not encoded in the MHC. The two chains are associated with one another on the cell surface by noncovalent bonds. The class I heavy chain displays short, branched-chained sugars, making this molecule a glycoprotein. The heavy chain is also a transmembrane polypeptide, anchoring the complex at the surface of the cell.

Class II molecules consist of two transmembrane polypeptides, an α chain with three domains, α_1, α_2, and α_3, and a β chain with two domains, β_1 and β_2. The two polypeptides associate, forming a groove between the α_1 and β_1 domains that will hold fragments of antigen that have been engulfed and processed by the cell (extracellular

Table 15.1 Genes of the Major Histocompatibility Locus

MHC Region	Gene Products	Tissue Location	Function
Class I	HLA-A, HLA-B, HLA-C	All nucleated cells	Identification and destruction of abnormal or infected cells by cytotoxic T cells
Class II	HLA-D	B lymphocytes, monocytes, macrophages, dendritic cells, activated T cells, activated endothelial cells, skin (Langerhans') cells	Identification of foreign antigen by helper T cells
Class III	Complement C2, C4, B	Plasma proteins	Defense against extracellular pathogens
Cytokine genes	TNF-α, TNF-β	Plasma proteins	Cell growth and differentiation

Outside of cell

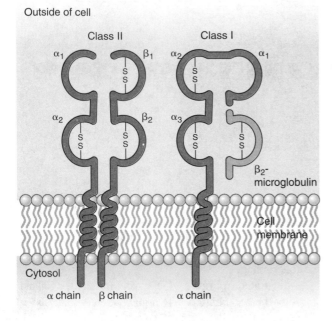

Figure 15-2 Class II (left) and class I (right) polypeptides. Class II antigens consist of two chains, α and β. Class I antigens consist of a heavy chain and a light chain associated together with a molecule of β-2 microglobulin.

Advanced Concepts

Class I and II molecules present fragments of antigens, usually about nine amino acids long, to T lymphocytes. Class I and II molecules vary from one another (are polymorphic), sometimes by a single amino acid. Due to these polymorphisms, different HLA molecules (HLA types) vary in their efficiency in binding antigen fragments, resulting in a range of immune responses to a given antigen. This distinction can affect symptoms of disease, for example, the likelihood of persons of a particular HLA type infected with HIV to develop full immunodeficiency.[18–20]

HLA Polymorphisms

Genes of the MHC are highly polymorphic. Polymorphisms in this locus were first defined phenotypically by acceptance or rejection of tissue or by reaction with defined antibodies (serological typing). Molecular typing methods reveal HLA polymorphisms as base changes in the DNA sequence (Fig. 15-3). The changes range from a single base pair (single nucleotide polymorphisms) to the loss or gain of entire genes. A particular sequence, or version, of an HLA gene is an **allele** of that gene. The **HLA type** is the collection of alleles detected by phenotypic or genotypic typing methods.

Thus, each HLA gene can differ in sequence from one individual to another, except for identical twins. A set of

antigens). In contrast, antigens bound to class I molecules (where the peptide-binding domain is formed between the α₁ and α₂ domains) are generated from the processing of macromolecules synthesized within the cell (intracellular antigens).

A

CGG	GCC	GCG	GTG	GAC	ACC	TAC	TGC	AGA	CAC	AAC	TAC	GGG	GTT	GGT	GAG	AGC	TTC ACA
CGG	GCC	GCG	GTG	GAC	ACC	TAT	TGC	AGA	CAC	AAC	TAC	GGG	GCT	GTG	GAG	AGC	TTC ACA
CGG	GCC	GCC	GTG	GAC	ACC	TAT	TGC	AGA	CAC	AAC	TAC	GGG	GCT	GTG	GNN	NNN	NNN NNN
CGG	GCC	GCG	GTG	GAC	ACC	TAC	TGC	AGA	CAC	AAC	TAC	GGG	GTT	GGT	GAG	AGC	TTC ACA

B

---	---	---	---	---	---	--T	---	---	---	---	---	---	-C-	-TG	---	---	--- ---
---	---	--C	---	---	---	--T	---	---	---	---	---	---	-C-	-TG	-**	***	*** ***

Figure 15-3 DNA polymorphisms in the HLA-DRB1 gene. The initial sequence (DRB1*01:01) is written at the top of panel A. Aligned underneath are two alleles of this region, DRB1*01:022 and DRB*01:03. The green bases are those that differ from DRB1*01:01. N indicates unknown or unsequenced bases. Panel B shows a different way of presenting the alleles. A dash indicates identity to the consensus sequence. Only the polymorphic bases are written. The asterisk indicates unknown or unsequenced bases.

alleles on the same chromosome is a **haplotype** (Fig. 15-4). These alleles are inherited together as a block of chromosomal sequence, unless a rare recombination within the region separates the alleles. An HLA haplotype is, therefore, the combination of polymorphic sequences or alleles in the HLA gene regions.

Polymorphisms are concentrated in exons 2 and 3 of the class I genes and in exon 2 of the class II genes. These exons code for the amino acids that interact with antigenic peptides, affecting the recognition of nonself peptides. Molecular methods target these exons in HLA-A, HLA-B, and HLA-C class I genes and mostly HLA-DRB class II genes. Other areas including introns have been investigated for potentially useful alleles.[21]

HLA Nomenclature

Polymorphisms are alterations in DNA and/or protein sequences shared by at least 2% of a population. Formally,

alterations present at lower frequencies are called mutations or variants. Structurally, mutations and polymorphisms are the same thing: changes from a consensus amino acid or nucleotide sequence. When these changes occur in a gene, the different versions of the gene are referred to as alleles. The polymorphic nature of the MHC, therefore, means that there are multiple alleles of each HLA gene present in the human population. These alleles differ by nucleotide sequence at the DNA level (polymorphisms) and by amino acid sequence and antigenicity at the protein level. Polymorphisms arise mostly as a result of gene conversion events and rare chromosomal recombinations. Each person will have a particular group of HLA alleles inherited from his or her parents (see Chapter 11 for details on human identification). The maternal and paternal HLA antigens are expressed codominantly on cells.

HLA alleles were first defined at the protein level by antibody recognition (serologically). A standard

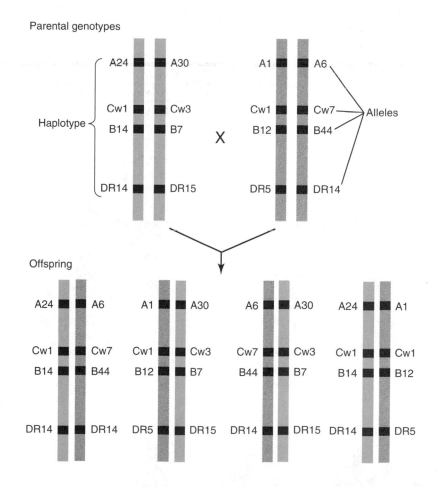

■ **Figure 15-4** A haplotype is the combination of alleles that are inherited together. In this example, parental genotypes (top) can produce four possible genotypes in the offspring (bottom).

nomenclature for expressing serologically defined antigens was established by the World Health Organization (WHO) Nomenclature Committee for Factors of the HLA System. In this system, "HLA" refers to the entire gene region, and "A, B, and D" refer to individual loci within the gene region, for example, HLA-A, HLA-B, or HLA-D. The HLA-D locus consists of subregions P, Q, M, O, and R, termed HLA-DP, HLA-DQ, HLA-DM, and so forth. Each of these subregions consists of genes that code for either an α or β chain polypeptide; for example, the first β polypeptide is encoded in the HLA-DRB1 gene (see Fig. 15-1).

A small "w" is included in the HLA-Cw, HLA-Bw4, and HLA-Bw6 allele nomenclature. The w denotation was originally a designation of alleles in "workshop" status or found in high prevalence in the population. Although the workshop designation is no longer required for the HLA-C locus, the w was retained for HLA-C alleles to distinguish them from the C designation used for complement genes. The w is retained in HLA-Bw4

and HLA-Bw6, which are considered "public" (high-prevalence) antigens.

A list of the serologically defined alleles of the HLA genes accepted by the WHO is shown in Table 15.2. The WHO official nomenclature refers to serologically defined alleles and a number follows the gene region name; for example, HLA-B51 denotes HLA-B antigen 51 (defined by reaction to a known antibody). Number designations of new alleles of a previously defined allele with broad specificity (parent allele) are followed by the number of the parent allele in parentheses. For example, HLA-A24(9) denotes the HLA-A antigen 24 from parent antigen 9. The derived antigens are called **split specificities**. Additional antigens have been defined by reactions between known antigens and serum antibodies (antiserum reactivity). For class I, there are 85, 188, and 42 HLA-A, B, and C alleles, respectively. For class II, there are 76, 32, and 221 HLA-DPB, DQB, and DRB alleles, respectively. These numbers will increase as new specificities are defined.

Table 15.2 **Serologically Defined HLA Specificities***

HLA-A	HLA-B	HLA-C	HLA-DR	HLA-DQ	HLA-DP
A1	B5	Cw1	DR1, DR103	DQ1	DPw1
A2, A203, A210	B51(5), B5102, B5103	Cw2	DR2	DQ5(1)	DPw2
A3	B52(5)	Cw3	DR15(2)	DQ6(1)	DPw3
A9	B7, B703	Cw9(w3)	DR15(2)	DQ2	DPw4
A23(9)	B8	Cw10(w3)	DR3	DQ3	DPw5
A24 (9), A2403	B12	Cw4	DR17(3)	DQ7(3)	DPw6
A10	B44(12)	Cw5	DR18(3)	DQ8(3)	
A25(10)	B45(12)	Cw6	DR4	DQ9(3)	
A26(10)	B13	Cw7	DR5	DQ4	
A34(10)	B14	Cw8	DR11(5)		
A66(10)	B64(14)		DR12(5)		
A11	B65(14)		DR6		
A19	B15		DR13(6)		
A74(19)	B62(15)		DR14(6), DR1403, DR1404		
A68(28)	B63(15)		DR7		
A69(28)	B75(15)		DR8		
A29(19)	B76(15)		DR9		
A30(19)	B77(15)		DR10		
A31(19)	B16		DR51		
A32(19)	B38(16)		DR52		
A33(19)	B39(16), B3901, B3902		DR53		
A36	B17				

Table 15.2 **Serologically Defined HLA Specificities*—cont'd**

HLA-A	HLA-B	HLA-C	HLA-DR	HLA-DQ	HLA-DP
A43	B57(17)				
A80	B58(17)				
	B18				
	B21				
	B49(12)				
	B50(12)				
	B22				
	B54(22)				
	B55(22)				
	B56(22)				
	B27, B2708				
	B35				
	B37				
	B40, B4005				
	B60(40)				
	B61(40)				
	B41				
	B42				
	B46				
	B47				
	B48				
	B53				
	B59				
	B67				
	B70				
	B71(70)				
	B72(70)				
	B73				
	B7801				
	B81				
	Bw4				
	Bw6				

*Alleles are listed in the order of the broad antigen groups, followed by split antigens for that group, with the broad antigen number in parentheses. Associated antigens, such as B40 and B4005, are listed together.

With the introduction of molecular biology techniques in the 1980s, HLA typing at the DNA level required nomenclature for specific DNA sequences.[22–24] Many new alleles have been and are currently being defined at this level and they are named in sequential order as they are discovered.[25–26] For denoting alleles defined by DNA sequence, a revised nomenclature is used. Parts of the allele name are delineated using colons (:) or field separators. The gene name, such as HLA-DRB1, is followed by an asterisk or separator (*), the allele sequence family number (allele group), and a number for the specific allele (DNA sequence encoding the HLA protein). For example, A*25:03 is the third specific allele, 03, of the HLA-A*25 family of alleles. Nucleotide substitutions that change the amino acid sequence are indicated by differences in these digits. Those changes in the DNA sequence that do not change the amino acid sequence (silent or **synonymous** substitutions) are designated by addition of a third group of digits. For example, A*03:01:02 indicates a synonymous allele, 02, of the first specific allele, 01, from the HLA-A*03 family of alleles. A fourth group of digits denotes nucleotide changes in untranslated regions and introns. Thus, A*26:07:01:01 is the 01 subtype allele of the HLA-A*26:07 allele, the second 01 indicating that the polymorphism is in an adjacent intron.

The letter N following the specific allele number indicates a **null allele**, or phenotypic absence of that antigen. For example, B*13:07N denotes the 07 allele of the 13 allele family in the HLA-B locus at the DNA level. At the protein level, however, the encoded protein does not react with any antibody. The B*13:07N null allele is due to a 15-bp deletion in the HLA-B gene. Null alleles can also result from nonsense, frameshift, splice site, or other premature stop mutations that prevent translation of the amino acids destined to bind to antibody.

Ambiguity is the recognition of two or more antigens by the same antibody, or cross-reaction, so that the exact allele cannot be called. Ambiguity is designated by "/" between the possible allele numbers or a dash for a series of alleles in which the first and last allele are named. For example, if a typing test results in either B*07:33 or B*07:35, the notation is B*07:33/B*07:35. If a typing test indicates that the allele is B*07:33, B*07:34, B*07:35, or B*07:36, the designation is B*07:33–B*07:36. Ambiguity also arises from the inability of some typing methods to assign heterozygous alleles to one or the other chromosome. A combination of methods may be used to resolve ambiguities. Family studies are also helpful in this regard.

Resolution is the level of detail to which the allele is determined. Low resolution identifies broad allele types or groups of alleles. A typing of A*26 is low resolution, which can be determined at the serological level. Typing methods that detect specific alleles in addition to identification of all serological types are at medium resolution. Typing result A*26:01/A*26:05/A*26:10/A*26:15 is medium resolution. High-resolution typing procedures can discriminate among almost all specific alleles. A*26:01 is high resolution as determined by DNA analysis. A range of methods from serological typing to direct DNA sequence analysis affords the laboratory a choice of low-, medium-, or high-resolution typing. Whereas low resolution is adequate for solid organ transplantation typing, bone marrow or stem cell transplants require high-resolution methods.

Molecular Analysis of the MHC

Over 1900 HLA alleles have been identified in all loci (Table 15.3). Genetic (DNA-based) typing concentrated on the HLA-A, -B, -C, and DRB1 genes has identified far more alleles for these genes than serological methods have. Over 400 new nucleotide sequences were defined in just 2 years, from 2002 to 2004, and the WHO Nomenclature Committee has devised rules for submitting new alleles for official numerical designation.[27] Allele sequences are stored in the GenBank, the European Molecular Biology Laboratory, and the DNA Data Bank of Japan databases. A list of newly reported alleles is published monthly in the journals *Tissue Antigens*, *Human Immunology*, and the *International Journal of Immunogenetics*. A comprehensive dictionary of antigen-DNA sequence allele equivalents is published periodically.[29–33]

Identification of alleles in the laboratory serves several purposes. In addition to the selection of organ donors, the extent of HLA-type matching between donor and recipient predicts the length of survival of the donor organ in the recipient. Furthermore, because disease genes are located in and around the MHC locus, certain HLA gene alleles are linked to disease, affording another aid in diagnosis or prediction of disease phenotypes.

There are three approaches to analysis of HLA alleles in the HLA laboratory: typing, screening, and **crossmatching**. Typing is the initial identification of the HLA alleles of a specimen through protein or DNA-based methods. Typing may be used both to define HLA haplotypes and to look for specific HLA types that are linked to disease states. Screening is the detection of antihuman antibodies in serum that match known HLA alleles. Crossmatching is more specific screening of recipient sera for antibodies against antigens displayed by potential organ donors.

Serological Analysis

Traditionally, HLA typing for organ transplantation was performed serologically, that is, by antigen-antibody recognition. Although serological testing yields only low-resolution typing results, it has some advantages. It is a relatively rapid method that reveals immunologically relevant epitopes. Also, serological studies can be used to resolve ambiguities or confirm null alleles detected by other methods. Serological tests include HLA phenotype determination, in which patient cells are tested with known antisera (HLA typing), and screening of patient sera for anti-HLA antibodies.

HLA Typing

Lymphocytes are HLA-typed using the **complement-dependent cytotoxicity** test (CDC; Fig. 15-5).[34] In this procedure, multiple alleles are determined using a panel

Table 15.3 **Number of HLA Alleles Identified Serologically and by DNA Sequence***

Gene	Serology	Genetic
Class I		
HLA-A	28	207
HLA-B	29	412
HLA-C	10	100
Class II		
HLA-DRA		2
HLA-DRB1	18	271
HLA-DRB2		1
HLA-DRB3	1	30
HLA-DRB4	1	10
HLA-DRB5	1	15
HLA-DRB6		3
HLA-DRB7		2
HLA-DRB8		1
HLA-DRB9		1
HLA-DQA1		20
HLA-DQB1	9	45
HLA-DMA		4
HLA-DMB		6
HLA-DPA1		19
HLA-DPB1		93
HLA-DOA		8
HLA-DOB		8
Extended MHC		
HLA-E		6
HLA-F		1
HLA-G		14
MICA		57
MICB		18
TAP1	6	6
TAP2	4	4

*The World Marrow Donor Association Quality Assurance and Working Group on HLA Serology to DNA Equivalents publishes a comprehensive dictionary of antigen and allele equivalents.

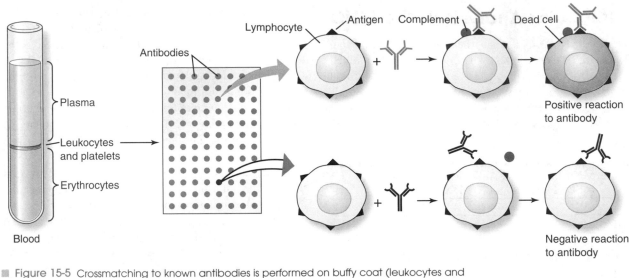

■ Figure 15-5 Crossmatching to known antibodies is performed on buffy coat (leukocytes and platelets, left) in a 96-well plate format where each well contains different known antibodies. If the antibody matches the cellular antigen (positive reaction, top), complement-dependent cytotoxicity will occur, and the dead cell will take up stain (green). If the antibody does not match the cellular antigen, there is no cytotoxicity.

of antibodies against known HLA types. These antibodies are prepared from cell lines or from donors or known HLA types. Plates preloaded with antibodies (**typing trays**) are commercially available, or laboratories may construct their own antibody panels. The collection of antibodies may be modified to represent ethnic populations or antigens of high prevalence in particular geographical areas. The repeated use of antibody preparations facilitates the recognition and recording of the antigen binding characteristics of the various antibodies. Experienced technologists have detailed documentation of antibody panels, including which antibodies bind antigen well and which antibodies bind less strongly.

To begin the typing procedure, different antibodies are placed in each well of a typing tray (a plastic plate with shallow wells). Donor or recipient lymphocytes to be typed are distributed to the wells. Cross-reactivity is assessed by the uptake of trypan blue or eosin red dye in cells that have been permeabilized due to reaction with the antibody and with the complement that is activated by the antigen-antibody complexes (Fig. 15-6). Cytotoxicity is scored by the estimated percentage of cells in a well that have taken up the dye. The American Society for Histocompatibility and Immunogenetics (ASHI) has developed guidelines for numerical description of the observed cytotoxicity (Table 15.4). High cytotoxicity

(reading >6) in a well of the plate indicates that the cells being tested have cell surface antigens matching the known antibody in that well. As reading is somewhat subjective, it is recommended that trays should be read by at least two technologists independently. An example of partial results from a CDC test is shown in Table 15.5.

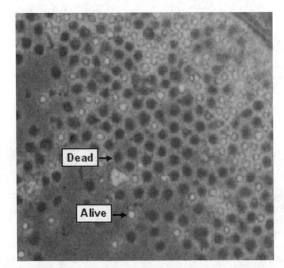

■ Figure 15-6 Cells stained for cytotoxicity. Dead cells take up dye, and live cells remain transparent. (Photo courtesy of Dr. Andres Jaramillo, Rush University Medical Center.)

Table 15.4 **Expression of CDC**

% Dead or Lysed (dyed)	Interpretation	Score
0–10	Negative	1
11–20	Doubtful negative	2
21–50	Weak positive	4
51–80	Positive	6
81–100	Strong positive	8
	Unreadable	0

The results indicate that the tested cells are HLA-type A28, B44.

Each HLA antigen has multiple epitopes, some unique to that HLA antigen and some **cross-reactive epitope groups (CREG)** shared by other HLA antigens. The CDC test can be performed with **private antibodies**, those that bind to one specific HLA type, or antibodies to broad CREG (or "**public**" **antigens**). Analysis of antibodies with shared specificities aids in narrowing the specificity of typing, as illustrated in Table 15.5. As shown, all antibodies with A28 or B44 specificity generated cytotoxicity, supporting the determination of an A28, B44 haplotype. CREG matching or residue matching (determined from the amino acid sequences of the antigens) is considered in kidney transplant screening in order to define the spectrum of HLA-specific antibodies more precisely. Some epitopes are more important than others with respect to organ rejection.[35] Certain mismatches, however, are allowable if the critical epitopes match.[36]

Table 15.5 **Example of Results from a CDC Assay**

Antibody	Score*
A2, A28, B7	8
A2, A28	6
A10	1
A10, A11	1
B7, B42	8
B7, B27	8
B7, B55	8
B44, B45, B21	6
B44, B45	8
B44	8
B45	1

*Scores are 1 to 8, depending on the percentage of dyed cells observed.

Screening

Successful organ transplant depends on minimal reaction of the recipient immune system to the antigens of the donor organ. Normally, serum does not contain antibodies against human antigens, termed **antihuman antibodies** or **alloantibodies**. Persons who have had a previous organ transplant, blood transfusions, or pregnancies, however, will have antihuman antibodies (termed **humoral sensitization**) that may react against a new donor organ. The chance of a successful transplant is improved by defining the specificity of the alloantibodies and selecting a suitable organ that does not have HLA antigens corresponding to the antibodies in the patient's sera.[37]

Humoral sensitization and the identity of alloantibodies present in the recipient serum are determined in a modified version of the CDC assay using the patient's serum as the source of antibodies and reference lymphocytes of known HLA types prevalent in the general population. The reference lymphocytes are defined by their recognition of **panel reactive antibodies (PRA)**. This test against PRA reveals the percentage of the general population with whom the patient will cross-react. The percentage of the panel of lymphocytes killed by the sera is referred to as %PRA. Patients with %PRA activity of more than 50% are considered to be highly sensitized; finding crossmatch-negative donors is more difficult in these cases.[38]

Screening of sera with microparticles (beads) is performed in laboratories with flow cytometry capability (Fig. 15-7). In this method, microparticles are attached to pools of antigens derived from cell lines of defined HLA types. The microparticles are exposed to test serum, and those beads carrying antigens that are recognized by antibodies present in the test serum will bind to those antibodies. After removal of unbound antibodies, a fluorescently labeled secondary reporter antibody is applied, and the antibody-bound beads are detected by flow cytometry. The advantages of this method over the CDC test are that the reaction is performed in a single tube and there is less subjectivity in the interpretation of results. Because this test uses pooled antigens, however, it can detect the prevalence of antihuman antibodies in the test serum but it cannot identify specifically which antibodies are present. A negative result does preclude further alloantibody assessment. A variation of this method developed by Luminex Corp. and MiraiBio utilizes beads that have their own internal fluorescence. By conjugating

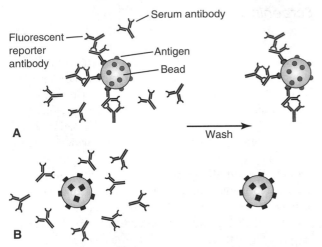

A

Fluorescent reporter antibody

Serum antibody

Antigen

Bead

Wash

B

■ **Figure 15-7** Detection of serum antibodies using bead arrays. In this illustration, separate preparations of beads are conjugated to two different known antigens. The patient serum tested contains an antibody to the antigen on the beads in (A) but not the antigen on the beads in (B). A secondary antibody targeting the bound serum antibody generates a fluorescent signal detected by flow cytometry. If a matching antibody is not present in the test serum, as in (B), no antibody will be bound.

known antigens to beads of different internal fluorescence, the positively reacting antibodies can be identified simultaneously in the same tube.

Crossmatching

The CDC test is also used for crossmatching potential organ donors and recipients. For crossmatching, recipient serum is the source of antibodies tested against donor lymphocytes (Fig. 15-8). If the recipient serum kills the donor lymphocytes, it is a positive crossmatch and a contraindication for using the crossmatched donor.

Other methods used for crossmatching include variations on the lymphocytotoxicity assay and nonlymphocytotoxic methods that utilize flow cytometry, such as the Luminex bead arrays. Alternative methods also include enzyme-linked immunosorbent assay (ELISA) using solubilized HLA antigens. ELISA can be used to monitor the change in antibody production over time or humoral sensitization developing after the transplant.

Mixed Leukocyte Culture

T lymphocytes are primarily responsible for cell-mediated organ rejection. The mixed leukocyte culture (MLC) is an in vitro method used to determine T-cell cross-reactivity between donor and recipient. The MLC assay measures

---

Advanced Concepts

More detailed crossmatch information is achieved by separate analysis of B and T donor lymphocytes. Unactivated T cells display class I antigens, and B cells display both class I and class II antigens. Therefore, if the B cells cross-react with the serum antibodies and the T cells do not, the serum antibodies are likely against class II antigens.

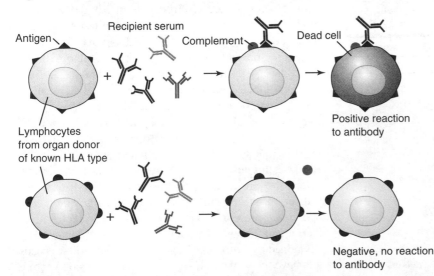

Antigen

Recipient serum

Complement

Dead cell

Positive reaction to antibody

Lymphocytes from organ donor of known HLA type

Negative, no reaction to antibody

■ **Figure 15-8** Crossmatch by CDC. In this assay, the recipient serum is the source of antibodies to type lymphocytes from potential organ donors. The antibodies in the recipient serum can be identified if the HLA type of the lymphocytes is known.

growth of lymphocytes activated by cross-reactivity as an indication of donor/recipient incompatibility. MLC can also test for cell-mediated cytotoxicity and cytokine production, by either the donor or recipient lymphocytes, so it can predict GVHD as well as recipient-mediated transplant rejection. For this test, cells must be incubated together for several days. Cell activation and growth are assessed by uptake of ^{3}H-thymine. Even though the MLC is more likely to detect HLA mismatches than serology techniques, the time and technical demands of the MLC preclude its routine use for pretransplant histocompatibility testing in the clinical laboratory.

Protein Gel Electrophoresis

The protein products of the HLA genes are distinguishable by mobility differences in one-dimensional gel isoelectric focusing or two-dimensional gel electrophoresis methods.[39,40] These typing methods have also been applied to forensic identification.[41] Protein methods are limited by the demands of the methodology and the ability to distinguish only those proteins that have different net charges. With the advent of proteomics, the use of protein markers to evaluate tissue and organ transplantation has been reevaluated.[42]

DNA-Based Typing

Many people are waiting for organ transplants. Typing, screening, and crossmatch analyses are critical in selecting potential donors and for successful engraftment. Methods differ in sensitivity. The choice and design of the method used, therefore, will affect the ability to predict rejection risk.

The limitations of serological and protein-based methods have led to the development of more refined molecular DNA typing with higher powers of resolution, especially for bone marrow transplantation typing. One of the first DNA molecular typing methods was restriction fragment length polymorphism (RFLP) analysis by Southern blot. This method was used to identify HLA class II alleles.[43,44] (See Chapter 6, "Analysis and Characterization of Nucleic Acids and Proteins," for a description of the Southern blot technique.) Studies showed that kidneys matched by RFLP typing survived longer than those matched by serological typing.[45,46]

Just as with other molecular testing applications, the development of amplification and direct sequencing methods greatly advanced the analysis of HLA polymorphisms at the DNA sequence level. DNA typing focuses on the most polymorphic loci in the MHC, HLA-B, and HLA-DRB. HLA-A, HLA-B, HLA-C, and HLA-DRB are all considered important for successful transplantation outcomes.[47] For this reason, the number of alleles identified in these particular loci has risen significantly compared to the number of serologically defined polymorphisms.

DNA-based typing uses whole-blood patient specimens collected in ethylene diamine tetra-acetic acid (EDTA) anticoagulant. Cell lines of known HLA type are used for reference samples. Standards and quality assurance for DNA-based assays have been established by ASHI (www.ashi-hla.org). DNA isolation (see Chapter 4, "Nucleic Acid Extraction Methods") is performed from white blood cell preparations (buffy coat) or from isolated nuclei treated with proteinase K.

Sequence-Specific Oligonucleotide Probe Hybridization

Hybridization of a labeled probe to immobilized amplicons of the HLA genes (dot blot) was one of the first methods that utilized polymerase chain reaction (PCR)–amplified DNA for HLA typing.[48] For **sequence-specific oligonucleotide probe hybridization** (SSOP; Fig. 15-9), the HLA region under investigation is amplified by PCR using primers flanking the polymorphic sequences. Because the majority of polymorphic sequences are located in exon 2 of the class II genes and exons 2 and 3 of the class I genes, primers are designed to target these regions.

An assay using 30 labeled probes requires approximately 70 µl of PCR product.[49] The amplicons are denatured by addition of NaOH and spotted onto a membrane in 1 to 2 µl volumes. Spotting is done manually with a multichannel pipette or by a vacuum manifold with a 96-well plate format. The spotted DNA is dried and then permanently attached to the membrane by ultraviolet cross-linking (exposure to ultraviolet light) or baking. Separate membranes are produced for each probe to be used. Every membrane should include reference amplicons complementary (positive control) and noncomplementary (negative control) to all probes in the assay. Spotting consistency may be checked using a consensus probe that will hybridize to all specimens on a membrane.

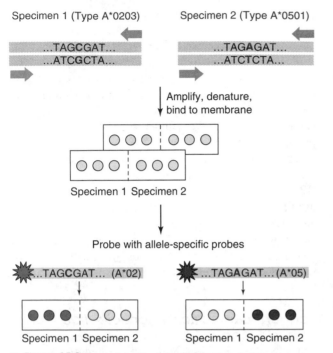

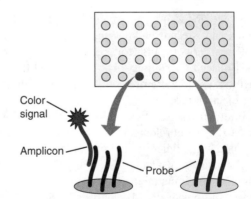

Specimen 1 (Type A*0203)   Specimen 2 (Type A*0501)

...TAGCGAT...
...ATCGCTA...

...TAGAGAT...
...ATCTCTA...

Amplify, denature, bind to membrane

Specimen 1 Specimen 2

Probe with allele-specific probes

..TAGCGAT... (A*02)   ...TAGAGAT...(A*05)

Specimen 1 Specimen 2   Specimen 1 Specimen 2

■ **Figure 15-9** The principle of the SSOP assay is shown. An HLA gene region is amplified from specimen DNA using generic primers (top). The amplicons are immobilized on a membrane and probed with labeled sequences complementary to specific alleles. Signal from the bound probe will indicate the allele of the immobilized DNA.

The probes used in this assay are short (19 to 20 bases), single-stranded DNA chains (oligonucleotides) designed to hybridize to specific HLA alleles. The oligonucleotide probes are labeled, that is, covalently attached to biotin or digoxygenin. (See Chapter 6 for a description of nonradioactive signal detection.) Probe sequences are based on sequence **alignments** of HLA polymorphic regions and are aligned so that the polymorphic nucleotide is in the middle of the sequence. Hybridization conditions depend on the optimal binding of the probe matching a test sequence in comparison to another sequence, differing from (not complementary to) the probe by at least one base. Spots of immobilized specimens bound to specific probes give a positive colorimetric or chemiluminescent signal. Panels of probes define specific alleles according to which probe binds to the immobilized, amplified DNA under investigation. The number of probes used depends on the design of the assay. For example, an intermediate-resolution assay of the HLA-DRB locus might use 30 to 60 probes.

Studies have achieved high-resolution identification of the majority of HLA-A, B, and C alleles using 67 HLA-A, 99 HLA-B, and 57 HLA-C probes and intermediate-resolution identification with 39 HLA-A and 59 HLA-B alleles.[50]

SSOP may also be performed in a reverse dot blot configuration in which the allele-specific probes are immobilized on the membrane (Fig. 15-10). In this method, the specimen DNA is labeled by PCR amplification using primers covalently attached to biotin or digoxygenin at the 5' end. In contrast to the SSOP described previously, in which amplicons from each specimen are spotted on multiple membranes, each specimen in a reverse dot blot is tested for multiple alleles on a single membrane. Therefore, instead of having a separate membrane of multiple specimens for each probe, a separate membrane of multiple probes is required for each specimen. Membranes with immobilized probes, such as Dynal RELI, SSO HLA-Cw, and DRB typing kits, are commercially available.

A bead array system where fluorescently distinct beads carry the oligonucleotide probes (LABType SSO, One Lambda, Inc.) has also been used in the reverse dot blot strategy. This system is commercially available for the typing of HLA-A, B, C class I, and HLA-DRB1, DRB3, DRB4, DRB5, and DQB1 antigens.

Color signal

Amplicon

Probe

■ **Figure 15-10** In reverse dot blot SSOP, the probe is immobilized on the membrane. Patient DNA is amplified using primers covalently bound to biotin or digoxygenin at the 5' end. The amplicons are then hybridized to panels of probes immobilized on a membrane (top). If the sequence of the amplicon matches and hybridizes to that of the probe, a secondary reaction with enzyme-conjugated avidin or antidigoxygenin will produce a color or light signal when exposed to substrate. If the sequence of the amplicon differs from that of the probe, no signal is generated (bottom right).

SSOP is considered low to intermediate resolution, depending on the number and types of probes used in the assay. The 13th International Histocompatibility Workshop lists probe panels at www.ikwg.org and the National Marrow Donor Program (NMDP) provides lists at www.nmdpresearch.org. Because some probes have multiple specificities, hybridization panels can be complex. Computer programs may be used for accurate interpretation of SSOP results.

Sequence-Specific PCR

A more rapid method of sequence-based typing, compared with SSOP, is the use of sequence-specific primers that will amplify only specific alleles (Fig. 15-11). As described in Chapter 7, the 3' end of a PCR primer must be complementary to the template for recognition and extension by DNA polymerase. By designing primers that end on the polymorphic sequences, successful generation of a PCR product will occur only if the test sequence has the polymorphic allele complementary to the primer. Detection of the PCR product is used to indicate specific alleles. Sequence-specific PCR (SSP-PCR) is faster and easier than SSOP in that no probes or labeling steps are required and the results of SSP-PCR are determined directly by agarose gel electrophoresis.

For SSP-PCR, isolated DNA is amplified using sets of primers designed to specifically amplify a panel of alleles. Reactions are set up in a 96-well plate format, with different allele- or sequence-specific primer sets in each well. In addition to the allele-specific primers, each PCR reaction mix contains amplification control primers in a multiplex format. The amplification control primers should yield a product for every specimen (except the reagent blank). The sequence-specific primers should yield a product only if the specimen has the allele complementary to (matching) the allele-specific primer sequence. The amplification primers are designed to produce a PCR product of a size distinct from the product of the allele-specific primers. The two amplicons are then resolved by agarose gel electrophoresis. An illustration of the results expected from SSP-PCR is shown in Figure 15-12. Specimens will yield two PCR products (amplification control and allele-specific product) only from those wells containing primers matching the specimen HLA allele. Wells containing primers that do not match the patient's HLA allele will yield a product only from the amplification control.

PCR plates preloaded with reaction mixes (typing trays) containing primers specific for class I and class II DRB and DRQ genes are commercially available (MicroSSP, One Lambda, Inc., and Pel Freez SSP UniTray). To use these products, specimen DNA is introduced into the individual wells, and the plates are placed in the thermal cycler. Plate maps of allele-specific primers are provided for interpretation of the HLA-type. SSP-PCR has become a commonly used method for testing potential donors before transplant.

Sequence-Based Typing

The most definitive way to analyze DNA at the nucleotide sequence level is by direct DNA sequencing. This is true for any DNA test, no less for discovery and identification of HLA types. (See Chapter 10, "DNA Sequencing," for a description of DNA sequencing

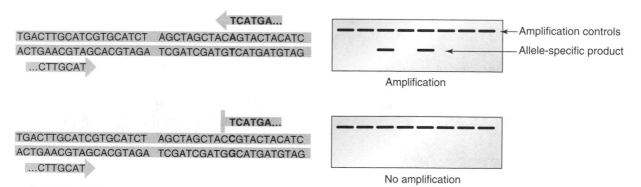

■ **Figure 15-11** The sequence-specific primer ending in AGTACT will be extended only from a template carrying the polymorphism shown.

Reagent blank

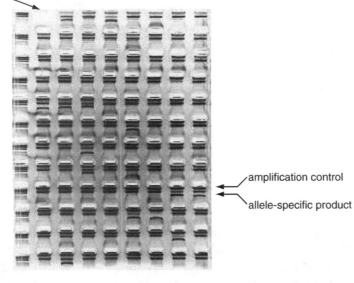

amplification control

allele-specific product

■ Figure 15-12 Results of an SSP-PCR of 95 primer sets detected by agarose gel electrophoresis. An amplification control is included with each reaction to avoid false-negative results due to amplification failure. Contamination is monitored by a reagent blank. (Photo courtesy of Christine Braun, Rush University Medical Center.)

methodology.) Sequence-based typing (SBT) involves amplification of polymorphic regions, for example, exons 2 and 3 of the HLA-B gene (Fig. 15-13). The amplicons are then purified and added to a sequencing reaction mix (Fig. 15-14). Following gel or capillary gel electrophoresis, the fragment patterns or electrophero-grams are examined for specific polymorphisms. Because HLA haplotypes are almost always heterozy-gous, the sequencing results often yield a heterozygous pattern at the site of the polymorphism (Fig. 15-15). Commercial systems including PCR and sequencing reaction mixes as well as software programs for inter-pretation of results are available.

Secondary structure and other artifacts may alter the mobility of some fragments and complicate interpreta-tion. Furthermore, a number of events can occur that will compromise sequence quality (see Chapter 10). Manu-facturers of sequencing reagents offer suggestions to

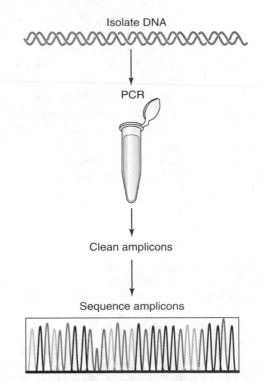

Isolate DNA

PCR

Clean amplicons

Sequence amplicons

■ Figure 15-14 For sequenced-based typing, HLA regions from patient DNA are amplified by PCR. The PCR products are then purified from unused PCR reaction components by alco-hol precipitation or column or gel purification methods. The amplicons are then sequenced to detect polymorphisms.

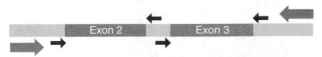

Exon 2   Exon 3

■ Figure 15-13 Example of primer placement for amplifica-tion and sequence analysis. PCR primers (outer large arrows) are used to amplify the region of interest. The PCR product is then sequenced using four different primers (inner small arrows) in separate sequencing reactions.

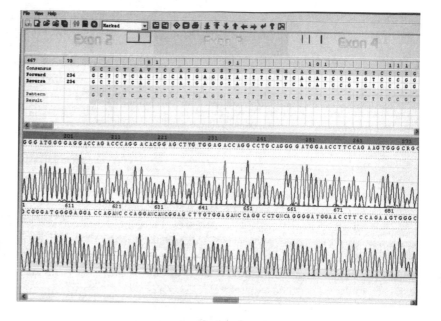

■ **Figure 15-15** A sequence-based typing result for the HLA-A gene. Software is designed to analyze the sequence of patient DNA, compare it with the consensus sequence, and identify the specific alleles by sequence polymorphisms. (Sequence courtesy of Christine Braun, Rush University Medical Center.)

correct most of these problems. As with any sequencing assay, it is useful to sequence both strands of the test DNA.

Other DNA-Based Methods

Almost any method that can determine DNA sequence or detect specific sequences or sequence differences can be applied to DNA-based HLA typing (see Chapter 9, "Gene Mutations"). Variations on SSOP, SSP, and SBT, such as nested PCR-SSP,[51] have also been proposed for HLA typing. Another example is allele-specific nested PCR-SSP, which has been applied to subtyping of highly polymorphic alleles.[52,53]

Heteroduplex (HD) analysis has been used for assessment of compatible bone marrow donors at the HLA-DR and HLA-DP loci.[54] Reference strand conformation polymorphism is a variation on the standard HD analysis; sample amplicons are mixed with fluorescently labeled reference DNA of known allele sequence before denaturation and renaturation to form heteroduplexes.[55] The homo- and heteroduplexes formed between the specimen amplicons and the reference strand are then resolved by capillary gel electrophoresis.

Single-strand conformation polymorphism (SSCP) has been applied to HLA-A, DR, DQ, and DP typing and subtyping, either alone[56,57] or coupled with allele-specific PCR.[58] High-performance liquid chromatography

(HPLC) has been proposed for HLA typing as well. However, conformation analyses, such as HD, SSCP, and HPLC, are limited by the complexity of the raw data and the strict demands on reactions and electrophoresis conditions; they are not routinely used in the clinical laboratory.

Other DNA-based typing approaches include array technology[59] and pyrosequencing.[60] Real-time PCR methods have been designed to assess specific HLA alleles[61] or blood groups.[62] No one method is without disadvantages with respect to technical demands, cost, or time consumption. To date, SSP, SSOP, and SBT are the DNA-based methods used in most clinical laboratories.[49,63]

Combining Typing Results

At the DNA level, HLA polymorphisms differ from one another by as little as a single nucleotide base. Serological typing does not always distinguish subtle genetic differences between types; it also requires the proper specimen. A specimen consisting of mostly T cells from a patient treated with chemotherapy, for example, will not provide B cells (which carry class II antigens) for testing of class II haplotypes. In contrast, DNA-based typing is not limited by specimen type, as all cells have the same HLA haplotype at the DNA level, regardless of whether the cell type expresses the antigens. Synonymous DNA changes and polymorphisms outside of the protein coding regions detected by sequencing, however, may not alter antigenicity at the protein level.

For DNA-based methods, the system design (primer and probe selection) determines the level of resolution. SSOP and SSP methods require specific primers and/or probes for each particular HLA type. Only those HLA types included in a given probe or primer set, therefore, will be identified. Sequence-based typing will only identify alleles included in the amplified regions that are sequenced.

Results from serological and DNA-based methods may be combined to improve resolution and further define HLA types. Sequential use of SSP-PCR and PCR-RFLP or SSOP-PCR and SSP-PCR increases the typing resolution of DNA-based tests.[49,64] Serological testing can be used to clarify or confirm the phenotype of alleles detectable by DNA-based methods. The resolution of results from various methods, therefore, reflects a range of resolution levels (Table 15.6). The choice of method will depend on the demand for high- or low-resolution typing.

HLA Test Discrepancies

HLA typing may produce discrepant results, especially if different methods are used to assess the same specimen. The most common discrepancies are those between serology and molecular testing results.[65] DNA sequence changes do not always affect protein epitopes. A serology type may represent several alleles at the DNA level. Also, a serology type may look homozygous (match to only one antibody) where the DNA alleles are heterozygous, the second allele not recognized by serology. For example, a serology type of A2 may be A*02, A*74 at the DNA level.

Discrepancies also arise when HLA types assigned to parent alleles based on DNA sequence homology differ from serology results that detect the same allele as a new antigen. For example, a DNA allele of B*40:05 is detected as a new antigen by serology and named B50. Similarly, split alleles (subtypes of serologically defined antigens) can differ between DNA and serology typing due to the cross-reactivity of antibodies used to define the HLA antigens. The identification of new alleles will result in discrepant retyping results based on the recognition of new alleles that were not defined at the time of an initial typing. These discrepancies may be difficult to resolve, especially if the original typing data are not accessible.

Coordination of HLA Test Methods

The choice of the appropriate method and resolution of HLA testing is influenced by the type of transplant. For solid organ transplants, antibody screening and cross-matching of recipient serum against donor antigens are routinely performed, although not always before transplantation. Pretransplant HLA typing is often determined for kidney and pancreas transplants, as the extent of HLA matching is directly proportional to time of survival of the donor organ.[66,67] Given the circumstances under which heart, lung, and liver transplants are performed, testing is frequently performed after the transplant. HLA typing for solid organs is usually done at the low-resolution serology level, although for heart and lung transplants, as for kidney transplants, studies have shown that matching HLA types are beneficial for organ survival.[68,69] For stem cell and bone marrow transplants, typing to high resolution (specific alleles) is preferred in order to decrease the risk of rejection and to avoid GVHD.[70,71]

Additional Recognition Factors

Minor Histocompatibility Antigens

Any donor protein that can be recognized as nonself by the recipient immune system can potentially affect engraftment. Proteins outside the MHC that influence graft failure are called **minor histocompatibility antigens (mHag)**, which were the first suspected cause of GVHD and graft rejection in MHC-identical transplants.[72–74] The H-Y antigen was the first characterized mHag.[75] Investigations using molecular methods have led to the

Table 15.6 **Resolution of HLA Typing Methods**

Low Resolution	Intermediate Resolution	High Resolution
CDC (serology)	PCR-SSP	PCR-SSP
PCR-SSP	PCR-SSOP	PCR-SSOP
PCR-SSOP	qPCR	qPCR
	PCR-RFLP	SSP-PCR + PCR-RFLP
		SSOP-PCR + SSP-PCR
		SBT

characterization of additional mHags, including HA-1, CD31, HPA-1, HPA-2, HPA-3, and HPA-5.[76] Comparative genomics have been proposed as a way to find mHags responsible for GVHD or graft-versus-tumor effects.[77,78] The evaluation of mHags in stem cell transplants is carried out by molecular methods such as SSP-PCR.[79]

Nonconventional MHC Antigens

Within the MHC locus are the related MHC class I *MICA* and *MICB* genes. Three pseudogene fragments, *MICC, MICD*, and *MICE*, are also found within the class I region. The products of the *MICA* and *MICB* genes along with those of the retinoic acid early transcript (RAET) gene cluster located on the long arm of chromosome 6 (6p21.3) bind to the receptor NKG2D on natural killer (NK) cells (killer cell lectin-like receptor, subfamily K, number 1, or KLRK1). These gene products participate in immune reactions against abnormal cells such as tumor cells through control of NK cells and cytotoxic T lymphocytes (CTL) expressing the γδ T-cell receptor. Virus- or bacteria-infected cells may also be recognized and eliminated in part by this system.

The *MICA* and *MICB* genes are highly polymorphic. According to the International ImMunoGeneTics information system (IMGT) HLA database (http://www.ebi.ac.uk/imgt/hla/), there are approximately 60 *MICA* and 30 *MICB* alleles. In contrast to the MHC class I alleles, polymorphisms in the *MIC* genes are distributed throughout the coding regions, with no hypervariable regions. Anti-MIC antibodies have been detected after organ transplantation, similar to anti-HLA alloantibodies, which is supportive of a role for these gene products in organ rejection.[80] Specific *MICA* and *MICB* alleles may also be associated with disease states.[81,82]

Killer Cell Immunoglobulin-like Receptors

NK cells and some memory T cells express killer cell immunoglobulin-like proteins (KIR). First observed as **"hybrid resistance"** in experiments with mice,[83] the mice with compromised immune systems were still capable of rejecting grafts from unrelated mice. That is, graft rejection still occurred even in the absence of a functional immune system. The KIR proteins, proposed as one source of nonself recognition outside of the MHC, interact with HLA antigens, specifically recognizing HLA-A, HLA-B, and HLA-C (class I) molecules. KIR proteins are also expressed on myelomonocytic lineage cells (leukocyte immunoglobulin-like receptor) and other leukocytes (leukocyte-associated immunoglobulin-like receptor). A cluster of genes coding for these receptor proteins has been found on chromosome 19q13.4, the leukocyte receptor cluster (Fig. 15-16).

Recipient KIR may participate in graft rejection, while donor KIR may be involved in GVHD.[84,85] Specific interactions between KIR and HLA genes are listed in Table 15.7. Just as with mHags, assessment of polymorphisms in KIR may be added to donor selection criteria in stem cell and bone marrow transplants, especially with unrelated donors.[86–88] In contrast to HLA typing, testing for KIR is aimed at finding donors and recipients who do *not* match. A KIR SSO commercial system using bead array technology is available for typing of 16 KIR genes and variants (One Lambda, Inc.). KIR may also be tested

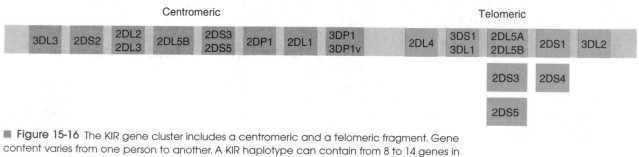

■ Figure 15-16 The KIR gene cluster includes a centromeric and a telomeric fragment. Gene content varies from one person to another. A KIR haplotype can contain from 8 to 14 genes in different combinations and gene orders. For example a haplotype may have a 2DL2 or 2DL3 gene between the 2DS2 and 2DL5B genes, or the order of 2DS1 and 2DS4 can be 2DS1–2DS4 or 2DS4–2DS1.

Table 15.7 **KIR and HLA Gene Interactions**

KIR	HLA Specificities
2DL1, 2DS1, (2DS4)	Cw*02, *03:07, *03:10, *03:15, *03:04, *03:05, *03:06, *07:07, *07:09, *12:04, *12:05, *15 (except *15:07), *16:02, *17, *18
2DL2, 2DL3, (2DS2)	Cw*01, *03, (except *03:07, *03:10, *03:15, *07 (except *07:07, *07:09), *07:08, *12 (except *12:04, *12:05), *13, *14, *15:07, *16 (except *16:02)
2DL4	G
2DL5	Unknown
3DL1	Bw4
3DL2	A3, A11
3DL3	Unknown
2DS3	Unknown
2DS5	Unknown
3DS1	Unknown

by SSP,[89] which is the basis of the Invitrogen™ KIR Genotyping Kit.

MHC Disease Association

Genetic diseases caused by single-gene disorders obey Mendelian laws. Their phenotypes are either dominant or recessive and are inherited in a predictable manner, illustrated in pedigrees (see Chapter 13, "Molecular Detection of Inherited Diseases"). Most diseases, however, are not caused by a single genetic lesion and therefore have complex segregation patterns. Multiple genes, epigenetics, and environmental factors combine to bring about these disease states. For such conditions as diabetes, high blood pressure, and certain cancers, genetic analysis yields results in terms of predisposition, probability, and risk of disease.

Autoimmune diseases, which affect 4% of the population, fall into this category. At least one of the genetic factors involved in autoimmunity is linked to the MHC, as autoimmune diseases have MHC associations. Rheumatoid arthritis, multiple sclerosis, diabetes mellitus type 1, and systemic lupus erythematosus are associated with particular HLA haplotypes. Determination of a disease-associated HLA haplotype aids in diagnosis or prediction of disease predisposition.[90]

The presence of a haplotype associated with disease is not diagnostic on its own, however. An example is the HLA-B27 type found in all cases of ankylosing spondylitis. HLA-B27 is also the most frequently found HLA-B allele. Therefore, many people with the B27 allele do not have this condition. The laboratory is usually asked to perform HLA typing of persons showing disease symptoms or with family histories of such a disease to aid or confirm the diagnostic decisions.

Normal states are also controlled by multiple genetic and environmental factors. The genes for olfactory sensation, histone genes, genes encoding transcription factors, and the butyrophilin (a constituent of milk in mammals) gene cluster are found in the MHC. The MHC may play a role not only in the predisposition to disease but in protection from disease as well, including some infectious diseases, notably HIV.[18,91,92] In this role, certain HLA types are considered "protective."

Summary of Laboratory Testing

Standard HLA testing includes a range of methods and test designs (Table 15.8). Determining donor and recipient compatibility is the primary goal of pretransplant

Table 15.8 **Summary of Testing for Pre- and Posttransplant Evaluation**

Purpose	Test Design	Methods
Determine HLA type	Determine HLA types with standard references or by DNA sequence	Serology
		DNA-based typing
Determine serum antibody status	Serum screening against known HLA antibodies	CDC
		ELISA
		Flow cytometry
Crossmatching	Compare serum of recipient with that of prospective donors	CDC
		ELISA
		Flow cytometry
Determine T-cell-mediated cytotoxicity between donor and recipient	Alloreactive T-cell characterization and quantitation	MLC
		Cytokine production

Advanced Concepts

HLA types are also associated with absence of inherited disease. Protection from genetic diseases is naturally enhanced by "**hybrid vigor**," or avoidance of inbreeding. The MHC may bring about such natural protection by controlling mating selection to ensure genetic mixing. For example, studies with mice have shown that olfactory sensation (sense of smell) may play a role in mate selection. In these studies, female mice were able to distinguish male mice with histocompatibility alleles different from their own.[93] This supports the idea of selective pressure to mate with immunogenetically dissimilar partners to increase genetic diversity. Another study in humans showed that women found the scent of T-shirts worn by some male subjects pleasant but others unpleasant. The odors detected as pleasant were from HLA-dissimilar males. The women were apparently able to distinguish HLA types different from their own through the sweat odors of the male test subjects.[94]

testing, especially bone marrow transplants from unrelated donors. The extent of HLA matching will increase the prospect of successful transplantation with minimal GVHD. For example, the NMDP requests HLA typing results for HLA-A, B, and C class I antigens and DRB1, DQB1, and DPB1 class II antigens for prospective bone marrow donors.

Combinations of molecular tests, serum screening, and crossmatching further define acceptable HLA mismatches, and the results are used to prevent hyperacute (almost immediate) rejection in organ transplants. Identification of HLA types associated with disease also provides important information, especially for disease caused by multiple genetic and environmental factors. Finally, mixed lymphocyte culture, although not generally part of routine clinical testing, can predict cellular factors involved in rejection.

Laboratory results are key for the selection of compatible donors, posttransplant evaluation, selection of the optimal treatment strategy, and predisposition to genetic disease. Molecular analysis has significantly increased the ease and ability to detect subtle differences in the MHC and associated regions. Nucleic acid analysis will play an expanding role in this area of laboratory analysis.

CASE STUDY 15 • 1

A 50-year-old man complained of digestive disorders and what he presumed was allergy to several foods. He consulted his physician, who collected blood samples for laboratory testing. The man was in a high-risk group for certain diseases, notably celiac disease, which would produce symptoms similar to those experienced by this patient. A specimen was sent to the laboratory to test HLA-DQA and -DQB alleles. Almost all (95%) people with celiac disease have the DQA1*05:01 and DQB1*02:01 alleles (DQ2 variant), compared to 20% in the general population. A second predisposing heterodimer, DQ8, is encoded by the DQA1*03:01and the DQB1*03:02 alleles. Most of the 5% of celiac patients who are negative for the DQ2 alleles display the DQ8 alleles. Serological results to detect the predisposing antigens, however, were equivocal. An SBT test was performed. The sequence results showed the following alleles at DQA1 and DQB1 loci:

DQA1*05:01

DQB1*02:01/DQB1*04:01

QUESTION: *Is it possible that this man has celiac disease based on his HLA haplotype?*

CASE STUDY 15 • 2

A 43-year-old man consulted his physician about a lump on his neck and frequent night sweats. A biopsy of the mass in his neck was sent to the pathology department for analysis. An abnormally large population of CD20-positive lymphocytes was observed by morphological examination. Flow cytometry tests detected a monoclonal B-cell population with co-expression of CD10/CD19 and CD5. This population was 88% kappa and 7% lambda. The results were confirmed by the observation of a monoclonal immunoglobulin heavy chain gene rearrangement that was also monoclonal for kappa light chain gene rearrangement. The patient was initially treated with standard chemotherapy, but the tumor returned before the therapeutic program was completed. The tumor persisted through a second treatment with stronger chemotherapy plus local irradiation. A nonmyeloablative bone marrow transplant was prescribed. To find a compatible donor, the man's HLA type and the types of five potential donors were compared. HLA-A and -B types were assessed by serology, and the HLA-DR type was determined by SSP-PCR and SSOP. The typing results are shown in the table.

Recipient	Donor 1	Donor 2	Donor 3	Donor 4	Donor 5
A*03:02	A*66:01/04	A*26:01	A*03:02	A*31:03/04	A*26:10
A*26:10	A*03:02	A*03:02		A*03:09	A*03:09
B*39:06	B*07:11	B*15:28	B*53:07	B*39:06	B*35:08
B*53:07	B*57:01	B*39:19	B*39:01	B*53:07	
DRB1* 08:01	DRB1* 07:01	DRB1* 13:17	DRB1* 08:01	DRB1* 07:01	DRB1* 13:17
	DRB1* 13:17	DRB1* 04:22		DRB1* 11:17	DRB1* 07:01

QUESTIONS:
1. *Which of the five donors is the best match for this patient?*
2. *Which mismatches are acceptable?*
3. *Using the donor bone marrow that matches most closely, is there more of a chance of graft rejection or GVHD?*

CASE STUDY 15 • 3

A 19-year-old woman reported to a local clinic with painful swelling in her face. Routine tests revealed dangerously high blood pressure that warranted hospitalization. Further tests were performed, which led to a diagnosis of systemic lupus erythematosus. Due to complications of this disease, her kidney function was compromised, and she would eventually suffer kidney failure. With an alternative of lifelong dialysis, a kidney transplant was recommended. Class I PRAs were assessed at 0% PRA. An additional screen for class II PRA was performed by flow cytometry.

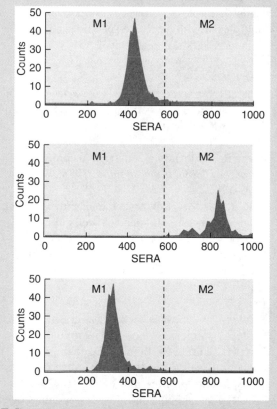

■ Flow cytometry analysis of HLA class II antigens in recipient serum. Top = negative control; middle = positive control; bottom = patient serum.

SSP-PCR results for HLA-A, -B, and -DR and their serological equivalents are shown in the table.

Crossmatching of the daughter's serum and mother's cells was performed by cytotoxicity and flow cytometry. Both test results were negative.

Class I and class II HLA typing was performed by SSP-PCR. An autocytotoxic crossmatch was also performed, revealing T-cell and B-cell positive antibodies, probably related to the lupus. The young woman's mother volunteered to donate a kidney to her daughter. Mother and daughter had matching blood group and HLA-DR antigens, which are the most critical for a successful organ transplant. The results from the typing tray are shown in the accompanying figure.

Daughter SSP-PCR	Serology	Mother SSP-PCR	Serology
A*24:19, A*34:01	A24(9), 34(10)	A*11:04, A*24:19	A11, A24(9)
B*08:02, B*56:03	B8, B22	B*08:04, B*56:03	B8, B22
DRB1*04:22, DRB1*14:11	DR4, DR14(6)	DRB1*04:22, DRB1*13:17	DR4, DR13(6)

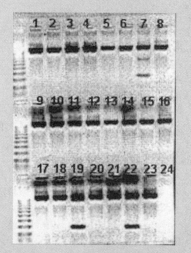

■ SSP-PCR results from an HLA-A typing tray for the daughter. Alleles were identified in lanes 7, 19, and 22.

QUESTIONS:

1. Is the mother a good match for the daughter? Based on the antibody and crossmatching studies, what is the risk of rejection?
2. Before performing the HLA studies, how many of the daughter's antigens would be expected to match those of her mother?

• STUDY QUESTIONS •

1. Which of the following is a high-resolution HLA typing result?
   a. B27
   b. A*02:02–02:09
   c. A*02:12
   d. A*26:01/A*26:05/A*26:01/A*26:15

2. Which of the following is a likely haplotype from parents with A25,Cw10,B27/A23,Cw5,B27 and A17,Cw4, B10/A9,Cw7,B12 haplotypes?
   a. A25,Cw10,B27
   b. A25,Cw5,B27
   c. A23,Cw4,B12
   d. A17,Cw4,B27

3. Upon microscopic examination, over 90% of cells are translucent after a CDC assay. How are these results scored according to the ASHI rules?

4. An HLA-A allele is a CTC to CTT change at the DNA level (leu → leu). How is this allele written?
   a. HLA-A*02
   b. HLA-A*02:01
   c. HLA-A2
   d. HLA-A*02N

5. A candidate for kidney transplant has a PRA of 75%. How might this affect eligibility for an immediate transplant?

6. An SSOP probe recognizes HLA-DRB*03:01–03:04. Another probe recognizes HLA-DRB*03:01/03:04, and a third probe hybridizes to HLA-DRB*03:01–03:03. Test specimen DNA hybridizes to all except the third probe in a reverse dot blot format. What is the HLA-DRB type of the specimen?

7. What is the relationship between alleles HLA-A10 and HLA-A26(10)?

8. A CDC assay yields an 8 score for sera with the following specificities: A2, A28 and A2, A28, B7, and a 1 score for serum with an A2 specificity. What is the HLA-A type?

9. HLA-DRB1*15:01 differs from DRB1*01:01 by a G to C base change. If the sequence surrounding the base change is: ...GGGTGCGGTTG̲CTGGAAA-GAT... (DRB1*01:01) or ...GGGTGCGGTTC̲CTG-GAAAGAT... (DRB1*15:01), which of the following would be the 3' end of a sequence-specific primer for detection of DRB1*15:01?
   a. ...ATCTTTCCAGG̲AACCC
   b. ...ATCTTTCCAGC̲AACCC
   c. ...ATCTTTCCAGC̲
   d. ...ATCTTTCCAGG̲

10. The results of an SSP-PCR reaction are the following: lane 1, one band; lane 2, two bands; lane 3 no bands. If the test includes an amplification control multiplexed with the allele-specific primers, what is the interpretation for each lane?

References

1. Dausset J, Nenna A. Présence d'une leuco-agglutinine dans le sérum d'un cas d'agranulocytose chronique. *Comptes Rendues des Societe de Biologie* 1952;146: 1539–1541.
2. Payne R. Fetomaternal leukocyte incompatibility. *Journal of Clinical Investigation* 1958;37: 1756–1763.
3. Bain B, Vaz MR, Lowenstein L. The development of large immature mononuclear cells in mixed lymphocyte cultures. *Blood* 1964;23:108–116.
4. Bach F, Hirschhorn K. Lymphocyte interaction: A potential histocompatibility test in vitro. *Science* 1964;142:813–814.
5. Jones E, Goodfellow PN, Bodmer JG, et al. Serological identification of HLA-linked human "Ia-type" antigens. *Nature* 1975;256:650–652.
6. Park M, Terasaki PI, Bernoco D, et al. Evidence for a second B-cell locus separate from the DR locus. *Transplantation Proceedings* 1978;10:823–828.
7. Tosi R, Tanigaki N, Centis D, et al. Immunological dissection of human Ia molecules. *Journal of Experimental Medicine* 1978;148:1592–1611.
8. Bover K. Homoisotransplantation van epidermis bei einigen Zwillingen. *Beitrage zur klinischen Chirurgica* 1927;141:393–453.
9. Gorer P. The genetic and antigenic basis for tumor transplantation. *Journal of Pathology and Bacteriology* 1937;44:691–697.

10. Snell G. Methods for the study of histocompatibility genes. *Journal of Genetics* 1948;49:87–108.

11. Inoko H, Trowsdale J. Linkage of TNF genes to the HLA-B locus. *Nucleic Acids Research* 1987;15:8957–8962.

12. Rosenthal A, Shevach E. Function of macrophages in antigen recognition by guinea pig T lymphocytes. I. Requirement for histocompatible macrophages and lymphocytes. *Journal of Experimental Medicine* 1973;138:1194–1212.

13. Kindred B, Shreffler DC. H-2 dependence of cooperation between T and B cells in vivo. *Journal of Immunology* 1972;109:940–943.

14. Ruddy DA, Lee VK, Mintier GA, et al. A 1.1-Mb transcript map of the hereditary hemochromatosis locus. *Genome Research* 1997;7:441–456.

15. Feder J, Gnirke A, Thomas W, et al. A novel MHC class I-like gene is mutated in patients with hereditary haemochromatosis. *Nature Genetics* 1996;13:399–408.

16. Powis S. Major histocompatibility complex class I molecules interact with both subunits of the transporter associated with antigen processing, TAP1 and TAP2l. *European Journal of Immunology* 1997;27:2744–2747.

17. van Endert P. Genes regulating MHC class I processing of antigen. *Current Opinion in Immunology* 1999;11:82–88.

18. Gao X, Bashirova A, Iversen AK, et al. AIDS restriction HLA allotypes target distinct intervals of HIV-1 pathogenesis. *Nature Medicine* 2005;11:1290–1292.

19. Ndung'u T, Gaseitsiwe S, Sepako E, et al. Major histocompatibility complex class II (HLA-DRB and -DQB) allele frequencies in Botswana: Association with human immunodeficiency virus type 1 infection. *Clinical and Diagnostic Laboratory Immunology* 2005;12:1020–1028.

20. Sahmoud T, Laurian Y, Gazengel C, et al. Progression to AIDS in French haemophiliacs: Association with HLA-B35. *AIDS* 1993;7:497–500.

21. Dunn P, Day S, Williams S, et al. HLA-DQB1 sequencing–based typing using newly identified conserved nucleotide sequences in introns 1 and 2. *Tissue Antigens* 2005;66:99–106.

22. Wake CT, Long EO, Mach B. Allelic polymorphism and complexity of the genes for HLA-DR beta-chains: Direct analysis by DNA-DNA hybridization. *Nature* 1982;300:372–374.

23. Owerbach D, Lernmark A, Rask L, et al. Detection of HLA-D/DR–related DNA polymorphism in HLA-D homozygous typing cells. *Proceedings of the National Academy of Sciences* 1983;80:3758–3761.

24. Marsh S, Bodmer JG, Albert ED, et al. Nomenclature for factors of the HLA system, 2000. *Tissue Antigens* 2001;57:263–283.

25. Hwang S, Cha CH, Kwon OJ, et al. Novel HLA-Cw*06 allele, Cw*0612, identified by sequence-based typing. *Tissue Antigens* 2005;66:330–331.

26. Longhi E, Frison S, Colombini I, et al. HLA-A*2626, a new allele identified through external proficiency-testing exercise. *Tissue Antigens* 2005;66:325–326.

27. Marsh S, Albert ED, Bodmer WF, et al. Nomenclature for factors of the HLA system, 2004. *Human Immunology* 2005;66:571–636.

28. Marsh SG, Albert ED, Bodmer WF, et al. An update to HLA nomenclature, 2010. *Bone Marrow Transplant* 2010;45:846–848.

29. Schreuder G, Hurley CK, Marsh SG, et al. The HLA dictionary 1999: A summary of HLA-A, -B, -C, -DRB1/3/4/5, -DQB1 alleles and their association with serologically defined HLA-A, -B, -C, -DR, and -DQ antigens. *Human Immunology* 1999;60:1157–1181.

30. Schreuder G, Hurley CK, Marsh SG, et al. The HLA Dictionary 2001: A summary of HLA-A, -B, -C, -DRB1/3/4/5, -DQB1 alleles and their association with serologically defined HLA-A, -B, -C, -DR and -DQ antigens. *Tissue Antigens* 2001;58:109–140.

31. Schreuder G, Hurley CK, Marsh SG, et al. The HLA Dictionary 2004: A summary of HLA-A, -B, -C, -DRB1/3/4/5 and -DQB1 alleles and their association with serologically defined HLA-A, -B, -C, -DR and -DQ antigens. *International Journal of Immunogenetics* 2005;32:19–69.

32. Schreuder G, Hurley CK, Marsh SG, et al. HLA dictionary 2004: Summary of HLA-A, -B, -C, -DRB1/3/4/5, -DQB1 alleles and their association with serologically defined HLA-A, -B, -C, -DR, and -DQ antigens. *Human Immunology* 2005;66:170–210.

33. Marsh SG. Nomenclature for factors of the HLA system, update August 2009. *Tissue Antigens* 2010;75:98–101.

34. Mittal KK, Mickey MR, Singal DP, et al. Serotyping for homotransplantation: Refinement of microdroplet lymphocyte cytotoxicity test. *Transplantation* 1968;6:913–927.

35. Thaunat O, Hanf W, Dubois V, et al. Chronic humoral rejection mediated by anti-HLA-DP alloantibodies: Insights into the role of epitope sharing in donor-specific and non-donor-specific alloantibodies generation. *Transplant Immunology* 2009;20:209–211.

36. Claas FH, Doxiadis II. Management of the highly sensitized patient. *Current Opinions in Immunology* 2009;21:569–572.

37. Laundy GJ, Bradley BA. The predictive value of epitope analysis in highly sensitized patients awaiting renal transplantation. *Transplantation* 1995;59:1207–1213.

38. Class F, Van Leeuwen A, Van Rood JJ. Hyperimmunized patients do not need to wait for an HLA-identical donor. *Tissue Antigens* 1999;34:23–29.

39. Westwood S, Sutton JG, Werrett DJ. Analysis of the common genetic variants of the human Gc system in plasma and bloodstains by isoelectric focusing in immobilized pH gradients. *Journal Forensic Science Society (London)* 1984;24:519–528.

40. Baldwin G, Mickelson EM, Hansen JA, et al. Electrophoretic variation between class II molecules expressed on HLA-DRw8 homozygous typing cells reveals multiple distinct haplotypes. *Immunogenetics* 1985;21:49–60.

41. Kido A, Oya M, Komatsu N, et al. A stability study on Gc subtyping in bloodstains: Comparison by two different techniques. *Forensic Science International* 1984;26:39–43.

42. Borozdenkova S, Westbrook JA, Patel V, et al. Use of proteomics to discover novel markers of cardiac allograft rejection. *Journal of Proteome Research* 2004;3:282–288.

43. Bidwell J. DNA-RFLP analysis and genotyping of HLA-DR and DQ antigens. *Immunology Today* 1988;9:18–23.

44. Bidwell J, Bidwell EA, Savage DA, et al. A DNA-RFLP typing system that positively identifies serologically well-defined and ill-defined HLA-DR and DQ alleles, including DRw10. *Transplantation* 1988;45:640–646.

45. Mytilineos J, Scherer S, Opelz G. Comparison of RFLP-DR beta and serological HLA-DR typing in 1500 individuals. *Transplantation* 1990;50:870–873.

46. Opelz G, Mytilineos J, Scherer S, et al. Analysis of HLA-DR matching in DNA-typed cadaver kidney transplants. *Transplantation* 1993;55:782–785.

47. Flomenberg N, Baxter-Lowe LA, Confer D, et al. Impact of HLA class I and class II high-resolution matching on outcomes of unrelated donor bone marrow transplantation: HLA-C mismatching is associated with a strong adverse effect on transplantation outcome. *Blood* 2004;104:1923.

48. Olerup O, Zetterquist H, Ohlson L, et al. Genomic HLA-DR and -DQ typing by Taq I RFLP analysis: An alternative to serologic tissue typing. *Transplantation Proceedings* 1990;22:144.

49. Rose N, Hamilton RG, Barbara D. Manual of Clinical Laboratory Immunology, 6th ed. Washington, DC: ASM Press, 2002.

50. Cao K, Chopek M, Fernandez-Vina MA. High and intermediate resolution DNA typing systems for class I HLA-A, B, C genes by hybridization with sequence-specific oligonucleotide probes (SSOP). *Reviews in Immunogenetics* 1999;1:177–208.

51. Bein G, Glaser R, Kirchner H. Rapid HLA-DRB1 genotyping by nested PCR amplification. *Tissue Antigens* 1992;39:68–73.

52. Krausa P, Brywka M, Savage D, et al. Genetic polymorphism within HLA-A*02: Significant allelic variation revealed in different populations. *Tissue Antigens* 1995;45:223–231.

53. Bunce M, O'Neill CM, Barnardo MC, et al. Phototyping: Comprehensive DNA typing for HLA-A, B, C, DRB1, DRB3, DRB4, DRB5 & DQB1 by PCR with 144 primer mixes utilizing sequence-specific primers (PCR-SSP). *Tissue Antigens* 1995; 46:355–367.

54. Clay T, Bidwell JL, Howard MR, et al. PCR fingerprinting for selection of HLA-matched unrelated marrow donors: Collaborating centres in the IMUST study. *Lancet* 1991;337:1049–1052.

55. Buchler T, Gallardo D, Rodriguez-Luaces M, et al. Frequency of HLA-DPB1 disparities detected by reference strand-mediated conformation analysis in HLA-A, -B, and -DRB1 matched siblings. *Human Immunology* 2002;63:139–142.

56. Carrington M, Miller T, White M, et al. Typing of HLA-DQA1 and DQB1 using DNA single-strand conformation polymorphism. *Human Immunology* 1992;33:208–212.

57. Hayashi T, Seyama T, Ito T, et al. A simple and rapid method for HLA-DQA1 genotyping by polymerase chain reaction–single strand conformation polymorphism and restriction enzyme cleavage analysis. *Electrophoresis* 1992;13:877–879.

58. Lo Y, Patel P, Mehal WZ, et al. Analysis of complex genetic systems by ARMS-SSCP: Application to HLA genotyping. *Nucleic Acids Research* 1992;20:1005–1009.

59. Bang-Ce Y, Xiaohe C, Ye F, et al. Simultaneous genotyping of DRB1/3/4/5 loci by oligonucleotide microarray. *Journal of Molecular Diagnostics* 2005;7:592–599.

60. Entz P, Toliat MR, Hampe J, et al. New strategies for efficient typing of HLA class-II loci DQB1 and DRB1 by using pyrosequencing. *Tissue Antigens* 2005;65:67–80.

61. Gersuk VH, Nepom GT. A real-time polymerase chain reaction assay for the rapid identification of the autoimmune disease-associated allele HLA-DQB1*0602. *Tissue Antigens* 2009;73:335–340.

62. Araujo F. Real-time PCR assays for high-throughput blood group genotyping. *Methods in Immunology* 2009;496:25–37.

63. Bunce M, Young NT, Welsh KI. Molecular HLA typing: The brave new world. *Transplantation* 1997;64:1505–1513.

64. Arguello R, Avakian H, Goldman JM, et al. A novel method for simultaneous high resolution identification of HLA-A, HLA-B, and HLA-Cw alleles. *Proceedings of the National Academy of Sciences* 1996;93:10961–10965.

65. Bozon MV, Delgado JC, Selvakumar A, et al. Error rate for HLA-B antigen assignment by serology: Implications for proficiency testing and utilization of DNA-based typing methods. *Tissue Antigens* 1997;50:387–394.

66. Opelz G, Mytilineos J, Scherer S, et al. Influence of HLA matching and DNA typing on kidney and heart transplant survival in black recipients. *Transplantation Proceedings* 1997;29:3333–3335.

67. Opelz G. Impact of HLA compatibility on survival of kidney transplants from unrelated live donors. *Transplantation* 1997;64:1473–1475.

68. Hosenpud J, Edwards EB, Lin HM, et al. Influence of HLA matching on thoracic transplant outcomes: An analysis from the UNOS/ISHLT thoracic registry. *Circulation* 1996;94:170–174.

69. Opelz G, Wujciak T. The influence of HLA compatibility on graft survival after heart transplantation: The Collaborative Transplant Study. *New England Journal of Medicine* 1994;330:816–819.

70. Rocha V, Cornish J, Sievers EL, et al. Comparison of outcomes of unrelated bone marrow and umbilical cord blood transplants in children with acute leukemia. *Blood* 2001;97:2962–2971.

71. Erlich H, Opelz G, Hansen J. HLA DNA typing and transplantation. *Immunity* 2001;14:347–356.

72. Miklos D, Kim HT, Miller KH, et al. Antibody responses to H-Y minor histocompatibility antigens correlate with chronic graft-versus-host disease and disease remission. *Blood* 2005;105:2973–2978.

73. Voogt P, Fibbe WE, Marijt WA, et al. Rejection of bone-marrow graft by recipient-derived cytotoxic T lymphocytes against minor histocompatibility antigens. *Lancet* 1990;335:131–134.

74. Warren EH, Fujii N, Akatsuka Y, et al. Therapy of relapsed leukemia after allogeneic hematopoietic cell transplantation with T cells specific for minor histocompatibility antigens. *Blood* 2010;115:3869–3878.

75. Goulmy E, Termijtelen A, Bradley BA, et al. Alloimmunity to human H-Y. *Lancet* 1976;2:1206.

76. O'Kunewick J, Kociban DL, Machen LL, et al. Effect of donor and recipient gender disparities on fatal graft-vs.-host disease in a mouse model for major histocompatibility complex–matched unrelated donor bone marrow transplantation. *Experimental Hematology* 1993;21:1570–1576.

77. Spaapen RM, de Kort RA, van den Oudenalder K, et al. Rapid identification of clinical relevant minor histocompatibility antigens via genome-wide zygosity-genotype correlation analysis. *Clinical Cancer Research* 2009;15:7137–7143.

78. Kamei M, Nannya Y, Torikai H, et al. HapMap scanning of novel human minor histocompatibility antigens. *Blood* 2009;113:5041–5048.

79. Wilke M, Pool J, den Haan JM, et al. Genomic identification of the minor histocompatibility antigen HA-1 locus by allele-specific PCR. *Tissue Antigens* 1998;52:312–317.

80. Bahram S, Inoko H, Shiina T, et al. MIC and other NKG2D ligands: From none to too many. *Current Opinion in Immunology* 2005;17:505–509.

81. Quiroga I, Lehmann DJ, Barnardo MC, et al. Association study of MICA and MICB in Alzheimer's disease. *Tissue Antigens* 2009;74:241–243.

82. Li Y, Xia B, Lu M, et al. MICB0106 gene polymorphism is associated with ulcerative colitis in central China. *International Journal of Colorectal Disease* 2010;25:153–159.

83. Cudkowicz G, Bennett M. Peculiar immunobiology of bone marrow allografts. I. Graft rejection by irradiated responder mice. *Journal of Experimental Medicine* 1971;134:83–102.

84. Tran T, Mytilineos J, Scherer S, et al. Analysis of KIR ligand incompatibility in human renal transplantation. *Transplantation* 2005;80: 1121–1123.

85. Venstrom JM, Gooley TA, Spellman S, et al. Donor activating KIR3DS1 is associated with decreased acute GVHD in unrelated allogeneic hematopoietic stem cell transplantation. *Blood* 2010;115: 3162–3165.

86. Witt C, Dewing C, Sayer DC, et al. Population frequencies and putative haplotypes of the killer cell immunoglobulin-like receptor sequences and evidence for recombination. *Transplantation* 1999; 68:1784–1789.

87. Dupont B, Hsu KC. Inhibitory killer Ig-like receptor genes and human leukocyte antigen class I ligands in haematopoietic stem cell transplantation. *Current Opinion in Immunology* 2004;16: 634–643.

88. Cooley S, Weisdorf DJ, Guethlein LA, et al. Donor selection for natural killer cell receptor genes leads to superior survival after unrelated transplantation for acute myelogenous leukemia. *Blood* 2010;[doi:10.1182/blood-2010-05-283051].

89. Ashouri E, Ghaderi A, Reed EF, et al. A novel duplex SSP-PCR typing method for KIR gene profiling. *Tissue Antigens* 2009;74:62–67.

90. Petukhova L, Duvic M, Hordinsky M, et al. Genome-wide association study in alopecia areata implicates both innate and adaptive immunity. *Nature* 2010;466:113–117.

91. Steck A, Bugawan TL, Valdes AM, et al. Association of non-HLA genes with type 1 diabetes autoimmunity. *Diabetes* 2005;54:2482–2486.

92. Kaur G, Mehra N. Genetic determinants of HIV-1 infection and progression to AIDS: Immune response genes. *Tissue Antigens* 2009;74:373–385.

93. Montag S, Frank M, Ulmer H, et al. "Electronic nose" detects major histocompatibility complex–dependent prerenal and postrenal odor components. *Proceedings of the National Academy of Sciences* 2001;98:9249–9254.

94. Santos P, Schinemann JA, Gabardo J, et al. New evidence that the MHC influences odor perception in humans: A study with 58 Southern Brazilian students. *Hormones and Behavior* 2005;47:384–388.

Chapter 16

Quality Assurance and Quality Control in the Molecular Laboratory

OBJECTIVES

- Describe proper specimen accession for molecular testing.
- Describe the optimal conditions for the holding and storage of various specimens, including nucleic acids.
- Explain the basic components of molecular test performance, including quality assurance and controls.
- Discuss instrument maintenance, repair, and calibration, particularly for instruments used in molecular analysis.
- Describe recommendations for the preparation and use of reagents in the molecular laboratory.
- Explain documentation and reporting of results, including gene sequencing results.

Congress passed the **Clinical Laboratory Improvement Amendments (CLIA)** in 1988 to establish quality testing standards to ensure consistent patient test results. CLIA specifies quality standards for proficiency testing, patient test management, quality control, personnel qualifications, and quality assurance for laboratories performing moderate- and/or high-complexity tests, including molecular testing. This chapter offers a brief overview of laboratory standards applied to molecular diagnostic tests.

Specimen Handling

Molecular tests, like any clinical laboratory tests, require optimal specimen handling and processing for accurate and consistent test results. The success of a test procedure is affected by the age, type, and condition of specimens. Therefore, specimen collection, transport, and handling in the laboratory require careful attention.

Preanalytical variables, both controllable and uncontrollable, must be taken into account for proper interpretation of test results. **Preanalytical error** is the consequence of erroneous or misleading results caused by events that occur prior to sample analysis. To minimize preanalytical error and maximize control of preanalytical variables, the Clinical and Laboratory Standards Institute (CLSI, formerly known as the National Committee for Clinical Laboratory Standards) provides recommendations for collection of specimens under standardized conditions.[1–3] Rules and recommendations for safe transport of potentially infectious or otherwise dangerous materials are available from the Centers for Disease Control and Prevention (CDC), the World Health Organization, and the U.S. Department of Transportation.

Criteria for Accepting Specimens

Each laboratory will have requirements for specimen handling, but general policies apply to all specimen collection. The condition of the specimen and, if necessary, the chain of custody is reviewed on receipt in the laboratory. If a specimen shows evidence of tampering or is otherwise compromised, the technologist must notify the supervisor. A specimen is not acceptable without proper labeling and identification on the specimen tube or container (placed by the person who collected the specimen). Also, if the labeling on the specimen does not match the identifying information on the accompanying requisition, it should not be accepted. In addition to relevant patient identification, the test requisition includes the type of specimen material (e.g., blood or bone marrow), ordered test, date and time of collection, and a contact (pager or telephone number) of the ordering physician. When required (for molecular genetics or parentage testing), patient consent forms, ethnicity, photo identification of the individuals tested, and transfusion history or a pedigree may also be supplied with the test specimen. Forensic specimens may require a documented chain of custody. Bar-coding of this information expedites specimen accession and decreases the chance for error.

The laboratory should have written procedures for documentation of specimen accession.[4] Accession books or electronic records are used to record the date of receipt, laboratory identifier, and pertinent patient information associated with the accession. If a specimen is unacceptable, the disposal or retention of the specimen is recorded in the patient report or laboratory quality assurance records. If not processed immediately, specimens are maintained in secure areas with limited access under the appropriate conditions for the analyte being tested (Fig. 16-1).

Molecular amplification methods have enabled laboratory professionals to perform nucleic acid–based testing on specimens with minimal cellular content, such as buccal cell suspensions and cerebrospinal fluids. These samples are centrifuged to collect the cells before DNA or RNA is extracted. For routine specimens tested by amplification methods, the entire specimen is often not used. In this case, or if more than one test is to be performed on the same specimen, cross-contamination of specimens must be carefully avoided. Cross-contamination can most likely occur from pipetting carryover. Moreover, an aliquot once removed from a specimen is never returned to the original tube or vessel.

Hemoglobin inhibits enzyme activity. Specimens received in the laboratory should therefore be inspected for visual signs of hemolysis. Hemoglobin and anticoagulants are removed effectively in most DNA and RNA isolation procedures; however, if white blood cell lysis has also occurred, DNA or RNA yield will be reduced. This could result in false-negative results in qualitative testing or inaccurate measurements in quantitative analyses. Buffers such as BloodDirect (Novagen) and Extract-N-Amp (Sigma) or resins such as Chelex have been designed to sequester anticoagulants or hemoglobin for more rapid nucleic acid isolation without the inhibitory effects of these substances. This process protects both the nucleic acid as well as gene expression patterns that may change upon sample storage.

Solid tissues are best analyzed from fresh or frozen samples (Fig. 16-2), especially for Southern blot or long-range polymerase chain reaction (PCR) methods that require relatively high-quality (long, intact) DNA. Surgical specimens designated for molecular studies, if not processed immediately, should be snap-frozen in liquid nitrogen. This process both preserves nucleic acid and preserves gene expression patterns that may change upon tissue storage. Snap freezing is routinely performed in the surgical pathology laboratory as it is a common process for preserving tissue morphology for microscopic examination. Fixed, paraffin-embedded tissues generally yield lower-quality DNA and RNA, depending on the type of fixative used, the amount of time of exposure of the tissue to the fixative, and how the specimen was handled prior to fixation. PCR and reverse transcription PCR (RT-PCR) amplification, however, are routinely performed on paraffin-embedded tissue samples. Methods such as Southern or northern blot, requiring large fragments of nucleic acids, are less likely to work consistently with fixed tissues.

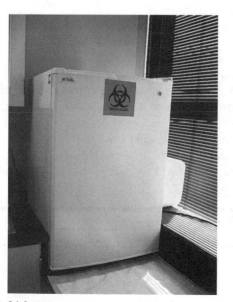

■ **Figure 16-1** Biohazard stickers are required for cabinets, refrigerators, or freezers that contain reagents or patient specimens.

Collection Tubes for Molecular Testing

Phlebotomy collection tubes are available with a number of different additives designed for various types of clinical tests. Table 16.1 lists a selection of collection tubes commonly used for molecular biology studies. Some anticoagulants used in blood and bone marrow collection may adversely affect analytical results. Heparin [and occasionally acid citrate dextrose (ACD)] has been shown to inhibit enzymes used in molecular analysis, such as reverse transcriptases and DNA polymerases in vitro.[5] The negative effect of this inhibition on molecular analysis is commonly accepted; however, heparinized samples

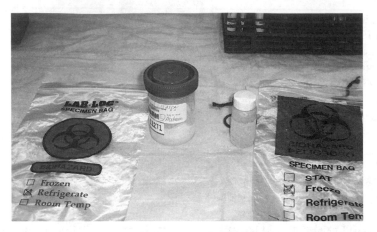

■ **Figure 16-2** Tissue is received in the laboratory in fresh (left) or frozen (right) form. Fresh tissue may be supplied as a specimen on gauze or other substrate or in saline. The vial shown on the right contains tissue that was flash-frozen in isopentane. The vial is stored immersed in liquid nitrogen, nitrogen vapors, or in a −70°C freezer.

have been processed successfully in many laboratories, and ACD tubes are also used routinely for molecular tests.

The various experiences with heparin may reflect levels of resistance of enzymes from different sources. The assay design can also have an effect on the amplification process. For instance, the inhibition of DNA polymerases compromises amplification of larger PCR products more than short ones. Due to the possible effects of heparin, trisodium EDTA (lavender top) or acid citrate dextrose (yellow top) tubes are recommended for most nucleic acid assays involving enzymatic treatment of the sample nucleic acid (Fig. 16-3).[6] High levels of disodium EDTA (royal-blue-capped tubes used for trace element studies) may also inhibit enzyme activity and should be avoided. One of the advantages of signal amplification methods such as bDNA technology is their decreased susceptibility to chemical effects of anticoagulants. When a specimen is received in the laboratory, the anticoagulant is not usually noted in the accompanying documentation; the technologist should be aware of the type of collection tube used, especially if a specimen is received in heparin or other additive that may affect the test results.

Tissue processing for molecular analysis requires caution to avoid contamination, especially where PCR or other amplification-based tests are to be performed. Recommendations for tissue processing for molecular diagnostic testing may be found in CLSI document MM13A, "Collection, Transport, Preparation, and Storage of Specimens for Molecular Methods; Approved Guideline."

In addition to the standard collection tubes, special collection tubes are designed particularly for stabilization of nucleic acids for molecular testing. These include the plasma preparation tubes (Vacutainer PPT, Becton Dickinson), which contain, in addition to the standard anticoagulants, a polymer gel that separates granulocytes and some lymphocytes from erythrocytes upon centrifugation. This type of tube is used for HIV and HCV analysis. The PPT tube is also used for separation of white cells for genetics and bone marrow engraftment testing. The tube stoppers have a black "tiger" pattern over the appropriate anticoagulant color designation. There are a variety of kit systems designed for specific procedures or target organisms with associated tubes or other collection

Table 16.1 A Selection of Collection Tubes Used in Nucleic Acid Testing

Additive	Color	Tests
None	Red	Chemistry, serum, viral antibody studies
Sodium heparin (freeze-dried)	Green	Immunology, virology studies
Sodium heparin	Brown	Cytogenetic studies, molecular studies
Tripotassium EDTA (7.5%–15% solution)	Lavender	Virology, molecular biology studies
Acid citrate dextrose solution	Yellow	Molecular biology studies

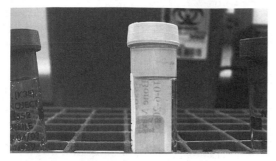

■ **Figure 16-3** For molecular analysis, blood or bone marrow specimens collected in EDTA or ACD tubes are preferred. Some immunology methods are performed on serum collected in tubes without coagulant. Fluorescent in situ hybridization studies are performed on specimens collected in heparin.

devices. Some tubes can be used with multiple kit systems; for example, the Wampole Isolator™ tubes used for collection and concentration of microbes in blood by centrifugation are used as part of the Isostat®/Isolator™ system or with other automated blood culture screening methods.

Stabilization of RNA in collected specimens has become increasingly important because of the increasing number of methods involving RNA transcript levels for measurement of gene expression. For example, quantitative RT-PCR analyses rely on transcript number to monitor the level of tumor cells or microorganisms in body fluids. Serial analysis requires that the specimens received in the laboratory at different times be handled as consistently as possible. Tubes such as the Tempus RNA Blood tube (Applied Biosystems) or the PAXgene Blood RNA tube (PreAnalytix) are designed to stabilize RNA. These tubes contain proprietary RNA stabilization agents that maintain the integrity of the RNA from collection through isolation.[7–9] Separated white blood cells from standard collection tubes can also be lysed in Trizol or TriReagent (Sigma) and the lysate stored at −70°C to stabilize RNA for several days. Immediate stabilization of the RNA is essential in order to produce comparable results.[10] As an alternative to standard collection tubes, methods involving impregnated paper matrices have been proposed for nucleic acid analysis.[11,12] These methods offer the convenience of immediate stabilization and room temperature storage; however, they are limited to methods that include PCR or other types of

amplification. Furthermore, humid conditions may compromise the sample integrity.

Precautions in Sample Processing

Standard precautions are recommended by the CDC for handling potentially infectious specimens. All specimens are potentially infectious and should be handled with standard precautions using proper personal protective equipment (PPE) to prevent disease transmission. **Transmission-based precautions** including respirators are used with airborne or contact-transmissible agents. **Contact precautions** are designed for direct patient care where there is the potential for direct exposure to infectious agents on or from the patient. In general, standard precautions including gloves and gowns as PPE are used by the molecular laboratory technologist who has no direct contact with patients. Eye protection or masks are required in cases where frozen tissue is being processed or where spraying or splashing of the sample may occur.

Properly fitting latex or latex-alternative gloves are highly recommended not only as part of standard precautions but also to protect nucleic acids from degradation by nucleases (Fig. 16-4). Gloves are absolutely required for the handling of RNA (Fig. 16-5). DNA is less susceptible to degradation from contaminating DNases; however, repeated handling of samples without gloves will

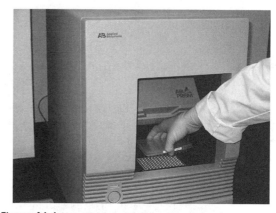

■ **Figure 16-4** Handling specimens with gloves is recommended to avoid possible exposure to infectious agents present in the sample and to protect the sample nucleic acids from degradation by nucleases and other contaminants.

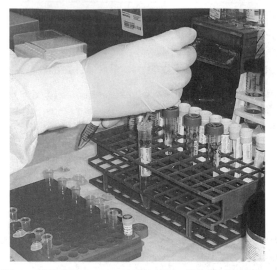

■ **Figure 16-5** Gloves are required for working with RNA.

adversely affect the integrity of the DNA over time. Standards and controls that are handled repeatedly are the most likely to be affected. Originally, having separate areas for isolating DNA and RNA was recommended. Some laboratories, however, isolate DNA and RNA on the same bench space. This requires maintenance of RNase-free conditions (see Chapter 4, "Nucleic Acid Extraction Methods") for all nucleic acid isolation. In a common isolation arrangement such as this, care must be taken that no inappropriate enzyme exposures occur if DNA samples are treated with RNase or RNA samples are treated with DNase.

Holding and Storage Requirements

Such methods as interphase and metaphase fluorescent in situ hybridization (FISH) and karyotyping require intact cellular structures or culturing of cells, so only fresh specimens are acceptable. Many molecular methods, however, do not require integrity of tissue or cellular structure, only that the nucleic acid remains intact. In either case, circumstances may arise that require the holding of specimens before analysis. DNA and RNA are stable when samples are collected and held under the proper conditions.[13,14] For example, multiple tests may

be performed on snap-frozen tissue specimens held at –70°C. Although most amplification methods are capable of successful analysis of limiting and challenging specimens, Southern or northern blot methods may not work consistently on improperly handled specimens or nucleic acids stored under less than optimal conditions. The College of American Pathologists (CAP), which provides accreditation standards for CAP-accredited laboratories, has published recommendations for sample and isolated nucleic acid storage (Table 16.2).

For long-term storage, isolated nucleic acid is preferred. Conditions for the storage of isolated nucleic acid have been recommended (Table 16.3). **Cryotubes** and specially designed labels are available for long-term nucleic acid storage at ultra-low temperatures (Fig. 16-6).

The general rules for holding specimens for processing differ depending on the analyte and its stability in the cell. Written procedures indicate the proper handling of specimens for optimal performance of that procedure. For example, room-temperature (22°C to 25°C) storage is recommended for viral RNA in whole blood. Refrigeration of blood will cause neutophils to degranulate, releasing enzymes that affect free virus particles. On the other hand, specimens in EDTA tubes held at 4°C may not show significant loss of human RNA stability, depending on the gene. Still, blood or bone marrow for human RNA testing should be processed within 24 hours. Blood and bone marrow specimens sent to outside laboratories for molecular analysis are shipped overnight at room temperature or kept cold with ice packs. Tissue is best shipped frozen on dry ice.

Isolated DNA of sufficient purity can be stored at room temperature for several months or at least 1 year in the refrigerator. Purified DNA can be stored at freezer temperatures (–20°C to –70°C) in tightly sealed tubes for up to 10 years or longer. Freezer temperatures are preferred for long-term storage; however, a clean DNA preparation in frequent use is better stored in the refrigerator to avoid DNA damage caused by multiple cycles of freezing/thawing. Note that shearing of DNA by freeze/thawing cycles will also occur in a frost-free freezer. As previously stated, PCR and methods that do not require large intact fragments of DNA are more forgiving with regard to the condition of the DNA.

Table 16.2 **Specimen Storage Requirements for Nucleic Acid Extraction**[33]

Nucleic Acid	Sample	Temperature	Time
DNA	Whole blood, buffy coat, bone marrow, fluids	22°–25°C	24 hours
		2°–8°C	72 hours*
		–20°C	At least 1 year*
		–70°C	More than 1 year*
	Tissue	22°–25°C	Not recommended
		2°–8°C	Up to 24 hours†
		–20°C	At least 2 weeks
		–70°C	At least 2 years
	Microorganisms in culture	22°–25°C	24 hours‡
		2°–8°C	72 hours‡
		–20°C	2–4 weeks‡
		–70°C	More than 1 year
	Cell lysates in GITC	22°–25°C	1–2 weeks§
RNA	Whole blood, buffy coat, bone marrow, fluids	22°–25°C	Not recommended§
		2°–8°C	2–4 hours*
		–20°C	2–4 weeks*
		–70°C	More than 1 year*
	Fluids collected in specialty RNA protection tubes	22°–25°C	5 days
		2°–8°C	7 days
		–20°C	2–4 weeks
		–70°C	At least 7 months
	Tissue	22°–25°C	Not recommended
		2°–8°C	Not recommended
		–20°C	Not recommended
		–70°C	At least 2 years
		–140°C (nitrogen vapor)	At least 2 years
	Cell lysates in GITC¶	22°–25°C	1–2 weeks§
	Cell lysates in RNA storage solution (Ambion)‖	22°–25°C	1 week
		2°–8°C	1 month
		–20°C	More than 1 year
	Microorganisms in culture	22°–25°C	24 hours‡
		2°–8°C	72 hours‡
		–20°C	2–4 weeks‡
		–70°C	More than 1 year

*Separation of white blood cells is recommended to avoid hemoglobin released upon hemolysis of red blood cells.
†Tissue types differ in stability and nuclease content.
‡Nucleic acid from cultured organisms is best isolated immediately on harvesting fresh cultures.
§RNA status depends on the type of cell or tissue and the gene under study.[34]
‖Depending on gene expression, adequate RNA may be isolated within a few hours. Storage of cell lysates in a stabilizing buffer is best for maintaining RNA.
¶GITC = guanidine isothiocyanate.

Table 16.3 **Nucleic Acid Storage Requirements**[33]

Nucleic Acid	Matrix	Temperature	Time
DNA	TE* buffer or DNase-free water	22°–25°C	Up to 4 months
	Freeze-dried or dried on collection paper[35]	22°–25°C	More than 15 years
	TE buffer or DNase-free water	2°–8°C	1–3 years[†]
	TE buffer or DNase-free water	–20°C	At least 7 years
	TE buffer or DNase-free water	–70°C	More than 7 years
RNA	TE buffer or RNase-free (DEPC[‡]-treated) water	22°–25°C	Not recommended
	TE buffer or RNase-free (DEPC-treated) water	2°–8°C	Not recommended
	TE buffer or RNase-free (DEPC-treated) water	–20°C	Up to 1 month
	RNA storage solution (Ambion)[§]	–20°C	More than 1 month
	Ethanol	–20°C	More than 6 months
	TE buffer or RNase-free (DEPC-treated) water	–70°C	Up to 30 days
	Ethanol	–70°C	More than 6 months

*10 mM Tris, 1 mM EDTA, pH 8.0
[†]1 year for Southern blot
[‡]DEPC = diethyl pyrocarbonate
[§]1 mM sodium citrate, pH 6.4

Storage of isolated RNA at room temperature or refrigerator temperature is not recommended in the absence of stabilization. RNA suspended in ethanol can be stored at –20°C for several months. Long-term storage is best in ethanol at –70°C, although RNA suspended in diethylpyrocarbonate (DEPC)-treated water is stable for at least 1 month. As with DNA, the long-term survival of the RNA depends on the quality of the initial isolation and handling of the specimen.

Test Performance

Many tests in the molecular laboratory are independently designed or are adaptations based on published methods. Development of new tests in the clinical laboratory requires validation of the performance of the method and reagents in accurately detecting or measuring the analyte.[15,16] Test performance is assessed by several criteria (Table 16.4), which are expressed as formulas.

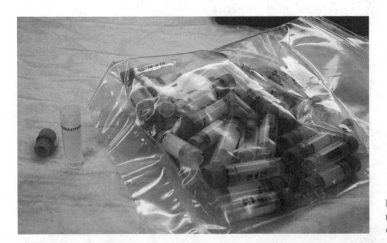

■ Figure 16-6 Cryotubes with tight-fitting lids are recommended for long-term freezer storage of DNA and RNA.

The **clinical sensitivity** of an assay equals:

$[TP/(TP + FN)] \times 100$

The **clinical specificity** of an assay equals:

$[TN/(TN + FP)] \times 100$

The accuracy of an assay equals:

$[(TN + TP)/(TN + TP + FN + FP)] \times 100$

where TN = true-negative, TP = true-positive, FN = false-negative, FP = false-positive.

True-positive and true-negative are determined using a gold standard, such as an established reference assay or a definitive clinical diagnosis. Note that the clinical sensitivity is different from the **analytical sensitivity** that may also be reported (Table 16.4). The analytical

Table 16.4 **Measurements of Test Performance**

Criteria	Definition	Example
Analytic sensitivity	Change in assay response with corresponding change in analyte	All positive reference standards tested positive with the new assay. The analytical sensitivity of the assay is 100%.
Clinical sensitivity	Ability of test result to predict a clinical condition	95 of 100 patients with a gene mutation have a disease state, a clinical sensitivity of 95%.
Detection limit	Lower limit of detection of the analyte	The t(14;18) translocation test can detect 1 translocated cell in 10,000 normal cells, a detection limit of 0.01%.
Analytic specificity	Ability to detect only the analyte and not nonspecific targets	The Invader assay for factor V Leiden successfully detected mutations in 18 positive specimens while yielding negative results for 30 normal specimens (no false-positive results).
Clinical specificity	Disease-associated results only in patients who actually have the disease conditions	1 of 100 normal specimens displayed a gene mutation (1 false-positive), a clinical specificity of 99%.
Precision	Agreement between independent test results	A quantitative method yields 99 results less than 1 standard deviation apart in 100 runs, a precision of 99%.
Reproducibility	Consistency of test results produced from the same procedure	A qualitative method yields 100 positive results when performed in 10 independent laboratories, a reproducibility of 100%.
Analyte measurement range	The range within which a specimen may be measured directly (without dilution or concentration)	A qPCR HSV assay yields reproducible linear results from 10 to 107 copies of HSV per 20 μL of CSF. Specimens within this range are measured directly.
Reportable range	The range within which test results are considered to be valid (with or without dilution)	A qPCR HCV assay yields reproducible results from 1 to 1000 copies of HCV per 1 mL of blood, requiring dilution for levels less than 100 copies. Specimens within this range are reportable.
Reference range	Expected analyte frequency or levels from a population of individuals	The reference range for prostatic specific antigen is 0 to 4 ng/mL.
Analytic accuracy	Production of correct results	99 of 100 specimens with mutations in the HCM gene are detected by sequencing, with no mutations detected in normal specimens.
Linearity	Quantitative correlation between test result and actual amount of analyte	A graph of test procedure results vs input analyte yields a straight line.

sensitivity is defined as the ability of the assay to detect the presence of the analyte, with changes in the assay response corresponding to changes in the amount of analyte present. Analytical sensitivity can further be refined by determining the **detection limit**, or lower limit of detection. The detection limit is the lowest level of analyte that is consistently detected by the assay. In qualitative assays, the analytical sensitivity and the limit of detection are practically equivalent. In quantitative assays, the analytical sensitivity is defined by differences in quantitative response with quantitative differences in the reference analyte. For tests with quantitative results reported qualitatively (positive/negative, for example), a cutpoint quantity must be established above which it is considered positive and below which it is negative. Thus, quantity may be determined empirically or statistically using probit or **logit analysis**.[17,18] These criteria, along with the analytical measurement range (Table 16-4), are documented as part of the test validation process.[19,20]

Test validation is performed on specimens of the types that will be encountered in the routine use of the test, such as frozen tissue, paraffin-embedded tissue, body fluids, and cultured cells. The number of specimens tested varies with the procedure and the availability of test material. Archived specimens are often used for this purpose. The results from the new test are compared with those of established procedures performed on these specimens or with the clinical diagnosis.[21–23] A standard form may be designed for preparation of reaction mixes according to the test parameters determined in the validation process (Fig. 16-7).

Predeveloped and U.S. Food and Drug Administration (FDA)–approved molecular methods are becoming increasingly available. According to the FDA, an *approved* test is one that has been accepted by the FDA as safe and effective for its intended use, based on the manufacturer's data. The manufacturer conducts studies to show that the test performs as claimed and does not present any unreasonable risk. The test is offered for sale after a premarket approval application has been reviewed and approved by the FDA. A test that has been *cleared* by the FDA has been shown to be similar to other tests already marketed, based on the manufacturer's data. For such a test, the manufacturer submits comparison results in a "premarket notification" that the FDA reviews and determines that the tests are substantially equivalent.

When FDA-approved or FDA-cleared methods are incorporated, the test performance is verified by using the purchased reagent sets to test validation specimens. This verification establishes that the results of the commercial test performed in the individual laboratory are as predicted by the developer. If the commercial test is modified, validation is required to show equal or superior performance of the modified procedure.

Once a procedure has been established, the method is documented in the laboratory according to CLSI guidelines.[24] The procedure description should include detailed information, for instance, primer and probe sequences, their purification conditions, and labeling. A copy of the standard form used to set up reaction mixes is included in the procedure description. A clear description of formulas and reporting units are required for quantitative results. Interpretation of qualitative data, acceptable ranges (such as band patterns), product sizes, melting temperatures, and reasons for rejecting results are required information. Methods used to score FISH or array results relative to internal control loci are also part of the written procedure. It is useful to incorporate pictures of gel patterns or instrument output data showing positive, negative, heterozygous, or other reportable results.

In the course of validation, the accuracy of a test will determine its correlation with disease, as performed in the testing laboratory. To account for biological variation, normal and abnormal ranges are established to define clinically useful results. The indications for ordering the test are determined, based on the validated clinical utility, and documented in the procedure manual. For forensic testing, all aspects of the test from validation to test reporting should adhere to guidelines established by the DNA Advisory Board Standards and the Scientific Working Group on DNA Analysis Methods.[25]

The procedure manual or standard operating procedure is maintained in the laboratory and reviewed at least annually. If a test is discontinued, the written procedure, noted with the dates of initial use and retirement, is kept for at least two years. Some laboratory professionals maintain retired procedures for longer periods.

Controls

Controls are samples of known type or amount that are treated like and run with patient specimens. Interpretation

PCR WORKSHEET

Run #_____ Tech_____   Date_____

Tube #	Patient name	Specimen/ treatment	µg/µl	µl DNA*	µl H₂O*
1					
2					
3					
4					
5					
6					
7	Positive control				
8	Sensitivity control				
9	Negative control				
10	Reagent blank				

* Dilute sample to 1µg/µl in a volume of 15µl.

PCR reaction mixture for test primers

	(#rxns)
DNAse-free water	28.8µl x_____ = _____µl
8 µM forward primer	2.5µl x_____ = _____µl
8 µM reverse primer	2.5µl x_____ = _____µl
1 mM dNTP	5.0µl x_____ = _____µl
10x PCR buffer	5.0µl x_____ = _____µl
750 µM $(NH_4)_2SO_4$	1.0µl x_____ = _____µl
Taq polymerase	0.2µl x_____ = _____µl

Place 45µl of mixture into PCR tubes. Add 5µl (5 µg) template to each PCR tube.

PCR mixture for internal control primers

DNAse water	30.8µl x_____ = _____µl
2 µM forward primer	1.25µl x_____ = _____µl
2 µM reverse primer	1.25µl x_____ = _____µl
1 mM dNTP's	5.0µl x_____ = _____µl
10x PCR buffer	5.0µl x_____ = _____µl
50mM $MgCl_2$	1.5µl x_____ = _____µl
Taq polymerase	0.2µl x_____ = _____µl

Place 45µl of mixture into the PCR tubes. Add 5µl template to each PCR tube.

■ **Figure 16-7** Example of a worksheet used to prepare home-brew PCR reaction mixes. A single reaction mix is made for multiple samples by multiplying the number of reactions by the volume of each reaction component and adding that amount to the master mix. Information regarding reagent lot numbers, PCR programs, and specimen dilutions may be included on the worksheet or documented separately.

of test results always includes inspection of controls and standards to verify acceptable test performance. With qualitative tests, a **positive**, **negative**, and, in some cases, a **sensitivity control** are required. The sensitivity control defines the lower limit of the analytical range for more meaningful interpretation of negative results. In PCR techniques, an **amplification control** is included as a target that should always amplify. The amplification control is used to distinguish true-negative amplification results from false-negatives due to amplification failure. In quantitative methods, high-positive, low-positive, and negative controls are included with each run. The high and low levels should be similar to critical points in the assay, such as the lowest detectable level of analyte. An acceptable range of variation for high- and low-positive controls may be established by repeated runs of each control sample on different days by different personnel. The average ± 2 or ± 3 standard deviations define the acceptable range for positive controls.

Quantitative PCR methods that automatically determine analyte levels require measurement of a **standard curve** or dilution series of analyte levels encompassing the levels expected from the patient specimens. On some instruments, the standard curve must be run simultaneously with the specimens, while in others, previously determined curves may be loaded into the software. Alternatively, results may be calculated manually by linear regression of the test results, using standard curve data in spreadsheet software.

In methods requiring detection of a target-specific product, or relative amounts of target, **internal controls** are run in the same reaction mix as the test specimen. For example, RNA from housekeeping genes is used for internal controls in methods quantifying infectious agents or detecting tumor cells by expression of tumor-specific transcripts.[26]

Centromere-specific probes serve as internal controls in FISH analyses, as do housekeeping gene probes on microarrays. In PCR, the internal control distinguishes false-negative results from failed amplifications (see Chapter 7, "Nucleic Acid Amplification"). The presence of an internal control also supplies a base for normalization of results. Internal controls that are amplified in the same tube with sample templates are designed to not interfere or inhibit target amplification, which could yield a false-negative result. Failed internal controls are documented and call for repeat of the assay.

The controls and standard curve should cover the critical detection levels or results of the method. Control results are continually monitored to spot trends or spikes outside of tolerance limits. Coefficients of variance or standard deviations of quantitative control levels should also be calculated at regular intervals. Laboratory professionals may establish criteria for control tolerance limits and document actions to be taken in the event of an unacceptable control result.

Controls are best prepared in larger quantities, aliquotted, and stored in conditions where they are most stable. Just as with new lots of other reagents, new aliquots are tested with old aliquots to verify consistent control results.

Quality Assurance

Periodic review and documentation of test results are required for all clinical testing, including molecular tests. Review might be, for example, in the form of numbers of positive and negative results compared with expected numbers from independent sources, such as published results, over time. This type of monitoring reveals trends or shifts in rates of positive or negative results. Critical values that require physician notification are established by validation and confirmed by monitoring.

As with all quantitative testing, molecular quantitative methods should have a defined dynamic range, sensitivity level, and accuracy.[27,28] For instance, a test that determines viral types by melt curves must include a defined narrow temperature range for the T_m of each viral type (Fig. 16-8). These values are established during the test validation and should be reviewed periodically. Test performance is monitored by inclusion of high/low sensitivity and negative standards in each run.

Band patterns, melt curves, and peak characteristics should be defined with regard to how the results of the test are to be interpreted. In assays such as single-strand conformation polymorphism (see Chapter 9, "Gene Mutations"), in which control patterns are not identical from run to run, normal controls for each scanned region are included in every run. Assay levels that distinguish positive from negative results (**cut-off values**) must be well defined and verified at regular intervals.

Quantitative results should be within the linear range of the assay. The linear range is established by measuring dilutions or known concentrations of a reference standard and establishing a direct correlation (standard curve)

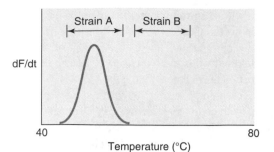

■ Figure 16-8 T_m ranges defined for two strains (A and B) of a theoretical microorganism are nonoverlapping. The melt curve shown would indicate that the test specimen contains strain A.

between test output and standard input. The technologist should observe that raw data are consistent with the final interpretation of the results. For example, if a viral load is interpreted as negative, the raw measurement should be below the cut-off value established for the test. Calculations and comparisons with standards used to verify test results should be described in the laboratory procedure manual.

Instrument Maintenance

Instruments used in the molecular laboratory must be monitored and maintained for consistent performance and accurate test results. Manufacturers supply recommendations for routine maintenance. Service contracts are used to provide support from professional service technicians. Laboratory scientists maintain a schedule

and instructions for all routine maintenance, such as checking temperature settings, timers, and background levels. Parts are replaced as required or as specified by the instrument manufacturer. Maintenance schedules should reflect the amount of use of the instrument.

In addition to routine maintenance and minor troubleshooting, such as replacing bulbs or batteries, repairs may be performed by the technologist with the aid of clear instructions from the manufacturer or as prepared by laboratory management. These instructions must be readily available to the technologist in the event of instrument malfunction. Technologists should be aware of the limits of user-recommended repairs and when service calls are indicated (Fig. 16-9). All maintenance, service calls, calibrations, and parts replacements must be documented.

Refrigerators and Freezers

Refrigerators and freezers used to store patient material and reagents are monitored at least daily (Fig. 16-10). Maximum/minimum thermometers register the highest and lowest temperature reached between monitoring points. During a busy shift, refrigerators and freezers may be opened frequently, causing the temperature to increase temporarily. This must be taken into account while monitoring. When out-of-range temperatures (e.g., more than ±2°C of the set temperature) are reported, confirmatory temperature checks at different times during the shift are required before further action is taken. Heat blocks, incubators, ovens, and water baths are also monitored for temperature stability and accuracy. U.S. National Institute of Standards and Technology (NIST)–certified standard

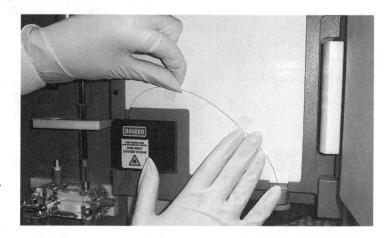

■ Figure 16-9 Routine maintenance, such as electrophoresis capillary replacement and instrument cleaning, is performed by the laboratory technologist. Dangerous or complex maintenance, such as repair or replacement of a laser source, is performed by service representatives.

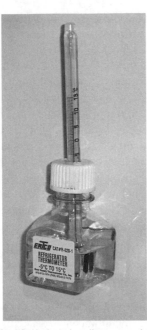

■ **Figure 16-10** Certified chamber thermometers are used for monitoring temperatures in incubators, refrigerators, ovens, and freezers. The thermometers are supplied in a variety of configurations, for example, resin bottles containing liquid glycol.

thermometers are used for this type of monitoring. Thermometers verified by a NIST thermometer are also acceptable for this purpose. Documentation of this verification is maintained in the laboratory. Specialized dry bath thermometers, which are encased in a 1.5-mL microfuge tube of mineral oil, are best for monitoring heat blocks.

All storage and incubation equipment is kept clean and free of contaminated specimens and expired reagents. If out-of-date reagents are used for research or other purposes, they should be well marked and/or maintained in an area separate from the clinical test reagents.

Thermal Cyclers

Although standard thermal cyclers have no automated moving parts, they decline in temperature control over time. This is especially true of block cyclers where hot and cold spots develop within the sample block. For this reason, thermal cyclers are checked periodically for proper temperature control. Thermometers with flexible probes (type K thermocouples) are convenient for checking representative wells in a block thermal cycler (Fig. 16-11). Approaches differ over whether each well should be

checked with each routine measurement or whether representative wells should be checked, with different wells checked each time. In some laboratories, test reactions are run in selected wells or all wells to demonstrate successful amplification at each position on the block (Cycler Check). More thorough and accurate temperature measurements are achieved with computer systems (e.g., Driftcon), with fixed or flexible probes designed to measure temperature in all wells throughout a PCR program, including ramping of the temperature up and down, overshooting set temperatures, and temperature drift during the hold phase of each step. Nonblock thermal cyclers, such as air-heated or modular instruments, are tested with probes modified to fit like the capillaries or tubes used in these instruments. Real-time thermal cyclers require additional maintenance of the detection system. Manufacturers supply materials for spectral calibrations. Background measurements are made using water or buffer samples. Each laboratory will establish the type and frequency of scheduled maintenance.

Centrifuges

Centrifuges and microcentrifuges are monitored at least annually using a tachometer. In some institutions, technologists perform this calibration. Alternatively, an institutional engineering department may do it. The actual speed of rotation is determined and recorded along with the set speed or setting number on the centrifuge. This information is then posted on the instrument (Fig. 16-12).

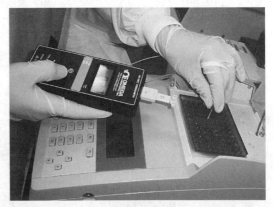

■ **Figure 16-11** Block thermal cyclers may be monitored using a thermometer with a flexible probe immersed in a PCR tube. More thorough monitoring is performed with multiple probes and software that follows the ramping temperatures as well as the holding temperatures.

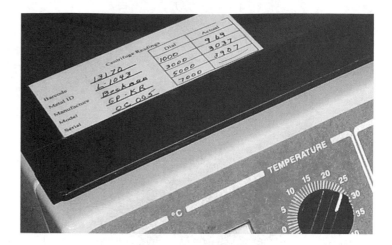

■ Figure 16-12 Centrifuge speeds are checked at least annually, and the results of actual and set speeds are posted on the instrument.

Power Supplies

Electrophoresis power supplies are tested at least annually to ensure delivery of accurate voltage and current. Personnel should be trained in safe operation. Leads and connectors to gel baths are kept free of precipitate (Fig. 16-13). Precipitation and corrosion are avoided by not leaving buffer in gel baths after electrophoresis runs. Capillary systems require cleaning of buffer and polymer delivery channels as well as replacing polymer at least twice per month or as recommended by the manufacturer. Capillaries are replaced according to their suggested life span in number of uses. Temperature-controlled electrophoresis equipment, such as capillary systems and those used for constant-temperature gel electrophoresis, is monitored for accurate temperature settings as recommended by the manufacturer.

Cameras and Detectors

Photographic equipment is frequently used in molecular laboratory procedures. Autoradiograms resulting from radioactive or chemiluminescent methods are developed in automated equipment or manually under dark room conditions. The processing equipment is maintained with fresh fixing and developing solutions free from debris or sediment. Digital systems have replaced film cameras for documenting gel data in most laboratories. Cameras should be firmly mounted and adjusted for optimal recording of gel data, free of shadows, dust, and other photographic artifacts (Fig. 16-14).

Periodically, background measurements are required on such instruments as fluorometric detectors (including real-time thermal cyclers), luminometers, and densitometers. Instrument manufacturers provide guidelines for

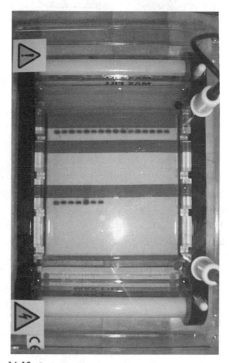

■ Figure 16-13 Gel electrophoresis equipment must be maintained free of precipitate and properly handled to avoid shock exposure.

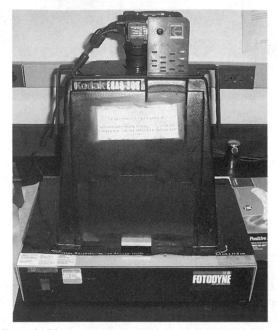

■ **Figure 16-14** Cameras should be mounted securely for gel photography. A digital camera, shown here, is mounted on a photographic hood. A mask shields the ultraviolet light source except for the area where the gel is illuminated.

acid standards, but wavelength scanning is unnecessary, as these instruments perform auto-calibration each time the software is started. Cuvette-less spectrophotometers (NanoDrop; Thermo Scientific) are calibrated with potassium dichromate standards to confirm that path lengths are within specifications.

Fume Hoods and Laminar Flow Hoods

Fume hoods and laminar flow (biological safety) hoods (Fig. 16-15) are monitored annually for proper air flow. Fume hood testing requires special equipment and is likely to be performed by building engineers. Laminar flow hoods are tested for proper filter performance and air displacement. This testing is performed at least annually or upon installation or movement of the hood. Professional service technicians or the hood manufacturers usually provide this type of certification.

For all detection systems, regular monitoring of functional characteristics will reveal any drift or trends that might affect test results. Tolerance limits should be

acceptable background levels. Laboratory professionals may use these measurements or establish their own acceptable background levels. Corrective action, such as cleaning or filter adjustment, is documented in the laboratory maintenance records. Ultraviolet (uv) illuminators should be kept free of dust and properly shielded while in use. The technologists should keep track of the life span of uv, xenon, laser, or other light sources and schedule replacement accordingly. Such specialty light sources, especially lasers, are replaced by instrument company representatives.

Spectrophotometers used to measure DNA, RNA, protein concentrations, and colorimetric assays and turbidity must be checked annually or as recommended by the manufacturer. Maintenance includes scanning through the range of wavelengths used (e.g., 200 to 800 nm) with supplied materials or filters. Operation manuals will include instructions for calibration and maintenance. Spectrophotometers dedicated to nucleic acid and protein measurement have fixed wavelengths at 260, 280, and 320 nm. These instruments may be checked for linearity of concentration measurements with reference nucleic

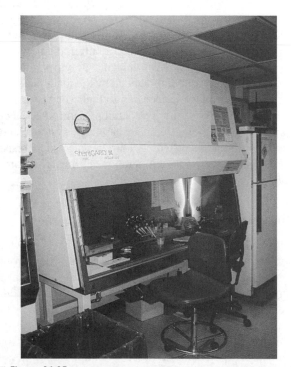

■ **Figure 16-15** Laminar flow hoods are used to protect against biological hazards and to help maintain a sterile environment.

established to warrant intervention by maintenance or recalibration of the instrument. Scheduled and unscheduled maintenance is documented in the laboratory records. These records should be readily available to the technologists using the equipment.

Liquid Handling

Pipettors used for dispensing specific quantities of reagents should be checked for accuracy before use and at 6-month intervals or as required according to manufacturer's recommendations. Gravimetric methods, in which measured samples of water are pipetted to a balance, have been used for many years.[29] The weights are converted to volumes using density values. The mean of several measurements from the same pipette reveals its accuracy. The standard deviation, or **coefficient of variance**, is calculated to determine the degree of reproducibility (imprecision) of the pipette. Commercial pipette monitoring systems along with software are also available.[30] Alternatively, some laboratory professionals prefer to hire service providers who clean and check pipettes on a per-pipette charge.

Many automated instruments have internal liquid handling systems. These are maintained according to manufacturer's recommendations. Tubing, filters, seals, valves, and other components may be monitored by a laboratory professional trained in the proper maintenance procedures or by manufacturer's representatives. The accurate function of these instruments is assured by calibration of their performance.

Calibrations

Calibration is adjusting an instrument or test system output to the actual concentration of a reference analyte by testing and making appropriate adjustments. In **calibration verification**, materials of known concentration throughout the **reportable range** are tested as patient samples to ensure the test system is accurate. If calibration verification fails, recalibration is required. CLIA-88 Regulations, 42CFR493.1255(b)(3), recommend performance of calibration verification at least every 6 months or when major components, instrument software, or lots of reagents of the test system are altered. Recalibration is also required if proficiency or other quality control testing fails or in the event of major instrument malfunction

and repair. Manufacturers of test systems may also provide calibration schedules and instructions on how to perform calibrations. Laboratory professionals must verify with reference standards the calibration of systems performed by the manufacturer.

A variety of materials may be used for calibration, including previously tested specimens, reference standards, and proficiency testing material. There must be independent assessment of the actual measurement of the calibration material. Once established, calibrator results should always be specified as ranges of values. Calibration materials should cover at least three levels of measurement: low, medium, and high points, based on the clinically important analyte levels. Standards used for calibration should be in the same matrix (e.g., plasma or urine) as the patient specimens.[26] Calibrators are prepared and used separately from quality control standards (e.g., positive, negative, and sensitivity controls) that are used for routine runs.

Reagents

When reagents are replaced in a test method, ideally the new lot is tested on a previously positive and negative specimen as well as on the run controls. Instructions for the preparation of reagents and the quantities used in each assay are included in the written laboratory protocol for each procedure. Lot numbers and working stocks of probes and primers used in amplification methods are documented and matched to test performance in the runs in which they were used. The sequences of primers and probes are also documented, as any sequence errors made during ordering or synthesis of primers or probes will adversely affect test specificity or even result in test failure.

Probes, particularly those used for linkage analysis and array technology are periodically updated as new markers are discovered. Probe sequences used for a given test should be noted, especially if new or additional probes are used in the assay. Primers are most conveniently supplied in lyophilized (freeze-dried) form from DNA synthesis facilities (Fig. 16-16). The supplier will also provide information on the quality, method of purification, molecular weight, and number of micrograms of dried primers. This information is used to rehydrate the primers to the required stock solution concentration. The stock solutions are then diluted into working stocks.

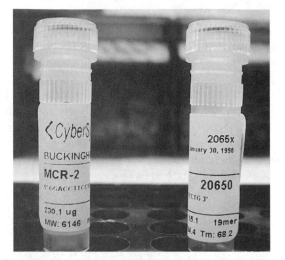

■ **Figure 16-16** Primers are often purchased from DNA synthesis facilities. On receipt in freeze-dried form, the primers are easily resuspended in nuclease-free water or buffer to make a stock solution. The stock solution is then diluted into working stocks.

Working stocks may be a combination of primers from stock solutions, for example, forward and reverse primers diluted into the same working stock.

Probes used for real-time PCR are supplied in solution, for example, a 100-μM stock solution that is diluted to 4- or 5-μM working stock before use. When new working stocks are prepared (diluted from the probe stocks or resuspended primers), they are treated as new reagent lots. Master mixes of primers, probe, buffer, nucleotides, and enzyme may be prepared or purchased and used as working stock.

As is required for all reagents, instructions on the preparation of primers, probes, and working stocks, along with the sequences and binding sites of primers and the expected size of the amplicons, are documented as part of the written laboratory protocol. Polymorphisms or translocation breakpoints that affect primer binding should be noted in terms of the expected frequency in the population or in the number of successful amplifications. Images displaying product sizes and band or peak patterns are useful for training purposes and for troubleshooting.

For hybridization procedures, labeled probe solutions are treated as working stock and diluted directly into hybridization buffer according to protocol. RNA probes are maintained under RNase-free conditions to protect their integrity. Stock solutions are verified by parallel analysis with old lots. FISH probes are validated and verified according to recommended procedures.[31] The quality of new microarray lots is verified by the manufacturer or by hybridizing labeled nucleotides that bind to all probes on a representative array from the lot.

It is important to document descriptive information on probes used in the laboratory. This information includes the type of probe (genomic, cDNA, oligonucleotide, plasmid, or riboprobe) and the species of origin of the probe sequence. The sequence of the probe, a GenBank number or other identification of the target sequence or gene region recognized by the probe, and a restriction enzyme map of that region are also useful information. Any known polymorphisms, sites resistant to endonuclease digestion, and cross-hybridizing bands should be noted. Recombination frequencies and map positions must be documented for linkage procedures. For inherited disease tests, chromosomal location of the target gene and known mutant alleles and their frequencies in various ethnic groups might be cited in published reports. Labeling methods and standards for adequacy of hybridization are included in the test procedure manual.

In multiplex reactions, primer and/or probe competition for substrates may affect results. Multiple fluorochrome signals in fluorescence assays may also cross into each other's detection ranges. For gel or capillary sizing, products of multiplex reactions should be reasonably different so that banding patterns do not complicate interpretation. For example, multiplex STR analysis by PCR includes 13 sets of primers that produce 13 amplicons labeled with three different fluorochromes (see Chapter 11, "DNA Polymorphisms and Human Identification"). The range of sizes of each amplified STR locus is designed not to overlap others labeled with the same fluorochrome. The instrument that detects the fluorescence is also calibrated to subtract any overlap of detection of one fluorochrome with another.

Reagent Categories

The Medical Device Amendment to the Federal Food, Drug, and Cosmetic Act (1938) authorized the FDA to regulate medical devices, including laboratory tests. Subsequent acts and amendments have further defined control, risk, safety, and performance of medical tests.

A growing list of categories defines the degree of endorsement of test performance and test components by the FDA.

Analyte-specific reagents (ASR) are probes, primers, antibodies, and other test components that detect a specific target, such as a cell surface protein or DNA mutation. ASRs comprise the active part of "home-brew" tests. ASRs, usually purchased from an outside manufacturer, are classified as I, II, or III. Most ASRs used in the molecular laboratory are class I. Several molecular tests are available as ASRs in infectious disease, tissue typing, and other areas of molecular diagnostics. Approved molecular methods include tests that utilize FISH, Hybrid Capture, PCR, and microarray technologies. Class II and III ASRs include those used by blood banks to screen for infectious diseases and those used in diagnosis of certain contagious diseases such as tuberculosis. Class I ASRs are not subject to special controls by the U.S. Food and Drug Administration. The test performance of class I ASRs is established during validation of individual laboratory-developed tests (LDT).

In the diagnostic laboratory, **in vitro diagnostic (IVD)** reagent sets are intended for use in the diagnosis of a specific disease or other condition. IVD reagent sets include products used to collect, prepare, and examine specimens collected from patients. They should be used strictly according to the manufacturer's protocol. IVD reagents are classified according to performance risk and requirements for surveillance and verification from class I (lowest risk) to class III (highest risk). Regardless of risk level, the performance (accuracy, precision, analytic sensitivity, reportable range, and **reference range**) of IVD tests must be verified by the laboratory in which they will be used. If an IVD protocol is modified, the procedure must be validated to show equivalent or improved performance compared to the original assay. A list of currently available FDA-approved tests is located on the Association for Molecular Pathology website (www.amp.org/FDATable/FDATable.doc).

In a proposed category of **in vitro analytical test (IVAT)** reagents, the FDA will approve only the analytical validity of the test, not claims of clinical utility. The medical laboratory would be responsible for any clinical claims. This category is intended to accommodate the use of promising high-complexity technologies facing long clearance processes. **Research Use Only (RUO)** and **Investigational Use Only (IUO)** reagents are not intended for diagnostic use. RUO reagents are not intended for use on patient samples; IUO reagent can be used on patient samples with proper institutional review and informed consent, for example, in clinical trials. RUO and IUO reagents are used to gather data that may result in the advancement of a product's status.

Chemical Safety

Most reagents used in current molecular diagnostic methods are not hazardous. Increased use of automated systems reduces exposure to reagents, especially those that can be harmful. Still, some manual procedures can present chemical hazards. The medical laboratory scientist should be familiar with the safe storage and handling of such reagents.

Volatile and flammable reagents are stored in properly vented and explosion-proof cabinets or refrigeration units (Fig. 16-17). The National Fire Protection Association (NFPA) has developed a series of warning labels for universal use on all chemical containers (Fig. 16-18).[32] Secondary or reinforced containers are required for transport and handling of dangerous chemicals, such as concentrated acids and phenol.

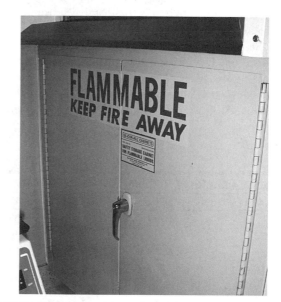

■ **Figure 16-17** Flammable and explosive materials are stored in designated protective cabinets or explosion-proof refrigerators.

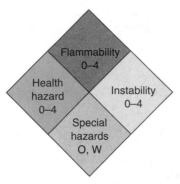

■ **Figure 16-18** NFPA hazard labels have three parts, labeled with numbers 0 to 4, depending on the amount of hazard, from none (0) to severe (4). The fourth section has two categories. O indicates a strong oxidizer, which greatly increases the rate of combustion. The stricken W symbol indicates dangerous reactivity with water, which would prohibit the use of water to extinguish a fire in the presence of this chemical.

Radioactive chemicals are used in some molecular methods (Table 16.5). Although methods involving radiation are being replaced by nonradioactive alternatives, some laboratory procedures still use these agents. The Nuclear Regulatory Commission requires that laboratory personnel working with radioactive reagents maintain a radiation safety manual providing procedures for the safe handling of radioactive substances in both routine and emergency situations. The Occupational Safety and Health Administration (OSHA) has also developed regulations regarding ionizing and nonionizing radiation.

Radioactive reagents and methods are used in designated areas. Working surfaces are protected with absorbent paper, drip trays, or other protective containers. Potentially volatile radioactive materials are handled under a fume hood. Radioactive waste is discarded in appropriate containers, separate from normal trash, according to regulations. Some isotopes with short half-lives may be stored over approximately seven half-lives, checked for residual emissions, and then discarded with regular waste. Containers and equipment used in designated areas should be labeled with "Caution Radioactive Material" signs (Fig. 16-19). Signs should be posted on the rooms where radioactive materials are used and cabinets or refrigerators/freezers where these materials are stored. OSHA has developed specifications for accident prevention signs and tags for radiation and other occupational hazards.

Laboratory personnel working with radioactive material should receive special training for safe handling, decontamination, and disposal of radioactive materials. Laboratory instructions for working with radiation should include inspection and monitoring of shipments as required by the U.S. Department of Transportation. Work spaces are decontaminated daily and checked at least monthly by swipe testing or by Geiger counter, depending on the type or radiation. Technologists wear gloves, lab coats, and safety glasses when handling radioactive solutions. Radiation badges are worn when handling 1.0 mCi or more of radioactive reagents. Exposure increases with decreasing distance from the radioactive reagent (see Table 16.5), so exposure at close distance, such as working over open containers, should be avoided. For isotopes such as ^{32}P, acrylic shielding is required for work, storage, and waste areas (Fig. 16-20).

Table 16.5 **Examples of Radionuclides Used in Laboratory Methods**

Radioisotope	Half-Life*	Radiation (MeV)[†]	Travel in Air	Critical Organs
^{32}P	14.29 days	β, 1.709	20 feet	Bone, whole body
^{33}P	25.3 days	β, 0.249	20 feet	Bone, whole body
^3H	12.35 years	β, 0.019	0.65 inches	Body water
^{14}C	5730 years	β, 0.156	10 inches	Whole body, fat
^{35}S	87.39 days	β, 0.167	11 inches	Whole body, testes
^{125}I	60.14 days	X,γ, 0.035	3 feet	Thyroid

*Time for half of the radiation emission to dissipate
[†]Million electron volts

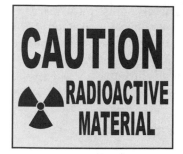

■ Figure 16-19 Rooms, cabinets, and equipment containing radioactive chemicals are identified with radiation safety labels.

Proficiency Testing

Proficiency testing refers to the analysis of external specimens supplied to independent laboratories from a reference source.[25] Such testing is done to assess the skills (competency) of laboratory personnel performing molecular assays as well as the performance of the assay itself. The availability of comprehensive test specimens in the rapidly expanding area of molecular diagnostics is sometimes problematic. The CAP supplies specimens in

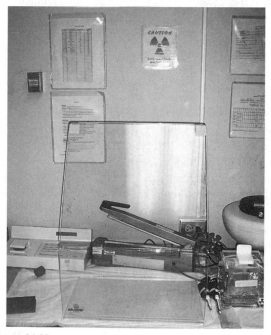

■ Figure 16-20 Acrylic shielding is required for working with gamma emitters, such as ^{32}P and ^{33}P.

the areas of molecular genetics, molecular oncology, and molecular microbiology testing, among others (www.cap.org). A number of analytes, however, are not available, especially for tests that are offered in a small number of laboratories. If proficiency specimens are not commercially available, laboratories must establish another proficiency testing procedure. One way is the exchange of split specimens between two or more laboratories; alternatively, specimens measured or documented by independent means such as chart review can be tested within a single laboratory.[33,34] Increasing numbers of reference standards for proficiency testing are commercially available. If at all possible, interlaboratory testing is preferable.

Proficiency testing is performed at least twice a year, with the proficiency samples tested within routine patient runs. The specific procedures should be defined and documented in the laboratory. Errors or incorrect responses for proficiency specimens are documented along with the corrective action taken, if necessary.

Technologists working in the area of molecular pathology will encounter tests in which the final details are determined empirically, such as in home-brew tests or commercial systems that are modified in the laboratory. As a result, a test procedure may differ from one laboratory to another. Even after the test procedure is established, troubleshooting is sometimes required as the procedure is used on a routine basis. Some reactions that work well for short-term research may prove to be less consistent and reproducible than is required in the clinical laboratory setting. In this situation, proficiency testing is especially important to assure that the accuracy and reproducibility of the test results are satisfactory for patient testing.

Documentation of Test Results

Test results in the form of electropherograms, gel images, and autoradiograms should be of sufficiently high quality that results are unequivocal. This includes clear bands or peaks without high background, cross-hybridization, distortions, or other artifacts. Controls should also be clear and consistent and reflect the expected size or level of analyte. Molecular-weight ladders on gels, autoradiograms, or electropherograms should cover the expected range of band or peak sizes produced from the specimen. For example, if primers used for a PCR test yield amplicons expected to range from 150 to 500 bp, the molecular-weight ladder used must range from less than 150 bp to more than 500 bp.

A record of the assay conditions and reagent lot numbers is kept with patient results. Identification of the technologist performing the assay may also be included. Documentation of the quality and quantity of the isolated DNA or RNA is also required, especially if designated amounts of nucleic acids are used for an assay. Quantity and quality are documented in the form of spectrophotometry or fluorometry data or quantity or gel photographs of high-molecular-weight DNA or ribosomal RNA quality (see Chapter 4). The quality of RNA analyzed by northern blot or RT-PCR may be assessed by monitoring a housekeeping gene, ribosomal RNA expression, or other calibrator.

If DNA is cut with restriction enzymes for Southern blot or PCR-restriction fragment length polymorphism, complete cutting by the restriction enzyme is verified on control targets and documented by photography of the cut DNA on the gel after electrophoresis. DNA digested with DNase for array analysis is also documented in this way to confirm proper fragment sizes. If specimen nucleic acid is labeled for hybridization arrays, labeling efficiency is assessed by measurement of the specific activity (signal per ng nucleic acid). For Southern blots, patient identification, gel lane (well) number, and probe target and type are also documented. It is also recommended that the test documentation should include pre-hybridization and hybridization conditions and probe and hybridization buffer lot numbers.

In situ results, such as FISH, are correlated with histological findings (stained sections) of tissue morphology. This is required when the molecular target detection is significant in specific cells, for example, with p53 detection in tumor cells. Documentation includes images of at least one normal cell with at least two abnormal cell results. These images are cross-referenced or retained together with photographs, films, and autoradiographs generated from additional testing of the same specimen. All these records are labeled with patient identification, sample numbers, target analyte, run identifiers, and the date of assay.

All of the raw data are retained with the final report and clinical interpretation of the test results. Careful documentation is important because molecular diagnostic results may differ from results of other laboratories or

from the clinical diagnosis. Such discrepancies occur most often with amplification methods because of their high sensitivity. If a molecular result is questioned, investigation of the discrepancy includes review of the raw data. Results of this investigation along with any corrective action taken are noted in the laboratory records.

Gene Nomenclature

Reporting of results from genetic testing requires unequivocal identification of the gene being tested. Gene names are sometimes not consistent, and multiple names can refer to the same gene. For example, the official HUGO Gene Nomenclature Committee (HGNC) gene name *ERBB2* is also called *HER2*, *HER-2*, and *EGFR2*. The official name can even be changed by the HGNC. Ongoing efforts to implement the universal usage of standard official gene names and symbols by molecular laboratory professionals are documented at www.genenames.org. Meanwhile, laboratory reports may refer to "also known as" names for the same gene, for example *ERBB2* (*HER2*). Gene name aliases can be found at the National Center for Biological Information (NCBI) Gene Database (http://www.ncbi.nlm.nih.gov/gene/). It is most important to use the gene name or symbol recognized by the laboratory's medical community.

Gene Sequencing Results

Direct sequencing is increasingly used in clinical applications to detect gene mutations or to type microorganisms. Sequence data must be of adequate quality with acceptably low baseline, especially if heterozygous target states are to be detected. Each nucleotide peak or band should be unequivocal. Sequencing is performed on both complementary strands of the template to confirm sequenced mutation or type. Repeated sequencing across the same area, or **resequencing**, for known sequence changes is sometimes performed only on one template strand; however, sequencing of both strands is recommended.

Criteria for acceptance of sequencing data include correct assignment of the nucleotide sequence in a defined region surrounding the critical area, not including the amplification primer binding sites, and a specified level of band or peak quality (intensity or fluorescence levels, respectively) with reasonably low background. Defined limits of fluorescence ratios are set to identify true heterozygous base positions. Ideally, a heterozygous position will have equal fluorescence contribution from the two genotypes, and the peak height will be approximately half that of a homozygous genotype at that position. Results are expressed in the standard nomenclature for DNA or protein sequences (see Chapter 9).

The utility of sequence data requires published normal or type-specific sequences. In the case of gene mutations, electronic or published databases of known mutations and polymorphisms are available for frequently tested genes. These records, especially Internet databases, are updated regularly. Newly discovered mutations are classified according to the type of mutation; the laboratory director or consultant uses published guidelines to determine if the mutation is clinically significant.[35] For example, a silent mutation will not affect protein function, whereas a frameshift mutation will.

Reporting Results

Test results are reported in terms that are unambiguous to readers who may not be familiar with molecular methods or terminology. The test report must include the method or manufactured kit used; the locus, mutation, or organism tested; the analytical interpretation of the raw data; and the clinical interpretation of the analytical result. This interpretation should include such interpretive complexities as the limit of detection of microorganisms, resistance factors, or the penetrance of inherited mutations, that is, the probability of having a mutation but not getting the associated disease.

The likelihood of false-positive or false-negative results is also included in a report. For example, detection of base changes in mutational analysis is not guaranteed, especially in large genes with hundreds of possible mutations that may or may not effectively compromise gene function. The mutation detection rate for this type of gene and the residual risk of undetected mutations are therefore included in the test report. Negative results are reported in terms of the sensitivity of the test, for example, less than 0.01% chance of detection or, alternatively, negative accompanied with the sensitivity levels of the test. For parentage reports, the combined paternity index, the probability of paternity as a percentage, prior probability of paternity used in calculations, and the population used for comparison are reported.

The laboratory director, pathologist, or other clinical expert reviews the analytical interpretation, determines the clinical interpretation, and verifies the final results with an actual or electronic signature on the test report. This verification will include coding for billing and reimbursement purposes. An internal laboratory summary sheet is often useful for compiling pertinent information (Fig. 16-21). Test results should not be released before they are reviewed by the director. Molecular diagnostic tests, in particular, may have technical complexities that influence the meaning of the test result. These results are included in the report along with the clinical significance of the laboratory findings.

When class I ASRs are used in an analytical method, the following disclaimer is included in the test report: "The FDA has determined that such clearance or approval is not necessary. This test is used for clinical purposes. It should not be regarded as investigational or for research. This laboratory is certified under the Clinical Laboratory Improvement Amendments of 1988 (CLIA-88) as qualified to perform high-complexity clinical laboratory testing."[36] The disclaimer is not required for tests using reagents that are sold together with other materials or instruments as a kit, nor for reagents sold with instructions for use. It is not necessary when FDA-approved tests are used.

Maintaining the confidentiality of molecular test results is essential. All results, including infectious disease and molecular genetic results, may affect insurability, employment, or other family members. Results are released only to the ordering physician or other authorized personnel, such as genetic counselors or nurse coordinators. Technologists should refer requests for patient data to supervisors. Data sent by facsimile must be accompanied by a disclaimer such as:

The documents accompanying this telecopy transmission contain confidential information belonging to the sender that is legally privileged. This information is intended only for the use of the individual or entity named above. The authorized recipient of this information is prohibited from disclosing this information to any other party and is required to destroy the information after its stated need has been fulfilled. If you are not the intended recipient, you are hereby notified that any disclosure, copying, distributing, or action taken in reliance on the contents of these documents is strictly prohibited. If you have received this telecopy in error, please notify the sender immediately to arrange for return or destruction of these documents.

PATIENT SAMPLE STORAGE AND RESULT SUMMARY

Date:

Patient ID Label   Sex: Diagnosis:

                          DOB: Specimen:

                          Age: Surgical Path #:

I.
Flow Cytometry Accession # _____ Date of Procedure:_____

Genetics Accession #_____ Date of Procedure:_____

Bone Marrow Aspirate #_____ Date of Procedure:_____

II. Tissue Storage: Freezer Box #_____ RNA Storage Box #_____Volume_____

III. RNA Isolation
O.D. Value   260/280   Volume   Concentration

IV.   DATA: RUN #_____

Previous Results:

Controls Acceptable: yes/no

__ Positive for BCR/ABL Translocation at M-bcr b2/a2 fusion
__ Positive for BCR/ABL Translocation at M-bcr b3/a2 fusion
__ Positive for BCR/ABL Translocation at m-bcr e1/a2 fusion
__ Negative for BCR/ABL Translocation

Pathology Result_____   Cytogenetics Result_____

V. Interpretation of lab results:_____
_____
_____
_____

Remarkable case:_____
_____

Verbal report to:_____ Date_____ By_____

VI. Physician's Interpretation:_____
_____
_____

Reviewed:_____ Date_____

■ Figure 16-21 Example of a patient result summary sheet used for documentation of test results of a BCR/ABL analysis by RT-PCR. Information included will differ depending on the disease and the type of test.

Test results are not released to employers, insurers, or other family members without the patient's documented consent. Any data discussed in a public forum are presented such that no patient or pedigree is identifiable by the patient or the general audience. Written consent from the patient may be required under some circumstances. Each institution will have a department that oversees the lawful use of confidential information.

Biotechnology is rapidly developing standard reagent sets and instrumentation for the most popular tests, but these also differ from one supplier to another. Furthermore, due to market demands, test reagent kits may be modified or discontinued. If replacement reagents are available, they may not be identical to those previously used. Ongoing tests then have to be optimized. This can be a concern where turnaround times are critical. It then becomes the responsibility of the technologist to perform and monitor tests on a regular basis to maintain consistency and accuracy of results. The technologist who understands the biochemistry and molecular biology of these tests will be better able to respond to these problems. In addition, with the ever-faster pace of evolution in the sciences, a knowledgeable technologist will recognize significant discoveries that offer potential for test improvement.

• STUDY QUESTIONS •

What actions should be taken in the following situations?

1. An unlabeled collection tube with a requisition for a factor V Leiden test is received in the laboratory.

2. After PCR, the amplification control has failed to yield a product.

3. An isolated DNA sample is to be stored for at least 6 months.

4. A bone marrow specimen arrives at the end of a shift and will not be processed for the *Bcl2* translocation until the next day.

5. The temperature of a refrigerator set at 8°C (±2°C) reads 14°C.

6. A PCR test for the BCR/ABL translocation was negative for the patient sample and for the sensitivity control.

7. A fragile X test result has been properly reviewed and reported.

8. A bottle of reagent alcohol with a 3 in the red diamond on its label is to be stored.

9. The expiration date on a reagent has passed.

10. Test results are to be faxed to the ordering physician.

11. Among a group of properly labeled containers, there is a container similar to the others, but unlabeled.

12. A blood sample is received in a serum tube for PML-RARa testing by PCR.

13. The laboratory is reporting a gene mutation replacing glycine at position 215 with alanine. The results are written 215G → A in the test report.

14. The laser on a complex instrument malfunctions.

15. A test result falls outside of the analytical measurement range of the validated method.

16. Reference standards are reading higher than their designated concentrations.

17. A new FDA-approved test does not perform as expected.

18. A solution containing radioactive waste has been stored in a properly protected area for 10 half-lives of the isotope.

19. There is no available proficiency test for a new method developed in the laboratory.

20. A research investigator asks for a patient specimen.

References

1. Calam R, Bessman JD, Ernst DJ, et al. Procedures for the Handling and Processing of Blood Specimens: Approved Guideline, H18-A3, 3rd ed. Clinical and Laboratory Standards Institute, Wayne, PA, 2004.
2. Rabinovitch A. Routine Urinalysis and Collection, Transportation, and Preservation of Urine Specimens: Approved Guideline, GP16-A3, 3rd ed. Clinical and Laboratory Standards Institute, Wayne, PA, 2009.
3. Arkin C, Bessman JD, Calam RR, et al. Tubes and Additives for Venous Blood Specimen Collection: Approved Standard, H1-A5, 5th ed. Clinical and Laboratory Standards Institute, Wayne PA, 2003.
4. Kiechle F, Chambers LM, Cox RS, et al. Patient preparation and specimen handling. In: Reference Guide for Diagnostic Molecular Pathology and Flow Cytometry. Fascicle VII: College of American Pathologists, Washington, DC, 1996.
5. Ghadessy F, Ong JL, Holliger P. Directed evolution of polymerase function by compartmentalized self-replication. *Proceedings of the National Academy of Sciences* 2001;98:4552–4557.
6. Lam N, Rainer TH, Chiu RWK, et al. EDTA is a better anticoagulant than heparin or citrate for delayed blood processing for plasma DNA analysis. *Clinical Chemistry* 2004;50:256–257.
7. Tanner M, Berk LS, Felten DL, et al. Substantial changes in gene expression level due to the storage temperature and storage duration of human whole blood. *Clinical and Laboratory Haematology* 2002;24:337–341.
8. Chai V, Vassilakos A, Lee Y, et al. Optimization of the PAXgene blood RNA extraction system for gene expression analysis of clinical samples. *Journal of Clinical Laboratory Analysis* 2005;19:182–188.
9. Elbeik T, Nassos P, Kipnis P, et al. Evaluation of the VACUTAINER PPT Plasma Preparation Tube for use with the Bayer VERSANT assay for quantification of human immunodeficiency virus type 1 RNA. *Journal of Clinical Microbiology* 2005;43:3769–3771.
10. Rainen L, Oelmueller U, Jurgensen S, et al. Stabilization of mRNA expression in whole blood samples. *Clinical Chemistry* 2002;48:1883–1890.
11. Rahman M, Goegebuer T, De Leener K, et al. Chromatography paper strip method for collection, transportation, and storage of rotavirus RNA in stool samples. *Journal of Clinical Microbiology* 2004;42:1605–1608.
12. Zhong K, Salas CJ, Shafer R, et al. Comparison of IsoCode STIX and FTA Gene Guard collection matrices as whole-blood storage and processing devices for diagnosis of malaria by PCR. *Journal of Clinical Microbiology* 2001;39:1195–1196.
13. Farkas D, Drevon A, Kiechle FL, et al. Specimen stability for DNA-based diagnostic testing. *Diagnostic Molecular Pathology* 1996;5:227–235.
14. Farkas D, Kaul KL, Wiedbrauk DL, et al. Specimen collection and storage for diagnostic molecular pathology investigation. *Archives of Pathology and Laboratory Medicine* 1996;120:591–596.
15. Statement AFMP. Recommendations for in-house development and operation of molecular diagnostic tests. *American Journal of Clinical Pathology* 1999;111:449–463.
16. Jennings L, van Deerlin VM, Gulley ML et al. Recommended principles and practices for validating clinical molecular pathology tests. *Archives of Pathology and Laboratory Medicine* 2009;133:743–755.
17. Pyne MT, Konnick EQ, Phansalkar A, et al. Evaluation of the Abbott investigational-use-only Real-Time hepatitis C virus (HCV) assay and comparison to the Roche TaqMan HCV analyte-specific reagent assay. *Journal of Clinical Pathology* 2009;47:2872–2878.
18. Goedel S, Rullkoetter M, Weisshaar S, et al. Hepatitis B virus (HBV) genotype determination by the COBAS AmpliPrep/COBAS TaqMan HBV Test, v2.0 in serum and plasma matrices. *Journal of Clinical Virology* 2009;45:232–236.
19. Bustin SA, Benes V, Garson JA. The MIQE guidelines: Minimum information for publication of quantitative real-time PCR experiments. *Clinical Chemistry* 2009;55:611–622.
20. Sloan LM. Real-time PCR in clinical microbiology: Verification, validation and contamination control. *Clinical Microbiology Newsletter* 2007;29:87–96.
21. Hirsh B, Brothman AR, Jacky PB, et al. Section E6 of the ACMG technical standards and guidelines: Chromosome studies for acquired abnormalities. *Genetics in Medicine* 2005;7:509–513.

22. Potter N, Spector EB, Prior TW. Technical standards and guidelines for Huntington disease testing. *Genetics in Medicine* 2004;6:61–65.

23. Ambros I, Benard J, Boavida M, et al. Quality assessment of genetic markers used for therapy stratification. *Journal of Clinical Oncology* 2003;21:2077–2084.

24. Berte L. Technical Procedure Manual, GP0A5, 4th ed., Clinical and Laboratory Standards Institute, Wayne, PA, 2006.

25. Clark G, Sarewitz SJ. Using Proficiency Testing (PT) to Improve the Clinical Laboratory: Approved Guideline, GP27-A2, 3rd ed. Clinical and Laboratory Standards Institute, 2007;

26. Beillard E, Pallisgaard N, van der Velden VH, et al. Evaluation of candidate control genes for diagnosis and residual disease detection in leukemic patients using "real-time" quantitative reverse-transcriptase polymerase chain reaction (RQ-PCR)—A Europe Against Cancer program. *Leukemia* 2003;17:2474–2486.

27. Madej R. Using standards and controls in molecular assays for infectious diseases. *Molecular Diagnostics* 2001;6:335–345.

28. Tse C, Brault D, Gligorov J, et al. Evaluation of the quantitative analytical methods real-time PCR for *HER-2* gene quantification and ELISA of serum *HER-2* protein and comparison with fluorescence in situ hybridization and immunohistochemistry for determining *HER-2* status in breast cancer patients. *Clinical Chemistry* 2005;51:1093–1101.

29. Stevenson G, Smetters GW, Copper JA. A gravimetric method for the calibration of hemoglobin micropipets. *American Journal of Clinical Pathology* 1951;31:489–491.

30. Bray W. Software for the gravimetric calibration testing of pipets. *American Clinical Laboratory* 995;14:14–15.

31. Enns R, Dewald G, Barker PE. Fluoresence in situ Hybridization (FISH) Methods for Medical Genetics: Approved Guideline MM7-A, Clinical and Laboratory Standards Institute, Wayne, PA, 2004.

32. Colonna PE, ed., Fire protection guide to hazardous materials. National Fire Protection Association, Quincy, MA, 2010.

33. Richards C, Grody WW. Alternative approaches to proficiency testing in molecular genetics. *Clinical Chemistry* 2003;49;717–718.

34. Sarewitz SJ, Harvey G, Miller WG, et al. Assessment of laboratory tests when proficiency testing is not available: Approved guideline, GP29-A, Clinical and Laboratory Standards Institute, Wayne, PA, 2008.

35. den Dunnen J, Antonarakis SE. Mutation nomenclature extensions and suggestions to describe complex mutations. *Human Mutation* 2000;15:7–12.

36. Molecular Pathology Checklist. College of American Pathologists, Washington, DC, 2009.

CHAPTER 1

DNA Structure and Function

1. What is the function of DNA in the cell?

   Answer: DNA is a storage system. The function of DNA is to store genetic information.

2. Compare the structure of the nitrogen bases. How do purines and pyrimidines differ?

   Answer: Purines have a double ring; pyrimidines have a single ring.

3. Write the complementary sequence to the following:

   5'AGGTCACGTCTAGCTAGCTAGA3'

   Answer: 5'TCTAGCTAGCTAGACGTGACCT3'

4. Which of the ribose carbons participate in the phosphodiester bond?

   Answer: The 5' ribose carbon carries the phosphate group that forms a phosphodiester bond with the hydroxyl group on the 3' ribose carbon.

5. Which of the ribose carbons carries the nitrogen base?

   Answer: The 1' carbon of the ribose carries the nitrogen base.

6. Why does DNA polymerase require primase activity?

   Answer: DNA polymerase cannot begin synthesis without a 3' OH group.

DNA Replication

1. What is the covalent bond between nucleotides catalyzed by DNA polymerase?

   Answer: The covalent bond between nucleotides is a phosphodiester bond.

2. Is DNA replication conservative or semi-conservative?

   Answer: DNA replication is semi-conservative.

3. What is the lagging strand in DNA synthesis?

   Answer: During DNA replication, the lagging strand is the strand positioned 5' to 3' with respect to the direction of synthesis, requiring the replication assembly to jump ahead and read 3' to 5' back toward the moving replication fork. The leading strand is read continuously 3' to 5'. Synthesis thus proceeds 5' to 3' on both strands.

4. Short pieces of DNA involved in DNA synthesis in replicating cells are called _____ fragments.

   Answer: Short pieces of DNA involved in DNA synthesis in replicating cells are called Okazaki fragments.

5. Name the function of the following enzymes:

   polymerase
   helicase
   primase
   exonuclease
   endonuclease

   Answer:

   Polymerase catalyzes formation of a phosphodiester bond between nucleotides.

   Helicase unwinds nucleic acids, relieving stress on the double helix by breaking and re-attaching phosphodiester bonds.

   Primase is an RNA polymerase that starts replication in the absence of a 3' OH group.

   Exonuclease digests phosphodiester bonds from the ends of nucleic acid molecules.

   Endonuclease breaks the phosphodiester bonds in nucleic acids within the polymer chains, rather than from the ends.

Restriction Enzyme Analysis

1. A plasmid was digested with the enzyme *Hpa*II. On agarose gel electrophoresis, you observe three bands: 100, 230, and 500 bp.

   a. How many *Hpa*II sites are present in this plasmid?

   b. What are the distances between each site?

   c. What is the size of the plasmid?

   d. Draw a picture of the plasmid with the *Hpa*II sites.

   A second cut of the plasmid with *Bam*H1 yields two pieces, 80 and *x* bp.

   e. How many *Bam*H1 sites are in the plasmid?

   f. What is *x* in base pairs (bp)?

Answers:
a. **There are three *Hpa*II sites in this plasmid.**
b. **The distances between the sites are 100, 230, and 500 bp.**
c. **The plasmid is 100 + 230 + 500 = 830 bp.**
d.

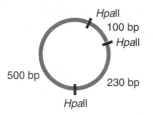

A second cut of the plasmid with *Bam*H1 yields two pieces, 80 and *x* bp.
e. **There are two *Bam*H1 sites in the plasmid.**
f. ***x* = 830 – 80 = 750 bp**

2. How would you determine where the *Bam*H1 sites are in relation to the *Hpa*II sites?
   Answer: Cut the plasmid with *Bam*H1 and *Hpa*II in the same reaction and note the fragments that are produced.

3. The plasmid has one *Eco*R1 site into which you want to clone a blunt-ended fragment. What type of enzyme could turn an *Eco*R1 sticky end into a blunt end?
   Answer: A single-strand exonuclease can digest the *Eco*R1 overhang, forming a blunt end. Alternatively, a polymerase could fill in the overhang to make a blunt end.

Recombination and DNA Transfer
1. Compare how DNA moves from cell to cell by (a) conjugation, (b) transduction, and (c) transformation.
   Answers:
   a. **For conjugation, DNA moves from cell to cell through physical contact.**
   b. **DNA moves from cell to cell through intermediary viruses or bacteriophages in transduction.**
   c. **In transformation, unprotected DNA moves from cell to cell without physical contact or viral carriers.**

2. Bacteria with phenotype A+ are mixed with bacteria with phenotype A– in a culture. Some of the A– bacteria become A+. When A+ bacteria are removed from the culture and A– bacteria are grown in the A+ cell culture medium only, they all remain A–. What type of transfer occurred in the mixed culture?
   Answer: Conjugation occurred in the mixed culture. If the A– bacteria became A+ through transformation or transduction, the cell culture medium from the A+ bacteria would contain DNA or phage, respectively, capable of transforming A– bacteria to A+.

3. What was the rationale for labeling bacteriophage with ^{35}S and ^{32}P in the Hershey and Chase "blender" experiment?
   Answer: ^{35}S labels protein, specifically since there is no S in nucleic acid. ^{32}P labels nucleic acid specifically, since there was no P in the phage proteins.

4. A plasmid that carries genes for its own transfer and propagation is called _____.
   Answer: A plasmid that carries genes for its own transfer and propagation is called self-transmissible.

5. What enzymes can convert a supercoiled plasmid to a relaxed circle?
   Answer: Helicases (topoisomerases) can digest the phosphodiester bond in one strand of the double-stranded DNA, allowing the twisted strands to unwind.

CHAPTER 2

RNA Secondary Structure

1. Draw the secondary structure of the following RNA. The complementary sequences (inverted repeat) are underlined.

5'CAU<u>GUUCA</u>GCUCAUG<u>UGAAC</u>GCU 3'

2. Underline *two* inverted repeats in the following RNA:

5'CUGAACUUCAGUCAAGCAAAGAGUUUGC
ACUG 3'

RNA Processing
1. Name three processing steps undergone by messenger RNA.
Answer: Three processing steps of mRNA are polyadenylation, capping, and splicing.

2. What is the function of polyadenylate polymerase?
Answer: Polyadenylate polymerase digests RNA and adds adenines to the 3' end of the transcript.

3. What is unusual about the phosphodiester bond formed between mRNA and its 5' cap?
Answer: The 5' cap is attached by an unusual 5'-to-5' pyrophosphate linkage.

4. The parts of the hnRNA that are translated into protein (open reading frames) are the _____.
Answer: 4. The parts of the hnRNA that are translated into protein (open reading frames) are the exons.

5. The intervening sequences that interrupt protein coding sequences in hnRNA are _____.
Answer: The intervening sequences that interrupt protein coding sequences in hnRNA are introns.

Gene Expression

1. Proteins that bind to DNA to control gene expression are called _____ factors.
Answer: Proteins that bind to DNA to control gene expression are called trans factors (or transcription factors).

2. The binding sites on DNA for proteins that control gene expression are _____ factors.
Answer: Proteins that bind to DNA to control gene expression are called cis factors.

3. How might a single mRNA produce more than one protein product?
Answer: A single RNA may be alternatively spliced to produce more than one product.

4. The type of transcription producing RNA that is continually required and relatively abundant in the cell is called _____ transcription.
Answer: The type of transcription producing RNA that is continually required and relatively abundant in the cell is called constitutive transcription.

5. A set of structural genes transcribed together on one polycistronic mRNA is called an _____.
Answer: A set of structural genes transcribed together on one polycistronic mRNA is called an operon.

The Lac Operon

Using the depiction of the lac operon in Figures 2-9 and 2-10, indicate whether gene expression (transcription) would be on or off under the following conditions (P = promoter, O = operator; R = repressor):
  a. P+ O+ R+, no inducer present — OFF
  b. P+ O+ R+, inducer present — ON
  c. P– O+ R+, no inducer present —
  d. P– O+ R+, inducer present —
  e. P+ O– R+, no inducer present —
  f. P+ O– R+, inducer present —
  g. P+ O+ R–, no inducer present —
  h. P+ O+ R–, inducer present —
  i. P– O– R+, no inducer present —
  j. P– O– R+, inducer present —
  k. P– O+ R–, no inducer present —
  l. P– O+ R–, inducer present —
  m. P+ O– R–, no inducer present —
  n. P+ O– R–, inducer present —
  o. P– O– R–, no inducer present —
  p. P– O– R–, inducer present —
Answers:
  a. P+ O+ R+, no inducer present — OFF
  b. P+ O+ R+, inducer present — ON
  c. P– O+ R+, no inducer present — OFF
  d. P– O+ R+, inducer present — OFF
  e. P+ O– R+, no inducer present — ON
  f. P+ O– R+, inducer present — ON
  g. P+ O+ R–, no inducer present — ON
  h. P+ O+ R–, inducer present — ON
  i. P– O– R+, no inducer present — OFF
  j. P– O– R+, inducer present — OFF
  k. P– O+ R–, no inducer present — OFF

l. P– O+ R–, inducer present — OFF
m. P+ O– R–, no inducer present — ON
n. P+ O– R–, inducer present — ON
o. P– O– R–, no inducer present — OFF
p. P– O– R–, inducer present — OFF

Epigenetics

1. Indicate whether the following events would increase or decrease expression of a gene:
   a. Methylation of cytosine bases 5' to the gene
   b. Histone acetylation close to the gene
   c. siRNAs complementary to the gene transcript
   Answers:
   a. Methylation of cytosine bases 5' to the gene will decrease expression.
   b. Histone acetylation close to the gene will increase expression.
   c. siRNAs complementary to the gene transcript will decrease expression.

2. How does the complementarity of siRNA to its target mRNA differ from that of miRNA?
   Answer: The complementarity of siRNA is exact. The complementarity of miRNA is imperfect.

3. What is imprinting in DNA?
   Answer: DNA imprinting is marking of selective areas of DNA usually by methylation.

4. What sequence structures in DNA, usually found 5' to structural genes, are frequent sites of DNA methylation?
   Answer: CpG islands are targets for DNA methylation 5' to structural genes.

5. What is the RISC?
   Answer: The RNA-induced silencing complex mediates the specific interaction between siRNA or miRNA and the target RNA.

CHAPTER 3

1. Indicate whether the following peptides are hydrophilic or hydrophobic:
   a. MLWILSS
   b. VAIKVLIL
   c. CSKEGCPN
   d. SSIQKNET
   e. YAQKFQGRT
   f. AAPLIWWA
   g. SLKSSTGGQ
   Answers:
   a. MLWILAA — hydrophobic
   b. VAIKVLIL — hydrophobic
   c. CSKEGCPN — hydrophilic
   d. SSIQKNET — hydrophilic
   e. YAQKFQGRT — hydrophilic
   f. AAPLIWWA — hydrophobic
   g. SLKSSTGGQ — hydrophilic

2. Is the following peptide positively or negatively charged at neutral pH?

   GWWMNKCHAGHLNGVYYQGGTY
   Answer: The peptide is positively charged.

3. Consider an RNA template made from a 2:1 mixture of C:A. What would be the three amino acids *most* frequently incorporated into protein?
   Answer: Proline (CCA), histidine (CAC), and threonine (ACC) would be most frequently incorporated.

4. What is the peptide sequence encoded in AUAUAUAUAUAUAUA . . .?
   Answer: The peptide sequence would alternate isoleucine (AUA) and tyrosine (UAU): IYIYI. . . .

5. Write the anticodons 5' to 3' of the following amino acids:
   a. L
   b. T
   c. M
   d. H
   e. R
   f. I
   Answers:
   a. L — UAA, CAA, AAG, GAG, UAG, CAG
   b. T — AGU, GGU, UGU, CGU
   c. M — CAU
   d. H — AUG, GUG
   e. R — ACG, GCG, UCG, CCG
   f. I — AAU, GAU

6. A protein contains the sequence LGEKKW-CLRVNPKGLDESKDYLSLKSKYLLL. What is the likely function of this protein? (Note: See Box A3-4.)

Answer: This protein has a leucine residue at sequential 7th positions forming a leucine zipper, found in transcription factors.

7. A histone-like protein contains the sequence: PKKGSKKAVTKVQKKDGKKRKRSRK. What characteristic of this sequence makes it likely to associate with DNA?

Answer: This protein is positively charged, which would facilitate association with negatively charged DNA.

8. A procedure for digestion of DNA with a restriction enzyme includes a final incubation step of 5 minutes at 95°C. What is the likely purpose of this final step?

Answer: The 95°C incubation will inactivate the protein, preventing its activity in subsequent steps of the assay.

9. What is a ribozyme?

Answer: A ribozyme is an RNA molecule that can metabolize other molecules like an enzyme.

10. Name the nonprotein prosthetic groups for the following conjugated proteins:

glycoprotein

lipoprotein

metalloprotein

Answers:
glycoprotein — sugars
lipoprotein — lipids
metalloprotein — metal atoms

CHAPTER 4

DNA Quantity/Quality

1. Calculate the DNA concentration in μg/mL from the following information:
   a. Absorbance reading at 260 nm from a 1:100 dilution = 0.307
   b. Absorbance reading at 260 nm from a 1:50 dilution = 0.307
   c. Absorbance reading at 260 nm from a 1:100 dilution = 0.172
   d. Absorbance reading at 260 nm from a 1:100 dilution = 0.088

   Answers:
   a. 0.307×50 ug/mL = 15.35 ug/mL
      15.35 ug/mL $\times 100$ = 1535 ug/mL
   b. 0.307×50 ug/mL = 15.35 ug/mL
      15.35 ug/mL $\times 50$ = 767.5 ug/mL
   c. 0.172×50 ug/mL = 8.60 ug/mL
      8.60 ug/mL $\times 100$ = 860 ug/mL
   d. 0.088×50 ug/mL = 4.40 ug/mL
      4.40 ug/mL $\times 100$ = 440 ug/mL

2. If the volume of the above DNA solutions was 0.5 mL, calculate the yield for (a) – (d).
   Answers:
   a. 1535 ug/mL $\times$ 0.5 mL = 767.5 ug
   b. 767.5 ug/mL $\times$ 0.5 mL = 383.8 ug
   c. 860 ug/mL $\times$ 0.5 mL = 430 ug
   d. 440 ug/mL $\times$ 0.5 mL = 220 ug

3. Three DNA preparations have the following A_{260} and A_{280} readings:

Sample	A_{260}	A_{280}
(i) 1	0.419	0.230
(ii) 2	0.258	0.225
(iii) 3	0.398	0.174

For each sample, based on the A_{260}/A_{280} ratio, is each preparation suitable for further use? If not, what is contaminating the DNA?
Answers:

Sample	A_{260}/A_{280}
1	0.419/0.230 = 1.82 This is suitable for use.
2	0.258/0.225 = 1.15 This is not suitable for use due to protein contamination.
3	0.398/0.174 = 2.23 This may be suitable for use if RNA contamination does not interfere with the subsequent assay.

4. After agarose gel electrophoresis, a 0.5 μg aliquot of DNA isolated from a bacterial culture produced only a faint smear at the bottom of the gel lane. Is this an acceptable DNA sample?

Answer: This amount of bacterial DNA should produce a bright smear near the top of the gel lane. This DNA is probagbly degraded and is therefore unacceptable.

5. Contrast the measurement of DNA concentration by spectrophotometry with analysis by fluorometry with regard to staining requirements and accuracy.
   Answer: Spectrophotometry requires no DNA staining. Fluorometry requires staining of DNA to generate a fluorescent signal. Fluorometry may be more accurate than spectrophotometry, since double-stranded DNA must be intact to stain and generate a signal, whereas single nucleotides will absorb light in spectrophotometry.

RNA Quantity/Quality

1. Calculate the RNA concentration in μg/mL from the following information:
   a. Absorbance reading at 260 nm from a 1:100 dilution = 0.307.
   b. Absorbance reading at 260 nm from a 1:50 dilution = 0.307.
   c. Absorbance reading at 260 nm from a 1:100 dilution = 0.172.
   d. Absorbance reading at 260 nm from a 1:100 dilution = 0.088.
   Answers:
   a. **0.307×40 ug/mL = 12.28 ug/mL**
      12.28 ug/mL $\times$ 100 = 1228 ug/mL
   b. **0.307×40 ug/mL = 12.28 ug/mL**
      12.28 ug/mL $\times$ 50 = 614 ug/mL
   c. **0.172×40 ug/mL = 6.88 ug/mL**
      6.88 ug/mL $\times$ 100 = 688 ug/mL
   d. **0.088×40 ug/mL = 3.52 ug/mL**
      3.52 ug/mL $\times$ 100 = 352 ug/mL

2. If the volume of the above RNA solutions was 0.5 mL, calculate the yield for (a)–(d).
   Answers:
   a. **1228 ug/mL $\times$ 0.5 mL = 614 ug**
   b. **614 ug/mL $\times$ 0.5 mL = 308 ug**
   c. **688 ug/mL $\times$ 0.5 mL = 344 ug**
   d. **352 ug/mL $\times$ 0.5 mL = 176 ug**

3. An RNA preparation has the following absorbance readings:

$A_{260} = 0.208$
$A_{280} = 0.096$

Is this RNA preparation satisfactory for use?
Answer: The A_{260}/A_{280} ratio is 0.208/0.096 = 2.17. This RNA preparation is satisfactory for use.

4. A blood sample was held at room temperature for 5 days before being processed for RNA isolation. Will this sample likely yield optimal RNA?
   Answer: This sample will likely not yield optimal RNA due to degradation and changes in gene expression at room temperature.

5. Name three factors that will affect yield of RNA from a paraffin-embedded tissue sample.
   Answer: Isolation of RNA from fixed tissue is especially affected by the type of fixative used, the age/length of storage of the tissue, and the preliminary handling of the original specimen.

CHAPTER 5

1. You wish to perform an electrophoretic resolution of your restriction enzyme–digested DNA. The size of the expected fragments ranges from 100 to 500 bp. You discover two agarose gels polymerizing on the bench. One is 0.5% agarose; the other is 2% agarose. Which one might you use to resolve your fragments?
   Answer: The 2% agarose is best for this range of fragment sizes.

2. After completion of the electrophoresis of DNA fragments along with the proper molecular-weight standard on an agarose gel, suppose (a) or (b) below was observed. What might be explanations for these?
   a. The gel is blank (no bands, no molecular-weight standard).
   b. Only the molecular weight standard is visible.
   Answers:
   a. **Since the molecular-weight standard is not visible, something is wrong with the general electrophoresis process. Most likely, staining with ethidium bromide was omitted.**
   b. **The presence of the molecular-weight standard indicates that the electrophoresis and staining were performed properly. In this case, the**

DNA fragments were not loaded, or the method used to produce the fragments was unsucessful.

3. How does PFGE separate larger fragments more efficiently than standard electrophoresis?
Answer: PFGE forces large fragments through the gel matix by repeatedly changing the direction of the electric current, thus realigning the sample with spaces in the gel matrix.

4. A 6% solution of 19:1 acylamide is mixed, deaerated, and poured between glass plates for gel formation. After an hour, the solution is still liquid. What might be one explanation for the gel not polymerizing?
Answer: The nucleating agent and/or the polymerization catalyst were not added to the gel solution.

5. A gel separation of RNA yields aberrantly migrating bands and smears. Suggest two possible explanations for this observation.
Answer: This RNA could be degraded. Alternatively, improper gel conditions were used to separate the RNA.

6. Why does DNA not resolve well in solution (without a gel matrix)?
Answer: Particles move in solution based on their charge/mass ratio. As the mass of DNA increases, slowing migration, its negative charge increases, counteracting the effect of mass.

7. Why is SyBr green I less toxic than EtBr?
Answer: SyBr green is a minor groove binding dye. It does not disrupt the nucleotide sequence of DNA. EtBr is an intercalating agent that slides in between the nucleotide bases in the DNA and can cause changes in the nucleotide sequence (mutations) in DNA.

8. What are the general components of loading buffer used for introducing DNA samples to submarine gels?
Answer: Gel loading buffer contains a density agent to facilitate loading of sample into the wells underneath the buffer surface and a tracking dye to follow the migration of the DNA during electrophoresis.

9. Name two dyes that are used to monitor migration of nucleic acid during electrophoresis.
Answer: Bromphenol blue and xylene cyanol green are two of several tracking dyes.

10. When a DNA fragment is resolved by slab gel electrophoresis, a single sharp band is obtained. What is the equivalent observation had this fragment been fluorescently labeled and resolved by capillary electrophoresis?
Answer: Capillary electrophoresis results will be a single peak on an electropherogram.

CHAPTER 6

1. Calculate the melting temperature of the following DNA fragments using the sequences only:
   a. AGTCTGGGACGGCGCGGCAATCGCA
      TCAGACCCTG CCGCG CCGTTAGCGT
   b. TCAAAAATCGAATATTTGCTTATCTA
      AGTTTTTAGCTTATAAACGAATAGAT
   c. AGCTAAGCATCGAATTGGCCATCGTGTG
      TCGATTCGTAGCTTAACCGGTAGCACAC
   d. CATCGCGATCTGCAATTACGACGATAA
      GTAGCGCTAGACGTTAATGCTGCTATT
   Answers:
   a. $(8 \times 2°C) + (17 \times 4°C) = 84°C$
   b. $(20 \times 2°C) + (6 \times 4°C) = 64°C$
   c. $(14 \times 2°C) + (14 \times 4°C) = 84°C$
   d. $(15 \times 2°C) + (12 \times 4°C) = 78°C$

2. What is the purpose of denaturation of double-stranded target DNA after electrophoresis and prior to transfer in Southern blot?
   Answer: Double-stranded target DNA is denatured to allow hybridization of the probe. Also, single-stranded DNA binds to nitrocellulose filters.

3. Name two ways to permanently bind nucleic acid to nitrocellulose following transfer.
   Answer: To permanently bind the nucleic acid, bake the filter at 80°C for 30 minutes. Alternatively, nucleic acid will be cross-linked to nitrocellulose upon exposure to ultra-violet light.

4. If a probe for Southern blot was dissolved in a hybridization buffer that contains 50% formamide, is the stringency of hybridization higher or lower than if there were no formamide?

Answer: The stringency is higher, since formamide facilitates denaturation of double-stranded DNA.

5. If a high concentration of NaCl were added to a hybridization solution, how would the stringency be affected?
Answer: The stringency would be decreased since high salt concentrations exclude nucleic acids, forcing them close together and promoting hybridization.

6. Does an increase in temperature from 65°C to 75°C during hybridization raise or lower stringency?
Answer: Increasing temperature raises stringency. Heat promotes separation of the hydrogen bonds holding the two single strands of double-stranded DNA together.

7. At the end of the Southern blot procedure, what would the autoradiogram show if the stringency was too high?
Answer: If the stringency is too high, faint or no bands will be present on the autoradiogram.

8. A northern blot is performed on an RNA transcript with the sequence GUAGGUATGUAUUUGGGCGC-GAACGCAAAA. The probe sequence is GUAGGUAT-GUAUUUGGGCGCG. Will this probe hybridize to the target transcript?
Answer: This probe will not bind to the target transcript. The sequences are identical and not complementary. Since RNA does not have a complementary partner, the probe must be complementary to the transcript sequence.

9. In an array CGH experiment, three test samples were hybridized to three microarray chips. Each chip was spotted with eight gene probes (Genes A–H). Below are results of this assay expressed as the ratio of test DNA to reference DNA. Are any of the eight genes consistently deleted or amplified in the test samples? If so, which ones?

Gene	Sample 1	Sample 2	Sample 3
A	1.06	0.99	1.01
B	0.45	0.55	0.43
C	1.01	1.05	1.06

Gene	Sample 1	Sample 2	Sample 3
D	0.98	1.00	0.97
E	1.55	1.47	1.62
F	0.98	1.06	1.01
G	1.00	0.99	0.99
H	1.08	1.09	0.90

Answer: Gene B is consistently deleted (test/reference < 1.0) and gene E is consistently amplified (test/reference > 1.0).

10. What are two differences between CGH arrays and expression arrays?
Answer: (a) CGH arrays are performed on DNA. Expression arrays are formed on RNA. (b) CGH arrays detect deletions and amplifications of chromosomal regions. Expression arrays detect changes in the RNA levels of specific genes.

CHAPTER 7

1. A master mix of all components (except template) necessary for PCR contains what basic ingredients?
Answer: Components of a standard PCR reaction mix include dNTPs, oligonucleotide primers, a buffer of proper pH and mono- and divalent cation concentration, and polymerase enzyme.

2. The final concentration of *Taq* polymerase is to be 0.01 units/μL in a 50 μL PCR. If the enzyme is supplied as 5 units/μL, how much enzyme would you add to the reaction?
   a. 1 μL
   b. 1 μL of a 1:10 dilution of *Taq*
   c. 5 μL of a 1:10 dilution of *Taq*
   d. 2 μL
Answer: Use VCVC to determine the volume of enzyme:

$$0.01 \times 50 = 5 \times x$$

$$x = (0.01 \times 50)/5 = 0.1 \text{ μL}$$

Option b would deliver 0.1 μL enzyme.

3. Primer dimers result from
   a. high primer concentrations
   b. low primer concentrations
   c. high GC content in the primer sequences
   d. 3' complementarity in the primer sequences

Answer: Primer dimmers occur when primers hybridize to each other at the 3' ends (option d).

4. Which control is run to detect contamination in PCR?
   a. Negative control
   b. Positive control
   c. Molecular-weight marker
   d. Reagent blank
   Answer: A reaction mix with all components except template (reagent blank, d) is used to monitor for contamination.

5. Nonspecific extra PCR products can result from
   a. mispriming
   b. high annealing temperatures
   c. high agarose gel concentrations
   d. omission of MgCl$_2$ from the PCR
   Answer: Nonspecific products occur when primers bind to regions other than the intended target (a). Omission of magnesium could possibly produce mispriming but more likely will prevent enzyme function.

6. Using which of the following is an appropriate way to avoid PCR contamination?
   a. High-fidelity polymerase
   b. Hot-start PCR
   c. A separate area for PCR setup
   d. Fewer PCR cycles
   Answer: PCR contamination is prevented by physical separation of pre- and post-PCR areas (c).

7. What are the three steps of a standard PCR cycle?
   Answer: The three steps of the PCR cycle are denaturation, annealing, and extension.

8. How many copies of a target are made after 30 cycles of PCR?
   a. 2 × 30
   b. 2^{30}
   c. 30^2
   d. 30/2
   Answer: PCR is a doubling reaction. Therefore, the number of products after 30 doublings would be 2^{30} (b).

9. Which of the following is a method for purifying a PCR product?
   a. Treat with uracil N glycosylase.
   b. Add divalent cations.
   c. Put the reaction mix through a spin column.
   d. Add DEPC.
   Answer: Spin columns (c) are used to purify PCR products from other components of the reaction mix.

10. In contrast to standard PCR, real-time PCR is
    a. quantitative
    b. qualitative
    c. labor-intensive
    d. sensitive
    Answer: Real-time PCR is quantitative (a).

11. In real-time PCR, fluorescence is *not* generated by which of the following?
    a. FRET probes
    b. TaqMan probes
    c. SYBR green
    d. *Tth* polymerase
    Answer: *Tth* polymerase (d) does not fluoresce.

12. Examine the following sequence. You are devising a test to detect a mutation at the underlined position.

    5' TATTTAGTTA TGGCCTATAC ACTATTTGTG
    AGCAAAGGTG ATCGTTTTCT GTTTGAGATT
    TTTATCTCTT GATTCTTCAA AAGCATTCTG
    AGAAGGTGAG ATAAGCCCTG AGTCTCAGCT
    ACCTAAGAAA AACCTGGATG TCACTGGCCA
    CTGAGGAGC TTTGTTTCAAC CAAGTCATGT
    GCATTTCCAC GTCAACAGAA TTGTTTATTG
    TGACAGTT<u>A</u>T ATCTGTTGTC CCTTTGACCT
    TGTTTCTTGA AGGTTTCCTC GTCCCTGGGC
    AATTCCGCAT TTAATTCATG GTATTCAGGA
    TTACATGCAT GTTTGGTTA AACCCATGAGA
    TTCATTCAGT TAAAAATCCA GATGGCGAAT 3'

    Design one set of primers (forward and reverse) to generate an amplicon containing the underlined base position.

    The primers should be 20 bases long.

    The amplicon must be 100 to 150 bp in size.

The primers must have similar melting temperatures (T_m), +/− 2°C.

The primers should have no homology in the last three 3′ bases.

a. Write the primer sequences 5′→ 3′ as you would if you were to order them from the DNA synthesis facility.

b. Write the T_m for each primer that you have designed.

Answers:
There are several choices that will satisfy the above conditions. One example is:

5′ TATTTAGTTA TGGCCTATAC ACTATTTGTG AGCAAAGGTG ATCGTTTTCT GTTTGAGATT TTTATCTCTT GATTCTTCAA AAGCATTCTG AGAAGGTGAG ATAAGCCCTG AGTCTCAGCT ACCTAAGAAA <u>AACCTGGATG TCACTGGCCA</u> CTGAGGAGC TTTGTTTCAAC CAAGTCATGT GCATTTCCAC GTCAACAGAA TTGTTTATTG TGACAGTT<u>AT</u> ATCTGTTGTC CCTTTGACCT TGTTTCTTGA AGGTTTCCTC <u>GTCCCTGGGC</u> <u>AATTCCGCAT</u> TTAATTCATG GTATTCAGGA TTACATGCAT GTTTGGTTA AACCCATGAGA TTCATTCAGT TAAAAATCCA GATGGCGAAT 3′

a. **5′ AACCTGGATG TCACTGGCCA 3′ (forward primer)**
5′ ATGCGGAATT GCCCAGGGAC 3′ (reverse primer)

b. **62°C (forward primer)**
64°C (reverse primer)
The product will be 150 bp in length.

13. How does nested PCR differ from multiplex PCR?
Answer: Nested PCR requires two rounds of replication. Multiplex PCR is a single PCR reaction where more than one product is made using multiple primer sets.

14. What replaces heat denaturation in strand displacement amplification?
Answer: In strand displacement amplification, a nick in the double-stranded product is used to prime replication, rather than denaturation and primer binding.

15. Prepare a table that compares PCR, LCR, bDNA, TMA, Qβ Replicase, and Hybrid Capture with regard to the type of amplification, target nucleic acid, type of amplicon, and major enzyme(s) for each.
Answer:

	PCR	LCR	bDNA	TMA	Qβ	HC
Amplification	DNA synthesis	Probe ligation	Hybridization	RNA synthesis	RNA synthesis	Hybridization
Target NA	DNA	DNA	RNA, DNA	RNA, DNA	DNA, RNA	RNA, DNA
Amplicon	Target	Probe	Signal	RNA	Probe	Signal
Enzyme	DNA polymerase	DNA ligase	Alkaline phosphatase	RNA polymerase	Qβ replicase	Alkaline phosphatase

CHAPTER 8

1. What chromosomal location is indicated by 15q21.1?
Answer: This location is on the long arm of chromosome 15, region 2, band 1, sub-band 1.

2. During interphase FISH analysis for the t(9;22) translocation, one nucleus was observed with two normal signals (one red for chromosome 22 and one green for chromosome 9) and one composite red/green signal. Five hundred other nuclei were normal. What is one explanation for this observation?

Answer: Since only 1 of 500 cells showed the composite signal, this observation may be due to overlap of the chromosomes on the slide, rather than a translocation. The presence of a translocation, however, cannot be ruled out.

3. Is 47;XYY a normal karyotype?
Answer: This is not a normal karyotype. There are two Y chromosomes.

4. Write the numerical and structural chromosomal abnormalities represented by the following genotypes:

   47,XY, +18

   46, XY,del(16)p(14)

   iso(Xq)

   46,XX del(22)q(11.2)

   45,X

   Answer:

   47,XY, +18 — trisomy 18.

   46,XY, del(16)p(14) — deletion in the short arm of chromosome 16 at region 1, band 4.

   iso(Xq) — isochromosome formed by centromeric joining of two long arms of the X chromosome.

   46,XX del(22)q(11.2) — a deletion in the long arm q of chromosome 22 at region 1, band 1, sub-band 2.

   45,X — deletion of one of the X or the Y chromosome.

5. A chromosome with a centromere located such that one arm of the chromosome is longer than the other arm, is called
   a. metacentric
   b. paracentric
   c. telocentric
   d. submetacentric
   Answer: A chromosome with a long and short arm is submetacentric (d).

6. A small portion from the end of chromosome 2 has been found on the end of chromosome 15, replacing the end of chromosome 15, which has moved to the end of chromosome 2. This mutation is called a
   a. reciprocal translocation
   b. inversion
   c. deletion
   d. robertsonian translocation
   Answer: Exchange of portions of chromosomes with no loss of genetic material is a reciprocal translocation (a).

7. Phytohemagglutinin is added to a cell culture when preparing cells for karyotyping. The purpose of the phytohemagglutinin treatment is to
   a. arrest the cell in metaphase
   b. spread out the chromosomes
   c. fix the chromosomes on the slide
   d. stimulate mitosis in the cells
   Answer: Phytohemagglutinin is a mitogen that stimulates mitosis in the cells (d).

8. A centromeric probe is used to visualize chromosome 21. Three fluorescent signals are observed in the cell nuclei when stained with this probe. These results would be interpreted as consistent with
   a. a normal karyotype
   b. Down syndrome
   c. Klinefelter syndrome
   d. technical error
   Answer: Down syndrome results from trisomy 13, which would lead to the observation above (b).

9. Cells were harvested from a patient's blood, cultured to obtain chromosomes in metaphase, fixed onto a slide, treated with trypsin, and then stained with Giemsa. The resulting banding pattern is called
   a. G banding
   b. Q banding
   c. R banding
   d. C banding
   Answer: The reproducible patterns in Giemsa-stained chromosomes is called G-banding.

10. A FISH test with a centromere 13 probe is ordered for a suspected case of Patau syndrome (trisomy 13). How many signals per nucleus will result if the test is positive for Patau syndrome?
    Answer: The FISH results would reveal three signals per nucleus with a probe to centromere 13.

11. What would be the results if a centromere 13 probe was used on a case of Edward syndrome (trisomy 18)?
    Answer: The FISH results would reveal two signals per nucleus with a probe to centromere 13. A probe to centromere 18 would yield three signals per nucleus.

12. Angelman syndrome is caused by a microdeletion in chromosome 15. Which method, karyotyping or metaphase FISH, is better for accurate detection of this abnormality? Why?
    Answers: Metaphase FISH is preferred for detection of microdeletions. The lower resolution of karyotyping makes detection of small deletions difficult.

13. The results of a CGH analysis of Cy3 (green)-labeled test DNA with Cy5 (red)-labeled reference DNA on a normal chromosome spread revealed a bright red signal along the short arm of chromosome 3. How is this interpreted?
    a. 3p deletion
    b. 3q deletion
    c. 3p amplification
    d. 3q amplification
    Answer: The red signal from the reference chromosome region indicates a loss or deletion of the test chromosome 3p (a).

14. A break-apart probe is used to detect a translocation. The results of FISH analysis show two signals in 70% of the nuclei counted and three signals in 30% of the nuclei. Is there a translocation present?
    Answer: A translocation is present, indicated by the cells in which three signals appear. The probe spans the translocation breakpoint, producing two separate signals when a translocation occurs. The third signal in these cells is the intact homologous chromosome.

15. What FISH technique is most useful for detection of multiple complex genomic mutations?
    Answer: Spectral karyotyping labels each chromosome with a different fluorescent color so that multiple complex genomic mutations are clearly identified.

CHAPTER 9

1. What characteristic of the genetic code facilitates identification of open reading frames in DNA sequences?
    Answer: Out-of-frame or chance coding sequences tend to be short, often ending in a stop codon.

2. Compare and contrast EIA with western blots for detection of protein targets.
    Answer: EIA is a liquid handling method and more easily automated than western blot. EIA is performed with immobilized antibodies exposed to test fluid. In western blot, antibodies or antigens are resolved by electrophoresis before exposure to test fluid.

3. On a size exclusion column, large molecules will elute _____ (before/after) small molecules.
    Answer: On a size exclusion column, large molecules will elute *before* small molecules.

4. MALDI methods separate ions by
    a. molecular volume
    b. mass
    c. charge
    d. mass and charge
    Answer: MALDI methods separate ions by mass and charge (d).

5. What is a heteroduplex?
    Answer: A heteroduplex is a double-stranded nucleic acid with one or more noncomplementary bases.

6. Exon 4 of the HFE gene from a patient suspected to have hereditary hemachromatosis was amplified by PCR. The G to A mutation, frequently found in hemachromatosis, creates an *RsaI* site in exon 4. When the PCR products are digested with *RsaI*, what results (how many bands) would you expect to see if the patient has the mutation and no other *RsaI* sites are naturally present in the PCR product?
    Answer: Digestion of *RsaI* would produce two bands if the patient has the mutation and if no other *RsaI* sites are naturally present in the PCR product.

7. Which of the following methods would be practical to use to screen a large gene for mutations?
    a. SSP-PCR
    b. SSCP
    c. PCR-RFLP
    d. DGGE
    e. FP-TDI
    Answer: DGGE (d) would be practical to use to screen a large gene for mutations as it can scan several hundred base pairs at a time. SSCP is limited by the size and GC content of fragments that can be accurately analyzed. The remaining methods are designed to detect known point mutations.

8. What is the effect on the protein when a codon sequence is changed from TCT to TCC?
Answer: There would be no effect on the protein as both TCT and TCC code for serine.

9. A reference sequence, ATGCCCTCTGGC, is mutated in malignant cells. The following mutations in this sequence have been described:

ATGC<u>G</u>CTCTGGC

ATGCCCTC—GC

AT<u>AG</u>CCTCTGGC

ATG<u>TCTCCC</u>GGC

Express these mutations using the accepted gene nomenclature (A = nucleotide position 1).

Answers:
ATGC<u>G</u>CTCTGGC   5C->G
ATGCCCTC_GC   9_10del or 9_10delTG
AT<u>AG</u>CCTCTGGC   3_4delGCinsAG or
                                3_4delinsAG or 3_4>AG
ATG<u>TCTCCC</u>GGC   4_9inv6

10. A reference peptide, MPSGCWR, is subject to inherited alterations. The following peptide sequences have been reported:
MPS<u>T</u>GCWR
MPSG<u>X</u>
MPSGCW<u>LVTG</u>X
MPSG<u>R</u>
MPSGCW<u>GCW</u>R

Express these mutations using the accepted nomenclature (M = amino acid position 1).
Answers:
MPSGCWR

MPS<u>T</u>GCWR   S3_G4insT or S3_G4ins1
MPSG<u>X</u>   C5X
MPSGCW<u>LVTG</u>X   R7insLVTGX or R7ins5 or
                    R7fs or R7LfsX5
MPSG<u>R</u>   C5Rdel2
MPSGCW<u>GCW</u>R   W6_R7insGCW or
                    W6_R7ins3

CHAPTER 10

1. Read 5' to 3' the first 15 bases of the sequence in the gel on the right in Figure 10-8 (pg. 229).
Answer: 5'ATCGTCCCTAAGTCA3'

2. After an automated dye primer sequencing run, the electropherogram displays consecutive peaks of the following colors:

red, red, black, green, green, blue, black, red, green, black, blue, blue, blue

If the computer software displays the fluors from ddATP as green, ddCTP as blue, ddGTP as black, and ddTTP as red, what is the sequence of the region given?
Answer: TTGAACGTAGCCC

3. A dideoxy sequencing electropherogram displays bright (high, wide) peaks of fluorescence, obliterating some of the sequencing peaks. What is the most likely cause of this observation? How might it be corrected?
Answer: The likely cause is the presence of unincorporated labeled dideoxynucleotides or dye blobs. Cleaning the sequencing ladder with spin columns, ethanol precipitation, or bead binding will correct this problem.

4. In a manual sequencing reaction, the sequencing ladder on the polyacrylamide gel is very bright and readable at the bottom of the gel, but the larger (slower-migrating) fragments higher up are very faint. What is the most likely cause of this observation? How might it be corrected?
Answer: The loss of longer products is caused by an overly high deoxynucleotide/deoxynucleotide ratio. The problem can be corrected by lowering the concentration of dideoxynucleotides in the sequencing reaction.

5. In an analysis of the *p53* gene for mutations, the following sequences were produced. For each sequence, write the expected sequence of the opposite strand that would confirm the presence of the mutations detected.

Normal: 5'TATCTGTTCACTTGTGCCCT3'

Homozygous substitution:
    5'TATCTGTTCATTTGTGCCCT3'

Heterozygous substitution:
    5'TATCTGT(T/G)CACTTGTGCCCT3'

Heterozygous Deletion:
    5'TATCTGTT(C/A)(A/C)(C/T)T(T/G)(G/T)(T/G)
    (G/C)CC(C/T)(T/...3'

Answers:

Homozygous substitution:

5'TATCTGTTCA̲TTTGTGCCCT3'
5'AGGGCACAAA̲TGAAVAGATA 3'

Heterozygous substitution:

5'TATCTGT(T̲/G̲)CACTTGTGCCCT3'
5'AGGGCACAAGTG(C̲/A̲)ACAGATA 3'

Heterozygous Deletion:

5'TATCTGTT(C/A)(A/C)(C/T)T(T/G)(G/T)(T/G)
(G/C)CC(C/T)(T/...3'

5'.../A)(A/G)GG(G/C)(C/A)(A/C)(C/A)A(A/G)
(G/T)(T/G)....3'

6. A sequence, TTGCTGCGCTAAA, may be methylated at one or more of the cytosine residues. After bisulfite sequencing, the following results are obtained:

   Bisulfite treated: TTGCTGTGCTAAA

   Untreated: TTGCTGCGCTAAA

   Write the sequences showing the methylated cytosines as C^{Me}.
   Answer: TTGC^{Me}TGCGC^{Me}TAAA

7. In a pyrosequencing readout, the graph shows peaks of luminescence corresponding to the addition of the following nucleotides:

   dT peak, dC peak (double height), dT peak, dA peak

   What is the sequence?
   Answer: TCCTA

8. Why is it not necessary to add adenosine residues in vitro to messenger RNA for sequencing?

Answer: mRNA already has a polyA 3' terminus required for immobilization by polyT hybridization. RNA species without a polyA-tail must be treated with poly(A) polymerase to add the 3' polyA-tail.

9. Which of the following is not next-generation sequencing?
   a. 454 sequencing
   b. tiled microarray
   c. SOLID system
   d. Illumina Genome Analyzer
   Answer: The tiled microarray (b) is not a next-generation sequencing procedure.

10. Which of the following projects would require mass array sequencing?
   a. Mapping the hemochromatosis gene
   b. Sequencing a viral genome
   c. Characterization of a diverse microbial population
   d. Typing a single bacterial colony
   Answer: Characterization of a diverse microbial population (c) would require high throughput sequencing.

CHAPTER 11

1. Consider the following STR analysis:

Locus	Child	Mother	AF1	AF2
D3S1358	15/15	15	15	15/16
vWA	17/18	17	17/18	18
FGA	23/24	22/23	20	24
TH01	6/10	6/7	6/7	9/10
TPOX	11/11	9/11	9/11	10/11
CSF1PO	12/12	11/12	11/13	11/12
D5S818	10/12	10	11/12	12
D13S317	9/10	10/11	10/11	9/11

   a. Circle the child's alleles that are inherited from the father.
   b. Which alleged father (AF) is the biological parent?

Answers:

a.

Locus	Child	Mother	AF1	AF2
D3S1358	15/*15*	15	15	15/16
vWA	17/*18*	17	17/18	18
FGA	23/*24*	22/23	20	24
TH01	*6/10*	6/7	6/7	9/10
TPOX	11/*11*	9/11	9/11	10/11
CSF1PO	12/*12*	11/12	11/13	11/12
D5S818	10/*12*	10	11/12	12
D13S317	*9*/10	10/11	10/11	9/11

b. AF2 is the biological parent.

2. The following evidence was collected for a criminal investigation:

Locus	Victim	Evidence	Suspect
TPOX	11/12	12, 11/12	11
CSF1PO	10	10, 9	9/10
D13S317	8/10	10, 8/10	9/12
D5S818	9/11	10/11, 9/11	11
TH01	6/10	6/10, 8/10	5/11
FGA	20	20, 20/22	20
vWA	15/17	18, 15/17	15/18
D3S1358	14	15/17, 14	11/12

The suspect is heterozygous at the amelogenin locus.
a. Is the suspect male or female?
b. In the evidence column, circle the alleles belonging to the victim.
c. Should the suspect be held or released?
Answers:
a. The suspect is male as indicated by the heterozygous amelogenin locus.
b.

Locus	Victim	Evidence	Suspect
TPOX	11/12	12, *11/12*	11
CSF1PO	10	*10*, 9/10	9/10
D13S317	8/10	10, *8/10*	9/12
D5S818	9/11	10/11, *9/11*	11
TH01	6/10	*6/10*, 8/10	5/11

Locus	Victim	Evidence	Suspect
FGA	20	*20*, 20/22	20
vWA	15/17	18, *15/17*	15/18
D3S1358	14	15/17, *14*	11/12

c. The suspect should be released.

3. A child and an alleged father (AF) share alleles with the following paternity index:

Locus	Child	AF	Paternity Index for Shared Allele
D5S818	9,10	9	0.853
D8S1179	11	11,12	2.718
D16S539	13,14	10,14	1.782

a. What is the combined paternity index from these three loci?
b. With 50% prior odds, what is the probability of paternity from these three loci?
Answers:
a. $0.853 \times 2.718 \times 1.782 = 4.131$
b. $(4.131 \times 0.5)/[(4.131 \times 0.5) + 0.5)] = 0.80$, or 80%

4. Consider the following theoretical allele frequencies for the loci indicated:

Locus	Alleles	Allele Frequency
CSF1PO	14	0.332
D13S317	9, 10	0.210, 0.595
TPOX	8, 11	0.489, 0.237

a. What is the overall allele frequency, using the product rule?
b. What is the probability that this DNA found at the two sources came from the same person?
Answers:
a. $0.332 \times 0.332 \times 0.21 \times 0.595 \times 0.489 \times 0.237 = 1.596 \times 10^{-3}$
b. $1/(1.596 \times 10^{-3}) = 626.5$. It is 626 times more likely that the two DNA samples came from the same person as from two random persons in the population.

5. STR at several loci were screened by capillary electrophoresis and fluorescent detection for informative

peaks prior to a bone marrow transplant. The following results were observed:

Locus	Donor Alleles	Recipient Alleles
LPL	7, 10	7, 9
F13B	8, 14	8
FESFPS	10	7
F13A01	5, 11	5, 11

Which loci are informative?
Answer: LPL and FESFPS are informative. F13B is donor-informative. F13A01 is not informative.

6. An engraftment analysis was performed by capillary gel electrophoresis and fluorescence detection. The fluorescence as measured by the instrument under the FESFPS donor peak was 28,118 units, and that under the FESFPS recipient peak was 72,691. What is the percent donor in this specimen?
Answer: 28,118/(28,118 + 72,691) = 28% donor

7. The T-cell fraction from the blood sample in Question 6 was separated and measured for donor cells. Analysis of the FESFPS locus in the T-cell fraction yielded 15,362 fluorescence units under the donor peak and 97,885 under the recipient peak. What does this result predict with regard to T-cell-mediated events such as graft-versus-host disease or graft-versus-tumor?
Answer: 15,362/(15,362 + 97,885) = 13.6% donor cells; GVDH or GVT is unlikely.

8. If a child had a Y haplotype including DYS393 allele 12, DYS439 allele 11, DYS445 allele 8, and DYS447 allele 22, what are the predicted Y alleles for these loci of the natural father?
Answer: The predicted alleles are DYS393 allele 12, DYS439 allele 11, DYS445 allele 8, and DYS447 allele 22.

9. Which of these would be used for a surname test: Y-STR, mini-STR, mitochondrial typing, or autosomal STR?
Answer: Y-STR would be used for a surname or paternal lineage test.

10. An ancient bone fragment was found and claimed to belong to an ancestor of a famous family. Living members of the family donated DNA for confirmation of the relationship. What type of analysis would likely be used for this test? Why?
Answer: Mitochondrial DNA typing might be indicated, because (1) the small circular, naturally amplified mitochondrial DNA is more likely to be attained from the old sample and (2) lineage across several generations can be determined using the maternal inheritance of mitochondrial type.

11. What are two biological exceptions to positive identification by autosomal STR?
Answer: Identical twins and clones have identical nuclear DNA profiles.

12. A partial STR profile was produced from a highly degraded sample. Alleles matched to a reference sample at five loci. Is this sufficient for a legal identification?
Answer: Five loci are not sufficient for a legal identification.

13. What is a SNP haplotype? What are tag SNPs?
Answer: Single nucleotide polymorphisms that are inherited together in a block without recombination between them comprise a SNP haplotype. SNP haplotypes are identifiable by two or three representative SNPS or tag SNPs within the haplotype.

14. Which of the following is an example of linkage disequilibrium?
   a. Seventeen members of a population of 1000 people have a rare disease and all 17 people have the same haplotype at a particular genetic location on chromosome 3.
   b. Five hundred people from the same population have the same SNP on chromosome 3.
   Answer: Example (a) is linkage disequilibrium.

15. Why are SNPs superior to STR and RFLP for mapping and association studies?
Answer: SNPs are more numerous in the genome and, therefore, offer higher resolution for mapping of precise genome locations.

CHAPTER 12

1. Which of the following genes would be analyzed to determine whether an isolate of *Staphylococcus aureus* is resistant to oxacillin?
   a. *mecA*
   b. *gyrA*
   c. *inhA*
   d. *vanA*
   Answer: (a) *mecA*. *S. aureus* developed resistance to antibiotics that target its penicillin-binding protein (PBP1) by replacing PBP1 with PBP2a encoded by the *mecA* gene. PBP2a found in methicillin-resistant *S. aureus* (MRSA) has a low binding affinity for methicillin.

2. Which of the following is a genotypic method used to compare two isolates in an epidemiological investigation?
   a. Biotyping
   b. Serotyping
   c. Ribotyping
   d. Bacteriophage typing
   Answer: (c) Ribotyping. There are many laboratory methods that can be used to determine the relatedness of multiple isolates, both *phenotypic* (e.g., by serology and antimicrobial susceptibility patterns) and *genotypic* (e.g., pulsed field gel electrophoresis and ribotyping).

3. For which of the following organisms must caution be exercised when evaluating positive PCR results because the organism can be found as normal flora in some patient populations?
   a. *Neisseria gonorrhoeae*
   b. HIV
   c. *Chlamydophila pneumoniae*
   d. *Streptococcus pneumoniae*
   Answer: (d) *Streptococcus pneumoniae*. Although PCR is specific for *S. pneumoniae*, the clinical significance of a positive PCR assay is questionable because a significant portion of the population (especially children) is colonized with the organism and PCR cannot discern between colonization and infection.

4. Which of the following controls are critical for ensuring that amplification is occurring in a patient sample and that the lack of PCR product is not due to the presence of inhibitors?
   a. Reagent blank
   b. Sensitivity control
   c. Negative control
   d. Amplification control
   Answer: (d) Amplification control. The amplification control should always generate a product, even in the absence of the target.

5. A PCR assay was performed to detect *Bordetella pertussis* on sputum obtained from a 14-year-old girl who has had a chronic cough. The results revealed two bands, one consistent with the internal control and the other consistent with the size expected for amplification of the *B. pertussis* target. How should these results be interpreted?
   a. False-positive for *B. pertussis*.
   b. The girl has clinically significant *B. pertussis* infection.
   c. *B. pertussis* detection is more likely due to colonization.
   d. Invalid because two bands were present.
   Answer: (b) The girl has clinically significant *B. pertussis* infection. Molecular-based assays are used almost exclusively for analysis of microorganisms such as *N. gonorrhoeae*, *C. trachomatis*, and *B. pertussis*.

6. Which of the following is a disadvantage of molecular-based testing?
   a. Results stay positive longer after treatment than do cultures.
   b. Results are available within hours.
   c. Only viable cells yield positive results.
   d. Several milliliters of specimen must be submitted for analysis.
   Answer: (a) Results stay positive longer after treatment than do cultures. Molecular-based results can detect both living and dead organisms. A positive result due to dead or dying organisms complicates interpretation of treatment efficacy.

7. A molecular-based typing method that has high typing capacity, reproducibility and discriminatory power, moderate ease of performance, and good-to-moderate ease of interpretation is
   a. repetitive elements
   b. PFGE
   c. plasmid analysis
   d. PCR-RFLP
   Answer: (b) PFGE. Observe the comparison of methods in Table 12.15.

8. A patient has antibodies against HCV and a viral load of 100,000 copies/mL. What is the next test that should be performed on this patient's isolate?
   a. Ribotyping
   b. PCR-RFLP
   c. Hybrid capture
   d. Inno-LiPA HCV genotyping
   Answer: (d) Inno-LiPA HCV genotyping. The viral load and the HCV genotype are used to determine the therapeutic protocol, both type of drug(s) as well as duration. Methods available in the laboratory for HCV genotyping are PCR with RFLP analysis and reverse hybridization (Inno-LiPA, Bayer), and direct DNA sequencing (HCV DupliType, Quest; TRUGENE®, Bayer; and ViroSeq™, Celera).

9. A positive result for HPV type 16 indicates
   a. high risk for antibiotic resistance
   b. low risk for cervical cancer
   c. high risk for cervical cancer
   Answer: (c) High risk for cervical cancer. Of the sexually transmitted types of HPV, 12 to 15 oncogenic genotypes have strong association with cervical cancers and are considered high-risk (HR) HPV types.

10. Which of the following is used to type molds?
    a. Sequence-specific PCR
    b. Microarray
    c. ITS sequencing
    d. Flow cytometry
    Answer: (c) ITS sequencing. Molds are typed by PCR and sequencing of Internal Transcribed Spacer (ITS) regions or 28S rRNA.

CHAPTER 13

1. Which of the following is not a triplet-repeat expansion disorder?
   a. Fragile X syndrome
   b. Huntington disease
   c. Factor V Leiden
   d. Congenital central hypoventilation syndrome
   Answer: (c) Factor V Leiden. Factor V Leiden is a single-nucleotide mutation (1691 A→G, R506Q).

2. A gene was mapped to region 3, band 1, sub-band 1, of the long arm of chromosome 2. How would you express this location from an idiogram?
   Answer: The designation of this location is 2q31.1.

3. Which of the following can be detected by PCR?
   a. Large mitochondrial deletions
   b. Full fragile X disorder
   c. Mitochondrial point mutations
   Answer: (b) Full fragile X disorder and (c) mitochondrial point mutations. With modern methods, both full fragile X disorder and mitochondrial point mutations are detectable by PCR.

4. A patient was tested for Huntington disease. PCR followed by PAGE revealed 25 CAG units.
   a. This patient has Huntington disease.
   b. This patient has a 1/25 chance of contracting Huntington disease.
   c. This patient is normal at the Huntington locus.
   d. The test is inconclusive.
   Answer: (c) This patient is normal at the Huntington locus. In the Huntington repeat expansion, the sequence CAG expands from 9 to 37 repeats to 38 to 86 repeats.

5. The factor V Leiden mutation can be detected by
   a. PCR-RFLP
   b. SSP-PCR
   c. invader technology
   d. all of the above methods
   Answer: (d) All of the above methods. There are several methods available for detection of the factor V Leiden mutation.

6. The most frequently occurring mutation in the HFE gene results in the replacement of cysteine (C) with tyrosine (Y) at position 282. How is this expressed according to the recommended nomenclature?
Answer: The recommended nomenclature is C282Y.

7. MELAS is a disease condition that results from an A to G mutation at position 3243 of the mitochondrial genome. This change creates a single *Apa*I restriction site in a PCR product, including the mutation site. What would you expect from a PCR-RFLP analysis for this mutation on a patient with MELAS?
  a. A single PCR product resistant to digestion with *Apa*I
  b. A single PCR product that cuts into two fragments upon digestion with *Apa*I
  c. A single PCR product only if the mutation is present
  d. Two PCR products
Answer: (b) A single PCR product that cuts into two fragments upon digestion with *Apa*I.

8. A father affected with a single gene disorder and an unaffected mother have four children (three boys and a girl), two of whom (one boy and the girl) are affected. Draw the pedigree diagram for this family.
Answer:

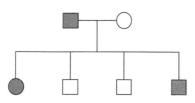

9. D16S539, an STR, was analyzed in the family described in Question 8. The result showed that the father had the 6,8 alleles, the mother had the 5,7 alleles. The affected children had the 5,6 and 6,7 alleles, and the unaffected children had the 5,8 and 7,8 alleles.
  a. If D16S539 is located on chromosome 16, where is the gene for this disorder likely to be located?
  b. To which allele of D16S539 is the gene linked?
Answers:
  a. Linkage with a specific D16S539 allele locates the gene on chromosome 16.
  b. The gene is linked to allele 6 of the D16S539 locus.

How might one perform a DNA analysis for the presence of the disorder?
  a. Analyze D16S539 for the 6 allele by PCR.
  b. Sequence the entire region of the chromosome where D16S539 was located.
  c. Test as many STRs as possible by PCR.
  d. Use Invader technology to detect the unknown gene mutation.
Answer: (a) Analyze D16S539 for the 6 allele by PCR. Linkage of this allele with the affected allele of the gene

10. Exon 4 of the *HFE* gene from a patient suspected of having hereditary hemochromatosis was amplified by PCR. The G to A mutation, frequently found in hemochromatosis, creates an *Rsa*I site in exon 4. When the PCR products are digested with *Rsa*1, which of the following results would you expect to see if the patient has the mutation?
  a. None of the PCR products will be cut by *Rsa*I.
  b. There will be no PCR product amplified from the patient DNA.
  c. The patient's PCR product will yield extra bands upon *Rsa*1 digestion.
  d. The normal control PCR products will yield extra *Rsa*1 bands compared with the patient sample.
Answer: (c) The patient's PCR product will yield extra bands upon *Rsa*1 digestion. An additional *Rsa*I site will result in additional fragmentation of the PCR product.

11. Almost all people with the C282Y or H63D *HFE* gene mutations develop hemochromatosis symptoms. This is a result of
  a. iron loss
  b. excessive drinking
  c. high penetrance
  d. healthy lifestyle
  e. glycogen accumulation
Answer: (c) High penetrance. The condition is frequently present as a result of the mutation.

12. The majority of disease-associated mutations in the human population are
  a. autosomal dominant
  b. autosomal recessive
  c. X-linked
  d. found on the Y chromosome

Answer: (b) Autosomal recessive. Most individuals carry recessive disease mutations that may result in affected offspring produced with close relatives.

13. Luminex bead array technology is most appropriate for which of the following?
    a. Cystic fibrosis mutation detection
    b. Chromosomal translocation detections
    c. STR linkage analysis
    d. Restriction fragment length polymorphisms
    Answer: (a) Cystic fibrosis mutation detection. Luminex bead arrays are used to detect multiple point mutations.

14. What chemical change in DNA is associated with imprinting?
    Answer: Addition of methyl groups to DNA nitrogen bases (methylation) silences genes and is associated with imprinting.

15. What accounts for the different phenotypes of Prader-Willi syndrome, del(15)(q11q13), and Angelman syndrome, del(15)(q11q13)?
    Answer: Dissimilar imprinting on paternal and maternal chromosomes is thought to account for phenotypic differences, depending on which chromosome 15 carries the deletion.

CHAPTER 14

1. What are the two important checkpoints in the cell division cycle that are crossed when the regulation of the cell division cycle is affected?
   Answer: The transition from unreplicated to replicated DNA (G1 to S) and from replicated DNA to cell division (G2 to M) are regulated checkpoints in the cell division cycle.

2. An *EWS-FLI-1* translocation was detected in a solid tumor by RT-PCR. Which of the following does this result support?
   a. Normal tissue
   b. Ewing sarcoma
   c. Inherited breast cancer
   d. Microsatellite instability
   Answer: (b) Ewing sarcoma. Ewing sarcoma is associated with the *EWS-FLI-1* t(11;22) translocation.

3. Mutation detection, even by sequencing, is not definitive with a negative result. Why?
   Answer: Mutations may be present outside of the sequenced area. Furthermore, mutations in genes coding for factors that interact with the target protein may affect its function in the absence of mutations in the target gene. In addition, epigenetic, post-transcriptional and post-translational events may affect gene function without changing the DNA sequence.

4. Which of the following predict efficacy of EGFR tyrosine kinase inhibitors?
   a. Overexpression of EGFR protein
   b. *EGFR*-activating mutations
   Answer: (b) *EGFR* activating mutations. Evidence suggests that, unlike the HER2 protein, overexpression of the EGFR protein does not predict efficacy of EGFR TKI.

5. What is the advantage of microdissection of tumor tissue in testing for tumor-specific molecular markers?
   Answer: Microdissection enriches the tested sample in tumor cells. This increases the sensitivity of testing, as normal cells may interfere with detection of tumor-specific markers.

6. Why are K-ras activating mutations and B-raf V600E mutually exclusive in colon cancer?
   Answer: K-ras and B-raf kinases are on the same signal transduction pathway. Once that pathway is activated through mutations in the *KRAS* or *BRAF* gene, there is no selective pressure to generate further activating mutations in genes in the same pathway.

7. What enzyme is responsible for continued sequence changes in the immunoglobulin heavy chain gene after gene rearrangement has occurred?
   Answer: Activation-induced cytidine deaminase alters C residues so that they base-pair with A instead of G residues, resulting in different amino acid substitutions in antibody proteins.

8. Why are translocation-based PCR tests more sensitive than IgH, IgL, and T-cell receptor gene rearrangement tests?

Answer: Gene rearrangements are not tumor-specific. Therefore, there will be a background from normal cells in gene rearrangement tests performed with consensus primers. Translocations are tumor-specific. The absence of background allows for more sensitive detection of tumor cells. Gene rearrangements may be detected with increased sensitivity using patient-specific primers that will detect only the gene rearrangement in the tumor cell population.

9. A PCR test for the Bcl-2 translocation is performed on a patient with suspected follicular lymphoma. The results show a bright band at 400 bp (amplification control) and another at about 300 bp for this patient. The negative control has only the 400 bp band. How would you interpret these results?
Answer: The results are positive for the presence of the Bcl-2 translocation, given that the 300-bp translocation-specific product is within the expected size range with the primers used.

10. Which of the following misinterpretations would result from PCR contamination?
a. False-positive for the t(15;17) translocation
b. False-negative for the t(15;17) translocation
c. False-negative for a gene rearrangement
Answer: (a) False-positive for the t(15;17) translocation. Contamination would result in a false-positive pattern.

11. After amplification of the t(12;21) breakpoint by RT-PCR, the PCR products were loaded and resolved on an agarose gel. What might be the explanation for each of the following observations when the gel is exposed to ultraviolet light? (Positive and amplification controls and a reagent blank control are included in the run.)
a. The gel is blank (no bands, no molecular weight standard).
b. Only the molecular-weight standard is visible.
c. The molecular-weight standard is visible; there are bands in every lane at 200 bp, even in the reagent blank lane.
Answers:
a. If the gel is blank (no bands, no molecular-weight standard), then the ethidium bromide

or SyBr green detection dye was omitted from the procedure.
b. The visible molecular-weight standard indicates that the electrophoresis process was adequate. The absence of sample bands suggests an error in the sample preparation or amplification.
c. Bands in every lane at 200 bp, even in the reagent blank lane, is an indication of contamination.

12. What is observed on a Southern blot for gene rearrangement in the case of a positive result?
a. No bands
b. Germline bands plus rearranged bands
c. Smears
d. Germline bands only
Answer: (b) Germline bands plus rearranged bands. The rearranged bands represent the gene rearrangement in the monoclonal population of tumor cells.

13. Cyclin D1 promotes passage of cells through the G1 to S cell division cycle checkpoint. What test detects translocation of this gene to chromosome 14?
a. t(14;18) translocation analysis (*BCL2, IGH*)
b. t(15;17) translocation analysis (*PML/RARA*)
c. t(11;14) translocation analysis (*BCL1/IGH*)
d. t(8;14) translocation analysis (*MYC/IGH*)
Answer: (c) t(11;14) translocation analysis (*BCL1/IGH*). Cyclin D1 is encoded by the *BCL1* gene located on chromosome 11.

14. What is one advantage of the Southern blot procedure over the PCR procedure for detecting clonal gene rearrangements?
a. Southern blot requires less sample DNA than does PCR.
b. The PCR procedure cannot detect certain gene rearrangements that are detectable by Southern blot.
c. Southern blot results are easier to interpret than PCR results.
d. PCR results are not accepted by the College of American Pathologists.
Answer: (b) The PCR procedure cannot detect certain gene rearrangements that are detectable by Southern blot. Although Southern blot can theoretically detect all possible gene

rearrangements, detection is limited by the sensitivity of the Southern blot method.

15. Interpret the following results from a translocation assay:

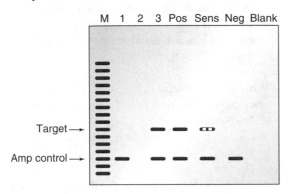

Are the samples positive, negative, or indeterminate?

Sample 1:

Sample 2:

Sample 3:

Answers:

Sample 1: Negative

Sample 2: Indeterminate

Sample 3: Positive

CHAPTER 15

1. Which of the following is a high-resolution HLA typing result?
   a. B27
   b. A*02:02–02:09
   c. A*02:12
   d. A*26:01/A*26:05/A*26:01/A*26:15
   Answer: (c) A*02:12. A*02 would be low resolution, determined at the serological level. A*26:01/A*26:05/A*26:01/A*26:15 is a medium resolution result.

2. Which of the following is a likely haplotype from parents with A25,Cw10,B27/A23,Cw5,B27 and A17, Cw4,B10/A9,Cw7,B12 haplotypes?
   a. A25,Cw10,B27
   b. A25,Cw5,B27
   c. A23,Cw4,B12
   d. A17,Cw4,B27

Answer: (a) A25, Cw10,B27 would be inherited together from one parent. A25,Cw5. B27 may occur as a result of a recombination event, but this would be infrequent.

3. Upon microscopic examination, over 90% of cells are translucent after a CDC assay. How are these results scored according to the ASHI rules?
   Answer: Negative for the presence of the test antigen or a score of 1. Less than 10% of the cells have taken up dye. Cytotoxicity (dye uptake) will only occur in those cells that carry antigens to the test antibodies.

4. A theoretical HLA-A*02 allele is a CTC to CTT change at the DNA level (leu → leu). How is this allele written?
   a. HLA-A*02:01
   b. HLA-A*02:01:01
   c. HLA-A2
   d. HLA-A*02N
   Answer: (b) HLA-A*02:01:01. Nucleotide substitutions that change the amino acid sequence are indicated by differences in the second group of digits. Those changes in the DNA sequence that do not change the amino acid sequence (silent or synonymous substitutions) are designated by addition of a third group of digits.

5. A candidate for kidney transplant has a PRA of 75%. How might this affect eligibility for immediate transplant?
   Answer: Transplant candidates with %PRA activity of more than 50% are considered to be highly sensitized. Finding a crossmatch-negative donor will be difficult in this case.

6. An SSOP probe recognizes HLA-DRB*03:01–03:04. Another probe recognizes HLA-DRB*03:01/03:04, and a third probe hybridizes to HLA-DRB*03:01–03:03. Test specimen DNA hybridizes to all except the third probe in a reverse dot blot format. What is the HLA-DRB type of the specimen?
   Answer: HLA-DRB*03:04. The test specimen hybridizes to the probes containing HLA-DRB*03:04 but not the probe containing HLA-DRB*03:01-03:03, eliminating the latter alleles.

7. What is the relationship between alleles HLA-A10 and HLA-A26(10)?
Answer: **HLA-A10 is the parent allele of HLA-A26(10). Number designations of new alleles of a previously defined allele with broad specificity (parent allele) are followed by the number of the parent allele in parentheses.**

8. A CDC assay yields an 8 score for sera with the following specificities: A2, A28 and A2, A28, B7, and a 1 score for serum with an A2 specificity. What is the HLA-A type?
Answer: **This is type HLA-A2. The high cytotoxicity (reading >6) in the wells containing A28 indicates that the cells being tested have cell surface antigens matching the A28.**

9. HLA-DRB1*15:01 differs from DRB1*01:01 by a G to C base change. If the sequence surrounding the base change is ...GGGTGCGGTTGCTGGAAAGAT... (DRB1*01:01) or ...GGGTGCGGTTCCTGGAAAGAT... (DRB1*15:01), which of the following would be the 3' end of a sequence-specific primer for detection of DRB1*15:01?
a. ...ATCTTTCCAGGAACCC
b. ...ATCTTTCCAGCAACCC
c. ...ATCTTTCCAGC
d. ...ATCTTTCCAGG
Answer: **(c) ...ATCTTTCCAGC. The primer should end on the complementary nucleotide of the polymorphic base.**

10. The results of an SSP-PCR reaction are the following: lane 1, one band; lane 2, two bands, lane 3 no bands. If the test includes an amplification control multiplexed with the allele-specific primers, what is the interpretation for each lane?
Answer: **Lane 1 is the expected result if the test allele and is not present; lane 2 indicates the presence of the allele; lane 3 is not interpretable as the amplification control is absent.**
G

CHAPTER 16

What actions should be taken in the following situations?

1. An unlabeled collection tube with a requisition for a factor V Leiden test is received in the laboratory.
Answer: **Notify the supervisor and reject the specimen.**

2. After PCR, the amplification control has failed to yield a product.
Answer: **Check the original DNA or RNA preparation. If it is adequate, repeat the amplification. If not, reisolate the nucleic acid.**

3. An isolated DNA sample is to be stored for at least 6 months.
Answer: **Store at −70°C in a tightly sealed tube.**

4. A bone marrow specimen arrives at the end of a shift and will not be processed for the Bcl-2 translocation until the next day.
Answer: **Place the specimen in the refrigerator.**

5. The temperature of a refrigerator set at 8°C (±2°C) reads 14°C.
Answer: **Recheck the temperature after a few hours. If it does not return to range, notify the supervisor.**

6. A PCR test for the BCR/ABL translocation was negative for the patient sample and for the sensitivity control.
Answer: **Repeat the PCR with the addition of a new sensitivity control.**

7. A fragile X test result has been properly reviewed and reported.
Answer: **File the test results, documents, and associated autoradiographs together in the laboratory archives.**

8. A bottle of reagent alcohol with a 3 in the red diamond on its label is to be stored.
Answer: **Place the alcohol bottle in a safety storage cabinet for flammable liquids.**

9. The expiration date on a reagent has passed.
Answer: **Discard the reagent. If it can be used for nonclinical purposes, label and store it in a separate area away from patient testing reagents.**

10. Test results are to be faxed to the ordering physician.
Answer: Fax the results with a cover sheet containing the proper disclaimer.

11. Among a group of properly labeled containers, there is a container similar to the others, but unlabeled.
Answer: Do not use the material in the unlabeled container. Consult the institutional safety representative for proper disposal of the contents.

12. A blood sample is received in a serum tube for PML-RARa testing by PCR.
Answer: Notify the supervisor that the specimen cannot be tested and explain the collection error (wrong/no anticoagulant).

13. The laboratory is reporting a gene mutation replacing glycine at position 215 with alanine. The results are written 215G→A in the test report.
Answer: Correct the test report to A215G before verification by the laboratory director.

14. The laser on a complex instrument malfunctions.
Answer: Call the instrument manufacturer. Do not try to access the laser.

15. A test result falls outside of the analytical measurement range of the validated method.
Answer: If the result exceeds the range, dilute the specimen and retest. If the results are below the range, report the results as less than the lower limit of the assay.

16. Reference standards are reading higher than their designated concentrations.
Answer: Calibrate the instrument/detection system using the reference standards.

17. A new FDA-approved test does not perform as expected.
Answer: Do not use the test. Contact the manufacturer. Consider an alternate test system.

18. A solution containing radioactive waste has been stored in a properly protected area for 10 half-lives of the isotope.
Answer: The solution may be safely discarded; however, contact the institutional safety department before discarding. Document all radioactive waste disposal.

19. There is no available proficiency test for a new method developed in the laboratory.
Answer: Establish an agreement with another laboratory to trade samples for testing. Use split samples from reference standards. Compare results with a reference in-house method, regional pools, previously assayed material, clinical evaluation, or other documented means.

20. A research investigator asks for a patient specimen.
Answer: Notify the supervisor. Do not release patient material without proper consent and patient safety review board approval.

CASE STUDY 11 • 1

A 32-year-old woman was treated for mantle cell lymphoma with a nonmyeloablative bone marrow transplant. Before the transplant and after a donor was selected, STR analysis was performed on the donor and the recipient to find informative alleles. One hundred days after the transplant, engraftment was evaluated using the selected STR alleles. The results from one marker, D5S818, are shown in the left panel. One year later, the patient was reevaluated. The results from the same marker are shown in the right panel.

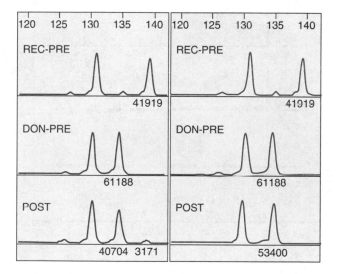

QUESTION: *Was the woman successfully engrafted with donor cells? Explain your answer.*

Interpretation for Case Study 11 • 1:

The woman was successfully engrafted. The recipient peak pattern has converted almost entirely to the donor peak pattern at 100 days. The percentage of residual recipient cells is calculated by analysis of the unshared alleles in this marker:

$$\%R = [R_{unshared}/(R_{unshared} + D_{unshared})] \times 100$$
$$= [3171/(40704 + 3171)] \times 100$$
$$= 7.2\%$$

At 1 year, no recipient peaks are detectable at the level of detection (0.5%—1%) of the instrument. The patient is, therefore, reported to have more than 99% donor cells and less than 1% recipient cells in the test specimen.

CASE STUDY 11 • 2

At the age of 26, M.K. reported to his doctor with joint pain and fatigue. Complete blood count and differential counts were indicative of chronic myelogenous leukemia. The diagnosis was confirmed by karyotyping, showing 9/20 metaphases with the t(9;22) translocation. Quantitative PCR was performed to establish a baseline for monitoring tumor load during and following treatment. Treatment with Gleevec and a bone marrow transplant were recommended. M.K. had a twin brother, R.K., who volunteered to donate bone marrow. The two brothers were not sure if they were fraternal or identical twins. Donor and recipient buccal cells were sent to the molecular pathology laboratory for STR informative analysis. The results are shown below.

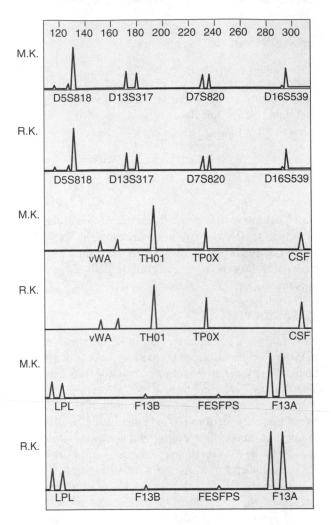

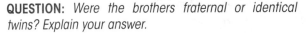

QUESTION: *Were the brothers fraternal or identical twins? Explain your answer.*

Interpretation for Case Study 11 • 2:

These results indicate that the two brothers are identical twins. This means that STR analysis cannot be used for monitoring engraftment after transplant in this case. There is less chance of graft-versus-host-disease with this transplant; however, there is also no graft versus tumor effect that can improve the chance of removing all of the tumor cells.

CASE STUDY 11 • 3

A fixed paraffin-embedded tissue section was received in the pathology department with a diagnosis of benign uterine fibroids. Slides were prepared for microscopic study. Only benign fibroid cells were observed on all slides, except one. A small malignant process was observed located between the fibroid and normal areas on one slide. As similar tissue was not observed on any other section, it was possible that the process was a contamination from the embedding procedure. To determine the origin of the malignant cells, DNA was extracted from the malignant area (T) and compared with DNA extracted from the patient's normal tissue (P). The results are shown below.

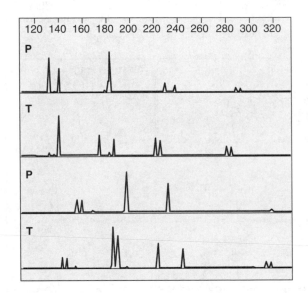

QUESTION: *Were the malignant cells seen in one section derived from the patient, or were they a contaminant of the embedding process? Explain your answer.*

Interpretation for Case Study 11 • 3:

The results show that the tissue was not of the same genetic origin as that of the patient. Apparently this microscopic fragment of tissue was introduced into one of the patient's sections during the fixing and embedding process.

CASE STUDY 12 • 1

During a holiday weekend at a luxury hotel, guests began to complain of stomach flu with nausea and vomiting. In all, more than 100 of the 200 guests who had dined at the hotel the previous evening described the same symptoms. Eight people had symptoms severe enough to warrant hospitalization. Most, however, recovered within 24 to 48 hours of the onset of symptoms. Health officials were notified. Interviews and epidemiological analyses pointed to a Norwalk-like virus, or norovirus, infection, probably foodborne. Stool specimens (1 to 5 mL) from hospitalized patients and samples of the suspected food sources (500 mg) were sent for laboratory analysis by RT-PCR. RNA extracted with 1,1,2 trichloro-1,2,2, trifluoroethane was mixed with a guanidium thiocyanate buffer and isolated by organic (phenol-chloroform) procedures. cDNA was synthesized using primers specific to the viral RNA polymerase gene. Strain-specific PCR primers were used to amplify the viral gene. The amplicons, resolved by agarose gel electrophoresis, are shown in the figure below.

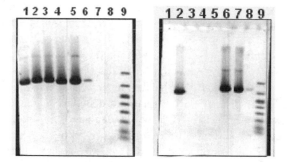

RT-PCR products were resolved on separate gels. Amplicons from four affected individuals (lanes 1–4, left). Lane 5, positive control; lane 6, sensitivity control; lane 7, negative control; lane 8, reagent blank. Specimens from suspected food served at the hotel (lanes 1–4, right). Lane 5, salad lettuce from the distributor; lanes 6–8, specimens from three hotel employees working the day of the outbreak; lane 9, molecular weight marker.

QUESTIONS:

1. Do these patients have norovirus?
2. What is the source of the organism?
3. When did the source get contaminated? Did the source come into the hotel infected, or was it infected inside the hotel?

Interpretation for Case Study 12 • 1:

The molecular evidence is consistent with norovirus. Norovirus cannot be cultured. Laboratory tests include electron microscopy, serology, and RT-PCR. Electron microscopy and immune electron microscopy require specialized equipment and technical expertise. Detection

of serum antibodies to the virus is not always straightforward, as most of the adult (but not child) population has serum antibodies to this virus. Furthermore, it can take several days after exposure to develop detectable IgM antibodies. RT-PCR, therefore, is the method of choice for detection of this RNA virus. The gene target is the viral RNA polymerase. Using this target, a broad spectrum of noroviral types can be detected. The results indicated that the virus was present in salad lettuce served at the hotel. Lettuce sampled directly from the distributor did not carry virus, indicating that the contamination occurred at the hotel. This assumption was supported by the discovery of viral RNA in hotel employees who had prepared the food. Direct sequencing of the RT-PCR products revealed identical sequences for all positive specimens, confirming that the guests, workers, and food source shared the same viral strain.

CASE STUDY 12 • 2

Five students from different local community high schools suffered recurrent skin infections with chronic wounds. Nasal swabs and skin specimens from the students were screened for MRSA by inoculation onto Mueller-Hinton agar supplemented with NaCl (0.68 mol/L) containing 6 µg/mL of oxacillin. The cultured organisms exhibited an MIC of more than 32 µg/mL vancomycin and a zone of inhibition of less than 14 mm in diameter. Isolates were sent to the CDC and referred for molecular testing. DNA isolated from the five cases and a control strain were embedded in agarose plugs and digested with SmaI for PFGE analysis. A depiction of the gel pattern is shown in the figure below.

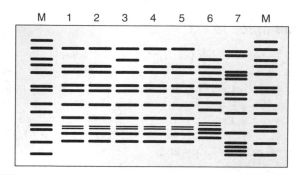

PFGE patterns of isolated strains. M, molecular weight markers. Lanes 1–5, isolates from the community infections; Lanes 6 and 7 unrelated hospital isolates.

Further PCR testing was performed on the isolates for virulence factors, particularly for *mecA* gene sequencing and detection of the Panton-Valentine leukocidin (PVL) genes, *lukS-PV* and *lukF-PV*. The results from these tests revealed that all five isolates contained the PVL genes and the type IV *mecA* element.

QUESTIONS:
1. Are all or some of the five isolates the same or different? Which isolates are the same, and which are different? What is the evidence to support your answer?
2. Was there a single source for these organisms or multiple sources?

Interpretation for Case Study 12 • 2:

Results from the culture of the isolates were consistent with MRSA. The results from the PFGE analysis indicated that all except one of the isolates from the students were the same strain. One isolate exhibited two differences from the others, indicating that it was closely related to these *S. aureus* isolates. Resistance to oxacillin/methicillin results from the expression of an altered penicillin-binding protein encoded by the *mecA* gene. All five isolates shared the type IV *mecA* gene, associated with MRSA. The toxin encoded by PVL, also produced by these isolates, is thought to be responsible for tissue necrosis in MRSA infections.

Further investigation into the cases revealed that all the students had participated in a wrestling meet at one of the high schools. Passage of the organism during this event was the likely source of the infection. The meet location was thoroughly cleaned according to CDC recommendations, and students were encouraged to always wash their hands and maintain good hygiene.

CASE STUDY 12 • 3

A 39-year-old HIV-positive male has been monitored closely since his diagnosis as HIV-positive 5 years ago. The man was on HAART and compliant. He was relatively healthy and had not even had a cold in the last 4 years. The man had HIV viral loads as determined by Amplicor RT-PCR that were consistently close to 10,000 copies/mL, never varying more than 0.2 $\log_{10}$ unit, until the last 6 months, when his viral loads were trending up to 25,500, then 48,900, with his most recent result being 55,000 copies/mL. Genotyping performed on virus

isolated from the patient revealed a mutation in the reverse transcriptase gene of M41L that is associated with resistance to zidovudine (AZT).

QUESTIONS:
1. What is the significance of the viral load results over the last 6 months?
2. What is the implication of the genotyping result for the patient's therapy?
3. How should this patient be monitored in the future?

Interpretation for Case Study 12 • 3:

The observation that the patient's viral loads were gradually increasing was a sign that the virus was developing resistance to the antiviral drugs. Slight variations of viral quantity within 0.3 $\log_{10}$ units are considered normal. This patient, however, was seeing significant increases in viral replication over the last 6 months.

This patient's virus has a mutation in the reverse transcriptase gene that has made the virus resistant to AZT. The patient's drug treatment needs to be changed immediately, with AZT being replaced by another reverse transcriptase inhibitor that would be unaffected by this mutation, such as didanosine or lamivudine. Viral load measurements should be taken regularly to make sure that the change in drug therapy causes a decrease in the viral load over the next few months. Genotyping should be performed again if the viral load starts to trend up.

CASE STUDY 13 • 1

A young mother was worried about her son. Having observed others, she was very aware of how her baby was expected to grow and acquire basic skills. As the child grew, however, he showed signs of slow development. His protruding ears and long face were becoming more noticeable as well. The pediatrician recommended chromosomal analysis for the mother and child. A constriction at the end of the X chromosome was found in the son's karyotype. The mother's karyotype was normal 46,XX. A Southern blot analysis for Fragile X was performed on a blood specimen from the mother, but showed no obvious abnormality. PCR analysis produced the following results:

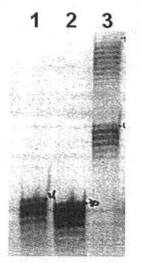

PCR analysis of the FMR promoter region showing two normal patterns (lanes 1 and 2) and the mother's pattern.

QUESTIONS:

1. *What do the PCR results in lane 3 indicate?*
2. *Why were there no abnormalities detected by Southern blot?*
3. *How would this result be depicted using triplet-primed PCR and capillary electrophoresis?*

Interpretation for Case Study 13 • 1:

The results in lane 3 show an expansion of the FMR1 promoter, suggesting the presence of a permutation in the mother. The full Fragile X expansion is not detected by standard PCR due to the size of the expanded products. The cytogenetic results, however, indicate the presence of the Fragile X expansion. Conversely, the size of the premutation expansion is not large enough for detection by Southern blot, but is apparent from the standard PCR results depicted. Capillary electrophoresis with triplet-primed PCR will show an extended peak pattern for the premutation. See Figure 13-24b.

CASE STUDY 13 • 2

A 14-year-old girl with muscle weakness and vision difficulties (retinopathy) was referred for clinical tests. A muscle biopsy was performed, and aberrant mitochondria were observed in thin sections. Histochemical analysis of the muscle tissue revealed cytochrome oxidase deficiency in the muscle cells. A skeletal muscle biopsy specimen was sent to the molecular genetics laboratory for analysis of mitochondrial DNA. Southern blot analysis of *Pvu*II cut mitochondrial DNA exhibited a band at 16,000 bp (arrow) in addition to the normal mitochondrial band at 16,500 bp, as shown below:

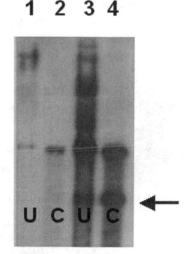

Southern blot of mitochondrial DNA uncut (U) and cut with *Pvu*II (C). Lanes 1 and 2, normal control; lanes 3 and 4, patient. Arrow points to a 16,000 kb band.

QUESTIONS:

1. *What is the 16,000 bp product? What is the 11,500 bp product?*
2. *What condition is associated with a 5-kb mitochondrial deletion?*
3. *Is this a case of homoplasmy or heteroplasmy?*

Interpretation for Case Study 13 • 2:

The 16,000 bp product is the linearized normal mitochondrial DNA (16,500 bp). The 16,000 bp product is the linearized mitochondrial circle with a 5,000 bp deletion. The 5-kb deletion is associated with Kearns Sayre syndrome (KSS), a rare neurological disorder affecting muscle function, stature, and hearing, among other symptoms. The results shown are a case of heteroplasmy as both normal and deleted mitochondria are present. The number of deleted mitochondria compared to the number of normal mitochondria will affect the severity of the disease symptoms.

CASE STUDY 13 • 3

A 40-year-old man was experiencing increasing joint pain, fatigue, and loss of appetite. He became alarmed when he suffered heart problems and consulted his physician. Routine blood tests revealed high serum iron (900 µg/dL) and 80% transferrin saturation. Total iron binding capacity was low (100 µg/dL). The man denied any extensive alcohol intake. A blood specimen was sent to the molecular genetics laboratory for detection of mutations in the hemachromatosis gene. The results are shown in lane 5 below:

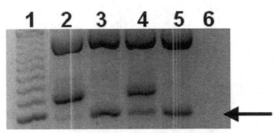

PCR-RFLP analysis of exon 4 of the *HFE* gene. The PCR product contains one recognition site for the restriction enzyme, *Rsa*I. An additional *Rsa*I site is created by the C282Y (G→A) mutation, the most common inherited mutation in hemochromatosis. This extra site results in a fragment of 240 bp, 110 bp (arrow) and ← 30 bp (not shown) instead of the 240 bp and 140 bp normal fragments. Lane 1, molecular weight markers; lane 2, normal control; lane 3, homozygous C282Y; lane 4, heterozygous C282Y; lane 5, patient specimen; lane 6, reagent blank.

QUESTIONS:

1. *Does this patient have the C282Y mutation?*
2. *Is this mutation heterozygous or homozygous?*
3. *Based on these results, what is the likely explanation for the patient's symptoms?*

Interpretation for Case Study 13 • 3:

The PCR-RFLP results in lane 5 indicate that the patient has the C282Y mutation, the most common inherited mutation in hemochromatosis. The G→A mutation produces an additional recognition site for the *Rsa*I restriction enzyme, 30 bp from one end of the 140 bp fragment in the normal sequence. The absence of the 140 bp fragment in lane 5 shows that the mutation is homozygous (although hemizygosity would also yield this pattern). The symptoms are likely due to iron overload caused by the loss of regulation of iron load through the *HFE* gene product.

CASE STUDY 13 • 4

A 30-year-old woman was brought to the emergency room with a painfully swollen left leg. She informed the nurses that she was taking contraceptives. Deep vein thrombosis was suspected, and compression ultrasound was ordered to look for pulmonary embolism. A clotting test for APC resistance resulted in a 1.5 ratio of clotting time with and without APC. An ELISA test for D-dimer was positive. The patient was immediately treated with heparin, and blood samples were taken. A blood sample was sent to the molecular genetics laboratory to test for the factor V Leiden 1691 G→A mutation and prothrombin 20210 G→A mutations. The results are shown below:

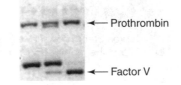

Agarose gel electrophoresis showing the band pattern for prothombin 20210/factor V Leiden mutation detection by multiplex SSP-PCR-RFLP. Specimens were cut with *Hind*III. Lane 1, molecular weight marker; lane 2, normal control (prothrombin, 407 bp + 99 bp, factor V, 241 bp); lane 3, heterozygous control, prothrombin (407, 384, 99, 23 bp)/factor V Leiden (241, 209, 323 bp); lane 4, homozygous factor V Leiden, normal prothrombin; lane 5, homozygous prothrombin 20210 mutation/normal factor V; lane 6, patient specimen; lanes 7 and 8, normal specimens.

QUESTIONS:

1. *Does this patient have a clotting disorder?*
2. *Is there a Factor V mutation? Is there a prothrombin mutation?*
3. *If present, is either mutation homozygous or heterozygous?*

Interpretation for Case Study 13 • 4:

The results of the physical and chemistry tests indicate that this patient has a thrombophilic clotting disorder (hypercoagulation). The molecular tests show a homozygous (or hemizygous) factor V Leiden 1691 G→A mutation. This nucleotide substitution will produce a *Hind*III site in the *F5* exon 10 PCR product with the primers used for this assay. Results for the prothrombin 20210 G→A mutation are negative (homozygous normal).

CASE STUDY 14 • 1

A 40-year-old woman with a history of non-Hodgkin's lymphoma reported to her physician for follow-up testing. Her complete blood cell count (CBC) was normal, including a white blood cell (WBC) count of 11,000/µL. Morphological studies on a bone marrow biopsy and a bone marrow aspirate revealed several small aggregates of mature and immature lymphocytes. Flow cytometry studies were difficult to interpret as there were too few B cells in the bone marrow aspirate specimen. No chromosomal abnormalities were detected by cytogenetics. A bone marrow aspirate tube was also sent for molecular analysis, namely, immunoglobulin heavy chain gene rearrangement and t(14;18) gene translocation analysis by PCR. The patient's results are shown in lanes 2 of the gel images below:

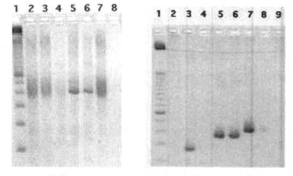

Immmunoglobulin heavy chain gene rearrangement results (left): lane 1, molecular weight marker; lanes 2 to 4, patient specimens; lane 5, positive control; lane 6, sensitivity; lane 7, negative control; lane 8, reagent blank. t(14;18) gene translocation test (right): lane 1, molecular weight marker; lanes 2 to 6, patient specimens; lane 7, positive control; lane 8, sensitivity; lane 9, negative control.

QUESTIONS:

1. *Is a monoclonal cell population with an amplifiable gene rearrangement present?*
2. *Are the translocation results at right consistent with those of cytogenetics?*
3. *What control is missing from the translocation analysis?*

Interpretation for Case Study 14 • 1:

The molecular results indicate that a small population of cells with the t(14;18) translocation is present in the bone marrow below the level of detection of the cytogenetics and flow cytometry tests for this specimen

with minimal B cells. The PCR translocation analysis, however, is lacking an amplification control. There may be a small monoclonal population representing part of the lymphoid aggregates observed in the morphological studies. The CBC result is apparently not representative of this tumor population. The immunoglobulin gene rearrangement results are indeterminate, indicating that the gene rearrangement in this small cell population is not amplifiable or is below the level of detection of the assay (1% of cells in the specimen). Although detection of the t(14;18) translocation is consistent with follicular lymphoma, the clinical significance of this cell population is not apparent from a single encounter. Patient history and subsequent analyses will provide important information as to whether this patient is going into remission or showing early signs of relapse.

CASE STUDY 14 • 2

A 54-year-old woman with thrombosis, a high platelet count (900,000/µL), and a decreased erythrocyte sedimentation rate was tested for polycythemia vera. Megakaryocyte clusters and pyknotic nuclear clusters were observed in a bone marrow biopsy. Overall cellularity was decreased. In the CBC, WBC and neutrophil counts were normal. Iron stores were also within normal range. A blood sample was submitted to the molecular pathology laboratory for JAK2 V617F mutation analysis by multiplex sequence-specific PCR (See Chapter 9, Figure 9-12). The results are shown below:

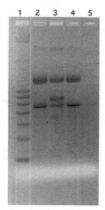

Agarose gel electrophoresis of SSP-PCR amplicons. Extension of a JAK2 V617F-specific primer produces a 270-bp band in addition to the normal 500- and 230-bp bands. Lane 1, molecular weight markers; lane 2, patient specimen; lane 3, V617F mutant control; lane 4, normal control; lane 5, reagent blank.

QUESTIONS:

1. *What is the source of the two bands in the normal control in lane 4?*
2. *What is the source of the additional band in the positive control in lane 3?*
3. *Does this patient have the JAK2 V617F mutation?*

Interpretation for Case Study 14 • 2:

The bands in the normal control lane are the products of the outer primers and the inner primer matching the normal *JAK2* sequence with one outer primer. The additional product in lane 3 is primed by the *JAK2* mutation-specific primer and one outer primer. The results in lane 2 indicate that the patient does not have the JAK2 V617F mutation. Only the products of the outer primers and the normal sequence-specific primer are present.

CASE STUDY 14 • 3

Paraffin-embedded sections were submitted to the molecular diagnostics laboratory for p53 mutation analysis. The specimen was a small tumor (intraductal carcinoma in situ) discovered in a 55-year-old woman. Lymph nodes were negative. Slides stained with hematoxylin and eosin were examined for confirmation of the location of tumor cells on the sections. These cells were dissected from the slide. DNA isolated from the microdissected tumor cells was screened by SSCP for mutations in exons 4 to 9 of the p53 gene. The results for exon 5 are shown below:

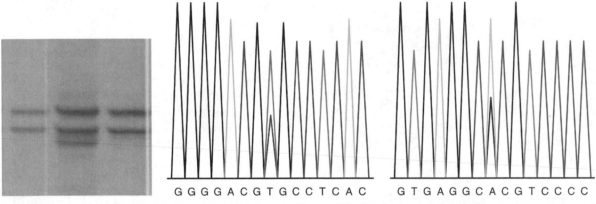

Polyacrylamide gel electrophoresis with silver stain detection of p53 exon 5 (left). Lane 1, normal; lane 2, patient; lane 3, normal. Direct sequencing (right) revealed a C→T (G→A) base change, resulting in a R→H amino acid change at position 175.

QUESTIONS:

1. *What information is gained from the SSCP results?*
2. *What is the source of the additional band in the patient SSCP lane?*
3. *What further confirmation/information is gained from direct sequencing?*

Interpretation for Case Study 14 • 3:

The SSCP banding pattern in lane 2 is different from that of the normal control in lane 3, indicating the presence of a sequence alteration in the patient DNA. The additional band represents the conformer formed by the folding of the altered sequence. While SSCP reveals the presence and the general location of the sequence alteration, direct sequencing identifies the exact sequence change. Since some DNA sequence changes do not change the amino acid sequence (silent mutations) and some sequence changes are benign polymorphisms, the sequencing information is valuable for interpretation of the actual effect of the sequence change.

CASE STUDY 14 • 4

Colon carcinoma and three polyps were resected in a right hemicolectomy of a 33-year-old man. Although there was no family history, the man's age and the location of the tumor warranted testing for hereditary nonpolyposis colorectal carcinoma. Histological staining was negative for MSH2 protein. Paraffin sections and a blood sample were submitted to the molecular pathology laboratory for microsatellite instability testing. DNA was isolated from tumor cells dissected from four paraffin sections and from the patient's white blood cells.

Both were amplified at the five microsatellite loci recommended by the National Cancer Institute. Results are shown below:

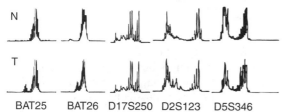

MSI analysis of normal cells (N, top row) and tumor cells (T, bottom row) at the five NCI loci.

BAT25   BAT26   D17S250   D2S123   D5S346

QUESTIONS:

1. *What are the indications for MSI analysis in this case?*
2. *What accounts for the difference in the peak patterns in the BAT25 and BAT26 loci?*
3. *How would you interpret the results of this analysis according to NCI recommendations?*

Interpretation for Case Study 14 • 4:

The MSI analysis shows instability in at least two of the five microsatellite markers tested (BAT25 and BAT26). The different peak patterns (additional alleles) in the tumor cells compared to the normal controls result from loss of nucleotide repeat units in the repeated sequences. Normally, these losses would be repaired by the mismatch repair system. When there are mutations that prevent this system from working properly, the new alleles remain in the DNA through subsequent rounds of replication. According to NCI recommendations, high microsatellite instability (MSI) is defined by instability in two of the five NCI loci. An alternative criterion for MSI when more than five loci are tested is more than 30% of the markers showing instability.

CASE STUDY 14 • 5

A 23-year-old college student was sent to the student health office with a painful bruise that persisted for several weeks. He was referred to the local hospital, where the physician ordered a bone marrow biopsy and a CBC. His WBC count was 28,000/µL; red blood cells, 2 million/µL; hemoglobin, 8; hematocrit, 20; platelets, 85,000/µL. Neutrophils were 7%, lymphocytes were 5%, and blasts were 95%. The pathologist who examined the bone marrow biopsy requested flow cytometry analysis of the aspirate. The cells expressed 84% CD20, 82% CD34, 92% HLA-DR, and 80% CD10/CD19. The results of these tests indicated a diagnosis of acute lymphoblastic leukemia. A blood specimen was sent to the cytogenetics laboratory for chromosomal analysis. Twenty metaphases examined had a normal 46,XY chromosomal complement. Interphase FISH was negative for t(9;22) in 500 nuclei.

QUESTIONS:

1. *What is the significance of the cytogenetic test results?*
2. *What other molecular abnormalities might be present in this type of tumor?*

Interpretation for Case Study 14 • 5:

The t(9;22) translocation is present in 95% of cases of chronic myelogenous leukemia (CML), 25% to 30% of adult acute lymphoblastic leukemia (ALL), and 2%–10% of pediatric ALL. The presence of the translocation is a negative prognostic marker in adult ALL. The t(1;19) translocation may be present in pre-B ALL. Monoclonal immunoglobulin heavy chain and light chain gene rearrangements may be used to monitor B-ALL. Monoclonal T-cell receptor gene rearrangements may be used to monitor T-ALL.

CASE STUDY 15 • 1

A 50-year-old man complained of digestive disorders and what he presumed was allergy to several foods. He consulted his physician, who collected blood samples for laboratory testing. The man was in a high-risk group for certain diseases, notably celiac disease, which would produce symptoms similar to those experienced by this patient. A specimen was sent to the laboratory to test HLA-DQA and -DQB alleles. Almost all (95%) people with celiac disease have the DQA1*05:01 and DQB1*02:01 alleles (DQ2 variant), compared with 20% of the general population. A second predisposing heterodimer, DQ8, is encoded by the DQA1*03:01 and the DQB1*03:02 alleles. Most of the 5% of celiac patients who are negative for the DQ2 alleles display the DQ8 alleles. Serological results to detect the predisposing antigens, however, were equivocal. An SBT test was performed. The sequence results showed the following alleles at DQA1 and DQB1 loci:

DQA1*05:01   DQB1*02:01, DQB1*04:01

QUESTION: *Is it possible that this man has celiac disease based on his HLA haplotype?*

Interpretation for Case Study 15 • 1:

This patient has the two DQ alleles, DQA1*05:01 and DQB1*02:01, that form the two parts (alpha chain and beta chain, respectively) of the DQ2 variant heterodimer found in most people with celiac disease. Although a diagnosis cannot be made based on the HLA haplotype alone, the presence of the variant allele is consistent with such a diagnosis made based on clinical and morphological evidence.

CASE STUDY 15 • 2

A 43-year-old man consulted his physician about a lump on his neck and frequent night sweats. A biopsy of the mass in his neck was sent to the pathology department for analysis. An abnormally large population of CD20-positive lymphocytes was observed by morphological examination. Flow cytometry tests detected a monoclonal B-cell population with co-expression of CD10/CD19 and CD5. This population was 88% kappa and 7% lambda. The results were confirmed by the observation of a monoclonal immunoglobulin heavy chain gene rearrangement that was also monoclonal for kappa light chain gene rearrangement. The patient was initially treated with standard chemotherapy, but the tumor returned before the therapeutic program was completed. The tumor persisted through a second treatment with stronger chemotherapy plus local irradiation. Non-myeloablative bone marrow transplant was prescribed. To find a compatible donor, the man's HLA type and the types of five potential donors were compared. HLA-A and -B types were assessed by serology, and HLA-DR type was determined by SSP-PCR and SSOP. The typing results are shown in the table.

Recipient	Donor 1	Donor 2	Donor 3	Donor 4	Donor 5
A*03:02	A*66:01/04	A*26:01	A*03:02	A*31:03/04	A*26:10
A*26:10	A*03:02	A*03:02		A*03:09	A*03:09
B*39:06	B*07:11	B*15:28	B*53:07	B*39:06	B*35:08
B*53:07	B*57:01	B*39:19	B*39:01	B*53:07	
DRB1*08:01	DRB1*07:01	DRB1*13:17	DRB1*08:01	DRB1*07:01	DRB1*13:17
	DRB1*13:17	DRB1*04:22		DRB1*11:17	DRB1*07:01

QUESTIONS:

1. *Which of the five donors is the best match for this patient?*
2. *Which mismatches are acceptable?*
3. *Using the donor bone marrow that matches most closely, is there more of a chance of graft rejection or GVHD?*

Interpretation for Case Study 15 • 2:

A successful transplant does not absolutely require a fully matched donor. In some cases, there may be more harm in delaying a transplant in search of a fully matched donor than in proceeding with the transplant earlier in the disease process. Mismatches at the HLA-B and C loci may be better tolerated than those at the HLA-A and HLA-DRB1 loci. Donor 3 is the closest match at the HLA-A, -B, and –DRB1 loci. Since donor 3 is homozygous for the A locus, only one determinate is displayed to the recipient immune system, which could lessen the likelihood of graft rejection. Conversely, when the graft does not have one of the recipient alleles, T cells in the donated bone marrow may react against the recipient and graft-versus-host disease may occur. In the present case, however, there is only one mismatch, and a single mismatch is less associated with GVHD than multiple mismatches in the class I and II antigen loci. The actual effect of an allele on the immune response will also depend on the location of the polymorphic amino acid in the protein. A mismatch may be tolerated if the polymorphic amino acid is not exposed on the outer surface of the folded protein.

CASE STUDY 15 • 3

A 19-year-old woman reported to a local clinic with painful swelling in her face. Routine tests revealed dangerously high blood pressure that warranted hospitalization. Further tests were performed, which led to a diagnosis of systemic lupus erythematosus. Due to complications of this disease, her kidney function was compromised, and she would eventually suffer kidney failure. With an alternative of life-long dialysis, a kidney transplant was recommended. Class I PRAs were assessed at 0% PRA for class I. An additional screen for class II PRAs was performed by flow cytometry. Class I and class II HLA typing was performed by SSP-PCR. An autocytotoxic crossmatch was also performed, revealing T-cell and B-cell positive antibodies, probably related to the lupus. The young woman's mother volunteered to donate a kidney to her daughter. Mother and daughter had matching blood group antigens and HLA-DR antigens, which are the most critical for successful organ transplant. The results from the typing tray are shown in the following figure:

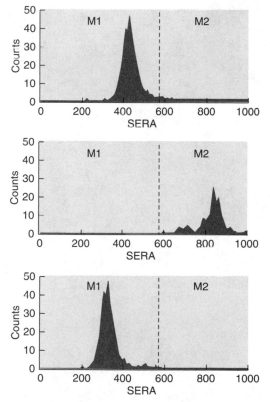

Flow cytometry analysis of HLA class II antigens in recipient serum. Top = negative control; middle = positive control; bottom = patient serum.

SSP-PCR results for HLA-A, -B, and -DR and their serological equivalents are shown in the table. Crossmatching of the daughter's serum and mother's cells was performed by cytotoxicity and flow cytometry. Both test results were negative.

Daughter

SSP-PCR	Serology
A*24:19, A*34:01	A24(9), 34(10)
B*08:02, B*56:03	B8, B22
DRB1*04:22, DRB1*14:11	DR4, DR14(6)

Mother

SSP-PCR	Serology
A*01:04, A*24:19	A1, A24(9)
B*37:03, B*08:04	B37, B8
DRB1*04:22, DRB1*13:17	DR4, DR13(6)

QUESTIONS:

1. *Is the mother a good match for the daughter? Based on the antibody and crossmatching studies, what is the risk of rejection?*
2. *Before performing the HLA studies, how many of the daughter's antigens would be expected to match those of her mother?*

Interpretation for Case Study 15 • 3:

A parent's alleles will not be a perfect match for an offspring. Even before typing, the mother will be expected to have at least half of the same alleles as her daughter. A fully matched sibling is the best donor type. Due to yet undefined factors that can affect organ rejection, fully matched siblings are better than unrelated fully matched donors who don't share these genetic factors. In the absence of a fully matched donor, the mother is an acceptable donor for her daughter. Crossmatching results were negative for antibodies in the daughter's serum against antigens displayed by the mother's organ, favoring successful transplantation.

A

A site adjacent site, location of incoming charged tRNA binding in the ribosome complex for acceptance of the growing peptide

abasic site position on the DNA sugar-phosphate backbone where the ribose sugar does not carry a nitrogen base

absorptivity constant characteristic tendency of a substance to absorb light at a given wavelength; used in quantifying nucleic acids, the absorptivity constants of DNA and RNA are (50 ug/mL)/absorbance unit and (40 ug/mL)/absorbance unit, respectively, at 260-nm wavelength

acrocentric having the centromere nearer one end of the chromosome than the other

activator in molecular biology, a protein that positively affects gene expression or function of other proteins

adaptors in recombinant DNA technology, synthetic short DNA fragments used to modify ends of DNA fragments

adenine one of the common nitrogen bases in DNA and RNA

adenosine one of the common nucleosides in DNA and RNA

affinity maturation selection of B cells expressing antibodies with greater affinity for the antigen

agarose polymer of agarobiose (1,4-linked 3,6-anhydro-α-L-galactopyranose) that, when hydrated, forms a gel frequently used for sieving nucleic acids

alignment comparison and lining up of two or more nucleic acid or protein sequences to achieve the maximal number of identical positions

alkaline phosphatase enzyme frequently used to generate signals from chemiluminescent or chromogenic substrates

allele different version of the same sequence, gene, or locus

allele-specific oligomer hybridization ASO; mutation/polymorphism detection technique using immobilized target and sequence-specific probes

allelic discrimination mutation/polymorphism detection using real-time PCR and fluorogenic probes

allelic exclusion gene rearrangement on only one of two homologous chromosomes

allelic ladders reference size standards used in short tandem repeat analysis representing all possible products (alleles) for a given locus

alloantibodies antibodies that recognize human antigens

allogeneic genetically from the different individuals

allograft transplanted organ from a genetically different donor

alpha helicases coiled secondary structural motif in proteins

alpha phosphate phosphate group closest to the ribose sugar in a nucleotide

alpha satellite highly repetitive sequences found at the centromere

alternative splicing removal of introns from RNA using different breakpoints

Alu elements short interspersed nucleotide sequences containing recognition sites for the *Alu* restriction enzyme

ambiguity recognition of two or more antigens by the same antibody

amelogenin locus gene located on the X and Y chromosome with an XY-specific polymorphism

amino acid tRNA synthetase one of twenty enzymes that attached the appropriate amino acid to its anticodon-containing tRNA

amino acids nitrogen-containing molecules with specific biochemical properties that are the building blocks of protein

aminoacyl tRNA synthetases enzymes that covalently attach the appropriate amino acid to its tRNA

amino terminal end of a protein or peptide containing the amino group of the amino acid, usually considered the beginning of the protein's amino acid sequence

ammonium persulfate APS; with TEMED, catalyzes polymerization of acrylamide gels

amplicon   product of a PCR reaction

amplification   replication, copying

amplification control   template sequences that are always present; used to confirm the functional competence of the reaction mix

amplification program   conditions under which a PCR reaction occurs, including denaturation, annealing and extension temperatures and times

amplified fragment length polymorphism   AFLP; analysis of polymorphic DNA by amplification of selected regions and resolving the amplified products by size

analyte measurement range   AMR; the range within which a specimen may be tested directly (without dilution or concentration) for an analyte

analyte-specific reagents   ASR; test components that detect a specific target

analytic accuracy   production of correct (true positive and true negative) results

analytical sensitivity   lower limit of detection of an analyte

analytic specificity   ability to detect only the analyte and not nonspecific targets

anaphase   mitosis or meiosis where replicated chromosomes separate

ancestral haplotype   haplotype in which a mutation originally occurred

Anderson reference   sequence of the mitochondrial hypervariable regions used as a reference for defining polymorphisms

aneuploid   having an aberrant number of chromosomes per nucleus, caused by genome mutations

aneuploidy   in diploid organisms, having other than two of each chromosome

anion   negatively charged atom or molecule

annealing   hybridization of complementary sequences

anode   positively charged electrode to which anions migrate

anticipation   in genetics, rising phenotypic severity through generations of a family

anticodon   trinucleotide sequence found in transfer RNA that is complementary to its amino acid codon

antihuman antibodies   AHA; alloantibodies; antibodies that recognize human antigens

antimicrobial agent   antibiotic; a substance that inhibits growth of or kills bacteria

antiparallel   two complementary single-stranded nucleic acids oriented so that when hydrogen bonded together through complementary bases, the 5' end of one molecule is next to the 3' end of the other

antisense strand   single strand of a DNA double helix that is used as a template for messenger RNA synthesis

apoptosis   self-directed cell death

arbitrarily primed PCR   PCR method using random priming with 6-10 b primers used for typing of organisms; also known as randomly amplified polymorphic DNA

arm   in cytogenetics, one end of a chromosome from the centromere to the telomere

array   in molecular biology, a set of probes or targets immobilized on the same substrate

array CGH   type of microarray used to detect deletions and amplifications in DNA

attenuation   mechanism of control of gene expression in prokaryotes that works through formation of stems and loops in the RNA transcript by intrastrand hydrogen bonding of complementary bases

autologous   genetically from the same individual

autophagy   degradation of intracellular substrates within the cell

autoradiography   detection of target as an image produced by exposing a light-sensitive film to a light- or radiation-emitting membrane

autosomal STR   short tandem repeats located on other than the X and Y chromosome

autosomal-dominant   inheritance pattern where the child of an affected and an unaffected individual has a 50% probability of being affected

autosomal-recessive   inheritance pattern where the child of an affected and an unaffected carrier has a 50% probability of being affected and where the child of two affected individuals has a 100% probability of being affected

autosome   any chromosome except for the X and Y sex chromosomes

avuncular testing   determination through genetic polymorphisms the probability of an aunt/uncle-niece/nephew relationship

B

bacteriocidal   kills bacteria

bacteriocins   proteins manufactured by bacteria that are toxic to other microorganisms

bacteriophage   viruses that infect bacteria

bacteriostatic   prevents growth of bacteria

balanced   in cytogenetics, genetic events that result in no gain or loss of genetic material

balanced polymorphism   DNA sequence difference, the phenotypic effect of which is counteracted by a second trait or polymorphism

band   in molecular biology, a pattern on a gel or autoradiogram representing a fragment of nucleic acid or protein

band compression   bunching of fragments in gel electrophoresis migration

banding   in cytogenetics, formation of microscopically visible bands on chromosomes by staining

Barr body   structure visible in the interphase nucleus formed by the inactive X chromosome

basal transcription complex   complex of protein factors required by RNA polymerase to initiate RNA synthesis

base   nitrogen base; also used as an expression of units of single-stranded nucleic acid

base extension sequence scanning   BESS; mutation/polymorphism scanning using dUTP incorporation into DNA followed by enzymatic cleavage at the dU sites, followed by electrophoretic resolution of the resulting fragments

base pair   expression of units of double-stranded nucleic acid

base pairing   association of adenine with thymine/uracil or guanine with cytosine through specific hydrogen bonds

Basic Local Alignment Search Tool   BLAST; a sequence comparison algorithm

bDNA amplification   branched DNA; a signal amplification system

bead array   probes attached to fluorescence-labeled beads

beta-2 microglobulin   12kD peptide associated at the cell membrane with the MHC heavy chain comprising the class I HLA

beta-lactam   cyclic protein found in antibiotics

beta-lactamase   enzyme produced by bacteria that are resistant to β-lactam containing antibiotics

beta-pleated sheets   pleated planar secondary structure found in proteins

betaine   *N,N,N*-trimethyl glycine; used in PCR reactions to increase specificity and yield by facilitating strand separation of the target double helix

bidirectional   reading or analysis of both forward and reverse strands of a double-stranded DNA

bilateral symmetry   having the same structure on two sides or ends, e.g., the recognition sites for type II restriction enzymes

bin   characteristic distribution of migration distances after electrophoretic resolution of the same allele multiple times

binning   in fragment analysis, collection of all peaks or band migration distances within a characteristic distribution in order to determine if two peaks or migration distances are representative of the same allele

bioinformatics   adaptation of information technology for the biological sciences; computational biology

biotin   vitamin that is used in the laboratory for nonradioactive probe detection

bisulfite DNA sequencing   nucleotide sequence analysis of DNA that has been treated with sodium bisulfite; a method to detect methylated cytosines in DNA

blank   reaction mix containing all components except for target; used to detect target contamination in test reagents

blast   basic local alignment search tool; a software program that compares nucleotide or protein sequences to find regions of similarity between them

blocking   covering nonspecific binding sites before probe hybridization

blot   transfer; the membrane carrying the transferred nucleic acid or protein

blunt   describing double-stranded nucleic acids that do not possess overhanging single strands on the ends

BOX   palindromic repetitive elements found in *Streptococcus pneumoniae*

branched DNA (bDNA) amplification   signal amplification method detecting target through a series of hybridizations

break-apart probe   FISH probes designed to detect translocations where there are multiple possible partners

buffer   ionic substance or solution that maintains specific pH

buffy coat   white blood cells separated by density centrifugation

C

C banding   centromere staining

calibration   fitting an instrument test output with the actual amount of a reference analyte

calibration verification   testing of materials of known amounts throughout the measurement range to ensure instrument accuracy

Cambridge reference sequence   sequence of the mitochondrial hypervariable regions used as a reference for defining polymorphisms

cancer   diseases that are caused by uncoordinated, rapid cell growth

cap   7-methyl G 5'ppp 5' G/A covalently attached to the 5' end of messenger RNA

capillary electrophoresis   separation of particles in solution inside of a glass capillary

capillary gel electrophoresis   separation of particles through a sieving polymer or gel inside of a glass capillary

capillary transfer   movement of nucleic acid or protein from a gel matrix to a membrane by capillary action

carboxy terminal   end of a protein or peptide containing the carboxyl group of the amino acid, usually considered the end of the protein's amino acid sequence

carcinoma   tumors of epithelial tissue origin

cathode   negatively charged electrode to which cations migrate

cation   positively charged atom or molecule

cell division cycle   the succession of events when a single cell divides, including prereplicative phase (G1), DNA synthesis (S), postreplication (G2), and separation (M)

centromere   repeated sequences in the area of each chromosome that attaches to the mitotic spindle through the kinetochore

centromeric probe   CEN, CEP; probes that bind to centromeres

chain   term sometimes used to describe a polymer of nucleotides comprising a single strand of nucleic acid

chaperone   specialized protein that protects growing peptides as they emerge from the ribosome

charging   attachment of an amino acid to tRNA

checkpoint   regulated places in the cell division cycle; between the G1 and S phases (G1 checkpoint) and between the G2 and M phases (G2 checkpoint)

chemical cleavage   breaking DNA chains with specific nonenzymatic substances

chimera (or chimerism)   an individual harboring cells or tissues from two different zygotes; describing such a state

chromatin   relaxed chromosomes found in interphase nuclei

chromosome   DNA double helix that carries genes

chromosome mutations   genetic alterations that result in structural changes in chromosomes

chromosome paint   cytogenetic probe analysis designed to visualize an entire metaphase chromosome

chromosome spread   array of intact chromosomes displayed upon hypotonic lysis of a nucleus

cis   on the same side; on the same molecule

cis factor   cis-regulatory element, cis-element; a DNA sequence that marks places on the DNA involved in the initiation and control of RNA synthesis

class switch recombination movement of the VDJ gene segment of a rearranged immunoglobulin gene to gene segments encoding IgG, IgE or IgA constant regions

cleavage-based amplification signal amplification system based on the proprietary cleavase enzyme

Clinical Laboratory Improvement Amendments CLIA; recommendations passed by Congress in 1988 to establish quality and testing standards

clinical sensitivity ability of a test result to predict a clinical condition

clinical specificity disease-associated results only in patients who actually have the disease conditions

clone two or more cells or individuals having the same genotype

***coa* typing** tandem repeat element in the 3' coding region of the *Staphylococcus aureus* coagulase gene, *coa*; analyzed by PFGE to identify MRSA

CODIS Combined DNA Indexing System; a set of 13 STR loci and amelogenin used for positive human identification

codon three nucleotide sequences that will guide the insertion of a specific amino acid into protein

coefficient of variance CV; normalized measure of dispersion about the mean; an expression of test precision determined through repeated tests of the same sample analyte

colicinogenic factors class of plasmid that carries genes coding for colicins, proteins with antibiotic properties

comb in electrophoresis, a device placed in melted agarose to mold wells or spaces for introducing samples to the gel

combined paternity index CPI; the product of the paternity indexes for a set of alleles

combined sibling index likelihood ratio generated by a determination whether two people share one or both parents; also called sibling index, kinship index

compaction Wrapping, folding, and coiling DNA to fit inside the nucleus

comparative genome hybridization CGH; microarray method to detect deletions or amplifications in DNA

comparative genomic array array hybridized to DNA in order to detect insertions or deletions

complement group of proteins that in combination with antibodies, cause the destruction of particulate antigens

complement-dependent cytotoxicity CDC; killing of cells based on HLA type using reference antigens

complementarity determining region CDR; domain in the immunoglobulin heavy chain gene variable region coding for amino acids that directly contact antigen

complementary term used to describe the order of two antiparallel single-stranded nucleic acids such that A on one strand is always across from T on the other strand and C is always across from G

complementary DNA double-stranded DNA synthesized using RNA as a template; cDNA

computational biology bioinformatics; life science based on mathematical and statistical applications

concatamers joined rings of DNA

conformation-sensitive gel electrophoresis resolution of homoduplexes from heteroduplexes under specified gel conditions

conformer three-dimensional structure formed by folding and intra-strand hybridization of a single strand of nucleic acid

congenital "born with"; having a genetic component

conjugate structure comprised of more than one type of molecule, such as a glycoprotein or lipoprotein, or an antibody with covalently attached alkaline phosphatase

conjugated proteins proteins with lipid, carbohydrate, metallic or other components

conjugation transfer of genetic information by physical association of cells

consensus in sequencing, a family of sequences representing different variations in a population

consensus primer primer directed to the immunoglobulin or T-cell receptor genes with sequences representing the most frequently occurring nucleotide at each position

consensus sequence family of sequences representing different variations in a population, but with similar motifs in nucleotide order

conservation   amino acid (or nucleotide) substitutions that preserve the biochemical and physical properties of the original residue or nucleotide sequence

conservative   (1) in DNA replication, a term used to describe replication of both strands of the parent double helix simultaneously, producing a daughter double helix comprised of two replicated strands; (2) in protein sequences, substitution of an amino acid with one of similar biochemical properties

conservative substitution   alteration in the nucleotide sequence that results in the substitution of an amino acid with one of similar properties

constitutive   transcription that is constantly active

contact precautions   protective equipment and/or clothing used for direct patient contact and potential exposure to airborne or contact-transmissible infectious agents from the patient

contamination   presence of unwanted materials; in PCR, presence of extraneous, non-template DNA in a reaction solution

contamination control   action taken to avoid or detect unwanted substrates or products of a reaction; in PCR, a reaction mix containing all components except target

continuous allele system   genetic structures that vary by increments and are defined by these incremental variations

control   analytes of known type and amount that are included with test specimens to monitor method systems

corepressor   component of a protein complex required for turning off gene transcription

CpG islands   regions of DNA rich in CG dinucleotides found in gene promoters

crossing over   breakage and rejoining of separate double helices, resulting in recombined products

crossmatching   analysis of the reaction between recipient serum antibodies and donor lymphocytes

cross-reactive epitope group   CREG; human leukocyte antigens recognized by antibodies that also recognize other HLAs

cryotube   plastic storage tube designed for storage at freezer temperatures

C_0t value   expression of the complexity of DNA sequences

$C_0t_{1/2}$ time required for half of a double-stranded sequence to anneal under a given set of conditions

cut-off value   quantitative assay levels that distinguish positive from negative results

cycle   in PCR, one series of extension, annealing and extension

cycling probe   signal amplification system based on RnaseH digestion of probe bound to target sequences

cycle sequencing   semi-automated method to determine the order of nucleotides in a nucleic acid using a thermal cycler

cytidine   one of the common nucleosides in DNA and RNA

cytochrome P-450   group of enzymes in the endoplasmic reticulum that participate in enzymatic hydroxylation reactions and also transfer electrons to oxygen

cytopathic effect   CPE; lysis, death, or growth inhibition of cells due to viral infection

cytosine   one of the common nitrogen bases in DNA and RNA

D

DAPI   4',6-diamidino-2-phenyl indole; DNA-specific dye used to visualize nuclei

de novo sequencing   determination of nucleotide order for the first time

deaza dGTP   modified nucleotide used to destabilize secondary structure in template DNA

deletion   loss of genetic material

denaturation   in nucleic acids, loss of hydrogen bonding between complementary strands; in protein, loss of tertiary structure

denatured alcohol   ethanol mixed with other components

denaturing agent   in electrophoresis, formamide or urea used to remove secondary structures from molecules

denaturing gel   polyacrylamide gel containing a substance that will separate double-stranded DNA into single strands

deoxyribonuclease   enzyme that digests DNA by catalyzing the breakage of phosphodiester bonds

deoxyribose   ribose without a hydroxyl group on the carbon in the 2 position on the sugar ring

depurination   removal of purines from the sugar-phosphate backbone of DNA

derivative chromosome   abnormal chromosome comprised of rearranged parts from two or more unidentified chromosomes joined to a normal chromosome

detection limit   lower limit of detection of the analyte

dideoxy chain termination   method using dideoxynucleotides to determine the order or sequence of nucleotides in a nucleic acid

dideoxy DNA fingerprinting   ddF; mutation/polymorphism screening using a one or two dideoxynucleotides and gel electrophoresis

dideoxynucleotide   ddNTP; a nucleoside triphosphate lacking a hydroxyl group at the 3' ribose position

diethyl pyrocarbonate   DEPC; ribonuclease inactivator; cross-links RNAse proteins

digoxygenin   steroidal compound used for nonradioactive probe detection

diploid   having two of each chromosome

discrete allele system   set of alleles that can be classified by a finite number of types

discriminatory capacity   DC; the power of a locus for use in identification, considering the number of different alleles of the locus and the total number individuals tested in a given population

discriminatory power   ability of typing methods to clearly distinguish strains

dispersive   term used to describe DNA replication where both strands of the parent double helix undergo simultaneous, discontinuous replication

DNA fingerprinting   genetic profiling; identification of the genetic alleles in multiple loci from an individual

DNA ligase   enzyme that catalyzes formation of a phosphodiester bond between preexisting fragments of DNA

DNA methyltransferase   enzyme that catalyzes the covalent attachment of a methyl group to a nitrogen base in DNA

dNTP   deoxyribose nucleotide triphosphate

domain   functional part of a protein

dot blot   hybridization technique with multiple targets spotted on a membrane all exposed to the same probe

double-stranded break   separation of both single strands of a double helix at the same location

dual fusion probe   dual color probes; FISH probes designed to detect translocations and their reciprocal products

dye blob   artifactual peak pattern caused by residual, unincorporated, labeled dideoxynucleotides in a sequencing reaction

dye primer   covalent attachment of fluorescent molecules to a sequencing primer

dye terminator   covalent attachment of fluorescent molecules to dideoxynucleotides

E

eastern blot   hybridization technique used to detect post-translational modification of immobilized proteins

electrode   metallic conductor of an electrical circuit that includes non-metallic parts

electroendosmosis   solvent flow toward an electrode in opposition to particle migration

electropherogram   data output from capillary electrophoresis where fluorescent signals are recorded as graphical peaks

electrophoresis   separation of particles through a solution or matrix under the force of an electric current

electrophoretic transfer   movement of nucleic acid or protein from a gel matrix to a membrane using an electric current

end labeling   incorporation of radioactive or otherwise labeled nucleotides on the 3' or 5' end of a nucleic acid

endonuclease   enzyme that separates DNA or RNA by cutting within the linear molecule

endpoint analysis   analysis or observation of a PCR product after the amplification program is complete

engraftment   establishment or repopulation of bone marrow cell lineages from a transplanted cell preparation

enhancer   DNA site that increases gene transcription, often located distal to the affected gene

enhanceosome   architectural and regulatory proteins assembled on an enhancer element

enterobacterial repetitive intergenic consensus (ERIC)   126-bp long genomic sequences found in some bacterial species that are highly conserved

enzyme adaptation   adjustment of metabolism by bacteria growing in media containing specific substrates in order to produce particular proteins

enzyme induction   stimulation of synthesis of RNA encoding enzymes or other factors from inducible genes

enzyme repression   active prevention of synthesis of RNA encoding enzymes or other factors from inducible genes

epidemic   disease or condition that affects many unrelated individuals at the same time

epigenetic regulation   heritable but sequence-independent control of gene expression and protein function

episome   genetic material within the cell not attached to the host chromosome(s)

epitope   specific antigenic sites on a protein

Eppendorf tube   plastic conical tubes with 0.5 mL to 2.0 mL capacity

ERIC   enterobacterial repetitive intergenic consensus; palindromic sequences found in gram-negative bacteria; typing of bacteria by analysis of PCR amplicons produced from primers homologous to these sequences

E site   position in the ribosome from which the "empty" tRNA is released

ER stress   cellular response to accumulation of unfolded proteins in the endoplasmic

ethidium bromide   intercalating agent that when bound to double-stranded DNA fluoresces under uv light

euchromatin   areas of chromosomes that are relatively open to transcription

euploid   having the proper number of chromosomes per nucleus

exclusion   in human identification, difference of at least one allele from a reference source

exon   sequences of DNA that code for protein

exonuclease   an enzyme that removes nucleotides from DNA or RNA from either end of the linear molecule

expression array   an array hybridized to RNA in order to measure gene expression

extended MHC locus   xMHC; an 8-Mb region of chromosome 6p including areas flanking the main MHC locus

extracellular   outside of the cell

F

F factor   a plasmid carrying instructions for physical association of cells and transfer of genetic information from cell to cell

factor V Leiden   a specific mutation in the gene coding for the factor V coagulation protein (F5 1691 A→G) resulting in the substitution of arginine at amino acid position 506 with glutamine

false negative   failure to detect an analyte present in a test sample; analogous to Type II or beta error

false positive   results suggesting the presence of an analyte that is not in a test sample; analogous to Type I or alpha error

fertility factor   a plasmid that carries genetic information from one cell to another, including genes responsible for establishing the physical connection between mating bacteria

fidelity   replication of template sequences without errors

field inversion gel electrophoresis (FIGE)   pulsed field gel separation that uses alternation of positive and negative electrodes to resolve large particles

fluorescent resonance energy transfer   FRET; a paired probe detection system for real-time PCR

fragment analysis   tests based on fragment sizes determined by electrophoretic migration

frameshift   insertion or deletion in the nucleotide sequence that throws the triplet code out of frame

frameshift mutation   deletion or insertion of other than a multiple of three base pairs in a coding sequence

framework region   FR; a domain in the immunoglobulin heavy chain gene variable region coding for amino acids that do not directly contact antigen

full chimerism   complete replacement of recipient bone marrow with donor bone marrow cells after a transplant

fungicidal   having the ability to destroy fungi

fungistatic   having the ability to inhibit the growth and reproduction of fungi without killing them

fusion gene   chimeric gene containing parts of two or more separate genes

G

G bands   banding patterns of chromosomes after staining with Giemsa

G0   a quiescent state of cells after mitosis without active progression through the cell cycle

G1   a phase of the cell cycle after mitosis and before chromosomes are copied

G2   a phase of the cell cycle after chromosomes are copied and before mitosis

gain-of-function   phenotype having a new, undesired trait; the new properties of the mutant allele are responsible for the phenotype even in the presence of the normal allele

gamete   a haploid reproductive cell

gap   discontinuity in one strand of a double-stranded nucleic acid; introduction of spacing used in sequence alignment

GC clamp   DNA sequences rich in guanosine and cytosine nucleotides that are more difficult to denature into single strands

gel   matrix formed from large hydrated polymers with variably sized spaces through which molecules can move

gel mobility shift assay   method used to detect specific peptides by changes in electrophoretic migration speed upon binding to specific antibodies

gene   order or sequence of nucleotides on a chromosome that contains all the genetic information to make a functional protein or RNA product

gene expression   production of RNA and protein using a DNA template

gene mutations   alterations in the primary DNA sequence

gene rearrangement   intrachromosomal deletion and ligation of gene segments in immunoglobulin and T-cell receptor genes

genetic code   relationship between DNA and amino acid sequence

genetic concordance   all alleles from two different sources are the same

genetic profiling   DNA fingerprinting; identification of the genetic alleles in multiple loci from an individual

genome   all of the genes in an organism

genome mutations   alterations in the number of chromosomes

genomics   study or analysis of the entire genetic component of an organism

genomic imprinting   enzymatic addition of methyl groups to specific nitrogen bases in a predicted pattern throughout the genome

genotype   genetic DNA composition of an organism

germline   having an innate, unmutated or unrearranged genotype or genetic structure

glycoproteins   polypeptides with covalently attached carbohydrate moieties

gonadal mosaicism   presence of more than one genotype in germ cells of an individual

gradient gel   gels with a range of concentrations of urea and polyacrylamide

graft failure   inability to detect donor bone marrow cells in a recipient after a bone marrow transplant

graft-versus-host disease   GVHD; phenotypic manifestations of immune reaction by donor cells (graft) to the recipient (host) after a bone marrow transplant

graft-versus-tumor (GVT) effect   immune reaction by donor cells (graft) on residual tumor cells after a bone marrow transplant for treatment of malignant disease

guanine   one of the common nitrogen bases in DNA and RNA

guanosine   one of the common nucleosides in DNA and RNA

gyrase   enzyme that untangles DNA by cutting and ligating both strands of the double helix; also called topoisomerase II

H

hairpin   fold in DNA or RNA that forms a short double strand along the single strand

haploid   having one of each chromosome

haplotype   genetically linked set of alleles that are inherited together

haplotype diversity   HD; calculated from the frequency of a given haplotype in a defined population

hapten   small molecule capable of causing an immune response when attached to a larger (carrier) molecule

Hardy-Weinberg equilibrium   constant relative frequency of two alleles in a population

helicase   an enzyme that untangles DNA by cutting and ligating one or both strands of the double helix

hematopoietic stem cells   HPC; undifferentiated white blood cells that can differentiate into multiple blood cell lineages

hemimethylated   having methyl groups covalently attached to one strand of a double helix

hemizygous   presence of only one of two possible alleles in a diploid genotype

heteresis   hybrid vigor; the biological advantages of animals produced from unrelated parents, compared with purebred animals

heterochromatin   transcriptionally silent chromosomal regions made up of more condensed nucleosome fibers

heteroduplex   double-stranded DNA in which the component strands are not completely complementary

heteroduplex analysis   HD; detection of sequence differences by denaturation and renaturation of test and reference double-stranded nucleic acids, forming heteroduplexes where test sequences differ from reference sequences

heterologous   non-complementary; also describes two double-stranded nucleic acids with different nucleotide sequences

heterologous extrinsic control   non-target templates added to a sample before amplification to assure proper sample purification and amplification

heterologous intrinsic control   non-target sequences naturally present in a sample such as eukaryotic genes in a test for microorganisms

heterophagy   intracellular degradation of extracellular substrates taken into the cell by phagocytosis or endocytosis

heteroplasmy   mitochondria with different sequences in the same cell

heterozygous   in diploid organisms, having different alleles on homologous chromosomes

Hfr bacteria   bacteria that can produce a high frequency of recombinants due the insertion of the F factor into the bacterial chromosome

hierarchal sequencing   determination of nucleotide order directed to known regions of the genome

high-density oligonucleotide array   large number of probes (more than 100,000) synthesized in place on the substrate

high-resolution banding   staining of less compacted chromosomes to produce a more detailed banding pattern

histocompatible   having the same alleles of the MHC locus

histone   basic protein that associates with DNA

histone code   the relationship between histone modification (methylation, acetylation, phosphorylation) and control of gene expression

HLA type   collection of alleles in the MHC locus detected by genotypic or phenotypic methods

Hoechst 33258   2'-[4-Hydroxyphenyl]-5-[4-methyl-1-piperazinyl]-2,5'-bi-1H-benzimidazole trihydrochloride pentahydrate; DNA-specific dye used in fluorometric quantification of DNA

holocentric   describing a chromosome the entire length of which acts as a centromere

holoenzyme   a multisubunit protein with enzymatic function

home-brew   describing a test system developed and validated within the clinical laboratory

homoduplex   double-stranded DNA in which the component strands are completely complementary

homologous   complementary; also describes two double-stranded nucleic acids with the same nucleotide sequence

homologous extrinsic control   a PCR template with primer binding sites matching test targets and a non-target insert

homoplasmy   all mitochondria in a cell having the same sequences

homozygous   in diploid organisms, having the same allele on both homologous chromosomes

hot-start PCR   preparation of PCR reaction mixes so that no enzyme activity is possible until after the mixes have gone through an initial heating in the thermal cycler

HPLC   high performance liquid chromatography or high pressure liquid chromatography; separation of components of a mixture in solution using a column packed with stationary phase material packed at high pressure

human genome   entire complement of genetic factors in a human cell

human leukocyte antigens   HLA; gene products of the major histocompatibility locus in humans

humoral sensitization   development of antihuman antibodies, often due to organ transplant, blood transfusion, or pregnancy

hybrid   a product of genetically unrelated parents

hybrid capture   an Elisa-like assay using antibodies to an RNA:DNA hybrid formed by hybridization of target RNA with a DNA probe

hybrid resistance   rejection of transplanted organs by immunocompromised mice

hybrid vigor   survival advantage observed in offspring of genetically unrelated parents over offspring of genetically similar parents

hybridization   in nucleic acids, formation of hydrogen bonds between complementary strands of DNA or RNA

hybridoma   hybrid cells, often used to make monoclonal antibodies

hydrogen bond   shared electrons between hydrogen atoms; the basis of base pairing in nucleic acids

hypervariable region   region found to have many different alleles (sequences) in a population

hypervariable region I, II   two polymorphic noncoding regions found in mitochondrial DNA

I

iatrogenic   infection caused by the actions of a physician

immobilized   in molecular biology, bound to a substrate such as a nitrocellulose based membrane or glass slide

imprinting   marking of DNA by enzymatic addition of methyl groups to specific nitrogen bases

in silico   analysis performed on a computer or by computer simulation

in vitro analytical tests   IVAT; reagent sets FDA-approved only for the detection of specific analytes with no claim to clinical utility

in vitro diagnostic tests   IVD; reagent sets intended for use in the diagnosis of specific diseases; these tests may be FDA-approved

in vitro synthesized protein   Or in vitro transcription/translation; product of in vitro cell-free transcription and translation of DNA

inclusion   in human identification, concordance of alleles with a reference source

indel   insertion in DNA with a concomitant deletion

inducible   transcription that is regulated by proteins and other factors

informative locus   genetic locus that differs between two individuals

induction   production of particular proteins by bacteria growing in media containing specific substrates

insertion   gain or duplication of genetic material

intercalating agents   chemicals that associate with nucleic acids by insertion between the planar nitrogen bases of a nucleic acid double helix

internal control   analytical target distinguishable from the test target but detectable with test reagents that is included in the reaction mix with the test target

internal labeling   incorporation of radioactive nucleotides in chain termination sequencing for visualization of the sequencing ladder

internal size standards   in electrophoresis, migration speed markers resolved in the same mixture as test fragments

internal transcribed spacer   ITS; conserved elements found in regions separating the ribosomal RNA genes; used for typing yeast and molds

interphase   cell state in between mitosis or meiosis

interphase FISH   cytogenetic probe analysis of mitotic nuclei

intervening sequences   noncoding sequences that interrupt coding sequences in DNA; introns

intracellular   inside of the cell

intron   noncoding sequences in DNA that interrupt coding sequences; intervening sequences

Invader assay   mutation/polymorphism detection using sequence-specific probes and a proprietary Cleavase enzyme

inversion   intrachromosomal breakage, reversal, and reunion of genetic material

inversion probe   mutation/polymorphism detection method based on sequence-specific probe hybridization, extension, ligation and amplification

investigational use only   IUO; reagents not intended for use on patient samples

isochromosome   chromosome containing two copies of the same arm and loss of the other arm

isotype   protein related to another through common function or structure; immunoglobulin classes directed against the same antigen

K

kappa deleting element   KDE; DNA sequence that determines deletion of the IgK constant region in cells producing the IgL light chains

karyotype   complete set of metaphase chromosomes of a cell

killer cell immunoglobulin-like receptors   KIR; proteins expressed on the surface of NK cells and some memory T cells that interact with HLA receptors

kinetochore   protein structure that attaches chromosomes to the spindle during cell division

kinship index   likelihood ratio generated by a sibling test used to determine if two individuals share at least one parent

Klenow fragment   the large fragment of DNA polymerase without its exonuclease activity

L

lagging strand   one strand of the parent double helix that is read 5' to 3' and replicated discontinuously

leading strand   one strand of the parent double helix that is read 3' to 5' and replicated continuously

leucine zipper   specialized secondary structure found in proteins that bind DNA with leucine residues at each seventh position for thirty residues

leukemia   neoplastic disease of blood in which large numbers of white blood cells populate the bone marrow and peripheral blood

leukocyte receptor cluster   a group of genes on the long arm of chromosome 19 coding for the killer cell immunoglobulin-like receptors

ligase   enzyme that forms one phosphodiester bond connecting two preexisting fragments of DNA

likelihood ratio   comparison of the probability that two genotypes come from the same source with the probability that they come from different sources

limit of detection   lowest concentration that can be detected 95% of the time in a test assay

linearity   quantitative correlation between test result and actual amount of analyte

linkage analysis   use of alleles or phenotypes from known locations in the genome to map genes

linkage disequilibrium (Chapter 11)   LD; simultaneous inheritance of genotypic/phenotypic markers more often than expected by random inheritance

linkage equilibrium   assumption that two alleles are not genetically linked

linker region   DNA between histones

lipoproteins   polypeptides with covalently attached lipid moieties

locked nucleic acid LNA; nucleic acid with modified sugar-phosphate backbone

locus in genetics, the site of a gene or other genetic structure in the genome

locus genotype number of repeats in alleles at a particular STR locus

locus-specific brackets definition of a high and low limit of migration within which alleles are identified with a given degree of certainty

locus-specific RFLP detection of polymorphisms in restriction sites within designated regions or genes; used for typing of microorganisms

logit analysis statistical method intended to translate a quantifiable measure to a predicted state or event, for example, level of gene expression and clinical state

long interspersed nucleotide sequences LINES; highly repeated DNA sequences of 6–8 kbp in length located throughout the human genome

loss of heterozygosity deletion or inactivation of a functional allele, leaving a mutated allele

loss-of-function phenotype lacking a desired trait; in diploid organisms, inactivation of the normal allele is responsible for the phenotype

lymphoma neoplasm of lymphocytes, capable of forming discrete tissue masses

Lyon hypothesis Lyon's hypothesis; only one X chromosome remains genetically active in females

lysosome cellular organelles in which cellular products are degraded

M

M M-phase; the mitotic phase of the cell cycle when duplicated chromosomes are compacted and segregated into daughter cells

M13 single-stranded DNA bacteriophage used in early procedures to make single-stranded templates for sequence analysis

M13 universal primer sequencing primer that could be used for all sequences cloned into the M13 RF plasmid

macroarray membrane containing multiple immobilized probes

major groove larger cleft in the double-stranded DNA helix

major histocompatibility complex MHC; a group of genes located on chromosome 6p in humans

marker site (gene or polymorphism) of known location in a genome

marker chromosome unknown chromosome or part of a chromosome of unknown origin

master mix preassembled components of a reaction solution

match identity or inheritance of one or a set of genetic alleles

match probability probability of identity or inheritance of a set of genetic alleles

matched unrelated donor MUD; a donor selected for a transplant from a pool based on HLA typing

Maxam-Gilbert method chemical sequencing method based on controlled breakage of DNA

mecA gene encoding the altered penicillin binding protein, PBP2a or PBP2', which has a low binding affinity for methicillin

meiosis replication and separation of DNA by reductional and equational divisions in diploid organisms, resulting in four haploid products

melt curve analysis MCA; mutation/polymorphism scanning based on changes in hybridization temperature

melting temperature Tm; the temperature at which DNA is 50% single-stranded and 50% double-stranded

messenger RNA ribonucleic acid that carries information from DNA in the cell nucleus to ribosomes in the cytoplasm

metacentric having the centromere in the middle of the chromosome

metalloproteins polypeptides with associated metal atoms

metaphase mitosis or meiosis where, replicated compacted chromosomes align and prepare to separate

metaphase FISH cytogenetic probe analysis of metaphase chromosomes

metastasis movement of tumor cells from the original (primary) site of the tumor to other locations

microarray   small glass slide or other substrate containing multiple immobilized probes

microdeletion   loss of a small amount of genetic material barely detectable, or undetectable, by karyotyping

microelectronic array   small substrate containing multiple immobilized probes subject to electrodes at each position on the array

microfuge   small centrifuge designed to accommodate 0.2-mL to 2.0-mL tubes

micro RNAs   short RNA species that negatively regulate gene expression

microsatellites   DNA from highly repeated short sequences (STR) such that it differs in density from nonrepeated DNA

microsatellite instability   MSI; contraction and expansion of mononucleotide and dinucleotide repeat sequences in DNA caused by lack or repair of replication errors

microvariant   repeated sequence in DNA missing part of the repeat unit

migration   in electrophoresis, movement of particles through a matrix under the force of a current

minisatellites   DNA from highly repeated sequences (VNTR) such that it differs in density from nonrepeated DNA

mini-STR   system of PCR amplification of short tandem repeat locus using primers that produce a smaller amplicon than standard STR systems

minimal haplotype   eight Y-STR loci used for paternal lineage testing and matching

minimum inhibitory concentration   MIC; least amount of antimicrobial agent that inhibits the growth of an organism

minor groove   smaller cleft in the double-stranded DNA helix

minor groove binding   MGB; the nature of association of a molecule with double-stranded DNA within the minor groove of the double helix

minor histocompatibility antigens   mHag; proteins outside of the main MHC locus that affect organ engraftment

mismatches   nucleotides in double-stranded nucleic acids that are not complementary

mismatch repair (MMR)   correction of replicative errors in DNA by a protein complex that binds to the resulting noncomplementary bases

misprime   aberrant initiation of DNA synthesis from a primer hybridized to template sequences different from the intended target

mitochondrion   subcellular organelle responsible for energy production in the cell

mitogen   substance that stimulates cells to divide

mitosis   separation of DNA in diploid organisms by equational division resulting in two diploid products

mixed chimerism   partial replacement of recipient bone marrow with donor bone marrow cells after a transplant

mixed lymphocyte culture   MLC; co-culturing of lymphocytes from unrelated individuals to determine HLA type

mobility   capacity for migration

Molecular Beacons   self-annealing probe detection system used in real-time PCR

monoclonal   having the same genotypic or phenotypic composition

monoclonal antibody   antibody preparation designed to recognize a defined antigen or epitope

monomer   single component of a complex of like parts

monomeric   single protein or peptide that can function alone

mosaic   individual harboring genotypically different cells or tissue arising from a single zygote

mosaicism   having genetically different cellular components arising from the same zygote

MRSA   methicillin resistant *Staphylococcus aureus*; a strain of *S. aureus* that has resistance to multiple antibiotics

multilocus sequence typing   MLST; characterization of bacteria using sequences of internal fragments of housekeeping genes

multiple displacement amplification   isothermal probe amplification method using restriction digestion and extension to detect a nucleic acid target

multiple locus probe   MLP; Southern blot probe set that hybridizes to more than one locus on the same blot

multilocus sequence typing (MLST)   characterization of bacterial isolates using sequences of internal fragments of housekeeping genes

multiplex PCR   amplification of more than one target in a single PCR reaction

mutation   a difference in DNA sequence found in less than 1% to 2% of a given population

myeloblative   in bone marrow transplants, removal of recipient bone marrow

N

NASBA   nucleic acid sequence based amplification; an isothermal DNA amplification process which includes an RNA intermediate

necrosis   cell and tissue destruction upon cell death

negative control   analytical target that does not react with reagent/detection systems; used to demonstrate that a procedure is functioning with proper specificity and without contamination

negative template control   template sequences that do not match the intended target

neoplasm   growth of tissue that exceeds and is not coordinated with normal tissue; tumor

nested PCR   amplification of the same target in two PCR reactions, using the product of the first amplification as the template for a second round of amplification with primers designed to hybridize within the amplicon formed by the first primer set

new mutation   spontaneous mutation arising in germ cells of an unaffected individual

nick   separation of one phosphodiester bond on one strand of a double-stranded DNA molecule

nick translation   addition of labeled nucleotides at nicks (single-strand breaks) in DNA

nitrocellulose   matrix material with high binding capacity for nucleic acids and proteins

nitrogen base   carbon-nitrogen ring structure that comprises part of a nucleoside

nonpolar   hydrophobic; water insoluble

nonconservative substitution   alteration in the nucleotide sequence that results in the substitution of an amino acid with one of dissimilar properties

nondisjunction   abnormal separation of chromosomes during cell division resulting on both of a chromosome pair in one daughter cell

nonhistone proteins   chromosome-associated proteins that maintain chromosomal compaction in the nucleus

noninformative locus   genetic locus which is identical in two individuals

nonisotopic RNA cleavage assay   NIRCA; a mutation/polymorphism screening and amplification method using RNase cleavage of heteroduplexes

nonsense codon   trinucleotide sequence that terminates translation; UAA, UAG, UGA

nonsense substitution   alteration in the nucleotide sequence that results in the substitution of a termination codon for an amino acid codon

nonsense-mediated decay   NMD; degradation of mRNA with premature stop codons

northern blot   method used to analyze specific RNA transcripts in a mixture of other RNA

nosocomial   hospital-caused infection

NTP   nucleotide triphosphate

nuclear organizing region (NOR) staining   using silver nitrate to highlight the constricted regions, or stalks, on the acrocentric chromosomes

nucleic acid   linear polymer of nucleotides

nucleic acid sequence-based amplification   NASBA: replication of a DNA or RNA target through an intermediate RNA product

nuclein   viscous substance isolated from nuclei by Miescher, later to be known as DNA

nucleolus   cellular organelle believed to be the location of ribosomal RNA synthesis

nucleoside   unit of nucleic acid comprised of a ribose sugar and a nitrogen base

nucleosome   eight histones wrapped in about 150 bp of DNA

nucleotide   unit of nucleic acid comprised of a phosphorylated ribose sugar and a nitrogen base

null allele   genetic type or variant with no phenotypic effect

O

Okazaki fragments   intermediate products of DNA synthesis on the lagging strand

oligoclone   small subpopulation with identical genotype or phenotype within a larger group

oligomer   proteins or peptides that function as components of more than one unit (dimer, trimer, tetramer); in nucleic acids, a short sequence of nucleic acid

oligonucleotide   short fragment of nucleic acid

oligonucleotide array   small glass slide or other substrate containing multiple immobilized probes synthesized directly on the substrate; high density oligonucleotide arrays.

oncogene   mutated gene that promotes proliferation and survival of cancer cells

oncology   study of cancer

ontogeny   course of development, for example of an individual organism

open reading frame   region of DNA comprised of codons coding for an amino acid sequence

operator   binding site of a repressor or other transcriptional control factor to DNA

operon   series of structural genes transcribed together on one mRNA and subsequently separated into individual proteins

Oxford sequence   sequence of the mitochondrial hypervariable regions used as a reference for defining polymorphisms

overhangs   unpaired single strands at the ends of a double-stranded nucleic acid

P

p   in cytogenetics, indicating the short arm of a chromosome

P site   peptidyl site, location of charged tRNA binding in the ribosome complex

palindromic   reading the same in both directions; in double-stranded DNA, reading the same 5' to 3' on both strands

pandemic   disease or condition found across wide geographical areas at the same time

panel reactive antibodies   PRA; set of reference antibodies used to define the HLA of reference lymphocytes

paracentric inversion   intrachromosomal breakage, reversal, and reunion of genetic material not including the centromere

paternity index   expression of how many times more likely a child's allele is inherited from an alleged father than from a random man in the population

pedigree   diagram of the inheritance pattern of a phenotype (or genotype) in a family

penetrance   frequency of expression of a disease phenotype in individuals with a gene lesion

peptide   polymer of a few amino acids

peptide bond   covalent carbon-nitrogen bonds that connect amino acids in proteins

peptide nucleic acid   PNA; nucleic acid with peptide bonds replacing the sugar-phosphate backbone

peptidyl transferase   ribozyme that catalyzes the formation of a peptide bond

pericentric inversion   intrachromosomal breakage, reversal, and reunion of genetic material including the centromere

pH drift   decrease of pH at the cathode and increase in pH at the anode during electrophoresis

phenotype   biological properties of an organism

phosphodiester bond   covalent attachment of the hydroxyl oxygen of one phosphorylated ribose (or deoxy ribose) sugar to the phosphate phosphorous of the next

phosphor   substance that glows after exposure to electrons or ultraviolet light

photobleaching   fading; photochemical destruction of a fluorescent molecule (fluorophore) by exposure to light

Phrap   sequence assembly tool

Phred   sequence quality assessment system

phylogeny   history and evolutionary development of a species or related group of organisms

plasmid   small, usually circular double-stranded DNA, often carrying genetic information that replicates independently or in synchrony with host cell replication

plasmid fingerprinting   isolation and restriction mapping of bacterial plasmid for epidemiological studies

plasma cells   mature white blood cells that produce antibodies

point mutation   DNA sequence alteration involving one or a few base pairs

polar   hydrophilic; water soluble

polarity   orientation of nucleic acid such that one end (5') has a phosphate group and the other end (3') has a hydroxyl group and is the site of extension of the molecule

poly A polymerase   enzyme that covalently adds adenosine nucleotides to the 3' end of messenger RNA

poly(A) tail   polyadenylic acid at the 3' terminus of messenger RNA

polyacrylamide gel   polymer of acrylamide and bis-acrylamide that, when hydrated, forms a gel frequently used for sieving proteins and nucleic acids

polyacrylamide gel electrophoresis (PAGE)   resolution of particles by size on a synthetic matrix of branched acrylamide polymer

polyadenylate polymerase   enzyme that catalyzes the formation of polyadenylic acid at the 3' terminus of messenger RNA

polyadenylation   addition of adenosines to the 3' end of a messenger RNA molecule

polyadenylation signal   site of activation of termination in eukaryotic RNA synthesis

polyadenylic acid   nucleic acid comprised only of adenosine nucleotides

polycistronic   having more than one protein encoded in a transcript

polyclonal   having a variety of genotypes or phenotypes

polyclonal antibody   collection of antibodies produced in vivo that recognize an antigen or epitope

polymerase   in nucleic acids, an enzyme that connects nucleotides by catalyzing the formation of phosphodiester bonds

polymerase chain reaction   PCR; primer-directed DNA polymerization in vitro resulting in amplification of specific DNA sequences

polymorphism   difference in DNA sequence found in 1% to 2% or more of a given population

polypeptide   a chain of amino acids; a protein

polyphred   sequence quality assessment designed to detect single nucleotide changes

polyploidy   in diploid organisms, having more than two of each chromosome

polythymine   nucleic acid comprised only of thymine nucleotides; poly T

polyuracil   nucleic acid comprised only of uracil nucleotides; poly U

position effect   differences in gene transcription depending on chromosomal location

positive control   analytical target known to react with reagent/detection systems; used to demonstrate that a procedure is functioning properly

post-PCR   laboratory areas and materials used for working with PCR products

preanalytical error   events occurring prior to sample analysis that adversely affect test results

precision   agreement between independent test results; reproducibility of test results

prehybridization   treatment of membranes before introduction of probe to minimize nonspecific binding

premutation   genetic lesion not manifesting a disease phenotype, but prone to advance to full mutation/disease status

pre-PCR   laboratory areas and materials not exposed to PCR products

preventive maintenance   routine review of instrument function with appropriate part replacement

primary antibody   antibody that directly binds a target molecule

primary resistance mutation   mutations that are specific for a given antibiotic or antiviral drug and make an organism less susceptible to that drug

primary structure   in proteins, the sequence of the amino acids; in nucleic acids the sequence of nucleotides

primase   the enzyme that produces short (~60 bp) complementary RNAs to prime DNA synthesis

primer   short single-stranded DNA fragment designed to prime synthesis of a specific DNA region

primer dimer   side product of PCR resulting from amplification of primers caused by 3' homology in primer sequences

prion   aberrantly folded proteins with capable of transferring their configuration to normal proteins

prior odds   initial probability of an event in the absence of a test effect

private antibodies   HLA type-specific antibodies

probability of paternity   number calculated from the combined paternity index and reported in paternity testing

probe   in blotting procedures, nucleic acid or protein with a detectable signal that specifically binds to complementary sequences or target protein

probe amplification   approach to increase sensitivity of target detection by protection and amplification of the probe, rather than the target

probit analysis   statistical method to form binary groups based on quantitative data; used to determine cutpoints for qualitative tests

processivity   ability of polymerase to stay with the template during replication of long sequences

product rule   the frequency of a genotype in a population is the product of the frequencies of its component alleles

proficiency testing   analysis of specimens supplied to independent laboratories from an external reference source

profile   set of markers, alleles, or other characteristics in an individual

promoter   DNA sequences that bind RNA polymerase and associated factors

proofreading   correction function of the DNA polymerase complex that repairs errors committed during DNA replication

prophase   early mitosis or meiosis

prosthetic group   non-protein moiety, such as a sugar or lipid group covalently attached to a protein

protease   enzyme that disassembles protein into its component amino acids

protein   polymer of amino acids with structural or functional capabilities

protein truncation test   mutation/polymorphism analysis using in vitro transcription-translation systems; also called in vitro synthesized protein or in vitro transcription/translation

proteome   all of the proteins that make up a cell

proteomics   study of the proteome, usually through array or mass spectrometry analysis

proto-oncogene   normal gene with potential to promote aberrant survival and proliferation if mutated

proximal   close to; next to

pseudoautosomal   describing homologous regions in the X and Y chromosomes that undergo crossing over during meiosis

pseudogene   intron-less nonfunctional copies of genes in DNA

psoralen(s)   substance from plants that covalently attach to DNA under ultraviolet light

public antigens   antigens to the common blood groups, found in almost all individuals

public antibodies   antibodies that recognize more than one HLA type

pulsed field gel electrophoresis   PFGE; a technique using alternating currents to move very large DNA fragments through an agarose gel

purine   nitrogen bases with a double ring structure; adenine and guanine are purines

pyrimidine   nitrogen bases with a single ring structure; cytokine, thymine, and uracil are pyrimidines

pyrimidine dimers   boxy structures resulting from covalent attachment of cytosine or thymine with an adjacent thymine in the same DNA strand; formed when DNA is exposed to uv light

pyrogram   luminescence data output from a pyrosequencer

pyrophosphate   ester of pyrophosphoric acid containing two phosphorous atoms, $P_2O_7^{4-}$

pyrosequencing   sequencing method based on release of pyrophosphates during DNA replication

Q

q   in cytogenetics, indicating the long arm of a chromosome

Q bands   banding patterns of chromosomes after staining with quinacrine fluorescent dyes

quantitative PCR   qPCR, real-time PCR

quaternary structure   functional association of separate proteins or peptides

quencher   molecule that takes fluorescent energy from a reporter dye

Q, replicase   RNA-dependent RNA polymerase from the bacteriophage, Qβ

R

R banding   modified G banding using acridine orange; the resulting pattern will be opposite that of G banding

R factors   bacterial plasmids that promote resistance to such common antibiotics as chloramphenicol, tetracycline, ampicillin, and streptomycin

R loop   hybrid structure formed between RNA and DNA such that the unpaired introns in the DNA form loops

random coils   chain of amino acids which has no ordered helical or sheet-like structure

random priming   template-directed synthesis of single strands of DNA carrying labeled nucleotides

randomly amplified polymorphic DNA   RAPD; a PCR method using random priming with 6-10 b primers used for typing of organisms; also known as arbitrarily primed PCR

rapid PCR   target amplification using small sample volumes in chambers that can be heated and cooled quickly

reagent alcohol   mixture of 90.25% ethanol, 4.75% methanol and 5% isopropanol

reagent blank   PCR reaction mix with all components except template

real-time PCR   PCR performed in an instrument that can measure the formation of amplicons in real time; also called quantitative PCR (qPCR)

reciprocal translocation   exchange of DNA between separate chromosomes with no gain or loss of genetic material

recognition site   sequences in DNA that are bound by proteins such as restriction enzymes or transcription factors

recombinant   new combination of DNA sequences that is produced from different preexisting (parent) sequences; a cell or organism containing a new combination of sequences

recombinant DNA technology   in vitro, directed formation of hybrid DNA molecules

recombine   to mix different DNA sequences such that a new combination of sequences is produced from different preexisting (parent) sequences

redundant tiling   design of probes on an array such that a predictable mutation is located at different places in the probe sequence

reference range   expected analyte frequency or levels from a population of individuals

REF-SSCP   mutation/polymorphism scanning by SSCP in combination with restriction enzyme fingerprinting; see single-strand conformation polymorphism

regulatory sequence   that part of a gene sequence that binds factors controlling expression of the gene

release factor   specialized protein required for the dissociation of the translation complex at the end of protein synthesis

replication fork   point of replication of double-stranded DNA where the parent strands are separated and copied into two double-stranded daughter strands

replisome   collection of enzymes and factors required for DNA replication in vivo

reportable range   range within which test results are considered to be valid (with or without dilution)

reporter dye   fluorescent dye whose signal indicates presence of target

REP-PCR   repetitive extragenic palindromic PCR; analysis of amplicons produced from primers homologous to interspersed recurring sequences in microorganisms

repressor   protein that downregulates transcription by binding to DNA

reproducible   consistency of test results produced from the same procedure

research use only   RUO; reagents not intended for use on patient samples

resequencing   analysis of a predetermined nucleotide order, usually to look for mutations within the region

resolution   level of detail at which an allele is determined; also the separation of particles by electrophoresis or chromatography

restriction endonuclease   enzyme that makes double-stranded cuts in DNA at specific sequences

restriction enzyme   endonuclease isolated from bacteria that will break single- or double-stranded nucleic acids at specific sequences

restriction fragment length polymorphism   RFLP; sequence variations that result in creating, destroying, or moving a restriction site

restriction map   diagram showing the linear placement of restriction enzyme recognition sites in DNA

restriction modification (rm) system   bacterial defense mechanism involving modifications of host DNA or foreign DNA and destruction of the foreign DNA

reverse dot blot   hybridization technique with multiple probes spotted on a membrane all exposed to the same target

reverse transcriptase   RNA-dependent DNA polymerase

reverse-transcriptase PCR   RT-PCR; polymerase chain reaction amplifying cDNA made from RNA by reverse transcriptase

reverse transcription   synthesis of DNA from an RNA template

RF   replicative form part of the M13 life cycle, where its genome is in the form of a double-stranded DNA circle

rho   protein factor that functions in termination of transcription in prokaryotes

ribonuclease   enzyme that separates RNA into its component nucleotides

ribonucleic acid   RNA; polymer of ribonucleotides

ribose   five-carbon sugar

ribosomal binding site   mRNA sequence that binds to ribosomes in preparation for protein synthesis

ribosomal RNA   ribonucleic acid that serves as a structural and functional component of ribosomes

ribosome   complex of RNA and proteins that catalyzes formation of peptide bonds

ribotyping   typing of microorganisms using restriction fragment polymorphisms in ribosomal RNA genes

ribozyme   RNA with enzymatic activity

ring chromosome   circular structure formed from fusion of the ends of a chromosome or chromosome fragment

RNA-dependent RNA polymerases   enzymes that synthesizes RNA using RNA as a template

RNA editing   posttranscriptional alteration of RNA sequences

RNA induced silencing complex (RISC)   complex of RNA and proteins that enables negative control of gene expression by siRNA and microRNA

RNA integrity control   an amplification control included in RT-PCR to distinguish negative and false-negative results

RNA interference   negative control of gene expression mediated by siRNA

RNA polymerase   enzyme that catalyzes the template-dependent formation of phosphodiester bonds between ribonucleotides forming ribonucleic acid

RNAse-free (RNF)   reagents, consumables, and facilities prepared or treated to protect RNA from RNA digesting enzymes

RNase protection   method used to detect transcripts by hybridizing test RNA with a labeled probe and removing unhybridized target and probe with single-strand–specific nucleus

RNAse H   exonuclease that digests RNA from RNA:DNA hybrids

RNA-SSCP   rSSCP; mutation/polymorphism scanning using RNA instead of DNA; see single-strand conformation polymorphism

robertsonian   movement of most of one entire chromosome to the centromere of another chromosome

S

S   sedimentation coefficient; used to describe the density (movement) of particles in a given medium under gravity or centrifugal force

S phase   S; the part of the cell cycle where chromosomes are replicated

S1 analysis   method used to detect transcripts by hybridizing test RNA with a labeled probe and removing un-hybridized target and probe with single-strand–specific nucleus

salting out   purification of nucleic acid by precipitating proteins and other contaminants with high salt at low pH

Sanger sequencing   dideoxy chain termination sequencing

sarcoma   tumors of bone, cartilage, muscle, blood vessels, or fat

satellite   used to describe repeated DNA sequences; based on the formation of satellite bands by repeated sequences in density gradient separation of DNA

Scorpion   self-annealing labeled primer detection system for real-time PCR

secondary antibody   antibody that binds primary antibody bound to a target molecule

secondary resistance mutation   secondary mutations that enable an organism with primary resistance mutations to replicate in the presence of a given antibiotic or antiviral drug

secondary structure   specific folding of protein or nucleic acid through interaction of amino acid side chains or nitrogen bases, respectively

selenocysteine   cysteine with selenium replacing the sulfur atom; the 21st amino acid

selenoprotein   protein containing selenocysteine

self-sustaining sequence replication   SSSR or 3SR: replication of a DNA or RNA target through an intermediate RNA product

semi-conservative   term used to describe DNA replication where one strand is conserved and serves as a template for a new strand, resulting in a new double helix comprised of one parent and one daughter strand

semi-nested PCR   amplification of the same target in two PCR reactions, using the product of the first amplification as the template for a second round of amplification with primers, one of which is the same as the first round and one of which is designed to hybridize within the amplicon formed by the first primer set

sense strand   single strand of a DNA double helix that is not used as a template for messenger RNA synthesis

sensitivity control   analytical target known to react with reagent/detection systems, but present in the lowest detectable concentration; used to demonstrate that the procedure is detecting the target down to the indicated input levels of testing

sequence   order of nucleotides in a nucleic acid polymer; the order of amino acids in a protein polymer

sequence complexity   length of nonrepetitive nucleic acid sequences

sequence (polymerization)-based typing   SBT; determination of HLA DNA polymorphisms by direct sequencing

sequence-specific (primer) PCR   SSP, SSP-PCR; detection of point mutations or polymorphisms in DNA with primers designed so that the 3'-most base of the primer hybridizes to the test nucleotide position in the template

sequence-specific oligonucleotide probe hybridization   SSOP, SSOPH; detection of DNA polymorphisms using amplified test DNA immobilized on a filter exposed to labeled probes that will hybridize to specific sequences

sequencing ladder   pattern of sequence reaction products on a polyacrylamide gel

serology   study of antigens or antibodies in serum

sex-linked   having genetic components located on the X or Y chromosome

shark's tooth comb   specialized comb used to generate lanes immediately adjacent to one another to facilitate lane-to-lane comparison

short interspersed nucleotide sequences   SINES; highly repeated sequences approximately 0.3 kbp in length located throughout the human genome

short tandem repeats   STRs; head-to-tail repeats of DNA sequences with fewer than 10 bp repeat units

shotgun sequencing   determination of nucleotide sequence by assembly of sequence data from a random collection of small fragments

sibling index   likelihood ratio generated by a determination whether two people share one or both parents

side chain   that portion of an amino acid with biochemical properties

sigma factor   protein that promotes accurate initiation of gene expression in prokaryotes

signal amplification   approach to increase sensitivity of target detection by amplification of the probe signal, rather than the target

signal-to-noise ratio   level of specific target detection compared with background or nonspecific activity

signal transduction   transfer of extracellular and intracellular stimuli through the cell cytoplasm to the nucleus, ultimately affecting gene expression patterns

silencers   sites in DNA that negatively control gene expression

silent substitution   alteration in the nucleotide sequence that does not change the amino acid sequence

silver stain   sensitive staining system for nucleic acids and proteins after gel electrophoresis

single locus probe   SLP; Southern blot probe that hybridizes to only one locus

single nucleotide polymorphism   SNP; one base-pair variation from a reference DNA sequence

single-strand conformation polymorphism   SSCP; method designed to detect sequence alterations in DNA through differences in secondary structure due to differences in the nucleotide sequence

slot blot   membrane containing multiple targets deposited in an elongated pattern, rather than a "dot"

Sm proteins   family of proteins that participate in splicing of RNA

solution hybridization   hybridization of a nucleic acid target and labeled probe in solution

somatic hypermutation   enzymatic alterations of nucleotide sequences in the variable region of the immunoglobulin heavy chain gene

Southern blot   method used to analyze specific regions of DNA in a mixture of other DNA regions

spa **typing**   tandem repeat elements in the 3' coding region of the *Staphylococcus aureus* protein A gene, *spa*, analyzed by PFGE to identify MRSA

spectral karyotyping   cytogenetic probe analysis designed to visualize the entire complement of metaphase chromosomes, with unique colors for each chromosome

spin column   small silica columns designed to fit within an Eppendorf tube, using centrifugal force to wash and elute bound substances

splicing   removal of intron sequences from messenger

splicesosome   complex in which the transesterification reaction linking the exons of RNA together takes place

split chimerism   differential replacement of specific recipient bone marrow cell lineages with donor bone marrow cells after a transplant

split specificity   antigenic types derived from a parent antigen

standard curve   graphical depiction of results from a dilution series of analyte encompassing levels predicted to result from unknown test specimens

standard precautions   recommendations by the Center for Disease Control and Prevention for handling potentially infectious specimens

standard tiling   organization of immobilized probes in high-density arrays such that the base substitution in the immobilized probe is always in the same position from its 3' end

star activity   digestion of DNA by a restriction enzyme outside of its recognition site

sticky ends   unpaired single strands of DNA on ends of double-stranded DNA molecules

Stoffel fragment   *Taq* polymerase lacking 289 N-terminal amino acids

stop codon   nonsense codon

STR analysis   short tandem repeat analysis; assessment of the size of sequences of DNA comprised of head-to-tail repeat units

strand   one molecule of nucleic acid, a double helix contains two strands of DNA

strand displacement amplification   SDA; an isothermal amplification reaction using nick translation and strand displacement

stringency   conditions under which a hybridization takes place

structural sequence   that part of a gene sequence that codes for amino acids

stutter   artifact that results in an additional product(s) when repeated sequences are amplified by PCR

submarine gel   agarose gels loaded under the buffer surface

submetacentric   describing a chromosome with a centrally located centromere closer to one end of the chromosome than the other

subpopulation   genetically defined groups within a population

sugar-phosphate backbone   chain of phosphodiester bonds that hold nucleotides together in a single strand of nucleic acid

suppressor tRNAs   transfer RNAs carrying amino acids that do not correlate to their anti-codons

surname test   test of paternal lineage using alleles on the Y chromosome

susceptibility testing   detection of resistance to given antimicrobial agents by ability to grow in the presence of the agent

SyBr green   fluorescent dye specific to double-stranded nucleic acid

synonymous   describing DNA sequence variants that do not change the reference amino acid sequence

T

tag SNP   one or two single nucleotide polymorphisms that can be used to define a haplotype or a ~10,000-bp block of DNA sequences

tailed primer   oligomer used for PCR carrying sequences at the 5' end that are not complementary to the target sequence

***Taq* polymerase**   heat stable polymerase isolated from *Thermus aquaticus*

TaqMan   probe detection system used in real-time PCR

target   specific sequences or regions that are detected in an analytical procedure

target amplification   replication of a specific target region of DNA

TE buffer   10 mM Tris, 1 mM EDTA buffer

telocentric   having the centromere at one end of the chromosome

telomere   end of chromosomes comprised of repeated DNA sequences and associated proteins

telomeric probe   probes that bind to telomeres

TEMED   *N,N,N',N'*-tetramethylethylenediamine, with APS catalyzes polymerization of acrylamide gels

template   single-stranded nucleic acid used as a guide for replication or synthesis of a complementary strand

teratocarcinoma   tumors comprised of multiple cell types

terminal transferase   enzyme that adds nucleotides to the end of a strand of nucleic acid without using a template

tertiary structure   configuration of folded proteins required for function

tetraploid   having four of each chromosome

thermal cyclers   Or thermocyclers; instruments designed to rapidly and automatically change incubation temperatures, holding at each one for designated periods

threshold cycle C_T, in real-time PCR, the PCR cycle at which the fluorescence from the PCR product surpasses as set cutpoint

thymidine   one of the common nucleosides in DNA and RNA

thymine   one of the common nitrogen bases in DNA and RNA

thymine dimers   boxy structures resulting from covalent attachment of adjacent thymines in the same DNA strand; formed when DNA is exposed to uv light

tissue typing   identification of HLA types

TMA   transcription mediated amplification; an isothermal amplification method using an RNA intermediate; also an abbreviation for tissue microarrays

topoisomerase   helicase that untangles DNA by cutting and ligating one or both strands of the double helix

touchdown PCR   modification of the polymerase chain reaction method to enhance amplification of desired targets by manipulation of annealing temperatures

tracking dye   in electrophoresis, a dye added to samples being separated to monitor the extent of migration through the matrix

trait   particular characteristic

transcription   template-guided synthesis of RNA by RNA polymerase

transcription-mediated amplification   TMA; replication of a DNA or RNA target through an intermediate RNA product

transcriptome   entire complement of transcripts in a cell or organism

transduction   transfer of genetic information from one cell to another through a viral intermediate

trans   on the opposite side; in nucleic acids, referring to a controlling element not covalently connected to its target

trans factor   in molecular biology, a protein factor that binds to specific sites in DNA to control gene expression; also a gene that codes for such a factor

transfer   in blotting, movement of DNA or protein resolved by electrophoresis from the gel matrix to a membrane

transfer RNA   adaptors that link codons in messenger RNA with amino acids

transformation   transfer of genetic information among cells without physical association, such that a new phenotype is produced in the recipient cells

translocation   breakage and fusion of separate chromosomes

transmembrane   spanning across the cell membrane

transmission pattern   mode of inheritance of a phenotype within a family

transmission-based precautions   protective equipment and/or clothing used with potential exposure to airborne or contact-transmissible infectious agents

transposon   fragment of DNA with the capacity to move from one genetic location to another

trimming   addition or deletion of nucleotides at the junctions between V, D, and J segments during immunoglobulin and T-cell receptor gene rearrangements

trinucleotide repeat   three base-pair tandem sequence repeats in DNA

triploidy   having three of each chromosome

tRNA charging   covalent attachment of an amino acid and its transfer RNA

true negative   lack of detection of a target marker that is not present in a test sample

true positive   accurate detection of a target marker present in a test sample

truncation   premature protein termination

Tth polymerase   a heat stable polymerase isolated from *Thermus thermophilus*

tumor suppressor gene   TSG; a gene that dampens proliferation and survival; TSG function is often lost in cancer cells

typing capacity   ability of a test to identify the target organism

typing trays   plates preloaded with reference antibodies used for study of HLA antigens

U

unbalanced   in cytogenetics, genetic events that result in gain or loss of genetic material

uniparental disomy   inheritance of chromosomal material from only one parent due to aberrant separation of chromosomes during meiosis

uracil   nitrogen base found in RNA

V

V(D)J recombination   normal intrachromosomal breaking and joining of DNA in the genes coding for immunoglobulins and T-cell receptors

vacuum transfer   movement of nucleic acid or protein from a gel matrix to a membrane using a vacuum

validation   series of analyte tests using a particular method to establish method characteristics

variable expressivity   range of phenotypes in individuals with the same gene lesion

variable number tandem repeats   VNTRs; head-to-tail repeats in DNA with 10–150 bp repeat units

variant   in genetics, an organism of genetic structure that differs from a reference standard

viral load   quantified presence of virus in a specimen

virus   microorganism dependent on host cell machinery for reproduction; also a sometimes deleterious electronic signal that can be passed among computers

W

well   in gel electrophoresis, an indentation or space molded into the gel to accommodate loading of molecules to be separated

western blot   method used to analyze specific proteins or peptides in a mixture of other proteins

whole chromosome paints   fluorescent probes that stain the entire length of a specific chromosome

X

X-linked   having genetic components located on the X chromosome

Y

Y-STR   short tandem repeats located exclusively on the Y chromosome

Y-STR/paternal lineage test   establishment of paternal ancestry using Y chromosome polymorphic short tandem repeat haplotypes

Z

zinc finger   specialized Zn-stabilized secondary structure found in proteins that bind DNA

zwitterion   molecule that can be completely positively or negatively charged at a given pH

Index

Numbers followed by *f* represent figures, numbers followed by *t* represent tables, and numbers followed by *b* represent boxes.